Adverse Drug Interactions

A Handbook for Prescribers

Adverse Drug Interactions
A Handbook for Prescribers

Lakshman Karalliedde DA FRCA
Visiting Senior Lecturer, Department of Public Health Sciences, King's College London School of Medicine;
Consultant Medical Toxicologist, Health Protection Agency, London, UK

Simon F.J. Clarke DA FRCS(Ed) FCEM
Consultant Emergency Medicine Physician, Frimley Park NHS Foundation Trust, UK;
Honorary Consultant Medical Toxicologist, Chemical Hazards and Poisons Division (London), Health Protection Agency, UK

Ursula Collignon BPharm MRPharmS
Senior Pharmacist, Guy's & St Thomas' NHS Foundation Trust, London, UK

Janaka Karalliedde MBBS MRCP
Clinical Lecturer in Diabetes and Endocrinology, King's College London School of Medicine, King's College London, UK

HODDER EDUCATION
AN HACHETTE UK COMPANY

First published in Great Britain in 2010 by
Hodder Arnold, an imprint of Hodder Education,
an Hachette UK company, 338 Euston Road, London NW1 3BH
http://www.arnoldpublishers.com/
http://www.hoddereducation.com

Whilst the advice and information in this book are believed to be true and accurate at the date of going to press, neither the authors nor the publisher can accept any legal responsibility or liability for any errors or omissions that may be made. In particular (but without limiting the generality of the preceding disclaimer) every effort has been made to check drug dosages; however it is still possible that errors have been missed. Furthermore, dosage schedules are constantly being revised and new side-effects recognized. For these reasons the reader is strongly urged to consult the drug companies' printed instructions before administering any of the drugs recommended in this book.

British Library Cataloguing in Publication Data
A catalogue record for this book is available from the British Library

Library of Congress Cataloging-in-Publication Data
A catalog record for this book is available from the Library of Congress

ISBN 9780340927694

1 2 3 4 5 6 7 8 9 10

Commissioning Editor: Philip Shaw
Project Editor: Joanna Silman
Production Controller: Karen Dyer
Indexer: Jan Ross

Typeset in 9/10.5 pt ITC Garamond Light BT by Macmillan Publishing Solutions, Chennai, India
Printed and bound in India

CONTENTS

About the authors ix
Preface x
Acknowledgements xi
Abbreviations xii
Index of drug names xiii

Introduction **lx**
Clinical features of some adverse drug interactions **lxix**

Part 1 **Cardiovascular drugs** **1**
- Introduction 1
- Aliskiren 7
- Antiarrhythmics 8
- Antihypertensives and heart failure drugs 34
- Antiplatelet drugs 54
- Beta-blockers 62
- Calcium channel blockers 78
- Cardiac glycosides 98
- Diuretics 107
- Ivabradine 119
- Lipid-lowering drugs 120
- Nitrates 130
- Peripheral vasodilators 133
- Potassium channel activators 137
- Selective phosphodiesterase inhibitors 138
- Sympathomimetics 138

Part 2 **Drugs acting on the nervous system** **147**
- Introduction 147
- Antidementia drugs 155
- Antidepressants 156
- Antiemetics 203
- Antiepileptics 209
- Antimigraine drugs 228
- Antiobesity drugs 236
- Antiparkinson's drugs 239
- Antipsychotics 251
- Anxiolytics and hypnotics 263
- CNS stimulants 274
- Drug dependence therapies 279
- Drugs used to treat neuromuscular diseases and movement disorders 283

Part 3 **Anticancer and immunomodulating drugs** **287**
Introduction 287
Cytotoxics 289
Hormones and hormone antagonists 346
Other immunomodulating drugs 350

Part 4 **Anticoagulants** **389**
Introduction 389
Anticoagulants – oral 390
Anticoagulants – parenteral 399
Thrombolytics 401

Part 5 **Antidiabetic drugs** **403**
Introduction 403
Insulin 405
Metformin 413
Sulphonylureas 421
Other diabetic drugs 433

Part 6 **Other endocrine drugs** **453**
Bisphosphonates 454
Danazol 454
Desmopressin 454
Diazoxide 454
Dutasteride 454
Female sex hormones 454
Gestrinone 454
Glucagon 454
Nandrolone 455
Somatropin (growth hormone) 455
Steroid replacement therapy 455
Strontium ranelate 455
Testosterone 455
Thyroid hormones 456
Trilostane 458

Part 7 **Analgesics** **459**
Introduction 459
Acetaminophen 461
Nefopam 461
Non-steroidal anti-inflammatory drugs (NSAIDs) 462
Opioids 470
Paracetamol 479

Part 8 **Musculoskeletal drugs** **481**
Introduction 481
Antigout drugs 482
Drugs affecting bone metabolism 488

Drugs treating inflammatory arthropathies 488
Skeletal muscle relaxants 488

Part 9 **Anaesthetic drugs 492**
Introduction 492
Anaesthetics – general 494
Anaesthetics – local 498
Anticholinesterases 502
Antimuscarinics 502
Benzodiazepines 502
Dantrolene 502
Muscle relaxants – depolarizing and non-depolarizing 502
Opioids 505

Part 10 **Drugs to treat infections 506**
Introduction 506
Antibiotics – aminoglycosides 510
Antibiotics – beta-lactams 513
Antibiotics – macrolides 515
Antibiotics – penicillins 525
Antibiotics – quinolones 526
Antibiotics – rifamycins 532
Antibiotics – sulphonamides 541
Antibiotics – tetracyclines 546
Other antibiotics 549
Antifungal drugs 561
Antimalarials 580
Other antiprotozoals 592
Antivirals – antiretrovirals 596
Antivirals – other 628

Part 11 **Drugs acting on the gastrointestinal tract 633**
Introduction 633
Antacids 634
Antidiarrhoeals 636
Antiemetics 637
Antimuscarinics 637
Drugs affecting bile 637
Drugs used to treat inflammatory bowel disease 637
H2 receptor blockers 638
Pancreatin 648
Proton pump inhibitors 649
Sucralfate 654
Tripotassium dicitratobismuthate 655

Part 12 **Respiratory drugs 656**
Introduction 656
Antihistamines 658

Bronchodilators ... 662
Doxapram ... 673
Leukotriene receptor antagonists ... 673

Part 13 **Metabolic drugs ... 675**
Agalsidase ... 676
Laronidase ... 676
Penicillamine ... 676
Sodium phenylbutyrate ... 676
Trientine ... 676

Part 14 **Drugs used in obstetrics and gynaecology ... 677**
Danazol ... 678
Ergometrine ... 678
Female hormones ... 678
Gestrinone ... 684
Mifepristone ... 684
Oxytocics ... 684
Prostaglandins ... 684
Raloxifene ... 685
Tibolone ... 685

Part 15 **Urological drugs ... 686**
Urinary retention ... 687
Urinary incontinence ... 687
Erectile dysfunction ... 688
Urinary alkalization ... 690

Part 16 **Drugs of abuse ... 691**
Cannabis ... 692
Amphetamines ... 699
Ecstasy (MDMA) ... 701
Cocaine ... 703
Heroin ... 704
Hallucinogens ... 704
Gamma hydroxybutyric acid ... 704
Amyl nitrite ... 704

Part 17 **Miscellaneous ... 705**
Introduction ... 705
Alcohol ... 713
Grapefruit juice ... 720
Minerals ... 733
Herbal drugs ... 742

Part 18 **Over-the-counter drugs ... 760**
Introduction ... 760

ABOUT THE AUTHORS

Lakshman Karalliedde is currently Visiting Senior Lecturer at the Division of Public Health Sciences, King's College London School of Medicine, King's College, London, UK; and Senior Collaborator at the South Asian Clinical Toxicology Research Collaboration, Faculty of Medicine, University of Peradeniya, Sri Lanka. He is also Consultant Medical Toxicologist, Chemical Hazards & Poisons Division (London), Health Protection Agency, UK.

Dr Karalliedde was formerly Senior Lecturer and Honorary Consultant Anaesthetist at the United Medical & Dental Schools of Guy's & St Thomas' Hospitals, London, UK; and Medical Toxicologist at Guy's Poisons Unit and National Poisons Information Service, Guy's & St Thomas' NHS Foundation Trust, London, UK.

Simon F. J. Clarke is Consultant Emergency Medicine Physician, Frimley Park NHS Foundation Trust, UK; and Honorary Consultant Medical Toxicologist, Chemical Hazards and Poisons Division (London), Health Protection Agency, UK.

Ursula Collignon is Senior Pharmacist at Guy's & St Thomas' NHS Foundation Trust, London, UK.

Janaka Karalliedde is Clinical Lecturer in Diabetes and Endocrinology in the Cardiovascular Division, King's College London School of Medicine, King's College London, UK.

PREFACE

Thirteen years ago, the journal of the American Medical Association (JAMA 1996) reported that 108, 000 Americans died in hospital from adverse drug reactions and 2.2 million Americans had reactions to FDA approved medications. In the UK an estimated 1.6 million bed days are due to in-patient adverse drug reactions and up to 6.5% of new patient admissions may be related to an adverse drug reaction. Recent estimates suggest that adverse drug reactions cost the NHS in England in excess of £637 million annually.

In 2009, in the UK, drugs are increasingly available over the counter and on-line without prescription. Furthermore, there is widespread use of numerous herbal medicines from relatively under-regulated suppliers and the constituents of such products are often not known. This clinical reality of the widespread use of potent medicines – be they allopathic or traditional – showed us the need for a practical hands-on guide that aims to be a compact, succinct and accessible source of information for practitioners, prescribers and the public about adverse drug interactions.

We are aware that there are numerous sources of information available to prescribers, pharmacists and users about adverse drug interactions and that new drug interactions are reported on a regular basis. This makes it difficult for the busy practicing health-care professional to keep up with the related literature. We have aimed to produce a user-friendly resource that not only describes the potential interactions themselves, but also gives practical advice about what clinical features to look out for, what to do to try to minimize their occurrence, and what to do if they occur. We aim to produce a source of information that can be used within the time frame of a consultation, to provide some guidance to prescribers, dispensers and users to minimize the risk of a drug interaction occurring.

Thus, this book intends to provide a source of easily accessible and concise information and guidance to busy prescribers, dispensers and users to minimize this avoidable or preventable hazard.

Note: The views expressed in this book are those of the authors, and not necessarily those of the Health Protection Agency.

ACKNOWLEDGEMENTS

The authors thank the following people for their specialized input which has contributed to this book:

Indika Gawarammana, Senior Lecturer in Medicine and Consultant Physician, Director of Clinical Research South Asian Clinical Toxicology Research Collaboration, Faculty of Medicine, University of Peradeniya, Sri Lanka; and Conjoint Senior Lecturer in Toxicology, University of Newcastle, Australia. He assisted LK in editing the book.

Edwin Chandraharan, Consultant Obstetrician and Gynaecologist, St George's Health Care NHS Trust, London, UK.

SAM Kularatne, Professor of Medicine, Faculty of Medicine, University of Peradeniya, Sri Lanka.

Karen Sturgeon, Medical Toxicology Information Service, Guy's and St Thomas' NHS Foundation Trust, London, UK.

Anomi Panditharatne, Division of Ophthalmology, University College London Hospital, London, UK.

Thilak Jayalath, Senior Lecturer in Medicine, Faculty of Medicine, University of Peradeniya, Sri Lanka.

Jean Sugathadasa, General Practitioner, London.

LK wishes to thank Ajayakumar Anandibhai Patel (B Pharmacy, King's College London), Karen Hogan, Penelope Dixie, Angela Dillaway and Louise Dowling for their assistance and advice. He is also very appreciative of the continuing encouragement of Philip Shaw at Hodder Arnold, without which the book would not have seen its completion.

ABBREVIATIONS

5-HT	5-hydroxytryptamine
ACE	angiotensin-converting enzyme
ACh	acetylcholine
ADH	antidiuretic hormone
AIDS	acquired immune deficiency syndrome
APTT	activated partial thromboplastin time
ATP	adenosine triphosphate
AUC	area under the curve
AV	atrioventricular
BCG	Bacille Calmette-Guerin
BP	blood pressure
BZD	benzodiazepine
CHM	Commission on Human Medicines
CHMP	Committee for Medical Products for Human Use
CK	creatine kinase
CNS	central nervous system
CSF	cerebrospinal fluid
CSM	Committee on Safety of Medicines
CYP	cytochrome P450
ECG	electrocardiogram
FBC	full blood count
FDA	Food and Drug Administration
GABA	gamma-amino butyric acid
GTN	glyceryl trinitrate
HbA_{1c}	glycated haemoglobin
HIV	human immunodeficiency virus
IL	interleukin
INR	international normalized ratio
LFT	liver function test
MAO	monoamine oxidase
MAOI	monoamine oxidase inhibitor
MDMA	methylenedioxymethamphetamine
MRP	multidrug resistance-associated protein
MSG	monosodium glutamate
NICE	National Institute for Health and Clinical Excellence
NMDA	*N*-methyl-D-aspartate
NNRTI	non-nucleoside reverse transcriptase inhibitor
NSAID	non-steroidal anti-inflammatory drug
OATP	organic anion-transporting polypeptide
OTC	over-the-counter
P-gp	P-glycoprotein
PR	pulse rate
PRN	... as required (pro re nata)
RNA	ribonucleic acid
SNRI	serotoinin–norepinephrine (noradrenaline) reuptake inhibitor
SSRI	selective serotonin reuptake inhibitor
TCA	tricyclic antidepressant
TFT	thyroid function test
TSH	thyroid-stimulating hormone
U&Es	urea and electrolytes
UDPGT	uridine diphosphate glucuronosyl transferase

INDEX OF DRUG NAMES

This index lists page numbers where the named drug appears as the **primary** drug in the interaction. Where interactions are in the book for a group of drugs (e.g. ace inhibitors), individual drug names in this index are referenced to the group (e.g. for fosinopril the reader is directed to '*see* ace inhibitors'). Herbal drugs (other than St. John's wort) are not listed here. The contents list gives the full page range for a particular drug group or category.

Drug (primary)	Page	Part of the Book	Category	Subcategory (drug groups only)
abacavir	603, 611	10. Drugs to treat infections	Antivirals – antiretrovirals	Nucleoside reverse transcriptase inhibitors
abciximab	*see* glycoprotein IIb/IIIa inhibitors 61			
acarbose	433–437	5. Antidiabetic drugs	Other antidiabetic drugs	
acebutolol	66	1. Cardiovascular drugs	Beta-blockers	
acemetacin	*see* non-steroidal anti-inflammatory drugs (NSAIDs) 462–470			
acenocoumarol	*see* anticoagulants – oral 390–399			
acetaminophen	*see* paracetamol			
acetazolamide	107–108	1. Cardiovascular drugs	Diuretics	Carbonic anhydrase inhibitors
aciclovir	628, 629	10. Drugs to treat infections	Antivirals – other	
acitretin	382	3. Anticancer and immunomodulating drugs	Other immunomodulating drugs	
actinomycin D	*see* dactinomycin			
adalimumab	351	3. Anticancer and immunomodulating drugs	Other immunomodulating drugs	

Drug (primary)	Page	Part of the Book	Category	Subcategory (drug groups only)
adefovir dipivoxil	630	10. Drugs to treat infections	Antivirals – other	
adenosine	8	1. Cardiovascular drugs	Antiarrhythmics	
adrenaline	*see* epinephrine			
agalsidase beta	676	13. Metabolic drugs	Agalsidase beta	
alcohol	713–719	17. Miscellaneous drugs	Alcohol	
aldesleukin	*see* interleukin-2			
alendronate	454	6. Other endocrine drugs	Bisphosphonates	
alfentanil	476, 478	7. Analgesics	Opioids	
alimemazine	660	12. Respiratory drugs	Antihistamines	
aliskiren	7	1. Cardiovascular drugs	Aliskiren	
allopurinol	482–483	8. Musculoskeletal drugs	Antigout drugs	
allopurinol	739	17. Miscellaneous drugs	Minerals	Other drug-mineral interactions
almotriptan	230, 231, 232, 233, 234, 235	2. Drugs acting on the nervous system	Antimigraine drugs	5-HT1 agonists – triptans
alprostadil	684	14. Drugs used in obstetrics and gynaecology	Prostaglandins	
alteplase	*see* thrombolytics 401–402			
amantadine	239–240	2. Drugs acting on the nervous system	AntiParkinson's drugs	
ambrisentan	*see* vasodilator antihypert-ensives 35, 36, 37, 38, 41, 42, 44–53			
amikacin	*see* aminogly-cosides 510–513			
amiloride	113	1. Cardiovascular drugs	Diuretics	Potassium-sparing diuretics and aldosterone antagonists
aminophylline	*see* theo-phyllines, 655			

Drug (primary)	Page	Part of the Book	Category	Subcategory (drug groups only)
amiodarone	9–14	1. Cardiovascular drugs	Antiarrhythmics	
amisulpride	253	2. Drugs acting on the nervous system	Antipsychotics	
amitriptyline	183, 187, 188, 189	2. Drugs acting on the nervous system	Antidepressants	Tricyclic antidepressants
amlodipine	*see* calcium channel blockers 78–98			
ammonium chloride	690	15. Urological drugs	Urinary alkalinization	
amobarbital	*see* barbiturates (as antiepileptics) 211–214			
amoxapine	187	2. Drugs acting on the nervous system	Antidepressants	Tricyclic antidepressants
amoxycillin	*see* penicillins 525			
amphetamines	699–700	16. Drugs of abuse		
amphotericin	561–562	10. Drugs to treat infections	Antifungal drugs	
ampicillin	525, 526	10. Drugs to treat infections	Antibiotics	Penicillins
amprenavir	620, 622, 626	10. Drugs to treat infections	Antivirals – antiretrovirals	Protease inhibitors
amyl nitrite	704	16. Drugs of abuse	Amyl nitrite	
anakinra	352	3. Anticancer and immunomodulating drugs	Other immunomodulating drugs	
anastrazole	346	3. Anticancer and immunomodulating drugs	Hormones and hormone antagonists	
antacids	634–636	11. Drugs acting on the gastrointestinal tract		
apomorphine	249, 250	2. Drugs acting on the nervous system	AntiParkinson's drugs	Dopaminergics
apraclonidine	*see* sympathomimetics 138			
aprazolam	264, 265, 266, 268, 269	2. Drugs acting on the nervous system	Anxiolytics and hypnotics	Benzodiazepines

Drug (primary)	Page	Part of the Book	Category	Subcategory (drug groups only)
aprepitant	203–204	2. Drugs acting on the nervous system	Antiemetics	
aripiprazole	253, 255, 257, 259	2. Drugs acting on the nervous system	Antipsychotics	
arsenic trioxide	290	3. Anticancer and immunomodulating drugs	Cytotoxics	
artemether	580–581	10. Drugs to treat infections	Antimalarials	
asparaginase	*see* crisantaspase			
aspirin	54–57	1. Cardiovascular drugs	Antiplatelet drugs	
astemizole	661	12. Respiratory drugs	Antihistamines	
atazanavir	620, 621, 622, 623, 626, 628	10. Drugs to treat infections	Antivirals – antiretrovirals	Protease inhibitors
atenolol	66	1. Cardiovascular drugs	Beta-blockers	
atomoxetine	274–276	2. Drugs acting on the nervous system	CNS stimulants	
atorvastatin	125, 126, 128	1. Cardiovascular drugs	Lipid-lowering drugs	Statins
atovaquone	582	10. Drugs to treat infections	Antimalarials	
atracurium	*see* muscle relaxants – depolarising, non-depolarising 502–505			
atropine	240, 241, 243	2. Drugs acting on the nervous system	AntiParkinson's drugs	Antimuscarinics
azapropazone	*see* non-steroidal anti-inflammatory drugs (NSAIDs) 462–270			
azathioprine	352–355	3. Anticancer and immunomodulating drugs	Other immunomodulating drugs	
azithromycin	515, 516, 522	10. Drugs to treat infections	Antibiotics	Macrolides
azithromycin	739	17. Miscellaneous drugs	Minerals	Other drug-mineral interactions

Drug (primary)	Page	Part of the Book	Category	Subcategory (drug groups only)
baclofen	488, 489, 490, 491	8. Musculoskeletal drugs	Skeletal muscle relaxants	
balsalazide	*see* aminosalicylates 351			
bambuterol	665	12. Respiratory drugs	Bronchodilators	Beta-2 agonists
bemiparin	*see* anticoagulants – parenteral, 399			
bendroflumethiazide	*see* thiazides 116–119			
benperidol	*see* antipsychotics 251–263			
betamethasone	*see* corticosteroids 367–374			
betaxolol	66	1. Cardiovascular drugs	Beta-blockers	
bethanechol	*see* antimuscarinics 240–247			
bexarotene	291	3. Anticancer and immunomodulating drugs	Cytotoxics	
bezafibrate	*see* fibrates 123–125			
bicalutamide	346	3. Anticancer and immunomodulating drugs	Hormones and hormone antagonists	
bisoprolol	66	1. Cardiovascular drugs	Beta-blockers	
bivalirudin	*see* hirudins 339, 401			
bleomycin	291	3. Anticancer and immunomodulating drugs	Cytotoxics	
bortezomib	291	3. Anticancer and immunomodulating drugs	Cytotoxics	
bosentan	41, 51, 52	1. Cardiovascular drugs	Antihypertensives and heart failure drugs	Vasodilator Antihypertensives

Drug (primary)	Page	Part of the Book	Category	Subcategory (drug groups only)
brimonidine	*see* sympatho-mimetics 138			
bromocriptine	244, 247, 250	2. Drugs acting on the nervous system	AntiParkinson's drugs	Dopaminergics
bumetanide	*see* loop diuretics 109			
bupivacaine	500	9. Anaesthetic drugs	Anaesthetics – local	
buprenorphine	476	7. Analgesics	Opioids	
bupropion	279–281	2. Drugs acting on the nervous system	Drug dependence therapies	
buspirone	270–272	2. Drugs acting on the nervous system	Anxiolytics and hypnotics	
busulfan	291–293	3. Anticancer and immunomodulating drugs	Cytotoxics	
butobarbital	*see* barbiturates (as antiepilep-tics) 211–214			
cabergoline	244, 247	2. Drugs acting on the nervous system	AntiParkinson's drugs	Dopaminergics
calcium	733–734	17. Miscellaneous drugs	Minerals	
calcium levofolinate	307	3. Anticancer and immunomodulating drugs	Cytotoxics	
candesartan	*see* angio-tensin-II receptor antagonists 34, 35, 26, 27, 38, 39, 41, 42, 43, 44, 46, 48, 49, 51, 52			
cannabis	692–699	16. Drugs of abuse	Cannabis	
capecitabine	293, 306	3. Anticancer and immunomodulating drugs	Cytotoxics	
capreomycin	511	10. Drugs to treat infections	Antibiotics	Aminoglycosides

Drug (primary)	Page	Part of the Book	Category	Subcategory (drug groups only)
captopril	*see* ACE inhibitors 34, 35, 36, 37, 38, 39, 40, 42, 43, 46, 48, 49, 50, 51, 52, 53			
carbamazepine	209, 215–219, 222	2. Drugs acting on the nervous system	Antiepileptics	
carbamazepine	740	17. Miscellaneous drugs	Minerals	Other drug-mineral interactions
carboplatin	331	3. Anticancer and immunomodulating drugs	Cytotoxics	
carisoprodol	491	8. Musculoskeletal drugs	Skeletal muscle relaxants	
carmustine	293	3. Anticancer and immunomodulating drugs	Cytotoxics	
carvedilol	66, 73	1. Cardiovascular drugs	Beta-blockers	
caspofungin	576	10. Drugs to treat infections	Antifungal drugs	
cefaclor	*see* cephalosporins 513–514			
cefadroxil	*see* cephalosporins 513–514			
cefalexin	*see* cephalosporins 513–514			
cefixime	*see* cephalosporins 513–514			
cefotaxime	*see* cephalosporins 513–514			
cefpodoxime	513	10. Drugs to treat infections	Antibiotics	Beta-lactams: Cephalosporins
cefradine	*see* cephalosporins 513–514			
ceftazidime	*see* cephalosporins 513–514			
ceftriaxone	*see* cephalosporins 513–514			

Drug (primary)	Page	Part of the Book	Category	Subcategory (drug groups only)
cefuroxime	513	10. Drugs to treat infections	Antibiotics	Beta-lactams: Cephalosporins
celecoxib	469	7. Analgesics	Non-steroidal anti-inflammatory drugs (NSAIDs)	
celiprolol	*see* beta-blockers 63–77			
cetirizine	*see* anti-histamines 658–662			
chloral hydrate	272	2. Drugs acting on the nervous system	Anxiolytics and hypnotics	
chlorambucil	293	3. Anticancer and immunomodulating drugs	Cytotoxics	
chloramphenicol	549–550	10. Drugs to treat infections	Other antibiotics	
chlordiazepoxide	266	2. Drugs acting on the nervous system	Anxiolytics and hypnotics	Benzodiazepines
chlormethiazole	272	2. Drugs acting on the nervous system	Anxiolytics and hypnotics	
chloroquine	583, 584, 585	10. Drugs to treat infections	Antimalarials	
chlorphenamine	659, 661	12. Respiratory drugs	Antihistamines	
chlorpheniramine	660	12. Respiratory drugs	Antihistamines	
chlorpromazine	254, 257, 259, 260, 261, 262	2. Drugs acting on the nervous system	Antipsychotics	
chlorpropamide	423, 431	5. Antidiabetic drugs	Sulphonylureas	
chlortalidone	*see* thiazides 116–119			
ciclosporin	355–367	3. Anticancer and immunomodulating drugs	Other immunomodulating drugs	
cidofovir	631	10. Drugs to treat infections	Antivirals – other	
cilastin (with imipenem)	514	10. Drugs to treat infections	Antibiotics	Beta-lactams
cilazapril	*see* ACE inhibitors 34, 35, 36, 37, 38, 39, 40, 42, 43, 46, 48, 49, 50, 51, 52, 53			

Drug (primary)	Page	Part of the Book	Category	Subcategory (drug groups only)
cilostazol	133–134	1. Cardiovascular drugs	Peripheral vasodilators	
cimetidine	638, 639, 640, 641, 642, 643, 644, 645, 646, 647, 648	11. Drugs acting on the gastrointestinal tract	H2 receptor blockers	
cinacalcet	734	17. Miscellaneous drugs	Minerals	
cinnarizine	*see* anti-histamines 658–662			
ciprofibrate	*see* fibrates 123–125			
ciprofloxacin	527, 528, 529, 530, 531	10. Drugs to treat infections	Antibiotics	Quinolones
ciprofloxacin	740	17. Miscellaneous drugs	Minerals	Other drug-mineral interactions
cisatracurium				
cisplatin	329–330	3. Anticancer and immunomodulating drugs	Cytotoxics	
citalopram	*see* selective serotonin reuptake inhibitors (SSRIs) 168–179			
clarithromycin	515, 516, 517, 518, 519, 520, 521, 522, 523, 524	10. Drugs to treat infections	Antibiotics	Macrolides
clemastine	*see* anti-histamines 658–662			
clindamycin	551	10. Drugs to treat infections	Other antibiotics	
clobazam	*see* benzodi-azepines (BZDs) 264–270			
clomipramine	183,187, 188, 189	2. Drugs acting on the nervous system	Antidepressants	Tricyclic antidepressants

Drug (primary)	Page	Part of the Book	Category	Subcategory (drug groups only)
clonazepam	266	2. Drugs acting on the nervous system	Anxiolytics and hypnotics	Benzodiazepines
clonidine	42	1. Cardiovascular drugs	Antihypertensives and heart failure drugs	Centrally acting antihypertensives
clopidogrel	58–59	1. Cardiovascular drugs	Antiplatelet drugs	
clozapine	252, 253, 254, 255, 256, 259, 260, 261, 262	2. Drugs acting on the nervous system	Antipsychotics	
clozapine	740	17. Miscellaneous drugs	Minerals	Other drug-mineral interactions
cocaine	703–704	16. Drugs of abuse	Cocaine	
codeine	476	7. Analgesics	Opioids	
colchicine	483–484	8. Musculoskeletal drugs	Antigout drugs	
colesevelam	*see* anion exchange resins 120–123			
colestipol	740			
colestyramine	740			
colistin	551–552	10. Drugs to treat infections	Other antibiotics	
cortisone	*see* cortico-steroids 367–374			
co-trimoxazole	542, 543–544, 545, 546	10. Drugs to treat infections	Antibiotics	Sulphonamides
crisantaspase	294	3. Anticancer and immunomodulating drugs	Cytotoxics	
cyclizine	*see* anti-histamines 658–662			
cyclopenthiazide	*see* thiazides 116–119			
cyclopentolate	*see* anti-muscarinics 240–247			
cyclophosphamide	294–295	3. Anticancer and immunomodulating drugs	Cytotoxics	
cycloserine	552	10. Drugs to treat infections	Other antibiotics	

Drug (primary)	Page	Part of the Book	Category	Subcategory (drug groups only)
cyproheptadine	659, 661	12. Respiratory drugs	Antihistamines	
cytarabine	296	3. Anticancer and immunomodulating drugs	Cytotoxics	
dacarbazine	296	3. Anticancer and immunomodulating drugs	Cytotoxics	
dactinomycin	296	3. Anticancer and immunomodulating drugs	Cytotoxics	
dalfopristin	558–559	10. Drugs to treat infections	Other antibiotics	
dalteparin	*see* heparins 400–401			
danaparoid	*see* heparins 400–401			
danazol	678	14. Drugs used in obstetrics and gynaecology	Danazol	
dantrolene	490, 491	8. Musculoskeletal drugs	Skeletal muscle relaxants	
dapsone	552–553	10. Drugs to treat infections	Other antibiotics	
daptomycin	553	10. Drugs to treat infections	Other antibiotics	
darifenacin	241, 242	2. Drugs acting on the nervous system	AntiParkinson's drugs	Antimuscarinics
darunavir	*see* protease inhibitors 611–628			
dasatinib	297	3. Anticancer and immunomodulating drugs	Cytotoxics	
daunorubicin	297	3. Anticancer and immunomodulating drugs	Cytotoxics	
deflazacort	*see* cortico-steroids 367–374			
demeclocycline	*see* tetracyclines 546–549			

Drug (primary)	Page	Part of the Book	Category	Subcategory (drug groups only)
desflurane	*see* anaesthetics – general 494, 496, 497			
desipramine	183, 190	2. Drugs acting on the nervous system	Antidepressants	Tricyclic antidepressants
desloratadine	*see* anti-histamines 658–662			
desmopressin	454	6. Other endocrine drugs	Desmopressin	
dexamethasone	368, 369, 371	3. Anticancer and immunomodulating drugs	Other immunomodulating drugs	Corticosteroids
dexamfetamine	146	1. Cardiovascular drugs	Sympathomimetics	
dexibuprofen	*see* non-steroidal anti-inflammatory drugs (NSAIDs) 462–470			
dexketoprofen	*see* non-steroidal anti-inflammatory drugs (NSAIDs) 462–470			
dextromethorphan	473	7. Analgesics	Opioids	
diamorphine	*see* opioids 470–479			
diazepam	264, 265, 266, 267, 268, 269	2. Drugs acting on the nervous system	Anxiolytics and hypnotics	Benzodiazepines
diazoxide	41	1. Cardiovascular drugs	Antihypertensives and heart failure drugs	Vasodilator Antihypertensives
diclofenac	*see* non-steroidal anti-inflammatory drugs (NSAIDs) 462–470			

Drug (primary)	Page	Part of the Book	Category	Subcategory (drug groups only)
dicycloverine	*see* anti-muscarinics 240–247			
didanosine	603, 604, 605, 606, 607, 609, 610, 611	10. Drugs to treat infections	Antivirals – antiretrovirals	Nucleoside reverse transcriptase inhibitors
digitoxin	98–107	1. Cardiovascular drugs	Cardiac glycosides	
digoxin	99–107	1. Cardiovascular drugs	Cardiac glycosides	
dihydrocodeine	476	7. Analgesics	Opioids	
diltiazem	90, 91, 92, 93, 94	1. Cardiovascular drugs	Calcium channel blockers	
dipipanone	*see* opioids 470–479			
dipivefrine	*see* sympatho-mimetics 138			
dipyridamole	59–60	1. Cardiovascular drugs	Antiplatelet drugs	
disodium etidronate	*see* bisphospho-nates 454			
disodium pamidronate	*see* bisphospho-nates 454			
disopyramide	15–18	1. Cardiovascular drugs	Antiarrhythmics	
distigmine	*see* antimus-carinics 240–247			
disulfiram	282–283	2. Drugs acting on the nervous system	Drug dependence therapies	
dobutamine	*see* sympatho-mimetics 138			
docetaxel	297–299	3. Anticancer and immunomodulating drugs	Cytotoxics	
dolasetron	*see* 5-HT3 antagonists 207–209			
domperidone	204, 205, 206	2. Drugs acting on the nervous system	Antiemetics	
donepezil	285	2. Drugs acting on the nervous system	Neuromuscular and movement disorders	Parasympathomimetics

Drug (primary)	Page	Part of the Book	Category	Subcategory (drug groups only)
dopamine	*see* sympatho-mimetics 138			
dopexamine	*see* sympatho-mimetics 138			
dosulepin	*see* tricyclic antidepres-sants 180–191			
doxazosin	*see* alpha blockers 34, 35, 47, 48, 50, 51			
doxapram	673	12. Respiratory drugs	Doxapram	
doxepin	187	2. Drugs acting on the nervous system	Antidepressants	Tricyclic antidepressants
doxorubicin	299–301	3. Anticancer and immunomodulating drugs	Cytotoxics	
doxycycline	546, 547, 548	10. Drugs to treat infections	Antibiotics	Tetracyclines
duloxetine	197, 198, 199	2. Drugs acting on the nervous system	Antidepressants	
dutasteride	687	15. Urological drugs	Urinary retention	
edrophonium	*see* parasympa-thomimetics 283–285			
efavirenz	596, 597, 598, 599, 600, 601, 602	10. Drugs to treat infections	Antivirals – antiretrovirals	Non-nucleoside reverse transcriptase inhibitors (NNRTIs)
eletriptan	230, 231, 232, 233, 234, 235	2. Drugs acting on the nervous system	Antimigraine drugs	5-HT1 agonists – triptans
emtricitabine	609, 610	10. Drugs to treat infections	Antivirals – antiretrovirals	Nucleoside reverse transcriptase inhibitors
enalapril	*see* ACE inhibitors 34, 35, 36, 37, 38, 39, 40, 42, 43, 46, 48, 49, 50, 51, 52, 53			

Drug (primary)	Page	Part of the Book	Category	Subcategory (drug groups only)
enoxaparin	*see* heparins 400–401			
enoximone	138	1. Cardiovascular drugs	Selective phosphodiesterase inhibitors	
entacapone	245, 249, 250	2. Drugs acting on the nervous system	AntiParkinson's drugs	Dopaminergics
ephedrine	*see* sympatho-mimetics 138			
epinephrine	142	1. Cardiovascular drugs	Sympathomimetics	
epinephrine (local anaesthetics with)	499	9. Anaesthetic drugs	Anaesthetics – local	
epirubicin	301–302	3. Anticancer and immunomodulating drugs	Cytotoxics	
eplerenone	*see* potassium-sparing diuretics and aldosterone antagonists 112–115			
eprosartan	*see* angiotensin-II receptor antagonists 34, 35, 26, 27, 38, 39, 41, 42, 43, 44, 46, 48, 49, 51, 52			
eptifibatide	*see* glycoprotein IIb/IIIa inhibitors 61			
ergotamine	229	2. Drugs acting on the nervous system	Antimigraine drugs	Ergot derivatives
erlotinib	302	3. Anticancer and immunomodulating drugs	Cytotoxics	
ertapenem	514	10. Drugs to treat infections	Antibiotics	Beta-lactams

Drug (primary)	Page	Part of the Book	Category	Subcategory (drug groups only)
erythromycin	515, 516, 517, 518, 519, 520, 521, 522, 523, 524	10. Drugs to treat infections	Antibiotics	Macrolides
escitalopram	177	2. Drugs acting on the nervous system	Antidepressants	Selective serotonin reuptake inhibitors (SSRIs)
esmolol	*see* beta-blockers 63–77			
esomeprazole	650, 652	11. Drugs acting on the gastrointestinal tract	Proton pump inhibitors	
estradiol	680	14. Drugs used in obstetrics and gynaecology	Female hormones	Oestrogens
estramustine	302	3. Anticancer and immunomodulating drugs	Cytotoxics	
etanercept	374	3. Anticancer and immunomodulating drugs	Other immunomodulating drugs	
ethambutol	553	10. Drugs to treat infections	Other antibiotics	
ethambutol	741	17. Miscellaneous drugs	Minerals	Other drug-mineral interactions
ethosuximide	209, 219	2. Drugs acting on the nervous system	Antiepileptics	
ethylestradiol	680	14. Drugs used in obstetrics and gynaecology	Female hormones	Oestrogens
etodolac	*see* non-steroidal anti-inflammatory drugs (NSAIDs) 462–470			
etomidate	*see* anaesthetics – general 494, 496, 497			
etoposide	303–304	3. Anticancer and immunomodulating drugs	Cytotoxics	

Drug (primary)	Page	Part of the Book	Category	Subcategory (drug groups only)
etoricoxib	*see* non-steroidal anti-inflammatory drugs (NSAIDs) 462–470			
etravirine	*see* non-nucleoside reverse transcriptase inhibitors (NNRTIs) 603			
ezetimibe	123, 127	1. Cardiovascular drugs	Lipid-lowering drugs	
famotidine	640, 642, 644, 647	11. Drugs acting on the gastrointestinal tract	H2 receptor blockers	
felodipine	93	1. Cardiovascular drugs	Calcium channel blockers	
fenbufen	*see* non-steroidal anti-inflammatory drugs (NSAIDs) 462–470			
fenofibrate	*see* fibrates 123–125			
fenoprofen	*see* non-steroidal anti-inflammatory drugs (NSAIDs) 462–470			
fenoterol	*see* beta-2 agonists 662–665			
fentanyl	476, 478	7. Analgesics	Opioids	
fexofenadine	660, 662	12. Respiratory drugs	Antihistamines	
flecainide	18–22	1. Cardiovascular drugs	Antiarrhythmics	
flucloxacillin	*see* penicillins 525			

Drug (primary)	Page	Part of the Book	Category	Subcategory (drug groups only)
fluconazole	563, 564, 566, 567, 568, 569, 571, 573, 574, 575	10. Drugs to treat infections	Antifungal drugs	Azoles
flucytosine	577	10. Drugs to treat infections	Antifungal drugs	
fludarabine	304	3. Anticancer and immunomodulating drugs	Cytotoxics	
flurbiprofen	*see* non-steroidal anti-inflammatory drugs (NSAIDs) 462–470			
fluoride	734	17. Miscellaneous drugs	Minerals	
fluorouracil	304–306	3. Anticancer and immunomodulating drugs	Cytotoxics	
fluoxetine	170, 175, 177	2. Drugs acting on the nervous system	Antidepressants	Selective serotonin reuptake inhibitors
flupentixol	254	2. Drugs acting on the nervous system	Antipsychotics	
fluphenazine	254	2. Drugs acting on the nervous system	Antipsychotics	
flurazepam	*see* benzodiazepines (BZDs) 264–270			
flutamide	346	3. Anticancer and immunomodulating drugs	Hormones and hormone antagonists	
fluvastatin	129	1. Cardiovascular drugs	Lipid-lowering drugs	Statins
fluvoxamine	171, 172, 173, 175, 176, 177, 178, 179	2. Drugs acting on the nervous system	Antidepressants	Selective serotonin reuptake inhibitors
folinate	307	3. Anticancer and immunomodulating drugs	Cytotoxics	
fondaparinux	399	4. Anticoagulants	Anticoagulants – parenteral	
formoterol	*see* beta-2 agonists 662–665			

Drug (primary)	Page	Part of the Book	Category	Subcategory (drug groups only)
fosamprenavir	*see* protease inhibitors 611–628			
foscarnet sodium	631–632	10. Drugs to treat infections	Antivirals – other	
fosinopril	*see* ACE inhibitors 34, 35, 36, 37, 38, 39, 40, 42, 43, 46, 48, 49, 50, 51, 52, 53			
fosphenytoin	220–225			
frovatriptan	*see* 5-HT1 agonists – triptans 230–236			
furosemide	*see* loop diuretics 109			
fusidic acid	553	10. Drugs to treat infections	Other antibiotics	
gabapentin	219	2. Drugs acting on the nervous system	Antiepileptics	
galantamine	283, 284	2. Drugs acting on the nervous system	Neuromuscular and movement disorders	Parasympathomimetics
ganciclovir	629, 630	10. Drugs to treat infections	Antivirals – other	
gemcitabine	307	3. Anticancer and immunomodulating drugs	Cytotoxics	
gemfibrozil	123, 124	1. Cardiovascular drugs	Lipid-lowering drugs	Fibrates
gentamicin	510	10. Drugs to treat infections	Antibiotics	Aminoglycosides
gestrinone	684	14. Drugs used in obstetrics and gynaecology	Gestrinone	
glibenclamide	*see* sulphony-lureas 421–423			
glicazide	*see* sulphony-lureas 421–423			
glimepiride	423, 432	5. Antidiabetic drugs	Sulphonylureas	
glipizide	423, 424, 427, 432	5. Antidiabetic drugs	Sulphonylureas	

Drug (primary)	Page	Part of the Book	Category	Subcategory (drug groups only)
glipizide	740	17. Miscellaneous drugs	Minerals	Other drug-mineral interactions
glucagon	454	6. Other endocrine drugs	Glucagon	
glyceryl trinitrate	*see* nitrates 130–133			
glycopyrronium	240	2. Drugs acting on the nervous system	AntiParkinson's drugs	Antimuscarinics
gold	374	3. Anticancer and immunomodulating drugs	Other immunomodulating drugs	
granisetron	*see* 5-HT3 antagonists 207–209			
grapefruit juice	720–732	17. Miscellaneous drugs	Grapefruit juice	
griseofulvin	577–579	10. Drugs to treat infections	Antifungal drugs	
guanethidine	35, 39	1. Cardiovascular drugs	Antihypertensives and heart failure drugs	adrenergic neurone blocking drugs
haloperidol	253, 254, 255, 258, 259, 260, 261, 262	2. Drugs acting on the nervous system	Antipsychotics	
halothane	495, 496, 497	9. Anaesthetic drugs	Anaesthetics – general	
heparin	*see* heparins 400–401			
homatropine	*see* anti-muscarinics 240–247			
hydralazine	*see* vasodilator antihyper-tensives 35, 36, 37, 38, 41, 42, 44–53			
hydrocortisone	*see* cortico-steroids 367–374			
hydroxycarbamide	307	3. Anticancer and immunomodulating drugs	Cytotoxics	
hydroxychloro-quine	583, 584	10. Drugs to treat infections	Antimalarials	

Drug (primary)	Page	Part of the Book	Category	Subcategory (drug groups only)
hydroxycobalamin	*see* vitamin B12			
hydroxyurea	*see* hydroxy-carbamide			
hydroxyzine	658, 659, 660	12. Respiratory drugs	Antihistamines	
hyoscine	*see* antimus-carinics 240–247			
ibandronate	*see* bisphospho-nates 454			
ibuprofen	*see* non-steroidal anti-inflammatory drugs (NSAIDs) 462–470			
idarubicin	308	3. Anticancer and immunomodulating drugs	Cytotoxics	
ifosfamide	308–309	3. Anticancer and immunomodulating drugs	Cytotoxics	
iloprost	*see* vasodilator antihyper-tensives 35, 36, 37, 38, 41, 42, 44–53			
imatinib	310–315	3. Anticancer and immunomodulating drugs	Cytotoxics	
imidapril	*see* ACE inhibitors 34, 35, 36, 37, 38, 39, 40, 42, 43, 46, 48, 49, 50, 51, 52, 53			
imipenem with cilastin	514	10. Drugs to treat infections	Antibiotics	Beta-lactams

Drug (primary)	Page	Part of the Book	Category	Subcategory (drug groups only)
imipramine	183, 187, 188, 190	2. Drugs acting on the nervous system	Antidepressants	Tricyclic antidepressants
indapamide	*see* thiazides 116–119			
indinavir	621, 623, 625, 628	10. Drugs to treat infections	Antivirals – antiretrovirals	Protease inhibitors
indometacin	462, 469	7. Analgesics	Non-steroidal anti-inflammatory drugs (NSAIDs)	
indoramin	*see* alpha blockers 34, 35, 47, 48, 50, 51			
infliximab	375	3. Anticancer and immunomodulating drugs	Other immunomodulating drugs	
inositol	*see* peripheral vasodilators 133–136			
insulin	405–412	5. Antidiabetic drugs	Insulin	
interferon	375	3. Anticancer and immunomodulating drugs	Other immunomodulating drugs	
interferon alfa	375	3. Anticancer and immunomodulating drugs	Other immunomodulating drugs	
interferon alpha	375	3. Anticancer and immunomodulating drugs	Other immunomodulating drugs	
interferon gamma	375	3. Anticancer and immunomodulating drugs	Other immunomodulating drugs	
interleukin-2	376	3. Anticancer and immunomodulating drugs	Other immunomodulating drugs	
ipratropium	241, 242	2. Drugs acting on the nervous system	AntiParkinson's drugs	Antimuscarinics
irbesartan	41	1. Cardiovascular drugs	Antihypertensives and heart failure drugs	Angiotensin-II receptor antagonists
irinotecan	315–316	3. Anticancer and immunomodulating drugs	Cytotoxics	

Drug (primary)	Page	Part of the Book	Category	Subcategory (drug groups only)
isocarboxacid	*see* monoamine oxidase inhibitors (MAOIs)			
isoflurane	*see* anaesthetics – general 494, 496, 497			
isometheptene	*see* sympathomimetics 138			
isoniazid	553–554	10. Drugs to treat infections	Other antibiotics	
isoprenaline	*see* sympathomimetics 138			
isosorbide dinitrate	*see* nitrates 130–133			
isosorbide mononitrate	*see* nitrates 130–133			
isradipine	*see* calcium channel blockers 78–98			
itraconazole	564, 565, 566, 567, 568, 569, 570, 571, 572, 573, 574, 575, 576	10. Drugs to treat infections	Antifungal drugs	Azoles
ivabradine	119–120	1. Cardiovascular drugs	Ivabradine	
kaolin	636	11. Drugs acting on the gastrointestinal tract	Antidiarrhoeals	
ketamine	494, 495, 498	9. Anaesthetic drugs	Anaesthetics – general	
ketoconazole	563, 564, 565, 566, 567, 568, 569, 570, 571, 572, 573, 574, 575	10. Drugs to treat infections	Antifungal drugs	Azoles

Drug (primary)	Page	Part of the Book	Category	Subcategory (drug groups only)
ketoprofen	*see* non-steroidal anti-inflammatory drugs (NSAIDs) 462–470			
ketotifen	661	12. Respiratory drugs	Antihistamines	
labetalol	68	1. Cardiovascular drugs	Beta-blockers	
lacidipine	93	1. Cardiovascular drugs	Calcium channel blockers	
lamivudine	605, 608, 610	10. Drugs to treat infections	Antivirals – antiretrovirals	Nucleoside reverse transcriptase inhibitors
lamotrigine	210, 219	2. Drugs acting on the nervous system	Antiepileptics	
lanreotide	346–347	3. Anticancer and immunomodulating drugs	Hormones and hormone antagonists	
lansoprazole	649, 653, 654	11. Drugs acting on the gastrointestinal tract	Proton pump inhibitors	
laronidase	676	13. Metabolic drugs	Laronidase	
leflunomide	377–378	3. Anticancer and immunomodulating drugs	Other immunomodulating drugs	
lepirudin	*see* hirudins 339, 401			
lercanidipine	93	1. Cardiovascular drugs	Calcium channel blockers	
letrozole	347	3. Anticancer and immunomodulating drugs	Hormones and hormone antagonists	
levamisole	592–593	10. Drugs to treat infections	Other antiprotozoals	
levobupivacaine	*see* anaesthetics – local 498			
levocetirizine	*see* anti-histamines 658–662			
levodopa	244, 245, 247, 248, 249, 250	2. Drugs acting on the nervous system	AntiParkinson's drugs	Dopaminergics
levodopa	741	17. Miscellaneous drugs	Minerals	Other drug-mineral interactions

Drug (primary)	Page	Part of the Book	Category	Subcategory (drug groups only)
levofloxacin	529	10. Drugs to treat infections	Antibiotics	Quinolones
levofloxacin	740	17. Miscellaneous drugs	Minerals	Other drug-mineral interactions
levomepromazine	*see* anti-psychotics 251–263			
levothyroxine	*see* thyroid hormones 456–458			
lidocaine	498, 499, 501, 502	9. Anaesthetic drugs	Anaesthetics – local	
linezolid	*see* monoamine oxidase inhibitors (MAOIs)			
liothyronine	*see* thyroid hormones 456–458			
lisinopril	*see* ACE inhibitors 34, 35, 36, 37, 38, 39, 40, 42, 43, 46, 48, 49, 50, 51, 52, 53			
lithium	156–159	2. Drugs acting on the nervous system	Antidepressants	
lofepramine	*see* tricyclic antidepres-sants 180–191			
lofexidine	283	2. Drugs acting on the nervous system	Drug dependence therapies	
lomustine	316	3. Anticancer and immunomodulating drugs	Cytotoxics	
loperamide	637	11. Drugs acting on the gastrointestinal tract	Antidiarrhoeals	
lopinavir	621, 622, 625	10. Drugs to treat infections	Antivirals – antiretrovirals	Protease inhibitors
loprazolam	*see* benzo-diazepines (BZDs) 264–270			

Drug (primary)	Page	Part of the Book	Category	Subcategory (drug groups only)
loratadine	661, 662	12. Respiratory drugs	Antihistamines	
lorazepam	266	2. Drugs acting on the nervous system	Anxiolytics and hypnotics	Benzodiazepines
lormetazepam	*see* benzo-diazepines (BZDs) 264–270			
losartan	36	1. Cardiovascular drugs	Antihypertensives and heart failure drugs	Angiotensin-II receptor antagonists
lovastatin	126, 128	1. Cardiovascular drugs	Lipid-lowering drugs	Statins
LSD	*see* hallucino-gens 704			
lumefantrine	580–581	10. Drugs to treat infections	Antimalarials	
lymecycline	*see* tetracyclines 546–549			
magnesium	734–735	17. Miscellaneous drugs	Minerals	
maprotiline	188	2. Drugs acting on the nervous system	Antidepressants	Tricyclic antidepressants
MDMA	701–703	16. Drugs of abuse	Methylenedioxymet hamphetamine (MDMA, Ecstasy)	
mebendazole	593	10. Drugs to treat infections	Other antiprotozoals	
mefenamic acid	*see* non-steroidal anti-inflammatory drugs (NSAIDs) 462–470			
mefloquine	585–587	10. Drugs to treat infections	Antimalarials	
meloxicam	*see* non-steroidal anti-inflammatory drugs (NSAIDs) 462–470			

Drug (primary)	Page	Part of the Book	Category	Subcategory (drug groups only)
melphalan	316	3. Anticancer and immunomodulating drugs	Cytotoxics	
memantine	155	2. Drugs acting on the nervous system	Antidementia drugs	
mepacrine	593	10. Drugs to treat infections	Other antiprotozoals	
meprobamate	272	2. Drugs acting on the nervous system	Anxiolytics and hypnotics	
meptazinol	*see* opioids 470–479			
mercaptopurine	317	3. Anticancer and immunomodulating drugs	Cytotoxics	
meropenem	514	10. Drugs to treat infections	Antibiotics	Beta-lactams
mesalazine	*see* aminosali-cylates 351			
mesna	317	3. Anticancer and immunomodulating drugs	Cytotoxics	
metaraminol	*see* sympatho-mimetics 138			
metformin	413–421	5. Antidiabetic drugs	Metformin	
methadone	470, 476, 477	7. Analgesics	Opioids	
methenamine	555	10. Drugs to treat infections	Other antibiotics	
methocarbamol	489, 490	8. Musculoskeletal drugs	Skeletal muscle relaxants	
methotrexate	318–325	3. Anticancer and immunomodulating drugs	Cytotoxics	
methyldopa	38, 39	1. Cardiovascular drugs	Antihypertensives and heart failure drugs	Centrally acting antihypertensives
methylphenidate	146	1. Cardiovascular drugs	Sympathomimetics	
methylpredni-solone	*see* cortico-steroids 367–374			
methysergide	229	2. Drugs acting on the nervous system	Antimigraine drugs	Ergot derivatives

Drug (primary)	Page	Part of the Book	Category	Subcategory (drug groups only)
metoclopramide	204, 205, 206	2. Drugs acting on the nervous system	Antiemetics	
metolazone	*see* thiazides 116–119			
metoprolol	64, 66, 67, 70	1. Cardiovascular drugs	Beta-blockers	
metronidazole	555–557	10. Drugs to treat infections	Other antibiotics	
mexiletine	22–25	1. Cardiovascular drugs	Antiarrhythmics	
mianserin	*see* tricyclic antidepres-sants 180–191			
miconazole	567, 568, 569, 574, 575	10. Drugs to treat infections	Antifungal drugs	Azoles
midazolam	264, 265, 266, 267, 269	2. Drugs acting on the nervous system	Anxiolytics and hypnotics	Benzodiazepines
mifepristone	684	14. Drugs used in obstetrics and gynaecology	Mifepristone	
milrinone	138	1. Cardiovascular drugs	Selective phosphodiesterase inhibitors	
minocycline	*see* tetracyclines 546–549			
minoxidil	*see* vasodilator antihyper-tensives 35, 36, 37, 38, 41, 42, 44–53			
mirtazapine	199–200	2. Drugs acting on the nervous system	Antidepressants	
mitomycin	325	3. Anticancer and immunomodulating drugs	Cytotoxics	
mitotane	326	3. Anticancer and immunomodulating drugs	Cytotoxics	
mitoxantrone	326	3. Anticancer and immunomodulating drugs	Cytotoxics	

Drug (primary)	Page	Part of the Book	Category	Subcategory (drug groups only)
mivacurium	*see* muscle relaxants – depolarising, non-depolarising 502–505			
mizolastine	658, 660, 661	12. Respiratory drugs	Antihistamines	
moclobemide	165, 166, 168	2. Drugs acting on the nervous system	Antidepressants	Monoamine oxidase inhibitors
modafinil	276–279	2. Drugs acting on the nervous system	CNS stimulants	
moexipril	*see* ACE inhibitors 34, 35, 36, 37, 38, 39, 40, 42, 43, 46, 48, 49, 50, 51, 52, 53			
montelukast	674	12. Respiratory drugs	Leukotriene receptor antagonists	
moracizine	25	1. Cardiovascular drugs	Antiarrhythmics	
morphine	473, 474	7. Analgesics	Opioids	
moxifloxacin	526	10. Drugs to treat infections	Antibiotics	Quinolones
moxisylyte	135	1. Cardiovascular drugs	Peripheral vasodilators	
moxonidine	*see* centrally acting hypertensives 38, 39, 40, 42–47, 50, 53	1. Cardiovascular drugs	Antihypertensives and heart failure drugs	Centrally acting antihypertensives
mycophenolate	379–381	3. Anticancer and immunomodulating drugs	Other immunomodulating drugs	
nabumetone	*see* non-steroidal anti-inflammatory drugs (NSAIDs) 462–470			
nadolol	*see* beta-blockers 63–77			

Drug (primary)	Page	Part of the Book	Category	Subcategory (drug groups only)
naftidrofuryl	*see* peripheral vasodilators 133–136			
nalidixic acid	527, 529	10. Drugs to treat infections	Antibiotics	Quinolones
nandrolone	455	6. Other endocrine drugs	Nandrolone	
naproxen	469	7. Analgesics	Non-steroidal anti-inflammatory drugs (NSAIDs)	
naratriptan	*see* 5-HT1 agonists – triptans 230–236			
natalizumab	381–382	3. Anticancer and immunomodulating drugs	Other immunomodulating drugs	
nateglinide	437–447	5. Antidiabetic drugs	Other antidiabetic drugs	Meglitinide derivatives
nebivolol	*see* beta-blockers 63–77			
nefopam	461–462	7. Analgesics	Nefopam	
nelfinavir	621, 622, 623, 625	10. Drugs to treat infections	Antivirals – antiretrovirals	Protease inhibitors
neomycin	510, 511	10. Drugs to treat infections	Antibiotics	Aminoglycosides
neostigmine	283, 284	2. Drugs acting on the nervous system	Neuromuscular and movement disorders	Parasympathomimetics
nevirapine	596, 598, 599, 601, 602, 603	10. Drugs to treat infections	Antivirals – antiretrovirals	Non-nucleoside reverse transcriptase inhibitors (NNRTIs)
nicardipine	93	1. Cardiovascular drugs	Calcium channel blockers	
nicorandil	*see* potassium channel activators 137–138			
nifedipine	92, 93, 94, 98	1. Cardiovascular drugs	Calcium channel blockers	
nimodipine	*see* calcium channel blockers 78–98			

Drug (primary)	Page	Part of the Book	Category	Subcategory (drug groups only)
nisoldipine	93	1. Cardiovascular drugs	Calcium channel blockers	
nitrazepam	*see* benzodiazepines (BZDs) 264–270			
nitrofurantoin	557	10. Drugs to treat infections	Other antibiotics	
nitrofurantoin	740	17. Miscellaneous drugs	Minerals	Other drug-mineral interactions
nitrous oxide	494	9. Anaesthetic drugs	Anaesthetics – general	
nizatidine	647	11. Drugs acting on the gastrointestinal tract	H2 receptor blockers	
noradrenaline	(*see* norepinephrine)			
norepinephrine	*see* sympathomimetics 138			
norethisterone	683	14. Drugs used in obstetrics and gynaecology	Female hormones	Progestogens
norfloxacin	528, 529, 530	10. Drugs to treat infections	Antibiotics	Quinolones
nortriptyline	183, 187	2. Drugs acting on the nervous system	Antidepressants	Tricyclic antidepressants
octreotide	347	3. Anticancer and immunomodulating drugs	Hormones and hormone antagonists	
oestrogens	678–682	14. Drugs used in obstetrics and gynaecology	Female hormones	
ofloxacin	529	10. Drugs to treat infections	Antibiotics	Quinolones
ofloxacin	740	17. Miscellaneous drugs	Minerals	Other drug-mineral interactions
olanzapine	254, 255, 256, 257, 259, 261, 262	2. Drugs acting on the nervous system	Antipsychotics	

Drug (primary)	Page	Part of the Book	Category	Subcategory (drug groups only)
olmesartan	*see* angiotensin-II receptor antagonists 34, 35, 26, 27, 38, 39, 41, 42, 43, 44, 46, 48, 49, 51, 52			
olsalazine	*see* amino-salicylates 351			
omeprazole	649, 650, 651, 652, 653	11. Drugs acting on the gastrointestinal tract	Proton pump inhibitors	
ondansetron	208,209	2. Drugs acting on the nervous system	Antiemetics	5-HT3 antagonists
orlistat	236–237	2. Drugs acting on the nervous system	Antiobesity drugs	
orphenadrine	*see* antimus-carinics 240–247			
oseltamivir	632	10. Drugs to treat infections	Antivirals – other	
oxaliplatin	*see* cytotoxics 289			
oxazepam	266	2. Drugs acting on the nervous system	Anxiolytics and hypnotics	Benzodiazepines
oxcarbazepine	210, 219	2. Drugs acting on the nervous system	Antiepileptics	
oxprenolol	*see* beta-blockers 63–77			
oxycodone	*see* opioids 470–479			
oxymetazoline	*see* sympatho-mimetics 138			
oxytetracycline	*see* tetracyclines 546–549			
oxytocin	*see* oxytocics 684			

Drug (primary)	Page	Part of the Book	Category	Subcategory (drug groups only)
paclitaxel	326–328	3. Anticancer and immunomodulating drugs	Cytotoxics	
paliperidone	*see* anti-psychotics 251–263			
palonosetron	*see* 5-HT3 antagonists 207–209			
pancreatin	648	11. Drugs acting on the gastrointestinal tract	Pancreatin	
pancuronium	504	9. Anaesthetic drugs	Muscle relaxants – depolarising, non-depolarising	
pantoprazole	*see* proton pump inhibitors 649–654			
papaveretum	*see* opioids 470–479			
paracetamol	479–480	7. Analgesics	Paracetamol	
parecoxib	462, 468	7. Analgesics	Non-steroidal anti-inflammatory drugs (NSAIDs)	
paroxetine	172, 173, 175, 177, 178	2. Drugs acting on the nervous system	Antidepressants	Selective serotonin reuptake inhibitors
pemetrexed	328	3. Anticancer and immunomodulating drugs	Cytotoxics	
penicillamine	382	3. Anticancer and immunomodulating drugs	Other immunomodulating drugs	
penicillamine	741	17. Miscellaneous drugs	Minerals	Other drug-mineral interactions
penicillin V	525	10. Drugs to treat infections	Antibiotics	Penicillins
pentamidine	595	10. Drugs to treat infections	Other antiprotozoals	
pentamidine isetionate	594–595	10. Drugs to treat infections	Other antiprotozoals	
pentazocine	*see* opioids 470–479			
pentostatin	328	3. Anticancer and immunomodulating drugs	Cytotoxics	

Drug (primary)	Page	Part of the Book	Category	Subcategory (drug groups only)
pentoxifylline	136	1. Cardiovascular drugs	Peripheral vasodilators	
pergolide	247	2. Drugs acting on the nervous system	AntiParkinson's drugs	Dopaminergics
pericyazine	*see* anti-psychotics 251–263			
perindopril	*see* ACE inhibitors 34, 35, 36, 37, 38, 39, 40, 42, 43, 46, 48, 49, 50, 51, 52, 53			
perphenazine	254, 255, 262	2. Drugs acting on the nervous system	Antipsychotics	
pethidine	473, 475, 477, 478	7. Analgesics	Opioids	
phenelzine	160, 165	2. Drugs acting on the nervous system	Antidepressants	Monoamine oxidase inhibitors
phenindione	*see* antico-agulants – oral 390–399			
phenobarbital	*see* barbitu-rates (as antiepilep-tics) 211–214			
phenoperidine	473	7. Analgesics	Opioids	
phenothiazines	251, 252, 253, 255, 256, 258, 261, 262	2. Drugs acting on the nervous system	Antipsychotics	
phenoxybenza-mine	*see* alpha blockers 34, 35, 47, 48, 50, 51			
phentolamine	*see* alpha blockers 34, 35, 47, 48, 50, 51			
phenylephrine	*see* sympatho-mimetics 138			

Drug (primary)	Page	Part of the Book	Category	Subcategory (drug groups only)
phenylpropanol amine	*see* sympatho-mimetics 138			
phenytoin	210, 220–225	2. Drugs acting on the nervous system	Anticonvulsants	
phenytoin	740	17. Miscellaneous drugs	Minerals	Other drug-mineral interactions
pilocarpine	284	2. Drugs acting on the nervous system	Neuromuscular and movement disorders	Parasympathomimetics
pimozide	251, 252, 253, 254, 255, 256, 259, 261, 262	2. Drugs acting on the nervous system	Antipsychotics	
pindolol	69	1. Cardiovascular drugs	Beta-blockers	
pioglitazone	447–452	5. Antidiabetic drugs	Other antidiabetic drugs	Thiazolidinediones
piperacillin	525	10. Drugs to treat infections	Antibiotics	Penicillins
pipotiazine	*see* anti-psychotics 251–263			
piracetam	285	2. Drugs acting on the nervous system	Neuromuscular and movement disorders	
piroxicam	*see* non-steroidal anti-inflammatory drugs (NSAIDs) 462–470			
pizotifen	236	2. Drugs acting on the nervous system	Antimigraine drugs	
porfimer	333	3. Anticancer and immunomodulating drugs	Cytotoxics	
posaconazole	563, 565, 566, 567, 569, 570, 572, 573, 574, 575	10. Drugs to treat infections	Antifungal drugs	Azoles
potassium	736–737	17. Miscellaneous drugs	Minerals	
pramipexole	248, 249	2. Drugs acting on the nervous system	AntiParkinson's drugs	Dopaminergics

Drug (primary)	Page	Part of the Book	Category	Subcategory (drug groups only)
pravastatin	*see* statins 125–129			
prazosin	*see* alpha blockers 34, 35, 47, 48, 50, 51			
prednisolone	741			
prilocaine	499	9. Anaesthetic drugs	Anaesthetics – local	
primaquine	587	10. Drugs to treat infections	Antimalarials	
primidone	740	2. Drugs acting on the nervous system	Antiepileptics	
probenecid	484–486	8. Musculoskeletal drugs	Antigout drugs	
procainamide	26–28	1. Cardiovascular drugs	Antiarrhythmics	
procaine	498, 501, 502	9. Anaesthetic drugs	Anaesthetics – local	
procarbazine	334–338	3. Anticancer and immunomodulating drugs	Cytotoxics	
prochlorperazine	261	2. Drugs acting on the nervous system	Antipsychotics	
procyclidine	241	2. Drugs acting on the nervous system	AntiParkinson's drugs	Antimuscarinics
progesterones	662–663	14. Drugs used in obstetrics and gynaecology	Female hormones	Progestogens
proguanil	587–588	10. Drugs to treat infections	Antimalarials	
promazine	*see* anti-psychotics 251–263			
promethazine	660	12. Respiratory drugs	Antihistamines	
propafenone	29–33	1. Cardiovascular drugs	Antiarrhythmics	
propanolol	66, 67, 68, 69, 71, 74	1. Cardiovascular drugs	Beta-blockers	
propantheline	242	2. Drugs acting on the nervous system	AntiParkinson's drugs	Antimuscarinics
propofol	495	9. Anaesthetic drugs	Anaesthetics – general	
pseudoephedrine	*see* sympatho-mimetics 138			
pyrazinamide	557	10. Drugs to treat infections	Other antibiotics	

Drug (primary)	Page	Part of the Book	Category	Subcategory (drug groups only)
pyridostigmine	283, 284	2. Drugs acting on the nervous system	Neuromuscular and movement disorders	Parasympathomimetics
pyrimethamine	588–589	10. Drugs to treat infections	Antimalarials	
quetiapine	*see* anti-psychotics 251–263			
quinagolide	*see* dopamin-ergics 243–250			
quinapril	*see* ACE inhibitors 34, 35, 36, 37, 38, 39, 40, 42, 43, 46, 48, 49, 50, 51, 52, 53			
quinine	590–592	10. Drugs to treat infections	Antimalarials	
quinupristin	558–559	10. Drugs to treat infections	Other antibiotics	
rabeprazole	*see* proton pump inhibitors 649–654			
raloxifene	685	14. Drugs used in obstetrics and gynaecology	Raloxifene	
raltitrexed	338	3. Anticancer and immunomodulating drugs	Cytotoxics	
ramipril	*see* ACE inhibitors 34, 35, 36, 37, 38, 39, 40, 42, 43, 46, 48, 49, 50, 51, 52, 53			
ranitidine	638, 642, 643, 644, 646, 647, 648	11. Drugs acting on the gastrointestinal tract	H2 receptor blockers	
rasagiline	244, 245, 246, 250	2. Drugs acting on the nervous system	AntiParkinson's drugs	Dopaminergics

Drug (primary)	Page	Part of the Book	Category	Subcategory (drug groups only)
reboxetine	201	2. Drugs acting on the nervous system	Antidepressants	
repaglinide	437–447	5. Antidiabetic drugs	Other antidiabetic drugs	Meglitinide derivatives
reteplase	*see* thrombolytics 401–402			
ribavirin	632	10. Drugs to treat infections	Antivirals – other	
rifabutin	536, 537, 538, 539, 540, 541	10. Drugs to treat infections	Antibiotics	Rifamycins
rifampicin	532, 533, 534, 535, 536, 537, 538, 539, 540, 541	10. Drugs to treat infections	Antibiotics	Rifamycins
rifapentine	537	10. Drugs to treat infections	Antibiotics	Rifamycins
riluzole	286	2. Drugs acting on the nervous system	Neuromuscular and movement disorders	
rimonabant	237–238	2. Drugs acting on the nervous system	Antiobesity drugs	
risedronate	*see* bisphospho-nates 454			
risperidone	254, 255, 256, 259, 262	2. Drugs acting on the nervous system	Antipsychotics	
ritonavir	614, 621, 622, 624, 625	10. Drugs to treat infections	Antivirals – antiretrovirals	Protease inhibitors
rituximab	383	3. Anticancer and immunomodulating drugs	Other immunomodulating drugs	
rivastigmine	*see* parasympa-thomimetics 283–285			
rizatriptan	231, 234	2. Drugs acting on the nervous system	Antimigraine drugs	5-HT1 agonists – triptans
rocuronium	*see* muscle relaxants – depolarising, non-depolarising 502–205			

Drug (primary)	Page	Part of the Book	Category	Subcategory (drug groups only)
ropinirole	244, 246, 249	2. Drugs acting on the nervous system	AntiParkinson's drugs	Dopaminergics
ropivacaine	500, 501	9. Anaesthetic drugs	Anaesthetics – local	
rosiglitazone	447–452	5. Antidiabetic drugs	Other antidiabetic drugs	Thiazolidinediones
rosuvastatin	126	1. Cardiovascular drugs	Lipid-lowering drugs	Statins
rotigoline	*see* dopaminergics 243–250			
salbutamol	664, 665	12. Respiratory drugs	Bronchodilators	Beta-2 agonists
salmeterol	*see* beta-2 agonists 662–665			
saquinavir	613, 621, 624, 625, 626	10. Drugs to treat infections	Antivirals – antiretrovirals	Protease inhibitors
secobarbital	*see* barbiturates (as antiepileptics) 211–214			
selegiline	244, 245, 246, 249, 250	2. Drugs acting on the nervous system	AntiParkinson's drugs	Dopaminergics
sertindole	253, 255, 259, 260, 262	2. Drugs acting on the nervous system	Antipsychotics	
sertraline	169, 170, 174, 175, 177, 178	2. Drugs acting on the nervous system	Antidepressants	Selective serotonin reuptake inhibitors
sevelamer	737	17. Miscellaneous drugs	Minerals	
sevoflurane	*see* anaesthetics – general 494, 496, 497			
sibutramine	238–239	2. Drugs acting on the nervous system	Antiobesity drugs	
sildenafil	688, 689	15. Urological drugs	Erectile dysfunction	Phosphodiesterase type 5 inhibitors
simvastatin	125, 126, 127, 128	1. Cardiovascular drugs	Lipid-lowering drugs	Statins
sirolimus	383–385	3. Anticancer and immunomodulating drugs	Other immunomodulating drugs	

Drug (primary)	Page	Part of the Book	Category	Subcategory (drug groups only)
sitaxentan	*see* vasodilator antihyper-tensives 35, 36, 37, 38, 41, 42, 44–53			
sodium bicarbonate	690	15. Urological drugs	Urinary alkalinization	
sodium clodronate	454	6. Other endocrine drugs	Bisphosphonates	
sodium nitroprusside	*see* vasodilator antihyper-tensives 35, 36, 37, 38, 41, 42, 44–53			
sodium oxybate	273	2. Drugs acting on the nervous system	Anxiolytics and hypnotics	
sodium phenylbutyrate	676	13. Metabolic drugs	Sodium phenylbutyrate	
sodium polystyrene sulphonate	735–736	17. Miscellaneous drugs	Minerals	Polystyrene sulphonate resins
solifenacin	242	2. Drugs acting on the nervous system	AntiParkinson's drugs	Antimuscarinics
somatropin	455	6. Other endocrine drugs	Somatropin	
sorafenib	339	3. Anticancer and immunomodulating drugs	Cytotoxics	
sotalol	62–63	1. Cardiovascular drugs	Beta-blockers	
spironolactone	*see* potassium-sparing diuretics and aldosterone antagonists 112–115			
St John's Wort	191–195	2. Drugs acting on the nervous system	Antidepressants	
stavudine	603, 604, 606, 610	10. Drugs to treat infections	Antivirals – antiretrovirals	Nucleoside reverse transcriptase inhibitors

Drug (primary)	Page	Part of the Book	Category	Subcategory (drug groups only)
streptokinase	*see* thrombolytics 401–402			
streptomycin	511	10. Drugs to treat infections	Antibiotics	Aminoglycosides
strontium ranelate	455	6. Other endocrine drugs	Strontium ranelate	
sucralfate	654	11. Drugs acting on the gastrointestinal tract	Sucralfate	
sulfadiazine	541	10. Drugs to treat infections	Antibiotics	Sulphonamides
sulfamethoxazole/ trimethoprim	542, 543–544, 545, 546	10. Drugs to treat infections	Antibiotics	Sulphonamides
sulfasalazine	*see* aminosalicylates 351			
sulfinpyrazone	486–487	8. Musculoskeletal drugs	Antigout drugs	
sulindac	*see* non-steroidal anti-inflammatory drugs (NSAIDs) 462–470			
sulpiride	253, 255, 263	2. Drugs acting on the nervous system	Antipsychotics	
sumatriptan	231	2. Drugs acting on the nervous system	Antimigraine drugs	5-HT1 agonists – triptans
sunitinib	339	3. Anticancer and immunomodulating drugs	Cytotoxics	
suxamethonium	503, 504, 505	9. Anaesthetic drugs		
tacrolimus	385–388	3. Anticancer and immunomodulating drugs	Other immunomodulating drugs	
tadalafil	688, 689	15. Urological drugs	Erectile dysfunction	Phosphodiesterase type 5 inhibitors
tamoxifen	348–349	3. Anticancer and immunomodulating drugs	Hormones and hormone antagonists	
tegafur	339	3. Anticancer and immunomodulating drugs	Cytotoxics	
teicoplanin	559	10. Drugs to treat infections	Other antibiotics	

Drug (primary)	Page	Part of the Book	Category	Subcategory (drug groups only)
telbivudine	632	10. Drugs to treat infections	Antivirals – other	
telithromycin	515, 516, 518, 519, 520, 522, 523	10. Drugs to treat infections	Antibiotics	Macrolides
telmisartan	*see* angiotensin-II receptor antagonists 34, 35, 26, 27, 38, 39, 41, 42, 43, 44, 46, 48, 49, 51, 52			
temazepam	266	2. Drugs acting on the nervous system	Anxiolytics and hypnotics	Benzodiazepines
temoporfin	339	3. Anticancer and immunomodulating drugs	Cytotoxics	
tenecteplase	*see* thrombolytics 401–402			
tenofovir	605, 606, 608, 609, 610	10. Drugs to treat infections	Antivirals – antiretrovirals	Nucleoside reverse transcriptase inhibitors
tenoxicam	*see* non-steroidal anti-inflammatory drugs (NSAIDs) 462–470			
terazosin	*see* alpha blockers 34, 35, 47, 48, 50, 51			
terbinafine	579	10. Drugs to treat infections	Antifungal drugs	
terbutaline	662	12. Respiratory drugs	Bronchodilators	Beta-2 agonists
terfenadine	658, 660, 661, 662	12. Respiratory drugs	Antihistamines	
testosterone	455–456	6. Other endocrine drugs	Testosterone	
tetrabenazine	286	2. Drugs acting on the nervous system	Neuromuscular and movement disorders	

Drug (primary)	Page	Part of the Book	Category	Subcategory (drug groups only)
tetracycline	546, 547, 548	10. Drugs to treat infections	Antibiotics	Tetracyclines
thalidomide	388	3. Anticancer and immunomodulating drugs	Other immunomodulating drugs	
theophylline	665–673	12. Respiratory drugs	Bronchodilators	Theophyllines
thioguanine	*see* tioguanine			
thiopentone	494, 495	9. Anaesthetic drugs	Anaesthetics – general	
thioridazine	262	2. Drugs acting on the nervous system	Antipsychotics	
thiotepa	339	3. Anticancer and immunomodulating drugs	Cytotoxics	
tiaprofenic acid	*see* non-steroidal anti-inflammatory drugs (NSAIDs) 462–470			
tibolone	685	14. Drugs used in obstetrics and gynaecology	Tibolone	
tigecycline	*see* tetracyclines 546–549			
tiludronate	*see* bisphosphonates 454			
timolol	67, 69, 71	1. Cardiovascular drugs	Beta-blockers	
tinidazole	595	10. Drugs to treat infections	Other antiprotozoals	
tinzaparin	*see* heparins 400–401			
tioguanine	340	3. Anticancer and immunomodulating drugs	Cytotoxics	
tiotropium	241	2. Drugs acting on the nervous system	AntiParkinson's drugs	Antimuscarinics
tipranavir	622, 624	10. Drugs to treat infections	Antivirals – antiretrovirals	Protease inhibitors
tirofiban	*see* glycoprotein IIb/IIIa inhibitors 61			

Drug (primary)	Page	Part of the Book	Category	Subcategory (drug groups only)
tizanidine	489, 490, 491	8. Musculoskeletal drugs	Skeletal muscle relaxants	
tobramycin	*see* aminoglycosides 510–513			
tolbutamide	423, 425, 426, 428, 432	5. Antidiabetic drugs	Sulphonylureas	
tolcapone	245, 249	2. Drugs acting on the nervous system	AntiParkinson's drugs	Dopaminergics
tolterodine	241, 242	2. Drugs acting on the nervous system	AntiParkinson's drugs	Antimuscarinics
tolterodine	687	15. Urological drugs	Urinary incontinence	
topiramate	226	2. Drugs acting on the nervous system	Antiepileptics	
topotecan	340	3. Anticancer and immunomodulating drugs	Cytotoxics	
torasemide	*see* loop diuretics 109			
toremifene	349–350	3. Anticancer and immunomodulating drugs	Hormones and hormone antagonists	
tramadol	470, 475, 476, 478	7. Analgesics	Opioids	
trandolapril	*see* ACE inhibitors 34, 35, 36, 37, 38, 39, 40, 42, 43, 46, 48, 49, 50, 51, 52, 53			
tranylcypromine	*see* monoamine oxidase inhibitors (MAOIs)			
trastuzumab	341	3. Anticancer and immunomodulating drugs	Cytotoxics	
trazodone	189	2. Drugs acting on the nervous system	Antidepressants	Tricyclic antidepressants

Drug (primary)	Page	Part of the Book	Category	Subcategory (drug groups only)
treosulfan	341	3. Anticancer and immunomodulating drugs	Cytotoxics	
tretinoin	383	3. Anticancer and immunomodulating drugs	Other immunomodulating drugs	
triamcinolone	*see* cortico-steroids 367–374			
triamterene	*see* potassium-sparing diuretics and aldosterone antagonists 112–115			
triazolam	264, 268	2. Drugs acting on the nervous system	Anxiolytics and hypnotics	Benzodiazepines
trientine	676	13. Metabolic drugs	Trientine	
trifluoperazine	*see* anti-psychotics 251–263			
trihexyphenidyl	*see* anti-muscarinics 240–247			
trilostane	458	6. Other endocrine drugs	Trilostane	
trimethoprim	542, 544, 545	10. Drugs to treat infections	Antibiotics	Sulphonamides
trimipramine	187	2. Drugs acting on the nervous system	Antidepressants	Tricyclic antidepressants
tripotassium dicitratobis-muthate	655	11. Drugs acting on the gastrointestinal tract	Tripotassium dicitratobismuthate	
tropisetron	208	2. Drugs acting on the nervous system	Antiemetics	5-HT3 antagonists
tryptophan	202	2. Drugs acting on the nervous system	Antidepressants	
urokinase	*see* thrombolytics 401–402			
ursodeoxycholic acid	637	11. Drugs acting on the gastrointestinal tract	Drugs affecting bile	

Drug (primary)	Page	Part of the Book	Category	Subcategory (drug groups only)
valaciclovir	628, 629	10. Drugs to treat infections	Antivirals – other	
valganciclovir	629, 630	10. Drugs to treat infections	Antivirals – other	
valproate	210, 226–227	2. Drugs acting on the nervous system	Antiepileptics	
valproate	740	17. Miscellaneous drugs	Minerals	
valsartan	*see* angiotensin-II receptor antagonists 34, 35, 26, 27, 38, 39, 41, 42, 43, 44, 46, 48, 49, 51, 52			
vancomycin	559–561	10. Drugs to treat infections	Other antibiotics	
vardenafil	689	15. Urological drugs	Erectile dysfunction	Phosphodiesterase type 5 inhibitors
vecuronium	505	9. Anaesthetic drugs		
venlafaxine	175, 196, 197, 198, 199	2. Drugs acting on the nervous system	Antidepressants	
verapamil	88, 89, 90, 91, 92, 93, 94	1. Cardiovascular drugs	Calcium channel blockers	
vigabatrin	210	2. Drugs acting on the nervous system	Antiepileptics	
vinblastine	342, 344, 345	3. Anticancer and immunomodulating drugs	Cytotoxics	
vincristine	342, 343, 344, 345	3. Anticancer and immunomodulating drugs	Cytotoxics	
vinorelbine	342, 343, 344	3. Anticancer and immunomodulating drugs	Cytotoxics	
vitamin A	737	17. Miscellaneous drugs	Minerals	Vitamins
vitamin B12	738	17. Miscellaneous drugs	Minerals	Vitamins
vitamin B6	737–738	17. Miscellaneous drugs	Minerals	Vitamins
vitamin C	738	17. Miscellaneous drugs	Minerals	Vitamins
vitamin D	738	17. Miscellaneous drugs	Minerals	Vitamins
vitamin E	738	17. Miscellaneous drugs	Minerals	

Drug (primary)	Page	Part of the Book	Category	Subcategory (drug groups only)
voriconazole	563, 564, 565, 566, 567, 568, 569, 571, 572, 573, 574, 575	10. Drugs to treat infections	Antifungal drugs	Azoles
warfarin	*see* anticoagulants – oral 390–399			
xipamide	*see* thiazides 116–119			
xylometazoline	*see* sympathomimetics 138			
zafirlukast	673–674	12. Respiratory drugs	Leukotriene receptor antagonists	
zalcitabine	608, 611	10. Drugs to treat infections	Antivirals – antiretrovirals	Nucleoside reverse transcriptase inhibitors
zaleplon	273	2. Drugs acting on the nervous system	Anxiolytics and hypnotics	
zidovudine	603, 604, 605, 606, 607, 610, 611	10. Drugs to treat infections	Antivirals – antiretrovirals	Nucleoside reverse transcriptase inhibitors
zidovudine	741	17. Miscellaneous drugs	Minerals	Other drug-mineral interactions
zinc	739	17. Miscellaneous drugs	Minerals	
zoledronate	*see* bisphosphonates 454			
zolmitriptan	230, 231, 234, 235	2. Drugs acting on the nervous system	Antimigraine drugs	5-HT1 agonists – triptans
zolpidem	273	2. Drugs acting on the nervous system	Anxiolytics and hypnotics	
zopiclone	273	2. Drugs acting on the nervous system	Anxiolytics and hypnotics	
zotepine	*see* antipsychotics 251–263			
zuclopenthixol	254, 262	2. Drugs acting on the nervous system	Antipsychotics	

INTRODUCTION

Factors that contribute to differences in drug response, which in some situations suggest that only 25–60% of patients show the expected response, also contribute to drug interactions. The estimated incidence of drug–drug interactions that have a clinical significance ranges from 3% to 20%, determined mainly by the number of drugs taken by a patient.[1] A commonly used concept is that with the use of four drugs the potential for drug–drug interactions is 6, increasing to 28 with eight drugs and to 35 with nine drugs. More than 2 million cases of adverse drug reactions occur annually in the USA, including 100 000 deaths; some reports in 1995 indicated that the cost of drug-related morbidity and mortality in the USA is $136 billion annually, which was more than the total cost of cardiovascular or diabetic care.[2]

The Institute of Medicine reported in January 2000 that between 44 000 and 98 000 deaths occur annually from medical errors and that an estimated 7000 deaths occur due to adverse drug reactions, which was in excess of the 6000 deaths that occurred annually from workplace injuries.[3]

The National Association of Chain Drug Stores reported that more than 3.5 billion prescriptions were filled in the USA in 2008,[4] which equates to an average of more than 11 prescriptions per head of the population. Efforts to reduce polypharmacy are important but, for many patients, the number of medications cannot always be reduced safely. Thus, it is important to understand the basis for drug interactions to enable the most appropriate choices in prescribing and avoid preventable adverse drug interactions.

It is not surprising that addressing the subtle and complex drug–drug interactions arising from exotic regimens exceeds the capabilities of most clinicians. Many clinicians and prescribers depend on office- or pharmacy-based computer software programs to help avert harmful drug interactions. These programs have unquestionable advantages over the human brain. However, limitations include the identification of interactions with variable accuracy, the inconsistent ranking of severity and the lack of sophistication to weed out trivial interactions, the latter often resulting in a surfeit of false alarms. No one can be faulted as most of the information comes from case reports and studies involving health volunteers. Thus, what does or could take place in disease states and real-world patients remains uncertain.

An essential preliminary step to prevent adverse drug–drug interactions is to obtain a comprehensive list of medications that a patient is taking. Unfortunately, there may be difficulties in taking an accurate drug history, often due to lack of time and especially when patients also take traditional/natural remedies, OTC drugs and nutrients, which patients often consider as unimportant to reveal.

This book, written with a definite clinical bias (as the editors and contributors are practising prescribers from a range of disciplines), is designed to be an easily accessible reference for busy prescribers/dispensers who may not have access to, or the time to search, the more comprehensive resources on adverse drug–drug interactions both in print and online. We have considered interactions which we considered to be important for clinicians and described the effects of such interactions, a summary of their probable mechanisms and factors that may influence the severity of interactions. Since the book is intended to be a practical guide for prescribers (doctors, nurses or pharmacists), we have also presented the following information:

- what precautions need to be taken;
- which alarm signals (symptoms and signs) to look out for;
- what sort of monitoring needs to be undertaken and how often;
- what interventions might prevent an adverse interaction.

Ours is a very simplistic approach to a subject associated with a varying range of uncertainties: mechanisms, grading of severity, predictability, individual susceptibility and interventions. The intent is to increase awareness, provide an easy-to-access information source and minimize the mistakes that busy prescribers may unintentionally make. To the best of our knowledge, we have described the consensus recommendations for managing each interaction. However, the evidence base for the recommendations given is variable so it should be recognized that, in some circumstances, it is difficult to provide an authoritative source of information with finite causations, clinical outcomes and predictability (e.g. when a serious interaction has a theoretical basis). However, we have pieced together succinct information that may assist in prescribing and assist clinicians who may be required to treat the consequences of adverse drug–drug interactions. There are also sections devoted to herbal medicines and to OTC medicines.

Factors influencing drug interactions

Patients tend to respond in different ways to the same medication. In several instances, this variability may be quite substantial as the differences in response can lead to drug-associated toxicity in some patients and to therapeutic failure in others. The beneficial and adverse effects of individual drugs are determined by pharmaceutical, pharmacokinetic and pharmacodynamic factors.

Pharmaceutical

Pharmaceutical interactions almost always occur when drugs are mixed outside the body prior to administration. Polycationic protamine binding to heparin inside the body is considered a pharmaceutical interaction. Mixing chemically incompatible drugs before intravenous infusion can result in precipitation or inactivation (e.g. incompatibility of phenobarbital with chlorpromazine or opioid analgesics, and of thiopentone when mixed with suxamethonium in the same syringe; in addition, phenytoin precipitates in dextrose solution, amphotericin precipitates in saline, and gentamicin is inactivated by most beta-lactam agents).

Pharmaceutical interactions are the least likely to cause problems in clinical practice, and there are no potentially hazardous interactions of this type with many drugs as precipitation, discoloration or any other physico-chemical reaction becomes obvious to the naked eye.

Pharmacokinetics

The concentration of the drug that reaches the site of action (target organs or receptors) is an important determinant of its clinical effect and, in particular, the balance between desired and adverse effects. Pharmacokinetics describes the processes that affect the concentration of drug at the receptor (i.e. what the human body does to the drug). It relates to the effects that occur during absorption (which can also be adjusted by manipulating certain *pharmaceutical* properties), distribution, metabolism and excretion. Pharmacokinetic interactions result in changes in the concentration of the drug at its site of action.

Absorption can be affected by changes to the transport proteins in the intestine (see the section on 'Transport proteins' below), due to drugs binding (chelating) with other drugs in the gut lumen, alterations of pH within the gut (particularly within the stomach) or alterations in gastrointestinal motility. The induction or inhibition of transport proteins will affect the amount of drug absorbed, as will agents that decrease salivary secretions affecting the absorption of sublingual tablets.

Distribution is essentially via the bloodstream, and any alterations in blood flow will affect distribution. This may occur due to decreased output from the heart (with myocardial depressants) and drugs that decrease blood flow (often due to vasoconstriction) to the liver and kidneys.

Metabolism may be altered by when drugs compete for the same metabolizing enzymes (e.g. in the liver or intestine) or excretory pathways in the kidney. As important is the induction and inhibition of metabolizing enzymes. See the section below on cytochrome enzymes for more details.

- *Excretion* may be altered by the induction or inhibition of transport proteins, and by decreases in blood flow to the organs where excretion takes place (liver and kidney).
- *First-pass metabolism.* All drugs absorbed from the gastrointestinal tract (the exception being drugs administered per rectum) pass through the liver, where a portion of the drug is metabolized before reaching the systemic circulation. Thus, the induction or inhibition of metabolizing enzymes in the liver will alter the amount of drug reaching the bloodstream after first-pass metabolism.

Displacement from protein-binding sites, increasing the plasma concentration of unbound, active drug, was considered to be associated with increased elimination, thus minimizing the clinical consequences. However, Sandson et al.[5] illustrated that drug displacement from protein-binding sites accompanied by an inhibition of metabolism results in an increased plasma concentrations of drugs (e.g. aspirin inhibits the beta-oxidation responsible for approximately 40% of valproate metabolism, the net result being increased free valproate plasma concentrations without a significant increase in total plasma valproate concentration). The clinical concerns are straightforward – the measurement or monitoring of only total concentrations of drugs during concomitant therapy runs the risk of failing to detect drug toxicities that often produce adverse clinical outcomes.

Pharmacodynamics

Pharmacodynamics describes the effect(s) of a drug on the human body, which is primarily determined by its concentration at the site of action (which in turn depends on its pharmacokinetics).The nature of change at target sites or receptors depends on the state of these sites, for example whether they are affected by disease states. Pharmacodynamic interactions may result in excessive therapeutic effects, diminished therapeutic effects or additive adverse effects (e.g. adding together two drugs that prolong the Q–T interval).

Antagonistic pharmacodynamic interactions, for example reversal of non-depolarizing muscle relaxants, or reversal of the toxic effects of opioids or of BDZs, are sometimes of value in critical situations.

Disease states shift the dose–response curve (i.e. concentration–response), usually to the left, which means that it is likely to be associated with an exaggerated response to a given dose at the site of action.

Therapeutic index

The range of concentrations within which a drug produces the desired effect without toxicity is important. If this range – the therapeutic index of the drug – is narrow (e.g. ciclosporin, digoxin, ergotamine, phenytoin, pimozide, quinidine, tacrolimus, terfenadine, theophylline), there is only a small difference between the level that produces the desired clinical effect and the concentration that results in undesired, adverse or toxic effects. Consequently, drugs with a narrow therapeutic index are more likely to be associated with clinically significant drug–drug interactions, because even small changes in concentration are likely to have significant clinical effects.

Common metabolizing enzymes

Cytochrome P450 superfamily

There are two recognized phases of drug metabolism:

1. phase I metabolism, in which drugs undergo hydrolysis, oxidation or reduction;
2. phase II metabolism, where drugs are bound to compounds (by glucuronidation or sulphuration) to facilitate excretion.

Phase I metabolism is mainly catalysed by a superfamily of enzymes, the cytochrome group (a group of nearly 30 related enzymes present in the endoplasmic reticulum of cells in the liver and intestine), which can be induced (producing increased activity) or inhibited (producing decreased activity).

Induction by drugs, food and herbal medicines is usually dose- and time-dependent, and in general reversible. The induction of enzymes increases the rate of synthesis and cellular content and activity of the enzymes. As induction involves protein synthesis, there is a delay in its onset (weeks with some drugs), and effects usually last longer after stopping the inducer (a long off-set time). Drug-induced inhibition is usually competitive and occurs immediately, but it is dependent on the concentration of the inhibitor. Thus, the half-life of the inhibitor will determine how long it has to be administered for before its full effects are observed and how long its effects last after discontinuation.

Following the oral administration of an enzyme/transport protein inhibitor, the intestinal CYP3A enzymes/transport proteins are exposed to higher levels of the interacting drug and are inhibited to a greater extent than are liver enzymes/transport proteins. The ability to induce or inhibit is not limited to the parent drug. Many products of metabolism (metabolites) may possess different inhibitory or inducing activity from the parent drug. Also, some drugs have different forms that have different activities. For example, warfarin is a racemic mixture: *S*-warfarin is metabolized by CYP2C9/10 and has the more potent anticoagulant effect. The relatively inactive enantiomer *R*-warfarin is metabolized by CYP1A2 but can inhibit CYP2C9/10 and thus produce an increased plasma concentration of *S*-warfarin. Fluvoxamine increases the activity of *R*-warfarin indirectly by inhibiting CYP1A2, which results in an inhibition of CYP2C9/10 and a build-up of *S*-warfarin.

CYP3A is the most abundant group in humans. Most pharmaceuticals are metabolized by CYP3A4, CYP2D6, CYP1A2, CYP2C, CYP2C10 and CYP2C19 isoenzymes. When a drug is metabolized by more than one set of isoenzymes, the clinical effect of an individual drug interaction depends upon a number of factors:

- the extent to which each CYP enzyme contributes to the metabolism of that drug;
- the potency of inducers/inhibitors for the drug's dominant metabolic pathway;
- changes in metabolizing activity that may result from genetic polymorphism (see later);
- metabolites possessing clinical activity.

In other words, an interaction may not follow the induction or inhibition of one of the isoenzymes provided the other isoenzyme metabolizes a considerable proportion of the drug and is not also affected by the inducers or inhibitors. The vast majority of drugs that may cause cardiac arrhythmias by prolonging the Q–T interval are metabolized by CYP3A.

Uridine diphosphate glucuronosyltransferases

UGTs are responsible for the metabolism of many anxiolytics, antidepressants, mood stabilizers and antipsychotics. Inhibition of the metabolism of carbamazepine by valproic acid in part results from an effect on UGTs. Amitriptyline and clomipramine decrease the metabolism of morphine by affecting UGTs.

Inducers of UGT include carbamazepine, phenobarbital, phenytoin and rifampin. Inhibitors of UGTs include amitriptyline, chlorpromazine, ciclosporin, clomipramine, diazepam, lorazepam, nitrazepam and valproic acid.

Transport proteins

Transport proteins are proteins present in cell membranes associated with movement of drugs into and out of the body and between body compartments (e.g. between the gut lumen and intestinal wall, from the intestinal wall into the endothelium, thence into the bloodstream, and from the bloodstream into the cells where the drug has its site of action).

P-glycoprotein and human *OATPs* play an important role in drug interactions by determining the concentration of a drug in the plasma/blood by influencing both the rate at which drugs are absorbed in to blood and the rate at which they are removed or excreted from the body. Transport systems have the greatest influence in the intestine, where they determine the rate at which drugs are absorbed, and in the kidney, where they determine the amount of drug excreted from the body. They also influence the amounts of drug lost in the bile. P-gp determines primarily the efflux of drug from the body, while OATPs determine the influx of a drug.

Drugs that are known to be substrates of P-gp include antihistamines (e.g. terfenadine), digoxin, ciclosporin, hydrocortisone and other steroids and drugs used in chemotherapy (e.g. paclitaxel, vinblastine). Ciclosporin, in addition to being a substrate of P-gp, is also an inhibitor of P-gp. Drugs known to induce P-gp include morphine, dexamethasone, phenobarbital, rifampin and St John's wort. Inhibitors of P-gp include amiodarone, amitriptyline, atorvastatin, chlorpromazine, ciclosporin, erythromycin, fluphenazine, haloperidol, quinidine, ritonavir and verapamil.

OATPs are found in the intestine, liver, kidney and brain. They tend to move or pump drugs from regions of high concentration to those of lower concentration. Examples of drugs that are influenced by the activity of OATPs include digoxin, enalapril, hydrocortisone, lovastatin and the anti-HIV protease inhibitor drugs saquinavir and ritonavir.

The metabolizing enzymes (cytochrome enzymes) P-gp and OATP have features in common:

- Their activity can be increased (induction) or decreased (inhibition).
- The are subject to genetic polymorphisms that affect their levels of activity.

Genetic polymorphisms

Pharmacogenetics is the relationship between genetic variations and individual differences in drug response. Sequence alterations (polymorphisms) in the genes involved in drug absorption and disposition (e.g. phase I and phase II enzymes and transport proteins) or with indirect effects on drug response contribute to genetic differences in drug response.

Population heterogeneities in alleles and phenotypes are present. Around 2–3% of white individuals and 4% of black individuals have poor metabolism with CYP2C19, whereas 10–25% of those in South-east Asia show poor metabolism. CYP2D6 polymorphisms affect drugs that are mainly used for cardiovascular and psychiatric diseases and that have a narrow therapeutic index and are usually used in the long term (e.g. antiarrhythmics, beta-adrenergic blockers, anticoagulants, antipsychotic agents, antidepressants, analgesics). Polymorphism of CYP2C9 isoenzyme influences the metabolism of nearly 100 commonly used drugs (e.g. fluoxetine, phenytoin, *S*-warfarin, losartan, several NSAIDs including celecoxib, tolbutamide).

The difference in enzyme activity that occurs due to polymorphisms results in individuals who are extensive metabolizers (with a subgroup of ultrarapid metabolizers) or poor metabolizers of drugs. Poor metabolizers have higher concentrations of drug for a given dose than extensive metabolizers. However, the slow metabolism results in lower levels of metabolites. The clinical effect of this depends upon the relative activity of the parent drug and its metabolite. For example, if a metabolite has no clinical activity, extensive metabolizers will show less clinical effect than poor metabolizers, while a therapeutic dose in an extensive metabolizer may result in toxicity for poor metabolizers – one man's medicine is literally another man's poison! Conversely, if the metabolite has more clinical activity than the parent drug (e.g. with a prodrug), extensive metabolizers will show more clinical effect than poor metabolizers, which may result in toxicity in extensive metabolizers or therapeutic failure in poor metabolizers. The consequences of genetic polymorphisms become clinically significant with drugs having a narrow therapeutic index.

Phenocopying results in the conversion of an extensive to a poor metabolizer. This has clinical relevance when SSRIs are used in combination with TCAs, when plasma levels of tricyclics may be increased by a factor of 2–4 after the co-administration of SSRIs.

In 2004, the FDA approved a microarray chip designed to routinely identify polymorphisms of drug-metabolizing enzymes related to cytochrome P450 drug metabolism.

Gender-related variability in drug response has also been suggested to be clinically important. For example, in treatment of HIV infections, mycophenolate metabolism is higher in male than female kidney transplant recipients.

Disease states

Infection can by itself affect activity of CYP isoenzymes (viral or bacterial pulmonary infections having been shown to depress CYP activity). Infection is likely to induce a global inhibition of cytochrome P450 catalytic activities (attributed to the release of endotoxin or interferon), thus predisposing to adverse drug–drug interactions. Adverse drug interactions are also important during the treatment of disease states considered to be 'serious' or life-threatening. Straubhaar et al.[6] concluded that accepted standard therapy for patients with heart failure has the potential to cause adverse drug interactions, with 25% of patients being exposed to possible severe interactions, and that drug combinations with the potential to cause changes in electrolytes (e.g. hyperkalaemia) and blood or fluid loss can cause adverse effects in the absence of careful monitoring.

Age

Older people tend to be more sensitive to drugs than younger people due to:

- *polypharmacy*, as older people (over 65 years of age) are often taking more prescribed and OTC medicines, and possibly traditional herbal remedies, than any other age group; also the risk of drug interactions increases exponentially with the number of drugs administered,[7] hence the need to inquire about OTC and herbal medicines;

- *altered pharmacodynamics*, due to alterations in physiological (reduced physiological reserve – diarrhoea may cause significant fluid depletion and electrolyte imbalance) and homeostatic (loss of elasticity in the blood vessels from arteriosclerosis) systems and the presence of narrowed blood vessels (atherosclerosis), including the autonomic nervous system (postural hypotension), the baroreceptors, thermoregulation and balance (falls may have serious consequences in elderly people);
- *altered pharmacokinetics*, as age-related hepatic or renal dysfunction may alter the ability to metabolize or excrete drugs, lowering the threshold for adverse drug interactions to occur. Loss of muscle mass also tends to produce higher plasma concentrations of an administered drug.

Adverse drug interactions may present in an unusual or non-specific manner in elderly people (e.g. the gradual onset of confusion), delaying their recognition. Effects such as hypotension, dizziness, blurred vision, sedation and ataxia should be avoided or detected and corrected early. Constipation and urinary retention tend to occur more frequently and cause considerable morbidity. It is advisable when starting therapy to use a lower dose (say 50% of the normal dose) and follow the adage to: 'start low and go slow'.

Although children as a rule have relatively large livers, this does not mean that they can metabolize drugs more efficiently (e.g. there is an impaired metabolism of chloramphenicol in neonates, causing toxicity). Furthermore, they have a developing nervous system and immune system, and adverse effects on such systems could have more deleterious effects than in young healthy adults. Different clinical scenarios occur in neonates, such as the presence of bilirubin and the displacement of bilirubin from binding sites by sulphonamides, predisposing to kernicterus.

Smoking and alcohol

Smoking induces CYP1A2, CYP2E1 and enzymes involved in glucuronidation so the metabolism of substrate drugs could be enhanced; there is even evidence that limited or passive smoking may have a measurable effect.[8] The clearance of these drugs may be increased by 60–90%, which could result in their plasma concentrations being decreased by 50% and would lead to therapeutic failure. It should be noted that this effect is reversed by stopping smoking, and Horn and Hansten[8] note that this can result in potential toxic effects that can be insidious in onset.

Examples of drugs affected by smoking[8] include: antiarrhythmics (flecainide, mexiletine), anticancer drugs (erlotinib), anticoagulants (warfarin), antidepressants (duloxetine, fluvoxamine, mirtazapine), antiparkinsonian drugs (rasagiline, ropinirole, selegiline), antipsychotics (chlorpromazine, clozapine, haloperidol, olanzapine), beta-blockers (propranolol), bronchodilators (theophylline), diuretics (triamterene), 5-hydroxytryptamine antagonists (frovatriptan, ondansetron) and skeletal muscle relaxants (tizanidine).

The acute ingestion of *alcohol* inhibits CYP2D6 and CYP2C19, whereas chronic use induces CYP2E1 and CYP3A4, which form the basis for adverse drug interactions with substrates of these isoenzymes.

Lysosomal trapping

This is a mechanism of drug interaction at cellular level. Tricyclic antidepressants, SSRIs and aliphatic phenothiazines are basic lipophilic compounds taken up by acidic compartments in the cell, which often principally involves association with phospholipids in the cell membrane, whereas others undergo lysosomal trapping within the cell. Tissues such as the lungs, liver and kidneys are rich in lysosomes (intracellular organelles containing lytic enzymes), and if a drug is susceptible to trapping, these tissues take up most of the drug in the body.

Drugs that are trapped compete with each other for uptake into the organelles. Mutual inhibition of lysosomal trapping results in higher plasma concentrations. This will have the greatest effect on tissues with a low density of lysosomes such as the heart. This interaction may contribute to the increased cardiotoxicity of drugs such as thioridazine when co-prescribed with antidepressants.

Within the brain, differences in lysosomal density among various cells may also predispose to adverse drug interactions. Lysosomes are more numerous in neurones than astrocytes, and decreased trapping may increase the exposure of cell surface receptors to the drug. Examples of this mechanism causing CNS effects are yet to be elucidated.

References

1. Brunton LL (ed.). *Goodman & Gilman's The Pharmacological Basis of Therapeutics*, 11th edn. London: McGraw-Hill, 2007.
2. Johnson JA, Bootman JL. Drug-related morbidity and mortality. A cost-of-illness model. *Arch Intern Med* 1995; **155**: 1949–56.
3. Committee on Quality of Health Care in America. Institute of Medicine. *To Err Is Human: Building a Safer Health System*. Washington, DC: National Academy Press, 2000.
4. National Academy of Chain Drug Stores. Chain Pharmacy Industry Profile Showcases Extraordinary Impact of Pharmacies as a Frontline Healthcare Provider, Significantly Impacting Economy. www.nacds.org/wmspage.cfm?parm1=5912 (accessed November 2008).
5. Sandson NB, Marcucci C, Bourke DL, Smith-Lamacchica R. An interaction between aspirin and valproate: the relevance of plasma protein displacement drug–drug-interactions. *Am J Psychiatry* 2006; **163**: 1891–6.
6. Straubhaar B, Krahenbuhl S, Schlienger RG. The prevalence of potential drug–drug interactions in patients with heart failure at hospital discharge. *Drug Saf* 2006; **29**: 79–90.
7. Milde AS, Motsch J. [Drug interactions and the anaesthesiologist]. *Anesthetist* 2003; **52**: 839–59.
8. Horn JR, Hansten P. Potential drug interactions in smokers and quitters. *Pharmacy Times* 2007; **5**: 56. Available online at: www.pharmacytimes.com/issues/articles/2007-05_4672.asp (accessed November 2008).

Further reading

DuBuske LM. The role of P-glycoprotein and organic anion-transporting polypeptides in drug interactions. *Drug Saf* 2005; **28**: 789–801.

Naguib M, Magboul MM, Jaroudi R. Clinically significant drug interactions with general anaesthetics – incidence, mechanisms and management. *Middle East J Anesthesiol* 1997; **14**: 127–83.

CLINICAL FEATURES OF SOME ADVERSE DRUG INTERACTIONS

General considerations

- If inducers of drug metabolism are used concurrently, be aware of a lack of therapeutic effect of the substrate (primary) drug and a risk of toxicity of the substrate drug when the inducer is discontinued, particularly if dose increases of the substrate drug have been made to obtain the desired therapeutic effect.
- If inhibitors of drug metabolism are used concurrently, be aware of and monitor for toxic/adverse effects of the substrate drug. Watch for a lack of therapeutic effect when the inhibitor is discontinued; the development of lack of therapeutic effect will depend on the half-life of the inhibitor.
- Be aware that OTC medications, nutritional supplements and herbal medications can interact in known and unknown ways to cause an inhibition/induction of metabolizing enzymes and transport mechanisms. The constituents can cause additive/antagonist effects and adverse life-threatening interactions, particularly in people on medications discussed in the main sections (e.g. MAOI antidepressants, opioids, corticosteroids, immunosuppressants, anticoagulants).

The clinical features of drug interactions are often non-specific, and therefore a high index of suspicion should be maintained if they are to be recognized promptly. When a new drug is started, a specific management plan should be made, which should include:

- which physiological parameters (e.g. PR, BP) should be measured and how often;
- which investigations (e.g. blood tests, ECG) should be undertaken and how often;
- educating patients (and carers when necessary) about the symptoms and signs of the potential interactions that may occur and when they should seek medical attention.

The following list of problems that may be the result of drug interactions is not exhaustive and does not include any recommendations about management; clinicians are advised to follow accredited national or local guidelines.

Blood glucose abnormalities

Home blood glucose monitoring is recommended for all patients on antidiabetic medications, particularly insulin. If values are below 4 mmol/L or persistently above 15 mmol/L, **patients should seek immediate medical advice**. Self-monitoring is usually offered to those with type 2 diabetes as an integral part of self-management education.

Hypoglycaemia

Hypoglycaemia (or a 'hypo') occurs when the blood glucose falls to below 4 mmol/L. The usual warning signs include tremor, sweating, paraesthesia, going pale, pounding heart, dizziness, slurred speech, confusion and irritability. It is likely that the longer a patient has had diabetes, the less obvious the warning symptoms will be. Beta-adrenergic blockers (e.g. propranolol, atenolol) may mask the symptoms of hypoglycaemia.

Hyperglycaemia

Common symptoms include thirst, polydipsia (increased oral fluid intake), a dry mouth, polyuria (increased urination), nocturia (increased passage of urine at night), weight loss, tiredness, fatigue and blurred vision. The glycosylated haemoglobin (HbA_{1c}) value indicates blood glucose levels for the previous 2–3 months and is usually measured at least twice a year. If there is an addition of medication(s) or significant dose changes, the HbA_{1c} is checked 2–3 months later. The current NICE target is below 6.5% for type 2 diabetes and less than 6.5% or less than 7.5% for type 1 diabetes depending on co-morbidities.

Severe hyperglycaemia may lead to diabetic ketoacidosis: polyuria, thirst, leg cramps, weakness, nausea, vomiting, abdominal pain, Kussmaul's respiration (increased depth and rate of breathing), drowsiness, confusion and coma.

Blood pressure changes

The British Hypertension Society and NICE recommend that BP should be measured with the patient sitting (the British Hypertension Society recommends for at least 3 minutes) with the arm supported in a horizontal position at the level of the mid-sternum. If the BP is found to be raised, a second measurement should be made after at least 1 minute (preferably at the end of the consultation). If there are symptoms suggestive of postural hypotension, BP should be measured with the patient standing up for at least 1 minute.

Blood pressure should be monitored monthly until stable (weekly if hypertension is severe) and ideally should be measured at the same time after taking antihypertensive medication.

Hypotension

Warn patients to report any symptoms suggestive of hypotension, for example light-headedness, dizziness, fainting while standing up (postural hypotension), blurred vision, confusion, tiredness, weakness or temporary loss of consciousness. Advise patients to keep properly hydrated (e.g. a minimum intake of 2 L of water a day). Hypotensive episodes are more likely in those with compromised compensatory mechanism such as in diabetic autonomic neuropathy and following myocardial infarction. Hypotensive episodes may also accompany arrhythmias.

Hypertension

Hypertension is usually asymptomatic; however, chronic headaches, dizziness/vertigo and blurred vision may occur with severe hypertension. Severe hypertensive crises may occur during concurrent treatment with MAOIs and drugs known to cause such an interaction (which is likely to occur for up to 2 weeks after discontinuing the MAOI or other offending drug; see section on MAOIs). An early warning sign is a throbbing headache, and immediate medical attention should be sought.

Severe hypertensive episodes (BP>180/110 mmHg, especially with papilloedema or retinal haemorrhages) need to be treated aggressively.

Q–T interval prolongation

It is necessary always to be aware of this adverse drug interaction, which has to be avoided as it leads to syncope and sudden death. Several classes of drug, as indicated in the tables throughout the book, are associated with this adverse interaction, predisposition being increased by the presence of electrolyte abnormalities (e.g. hypokalaemia, hypomagnesaemia).

This dangerous adverse interaction may occur with some OTC drugs and with commonly prescribed/dispensed antibiotics (usually short-term courses) for common infections (e.g. coughs, fungal infection), particularly when the patient is on a drug that belongs to a class known to be associated with the causation of QT prolongation. Thus, a history of current medications is needed.

Potassium abnormalities

Hyperkalaemia

Hyperkalaemia (defined as serum potassium >5.3 mEq/L) is rare in healthy individuals. Levels over 7 mmol/L indicate a medical emergency as cardiac arrest may occur. Drugs are implicated in the development of hyperkalaemia in as many as 75% of cases.

Hyperkalaemia is often asymptomatic; symptoms when they occur are non-specific, such as fatigue, weakness, paraesthesia and palpitations. Therefore, it is vitally important to monitor serum potassium levels in all patients who take medications that may cause hyperkalaemia.

Symptoms suggestive of hyperkalaemia require immediate medical attention. Note that in one study, all patients who died of hyperkalemia had normal potassium levels within the 36 hours prior to death.

Hypokalaemia

This is probably the most common electrolyte abnormality affecting hospitalized patients. Again, the symptoms are relatively non-specific, so regular monitoring of serum potassium levels is extremely important.

Features include muscle weakness and cramps, paraesthesia, nausea, vomiting, constipation, abdominal pain, polyuria, polydipsia, depression, confusion and psychosis. Hypokalaemia may cause brady/tachyarrhythmias, hypotension, respiratory failure, ileus and altered mental state. It also increases the toxicity of cardiac glycosides. There are several associated disease states (e.g. diarrhoea, vomiting, renal tubular acidosis types I and II, hypomagnesaemia, Conn's syndrome, Cushing's disease, Gitelman's syndrome, villous adenoma, pyloric stenosis, intestinal fistulae).

Serotonin toxicity and serotonin syndrome

This is caused by excessive stimulation of CNS and peripheral serotonin receptors and is characterized by changes in mental state, autonomic hyperactivity (hypertension, tachycardia, hyperthermia, may be up to 41°C, hyperactive bowel sounds, mydriasis, excessive sweating) and neuromuscular abnormality (tremor, clonus, ocular clonus, hypertonicity, hyperreflexia); the latter may lead to rhabdomyolysis with consequent risk of renal failure, hyperkalaemia and hypocalcaemia. Symptoms usually occur within 6 hours of taking the provoking drug. Tremor, akathisia and diarrhoea are early features.

This is a very serious adverse interaction and immediate medical attention is necessary, usually in a critical care setting.

Immunosuppression and blood dyscrasias

Leukocyte and differential counts (including platelet counts) must be normal before starting treatment with drugs that have the potential to cause blood dyscrasias or bone marrow suppression.

Patients and their carers should be told to recognize signs of blood disorders and advised to seek immediate medical treatment if symptoms such as fever, sore throat, flu-like illnesses, rashes, mouth ulcers, purpura, bleeding or bruising develop, or the individual feels unduly tired, weak or unwell (fatigue, lethargy or malaise). Bleeding can be indicated by gum bleeding while brushing the teeth, nosebleeds of no apparent cause, bruising with no or minimal trauma, dark urine and/or tarry stools.

Neutropenia, lymphopenia and pancytopenia are likely to occur when two drugs causing such effects are co-administered or can arise from increased concentrations of such a drug due to impaired metabolism or impaired excretion.

With neutropenia, symptoms may be absent but there may be signs of severe life-threatening infection. Neutrophil counts below 0.5×10^9/L are associated with the highest risk of severe infections. The clinical features of infection may be modified.

Bleeding disorders

Excessive anticoagulation

The likely causes of this are increased plasma concentrations of warfarin (see warfarin interactions) and/or the concurrent use of drugs with effects on coagulation (e.g. drugs with antiplatelet or anti-thrombolytic activity). Assess clotting screen (INR for warfarin, APTT for unfractionated heparin; low molecular weight heparins are not routinely monitored), liver function and FBC (for platelet count) prior to initiating anticoagulant therapy. Local guidelines may vary, but it would seem safe to measure INR every other day until stable during concurrent administration with a drug that has the potential to interact.

Underanticoagulation

This is usually asymptomatic, but it may have potentially life-threatening consequences (e.g. pulmonary embolism, catastrophic heart failure) as anticoagulants are mainly used for the treatment and prevention of venous thromboembolic disease and after heart valve replacement. When a drug is added that may reduce the effect of anticoagulants (and when it is stopped), the INR should be measured every other day until it stabilizes.

Central nervous system depression

Many drugs are known depressants of the CNS, for example opioids, anxiolytics and hypnotics, older antihistamines, antipsychotic drugs and antidepressants. Other drugs may cause fatigue or lethargy by other mechanisms, as is seen with calcium channel blockers. Even minor degrees of sedation can be dangerous, for example:

- for everyday activities such as driving or cooking;
- if the patient's occupation requires operating machinery, the use of sharp implements or working at heights;
- for individuals at risk of falling, such as elderly people and those with pre-existing balance impairments.

It is important to remember that the sedative effects of all of these drugs are exacerbated by even small amounts of alcohol.

Some of these CNS depressants, particularly opioid analgesics, may be administered topically. Patients/carers should be warned about the following/signs and be advised to seek immediate medical attention if they occur:

- excessive drowsiness;
- laboured breathing;
- impairment of mental acuity (cognition).

Antimuscarinic effects

Antagonism of the muscarinic receptors of the parasympathetic nervous system causes a wide range of symptoms and signs, including dry mouth, blurred vision, constipation, difficulty in passing urine, dizziness, confusion, palpitations and tachycardia.

Many drugs used in elderly patients have antimuscarinic effects, such as drugs used to treat urinary incontinence, depression, Parkinson's disease and gastrointestinal disorders, and those given topically for some eye disorders. Additive antimuscarinic effects such as confusion, retention of urine and blurring of vision are potentially dangerous in the elderly as they increase the risk of accidents and falls. If the individual has been prescribed drugs to be taken sublingually (e.g. GTN tablets), a dry mouth would result in reduced dissolution of these tablets and decreased effect of the drug, which is undesirable, for example during an angina attack.

Both patients and their carers should be advised to look out for early features of confusion, unstable gait and visual symptoms. In order to minimize patient discomfort, immediate measures should be taken to relieve these symptoms, for example using mild laxatives for constipation, ensuring adequate hydration and ensuring assistance is available when patients wish to be mobile. Some OTC drugs (e.g. antihistamines) have antimuscarinic effects.

Gastrointestinal adverse effects – risk of ulcers and haemorrhage

Symptoms and warning signs include gastrointestinal (stomach) discomfort such as dyspepsia/indigestion, nausea or vomiting (with or without fresh or altered blood), and dark, tarry stools.

Additive gastrointestinal side-effects are likely to occur with combinations of:

- more than one NSAID;
- high-dose aspirin (>100 mg) with NSAIDs;
- corticosteroids with NSAIDs.

Renal toxicity

The kidneys are an important pathway for elimination of drugs, and any impairment of renal function (e.g. decreased renal blood flow, renal damage) can cause marked increases in plasma concentrations of drugs eliminated primarily by renal mechanisms.

Additive renal toxic effects may occur with immunosuppressants (e.g. azathioprine, ciclosporin, tacrolimus), ACE inhibitors, penicillamine, irinotecan and aminoglycoside antibiotics. A deterioration of renal function may even occur after the topical use of NSAIDs. Guidelines are variable for the use of NSAIDs with differing degrees of renal function, as assessed by creatinine clearance measurements.

Drugs to be avoided in renal insufficiency

These include mesalazine, metformin, NSAIDs, tetracyclines (except doxycycline and minocycline), chloramphenicol, lithium, methotrexate, chloroquine, fibrates, chlorpropamide and glibenclamide. Clinically, it is useful to measure urine output per hour or per 24 hours as a fall in urine output in the presence of adequate fluid intake often indicates or warns of some impairment of renal function. Furthermore, it is neither expensive nor time-consuming to perform a quick test for albumin, casts and red cells in the urine, and to measure pH. Creatinine clearance values are often used to determine the 'safe' doses for several drugs (e.g. NSAIDs, ciclosporin).

Inadequate control of seizures with antiepileptics

Patients and carers are recommended to keep a diary indicating frequency of attacks, occurrence of déjàvu and ja nuvis phenomena, blank spells, flashing lights and episodes of abnormal behaviour. An increased occurrence of any of the above or a lack of decrease in occurrence indicates inadequate therapeutic control, and dose adjustments are necessary.

Toxic profiles of the common antiepileptics vary. Of these, phenytoin has the narrowest therapeutic index, and toxicity is likely to cause ataxia, diplopia and dysarthria. Measurement of blood levels is necessary. With carbamazepine, patients and carers should report any skin reactions or eruptions, tremor or weight gain. For adverse effects with add-on antiepileptics, see the relevant sections in the text.

Therapeutic drug monitoring is as essential as clinical and biochemical monitoring in the drug treatment of epilepsy.

Failure of therapeutic response to antibacterials

Drug interaction-induced failure of antibiotics for common infections is invariably a result of inadequate blood concentrations (increased metabolism or reduced absorption, and infrequently increased elimination). The persistence of symptoms such as fever, shivering, pain or altered mental state should be reported immediately. In children, persistent crying or irritability and going off feeds may be early features of failure of therapy.

Haematological measurements (e.g. white cell count, C-reactive protein) may not reveal the necessary changes of response to antibiotics, so repeat blood cultures are necessary as there is a theoretical risk that inadequate antibacterial therapy will promote the development of drug-resistant strains of bacteria.

Liver dysfunction and liver failure

Common signs of liver damage include nausea, a yellow colouring (jaundice) of the skin or whites of the eyes, the passage of dark urine, tenderness below the ribs on the right side and flu-like symptoms. Jaundice, ascites, a prolonged prothrombin time, hypoalbuminaemia, malnutrition or encephalopathy indicates severe liver dysfunction, and there will be considerable impairment of drug metabolism. Impairment of drug metabolism may also occur with acute hepatitis, congestion of the liver in heart failure and cirrhosis.

Examples of some drugs whose activity is increased in liver disease include oral anticoagulants, metformin, chloramphenicol, NSAIDs and sulphonylureas. It is well known that drugs such as opioids should be used in reduced dosage in patients with hepatic dysfunction; doses need to be titrated. Therefore, if adverse drug interactions with opioids occur in patients with liver dysfunction, the consequences such as respiratory depression could be life-threatening.

Thus, in patients who have liver disease, the combination of drugs that are primarily metabolized and excreted by the liver with drugs that have the potential to interfere with their hepatic metabolism/excretion can give rise to dangerous and often unpredictable adverse/toxic effects.

Therapeutic and toxic plasma concentrations of some drugs

	Time for sampling	Concentration below which a therapeutic effect is unlikely	Concentration above which a toxic effect is more likely
Carbamazepine	Before next dose	4 mg/L (17 μmol/L)	10 mg/L (42 μmol/L)
Digoxin	11 hours after last dose	0.8 μg/L (1.0 nmol/L)	2 μg/L (2.6 nmol/L)
Ciclosporin	Just before next dose	125 μg/L (104 nmol/L)	200 μg/L (166 nmol/L)
Lithium	12 hours after last dose	0.4 nmol/L	1.0 nmol/L
Phenytoin	Just before next dose	10 mg/L (40 μmol/L)	20 mg/L (80 μmol/L)
Theophylline	Just before next dose	10 mg/L (55 μmol/L)	20 mg/L (110 μmol/L)

Part 1 CARDIOVASCULAR DRUGS

Aliskerin

Aliskerin is a direct inhibitor of renin, preventing the conversion of angiotensinogen to angiotensin. It is predominantly eliminated unchanged via the biliary route, is metabolized to a limited extent by CYP3A4 and is a substrate of P-gp.

Antiarrhythmics

Antiarrhythmics act by blocking the membrane sodium, potassium and calcium ion channels, but no agent has an exclusive action on a given type of channel. Additive effects may occur from drugs that affect different channels.

The metabolism of propafenone is complex. The primary pathway involves CYP2D6, with some people having higher activity than others; those with less extensive activity are more susceptible to the effects of CYP2D6 inhibitors. CYP3A4 acts as a back-up pathway.

Antihypertensives and heart failure drugs

This category includes ACE inhibitors, adrenergic neurone blockers, alpha-blockers, angiotensin II receptor antagonists and centrally acting vasodilatory antihypertensives.

Beta-blockers, calcium channel blockers and diuretics have their own sections in the text because their use extends beyond their role in hypertension and heart failure.

A wide variation in the metabolism of these drugs occurs both within and between different classes. Individual drugs have complex metabolisms involving a number of pathways. The effect of inhibition or induction of an individual enzyme will depend on the contribution of the alternative metabolic pathways for each drug. However, many of the interactions result from the additive effect on lowering BP (which of course may be used therapeutically).

Bosentan

This vasodilatory antihypertensive used in the treatment of pulmonary hypertension is metabolized by CYP3A4 and CYP2C9 isoenzymes and is a weak inducer of CYP2C8/9 and CYP3A4. Importantly, bosentan is a substrate of OATP1B1 and OATP1B3.

Antiplatelet agents

Aspirin

Aspirin inhibits cyclooxygenase, thus impairing platelet aggregation. This may be additive to other drugs with a similar effect and to those which affect other aspects of blood clotting. The risk of interactions and adverse effects is reduced by using a lower dose (e.g. 75 mg); fortunately, a full antiplatelet effect is seen at this dose.

Clopidogrel

Clopidogrel is converted to an active thiol metabolite by several CYP isoforms, including 3A4; this then binds rapidly and irreversibly with platelet adenosine diphosphate receptors, thus inhibiting platelet aggregation. At present, inhibition of the antiplatelet effects of clopidogrel by atorvastatin represents a formulated but untested hypothesis, and these agents may be administered concurrently.

Dipyridamole

Dipyridamole inhibits platelet aggregation. Its absorption is pH-dependent and is therefore affected by changes in gastric pH.

Glycoprotein IIa and IIIb inhibitors

These are potent platelet inhibitors used to prevent the binding of fibrinogen to glycoprotein receptors on the platelet surface that inhibit the final common pathway for platelet aggregation. It is given in combination with aspirin and heparin to prevent clotting before and during invasive heart procedures.

Beta-blockers

Systemic absorption may occur when eye drops containing beta-blockers are administered. Beta-receptors are found in heart muscle (predominantly beta-1) and the smooth muscle of the blood vessels and bronchioles (mainly beta-2). Selective beta-blockers (atenolol, bisoprolol, metoprolol, nebivolol, acebutolol) primarily (but not exclusively) antagonize beta-1 receptors, while the non-selective drugs (carvedilol, celiprolol, esmolol, labetalol, nadolol, oxprenolol, pindolol, propanolol, sotalol, timolol) block both beta-1 and beta-2 receptors.

Some beta-blockers have additional vasodilating properties by a variety of mechanisms such as beta-1 agonism or alpha-1 antagonism (e.g. carvedilol, celiprolol, labetalol, nebivolol). These seem to increase insulin sensitivity (whereas non-vasodilating beta-blockers reduce it) so may be preferable in patients with diabetes mellitus.

Sotalol

Sotalol is a beta-blocker that also has class III antiarrhythmic effects. It causes prolongation of the Q–T interval and is recommended solely as an antiarrhythmic. It is included in this section because it is subject to interactions from its beta-blocking properties as well as its Q–T prolongation

For Q–T prolongation, see Clinical Features of Some Adverse Drug Reactions, Q–T interval prolongation.

Calcium channel blockers

There are two groups: dihydropyridines and diltiazem/verapamil. Both groups are metabolized by the CYP3A family of isoenzymes (especially CYP3A4), which are the sites of many of the pharmacokinetic interactions involving this class. Some drugs are substrates for P-gp.

Cardiac glycosides – digoxin and digitoxin

These are both negative chronotropes and positive inotropes, and have a narrow therapeutic index and relatively long-half life of elimination (digoxin 14–60 hours, digitoxin 30–40 hours).

The side-effects are associated with vagal effects on the gastrointestinal tract (anorexia, abdominal discomfort/pain, vomiting and diarrhoea), while cardiotoxic effects include premature ventricular depolarizations, nodal rhythms and AV dissociation. Toxicity is enhanced by hypokalaemia, and this may predispose to more complex arrhythmias.

Lipid-lowering drugs

Anion exchange resins

Colestipol and colestyramine bind bile sodium and acidic drugs in the intestine. Interference with the absorption of acidic drugs is minimized by the separating doses (the secondary drug should be taken at least 1 hour before or 4–6 hours after the anion exchange resin).

Interactions are only included in this section if:

- the interaction does not involve this mechanism;
- dose separation does not minimize the effect;
- the recommended period of dose separation varies from the standard.

Ezetimibe

Ezetimibe reduces the absorption of cholesterol from the gastrointestinal tract.

Fibrates

Fibrates activate peroxisome proliferator-activated receptors, which are intracellular receptors that cause the transcription of a number of genes on the DNA that facilitate lipid metabolism. They are well absorbed from the gastrointestinal tract (with the exception of medium-acting fenofibrate), display a high degree of binding to albumin, are metabolized by CYP3A4 and are primarily excreted via kidneys; there is thus some increase in half-life in patients with severe renal impairment.

Statins

Atorvastatin and simvastatin are primarily metabolized by CYP3A4. They are both transported by P-gp, and atorvastatin is also transported by OATP1B1. Fluvastatin is metabolized primarily by CYP2C9. Pravastatin has not been shown to be metabolized by CYP3A4 to a clinically significant degree, although it is enzymatically broken down in the liver. Nor is pravastatin a known substrate of P-gp.

Rosuvastatin is a substrate of OATP2 and is metabolized slowly and to a limited extent by CYP2C9 and CYP2C19.

Sympathomimetics: inotropes and vasopressors

Sympathomimetics act directly on receptors at nerve endings (direct acting) or indirectly by stimulating the release of norepinephrine from the nerve terminals (indirect acting). Some act by both mechanisms (mixed). For the purposes of this section, mixed sympathomimetics will be considered as direct acting.

- **Indirectly acting sympathomimetics** include dexamfetamine, ephedrine (mixed), isometheptene, methylphenidate, oxymetazoline, phenylpropanolamine (mixed), pseudoephedrine (mixed) and xylometazoline.
- **Directly acting sympathomimetics** include epinephrine and dipivefrine (alpha and beta respectively); phenylephrine, metaraminol, norepinephrine, brimonidine and apraclonidine (alpha); dopamine and dobutamine (beta-1); and dopexamine and isoprenaline (cardiac beta-2).

Diuretics

Osmotic

Glucose (metabolized), mannitol, urea, glycerin (non-metabolized) and iodine radiocontrast media (incidental) produce an overexpansion of the extracellular fluid and circulatory overload (and are therefore contraindicated in congestive cardiac failure). This is often accompanied by dilutional hyponatraemia, and hyperkalaemia is also possible. Elimination is renal (80–90%).

Carbonic anhydrase inhibitors

Acetazolamide, dichlorphenamide, methazolamide and ethoxzolamide facilitate the excretion of hydrogen ions and the recovery of bicarbonate. They are never used as diuretics but are employed to reduce the production of aqueous humour in they eye (in glaucoma).

Thiazides

Thiazides cause potassium ion loss (aggravating hypokalaemia and increasing the toxicity of digoxin and the effects of muscle relaxants). They increase calcium ion reabsorption and so are dangerous in hypercalcaemia or with drugs causing increased calcium absorption. Thiazides can cause additive agranulocytosis, hyperuricaemia (decreasing the effect of antigout medications), thrombocytopenia (possibly increasing the bleeding tendency with antiplatelet drugs or anticoagulants) and hyperglycaemia (antagonizing the effects of hypoglycaemic agents). They are eliminated unchanged in the urine.

Loop diuretics

Furosemide is eliminated in equal portions by renal and non-renal (glucuronidation) routes. Its half-life is prolonged in renal failure, but hepatic failure has little effect. Bumetanide and torasemide are eliminated via CYP isoenzymes and so their half-life is affected by hepatic disease more than renal disease. They are known to cause thrombocytopenia (but decrease activity of oral anticoagulants), ototoxicity and nephrotoxicity.

Sildenafil and other phosphodiesterase type 5 inhibitors

These drugs enhance the effect of nitric oxide by inhibiting phosphodiesterase type 5. Tadalafil has cross-reactivity with phosphodiesterase type 11, which may cause back pain and myalgia. The approximately 4000-fold selectivity for phosphodiesterase type 5 versus type 3 is important because type 3 is involved in the control of cardiac contractility.

Sildenafil, tadalafil and vardenafil have similar, although not identical, mechanisms of action and structural similarity, and are metabolized primarily by the CYP3A4 isoenzymes. Vardenafil is 32-fold more potent than sildenafil in inhibiting phosphodiesterase type 5. Tadalafil has a quicker onset of action and a longer duration of action – around 36 hours – hence the need to be aware of the potential for adverse drug interactions for nearly 2 days after the intake of a single tablet.

Sildenafil and vardenafil inhibit phosphodiesterase types 6 and 1 (found in the brain, heart and vascular smooth muscle) more than tadalafil. Type 5 inhibition can result in an increase of the Q–T interval and a risk of life-threatening ventricular arrhythmias with class 1A and class III antiarrhythmics, this risk being greater with tadalafil and vardenafil.

Sildenafil is a weak inhibitor of the CYP450 isoforms 1A2, 2C9, 2C19, 2D6, 2E1 and 3A4.

Note from FDA approvals April 2009

Everolimus

The most frequently reported adverse effects (with an incidence of 20% more) are stomatitis, asthenia, diarrhoea, poor appetite and fluid build-up in the extremities (note this effect with drugs tending to cause fluid retention, e.g. NSAIDs). More than 50% of cases developed hyperglycaemia, hypercholesterolaemia, lymphopenia or increased creatinine levels.

Live vaccinations and close contact with people who have received live vaccines should be avoided during treatment with everolimus.

The concomitant use of strong or moderate CYP3A4 or P-gp inhibitors should be avoided in patients receiving everolimus therapy. Dose increases are recommended for co-administered strong CYP3A4 inducers.

Nitrofurantoin

The FDA warns that rare and sometimes fatal hepatic reactions to nitrofurantoin may occur and that the onset of chronic active hepatitis may be insidious. Patients should therefore be monitored periodically using LFTs. The development of hepatitis warrants permanent discontinuation.

ACE inhibitors and injectable gold

Nitritoid reactions have been reported rarely in patients receiving therapy with injectable gold (sodium aurothiomalate) and concomitant ACE inhibitor therapy. Symptoms may include facial flushing, nausea, vomiting and hypotension. Be aware.

Primary drug	Secondary drug	Effect	Mechanism	Precautions
ALISKIREN				
Aliskiren is a direct inhibitor of renin, preventing the conversion of angiotensinogen to angiotensin I It is predominantly eliminated unchanged via the biliary route. It is metabolized to a limited extent by CYP3A4 and is a substrate of P-gp				
ALISKIREN	ANTICANCER AND IMMUNOMODULATING DRUGS – CICLOSPORIN	Likely to ↑ plasma concentrations of aliskiren	Uncertain	Avoid co-administration
ALISKIREN	ANTICOAGULANTS – PARENTERAL	Risk of hyperkalaemia with heparin	Additive effect	Monitor serum potassium closely
ALISKIREN	ANTIFUNGALS	Aliskiren levels ↑ by ketoconazole	Uncertain	Monitor BP and serum potassium at least weekly until stable
ALISKIREN	ANTIHYPERTENSIVES AND HEART FAILURE DRUGS – ANGIOTENSIN II RECEPTOR ANTAGONISTS	Aliskiren levels possibly ↓ by irbesartan. Risk of hyperkalaemia	Uncertain	Monitor BP at least weekly until stable
ALISKIREN	**DIURETICS**			
ALISKIREN	LOOP DIURETICS	↓ plasma levels of furosemide	Uncertain	Watch for poor response to furosemide
ALISKIREN	POTASSIUM-SPARING DIURETICS AND ALDOSTERONE ANTAGONISTS	Risk of hyperkalaemia	Additive effect	Monitor serum potassium every week until stable, then every 3–6 months
ALISKIREN	POTASSIUM	Risk of hyperkalaemia	Additive effect	Avoid co-administration

CARDIOVASCULAR DRUGS ALISKIREN

Primary drug	Secondary drug	Effect	Mechanism	Precautions
ANTIARRHYTHMICS				
ADENOSINE				
ADENOSINE	ANAESTHETICS – LOCAL	↑ myocardial depression	Additive effect; local anaesthetics and adenosine are myocardial depressants	Monitor PR, BP and ECG closely
ADENOSINE	ANTIARRHYTHMICS	Risk of bradycardia and ↓ BP	Additive myocardial depression	Monitor PR, BP and ECG closely
ADENOSINE	ANTIPLATELET AGENTS – DIPYRIDAMOLE	↑ effect of adenosine; ↓ doses needed to terminate supraventricular tachycardias; case report of profound bradycardia when adenosine infusion was given for myocardial stress testing	Dipyridamole inhibits adenosine uptake into cells	↓ bolus doses of adenosine by up to fourfold when administering it for treating supraventricular tachy-cardias. Some recommend avoiding adenosine for patients taking dipyridamole. Advise patients to stop dipyridamole for 24 hours before using adenosine infusions
ADENOSINE	ANTIPSYCHOTICS	Risk of ventricular arrhythmias, particularly torsades de pointes, with phenothiazines and pimozide. There is also a theoretical risk of Q–T prolongation with the atypical antipsychotics	All of these drugs prolong the Q–T interval	Avoid co-administration of phenothiazines, amisulpride, pimozide or sertindole with adenosine. Monitor the ECG closely when adenosine is co-administered with atypical antipsychotics
ADENOSINE	BRONCHODILATORS – THEOPHYLLINE	↓ efficacy of adenosine	Theophylline and other xanthines are adenosine receptor antagonists	Watch for poor response to adenosine; higher doses may be required

AMIODARONE				
Amiodarone has a long half-life and therefore interactions may persist for weeks after stopping therapy				
AMIODARONE	**DRUGS THAT PROLONG THE Q–T INTERVAL**			
AMIODARONE	1. ANTIARRHYTHMICS – disopyramide, procainamide, propafenone 2. ANTIBIOTICS – macrolides (especially azithromycin, clarithromycin, parenteral erythromycin, telithromycin), quinolones (especially moxifloxacin), quinupristin–dalfopristin 3. ANTI-CANCER AND IMMUNOMODULATING DRUGS – arsenic trioxide 4. ANTI-DEPRESSANTS – TCAs, venlafaxine 5. ANTIEMETICS – dolasetron 6. ANTI-FUNGALS – fluconazole, posaconazole, voriconazole 7. ANTIHISTAMINES – terfenadine, hydroxyzine, mizolastine 8. ANTIMALARIALS – artemether with lumefantrine, chloroquine, hydroxy-chloroquine, mefloquine, quinine 9. ANTIPROTOZOALS – pentamidine isetionate 10. ANTIPSYCHOTICS – atypical agents, phenothiazines, pimozide 11. BETA-BLOCKERS – sotalol 12. BRONCHODILATORS – parenteral bronchodilators 13. CNS STIMULANTS – atomoxetine	Risk of ventricular arrhythmias, particularly torsades de pointes	Additive effect; these drugs cause prolongation of the Q–T interval. In addition, procainamide levels may be ↑ by amiodarone (uncertain mechanism). Also, amiodarone inhibits CYP2C9 and CYP2D6, which have a role in metabolizing TCAs	Avoid co-administration

Primary drug	Secondary drug	Effect	Mechanism	Precautions
AMIODARONE	AGALSIDASE BETA	↓ clinical effect of agalsidase beta	Uncertain	Avoid co-administration
AMIODARONE	ANAESTHETICS – GENERAL	Amiodarone may ↑ the myocardial depressant effects of inhalational anaesthetics	Additive effect	Monitor PR, BP and ECG closely
AMIODARONE	ANAESTHETICS – LOCAL	Risk of ↓ BP	Additive myocardial depression	Particular care should be taken to avoid inadvertent intravenous administration during bupivacaine infiltration; monitor PR, BP and ECG during epidural administration of bupivacaine
AMIODARONE	**ANTIARRHYTHMICS**			
AMIODARONE	ANTIARRHYTHMICS	Risk of bradycardia and ↓ BP	Additive myocardial depression	Monitor PR and BP closely
AMIODARONE	FLECAINIDE	↑ plasma levels of flecainide	Amiodarone is a potent inhibitor of the CYP2D6-mediated metabolism of flecainide	↓ the dose of flecainide (by up to 50%)
AMIODARONE	**ANTIBIOTICS**			
AMIODARONE	CO-TRIMOXAZOLE	Risk of ventricular arrhythmias	Uncertain	Avoid co-administration
AMIODARONE	RIFAMPICIN	↓ levels of amiodarone	Uncertain, but rifampicin is a known enzyme inducer and therefore may ↑ metabolism of amiodarone	Watch for a poor response to amiodarone
AMIODARONE	**ANTICANCER AND IMMUNOMODULATING DRUGS**			
AMIODARONE	CICLOSPORIN	Ciclosporin levels may be ↑ by amiodarone; risk of nephrotoxicity	Uncertain; ciclosporin is metabolized by CYP3A4, which is markedly inhibited by amiodarone. Amiodarone also interferes with renal elimination of ciclosporin and inhibits intestinal P-gp, which may ↑ the bioavailability of ciclosporin	Monitor renal function closely; consider reducing the dose of ciclosporin when co-administering amiodarone

AMIODARONE	CYTOTOXICS	↑ risk of photosensitivity reactions	Attributed to additive effects	Avoid exposure of skin and eyes to direct sunlight for 30 days after porfimer therapy
AMIODARONE	ANTICOAGULANTS – ORAL	Cases of bleeding within 4 weeks of starting amiodarone in patients previously stabilized on warfarin. The effect was seen to last up to 16 weeks after stopping amiodarone	Amiodarone inhibits CYP2C9- and CYP3A4-mediated metabolism of warfarin	↓ the dose of anticoagulant by 30–50% and monitor INR closely for at least the first month of starting amiodarone and for 4 months after stopping amiodarone. If the INR suddenly ↑ after being initially stabilized, check TSH level
AMIODARONE	**ANTIDEPRESSANTS**			
AMIODARONE	LITHIUM	1. Rare risk of ventricular arrythmias, particularly torsades de pointes 2. Risk of hypothyroidism	1. Additive effect; lithium rarely causes Q–T prolongation 2. Additive effect; both drugs can cause hypothyroidism	1. Manufacturer of amiodarone recommends avoiding co-administration 2. If co-administration is thought to be necessary, watch for symptoms/signs of hypothyroidism; check TFTs every 3–6 months
AMIODARONE	SSRIs – SERTRALINE	Sertraline may ↑ amiodarone levels	Sertraline may inhibit CYP3A4-mediated metabolism of amiodarone	Watch for amiodarone toxicity; for those taking high doses of amiodarone, consider using an alternative SSRI with a lower affinity for CYP3A4
AMIODARONE	ANTIEPILEPTICS – PHENYTOIN	Phenytoin levels may be ↑ by amiodarone; conversely, amiodarone levels may be ↓ by phenytoin	Uncertain; amiodarone inhibits CYP2C9, which plays a role in phenytoin metabolism while phenytoin is a known hepatic enzyme inducer. Also, amiodarone inhibits intestinal P-gp, which may ↑ the bioavailability of phenytoin	↓ phenytoin dose by 25–30% and monitor levels; watch for amiodarone toxicity. Note that phenytoin and amiodarone share similar features of toxicity, such as arrhythmias and ataxia

Primary drug	Secondary drug	Effect	Mechanism	Precautions
AMIODARONE	ANTIOBESITY DRUGS – ORLISTAT	Possible ↓ amiodarone levels	↓ absorption of amiodarone	Watch for poor response to amiodarone
AMIODARONE	ANTIVIRALS	Amiodarone levels may be ↑ by protease inhibitors	Uncertain, but postulated to be due to ↓ metabolism of amiodarone	Watch closely for amiodarone toxicity; for those taking high doses of amiodarone, consider reducing the dose when starting protease inhibitor anti-HIV therapy
AMIODARONE	BETA-BLOCKERS	Risk of bradycardia (occasionally severe), ↓ BP and heart failure. Also, ↑ plasma levels of metoprolol	Additive negative inotropic and chronotropic effects. In addition, high-dose amiodarone is associated with ↑ plasma levels of metoprolol due to inhibition of CYP2D6	For patients on beta-blockers, monitor BP closely when loading with amiodarone
AMIODARONE	BRONCHODILATORS – THEOPHYLLINE	Theophylline levels may be ↑ by amiodarone (single case report of theophylline levels doubling)	Uncertain; amiodarone probably inhibits the metabolism of theophylline	Watch for theophylline toxicity; monitor levels regularly until stable
AMIODARONE	CALCIUM CHANNEL BLOCKERS	Risk of bradycardia, AV block and ↓ BP when amiodarone co-administered with diltiazem or verapamil	Additive negative inotropic and chronotropic effect. Also, amiodarone inhibits intestinal P-gp, which ↑ the bioavailability of diltiazem and verapamil	Monitor PR, BP and ECG closely; watch for heart failure
AMIODARONE	**CARDIAC GLYCOSIDES**			
AMIODARONE	DIGOXIN	Amiodarone may ↑ plasma levels of digoxin (in some cases up to fourfold)	Uncertain; thought to be due to inhibition of P-gp-mediated renal clearance of digoxin. Amiodarone is also known to inhibit intestinal P-gp, which may ↑ the bioavailability of digoxin	↓ digoxin dose by one-third to one-half when starting amiodarone. Monitor digoxin levels; watch for digoxin toxicity, especially for 4 weeks after initiating or adjusting amiodarone therapy

AMIODARONE	DIGITOXIN	Reports of digitoxin toxicity in two patients on digitoxin after starting amiodarone	Uncertain; thought to be due to inhibition of P-gp-mediated renal clearance of digoxin	Watch for digitoxin toxicity
AMIODARONE	**DIURETICS**			
AMIODARONE	CARBONIC ANHYDRASE ANTAGONISTS, LOOP DIURETICS, THIAZIDES	Risk of arrhythmias	Cardiac toxicity directly related to hypokalaemia	Monitor potassium levels every 4–6 weeks until stable, then at least annually
AMIODARONE	POTASSIUM-SPARING DIURETICS	Risk of ↑ levels of eplerenone with amiodarone; risk of hyperkalaemia directly related to serum levels	Calcium channel blockers inhibit CYP3A4-mediated metabolism of eplerenone	Restrict dose of eplerenone to 25mg/day. Monitor serum potassium concentrations closely; watch for hyperkalaemia
AMIODARONE	DRUG DEPENDENCE THERAPIES – BUPROPION	↑ plasma concentrations of amiodarone, with risk of toxic effects	Bupropion and its metabolite hydroxybupropion inhibit CYP2D6	Initiate therapy of these drugs at the lowest effective dose
AMIODARONE	GRAPEFRUIT JUICE	Possibly ↓ effect of amiodarone	Inhibition of CYP3A4-mediated metabolism of amiodarone to its active metabolite	Warn patients to avoid grapefruit juice; if amiodarone becomes less effective, ask the patient about grapefruit juice ingestion
AMIODARONE	H2 RECEPTOR BLOCKERS	Cimetidine may ↑ amiodarone levels	Uncertain	Monitor PR and BP at least weekly until stable. Warn patients to report symptoms of hypotension (light-headedness, dizziness on standing, etc.). Consider alternative acid suppression therapy
AMIODARONE	IVABRADINE	Risk of arrhythmias	Additive effect	Monitor ECG closely

Primary drug	Secondary drug	Effect	Mechanism	Precautions
AMIODARONE	LIPID-LOWERING DRUGS			
AMIODARONE	ANION EXCHANGE RESINS	Colestyramine ↓ amiodarone levels	Colestyramine binds amiodarone, reducing its absorption and interrupting its enterohepatic circulation	Avoid co-administration
AMIODARONE	SIMVASTATIN	↑ risk of myopathy with high doses (>40 mg daily) of simvastatin	Uncertain; amiodarone inhibits intestinal P-gp, which may ↑ the bioavailability of statins	Avoid >20 mg daily doses of simvastatin in patients taking amiodarone; if higher doses are required, switch to an alternative statin
AMIODARONE	OXYGEN	Risk of pulmonary toxicity (adult respiratory distress syndrome) in patients on amiodarone who were ventilated with 100% oxygen during surgery	Uncertain	Manufacturers recommend that, for patients on amiodarone undergoing surgery, the lowest possible oxygen concentrations to achieve adequate oxygenation should be given
AMIODARONE	THYROID HORMONES	Risk of either under- or overtreatment of thyroid function	Amiodarone contains iodine and has been reported to cause both hyper- and hypothyroidism	Monitor triiodothyronine, thyroxine and TSH levels at least 6 monthly

CARDIOVASCULAR DRUGS ANTIARRHYTHMICS

DISOPYRAMIDE				
DISOPYRAMIDE	DRUGS THAT PROLONG THE Q–T INTERVAL			
DISOPYRAMIDE	1. ANTIARRHYTHMICS – amiodarone, procainamide, propafenone 2. ANTIBIOTICS – macrolides (especially azithromycin, clarithromycin, parenteral erythromycin, telithromycin), quinolones (especially moxifloxacin), quinupristin/dalfopristin 3. ANTICANCER AND IMMUNOMODULATING DRUGS – arsenic trioxide 4. ANTIDEPRESSANTS – TCAs, venlafaxine 5. ANTIEMETICS – dolasetron 6. ANTIFUNGALS – fluconazole, posaconazole, voriconazole 7. ANTIHISTAMINES – terfenadine, hydroxyzine, mizolastine 8. ANTIMALARIALS – artemether with lumefantrine, chloroquine, hydroxychloroquine, mefloquine, quinine 9. ANTIPROTOZOALS – pentamidine isetionate 10. ANTIPSYCHOTICS – atypicals, phenothiazines, pimozide 11. BETA-BLOCKERS – sotalol 12. BRONCHODILATORS – parenteral bronchodilators 13. CNS STIMULANTS – atomoxetine	Risk of ventricular arrhythmias, particularly torsades de pointes	Additive effect; these drugs prolong the Q–T interval. Also, macrolides ↑ the levels of disopyramide by inhibiting its metabolism (probably CYP3A mediated)	Avoid co-administration

Primary drug	Secondary drug	Effect	Mechanism	Precautions
DISOPYRAMIDE	**DRUGS WITH ANTIMUSCARINIC EFFECTS**			
DISOPYRAMIDE	1. ANALGESICS – nefopam 2. ANTIARRHYTHMICS – propafenone 3. ANTIDEPRESSANTS – TCAs 4. ANTIEMETICS – cyclizine 5. ANTIHISTAMINES – chlorphenamine, cyproheptadine, hydroxyzine 6. ANTIMUSCARINICS – atropine, benzatropine, cyclopentolate, dicycloverine, flavoxate, homatropine, hyoscine, orphenadrine, oxybutynin, procyclidine, propantheline, tolterodine, trihexyphenidyl, tropicamide 7. ANTI-PARKINSON'S DRUGS – dopaminergics 8. ANTIPSYCHOTICS – phenothiazines, clozapine, pimozide 9. MUSCLE RELAXANTS – baclofen 10. NITRATES – isosorbide dinitrate	↑ risk of antimuscarinic side-effects. **NB ↓ efficacy of sublingual nitrate tablets**	Additive effect; both drugs cause antimuscarinic side-effects. **Antimuscarinic effects ↓ salivary production, which ↓ dissolution of the tablet**	Warn patient of this additive effect. **Consider changing the formulation to a sublingual nitrate spray**

CARDIOVASCULAR DRUGS ANTIARRHYTHMICS

DISOPYRAMIDE	ANAESTHETICS – LOCAL	Risk of ↓ BP	Additive myocardial depression	Particular care should be taken to avoid inadvertent intravenous administration during bupivacaine infiltration; monitor PR, BP and ECG during epidural administration of bupivacaine
DISOPYRAMIDE	ANALGESICS	Disopyramide may slow the onset of action of intermittent dose paracetamol	These drugs have anticholinergic effects that include delayed gastric emptying. This will delay absorption	Warn patients that the action of paracetamol may be delayed. This will not be the case when paracetamol is taken regularly
DISOPYRAMIDE	ANTIARRHYTHMICS	Risk of bradycardia and ↓ BP	Additive effects; antiarrhythmics are myocardial depressants	Monitor PR, BP and ECG closely
DISOPYRAMIDE	ANTIBIOTICS – RIFAMPICIN	Disopyramide levels are ↓ by rifampicin	Rifampicin induces hepatic metabolism of disopyramide	Watch for poor response to disopyramide; check serum levels if necessary
DISOPYRAMIDE	ANTIDIABETIC DRUGS	↑ risk of hypoglycaemic episodes, particularly in patients with impaired renal function. Hypoglycaemic attacks may occur even when plasma levels of disopyramide are within the normal range (attacks occurring with plasma disopyramide levels of 1–4 ng/mL)	Disopyramide and its metabolite mono-isopropyl disopyramide ↑ secretion of insulin (considered to be due to inhibition of potassium-ATP channels). Suggestion that disopyramide causes an impairment of the counterregulatory (homeostatic) mechanisms that follow hypoglycaemia	In patients receiving antidiabetic drugs, start with the lowest dose of disopyramide if there is no alternative. Measure creatinine clearance. If creatinine clearance is 40 mL/min or less, the dose of disopyramide should not exceed 100 mg and should be administered once daily if creatinine clearance is less than 15 mL/min ➢ ***For signs and symptoms of hypoglycaemia, see Clinical Features of Some Adverse Drug Interactions, Hypoglycaemia***

CARDIOVASCULAR DRUGS ANTIARRHYTHMICS

Primary drug	Secondary drug	Effect	Mechanism	Precautions
DISOPYRAMIDE	ANTIEPILEPTICS – BARBITURATES, PHENYTOIN	Disopyramide levels are ↓ by phenobarbital and primidone	Phenobarbital and primidone induce the hepatic metabolism of disopyramide	Watch for poor response to disopyramide; check serum levels if necessary
DISOPYRAMIDE	ANTIVIRALS	Disopyramide levels may be ↑ by protease inhibitors	Inhibition of CYP3A4-mediated metabolism of disopyramide	Watch closely for disopyramide toxicity
DISOPYRAMIDE	BETA-BLOCKERS	Risk of bradycardia (occasionally severe), ↓ BP, and heart failure	Additive negative inotropic and chronotropic effects	Monitor PR, BP and ECG at least weekly until stable; watch for development of heart failure
DISOPYRAMIDE	CALCIUM CHANNEL BLOCKERS	Risk of myocardial depression and asystole when disopyramide is co-administered with verapamil, particularly in the presence of heart failure	Disopyramide is a myocardial depressant like verapamil and can cause ventricular tachycardia, ventricular fibrillation or torsades de pointes	Avoid co-administering verapamil with disopyramide if possible. If single-agent therapy is ineffective, monitor PR, BP and ECG closely; watch for heart failure
DISOPYRAMIDE	DIURETICS – CARBONIC ANHYDRASE INHIBITORS, LOOP DIURETICS, THIAZIDES	Risk of ↑ myocardial depression	Cardiac toxicity directly related to hypokalaemia	Monitor potassium levels closely
DISOPYRAMIDE	GRAPEFRUIT JUICE	Possibly ↓ effect of disopyramide	Unclear	Monitor ECG and side-effects more closely
DISOPYRAMIDE	IVABRADINE	Risk of arrhythmias	Additive effect	Monitor ECG closely
FLECAINIDE				
FLECAINIDE	AMMONIUM CHLORIDE	Urinary acidification ↓ flecainide levels	Flecainide excretion is ↑ in the presence of an acidic urine; flecainide exists in predominantly ionic form, which is less readily reabsorbed from the renal tubules	Watch for a poor response to flecainide

FLECAINIDE	ANAESTHETICS – LOCAL	Risk of ↓ BP	Additive myocardial depression	Particular care should be taken to avoid inadvertent intravenous administration during bupivacaine infiltration; monitor PR, BP and ECG during epidural administration of bupivacaine
FLECAINIDE	**ANALGESICS**			
FLECAINIDE	NSAIDs	Parecoxib may ↑ flecainide levels	Parecoxib weakly inhibits CYP2D6-mediated metabolism of flecainide	Monitor PR and BP closely. If possible, use only short courses of NSAID
FLECAINIDE	OPIOIDS	Methadone and tramadol may ↑ flecainide levels	Methadone and tramadol inhibit CYP2D6-mediated metabolism of flecainide	Monitor PR and BP closely
FLECAINIDE	**ANTIARRHYTHMICS**			
FLECAINIDE	ANTIARRHYTHMICS	Risk of bradycardia and ↓ BP	Additive myocardial depression	Monitor PR and BP closely; watch for flecainide toxicity
FLECAINIDE	AMIODARONE	↑ plasma levels of flecainide	Amiodarone is a potent inhibitor of CYP2D6-mediated metabolism of flecainide	↓ the dose of flecainide (by up to 50%)
FLECAINIDE	ANTICANCER AND IMMUNOMODULATING DRUGS – IMATINIB	Imatinib may cause an ↑ in plasma concentrations of flecainide with a risk of toxic effects, e.g. visual disturbances, dyspnoea, liver dysfunction	Imatinib is a potent inhibitor of CYP2D6 isoenzymes, which metabolize flecainide	Monitor for clinical efficacy and toxicity of flecainide. Monitor liver function and BP, and do FBCs if toxicity is suspected
FLECAINIDE	**ANTIDEPRESSANTS**			
FLECAINIDE	DULOXETINE	Duloxetine may ↑ flecainide levels	Duloxetine moderately inhibits CYP2D6, which metabolizes flecainide	Monitor PR and BP at least weekly until stable

Primary drug	Secondary drug	Effect	Mechanism	Precautions
FLECAINIDE	SSRIs	SSRIs may ↑ flecainide levels	SSRIs inhibit CYP2D6-mediated metabolism of flecainide	Monitor PR and BP closely; watch for flecainide toxicity
FLECAINIDE	TCAs	Risk of arrhythmias	Additive effect; both drugs may be proarrhythmogenic. In addition, amitriptyline and clomipramine may inhibit CYP2D6-mediated metabolism of flecainide	Monitor PR, BP, and ECG closely; watch for flecainide toxicity
FLECAINIDE	ANTIEMETICS – 5-HT3-ANTAGONISTS	Risk of arrhythmias	Additive effect	Manufacturers recommend avoiding co-administration of flecainide with dolasetron. Caution with other 5-HT3-antagonists; monitor ECG closely
FLECAINIDE	ANTIHISTAMINES – TERFENADINE, HYDROXYZINE, MIZOLASTINE	Risk of arrhythmias	Additive effect	Avoid co-administration
FLECAINIDE	**ANTIMALARIALS**			
FLECAINIDE	ARTEMETHER/LUMEFANTRINE	Risk of arrhythmias	Additive effect	Avoid co-administration
FLECAINIDE	QUININE	Quinine may ↑ flecainide levels	Quinine inhibits CYP2D6-mediated metabolism of flecainide	The effect seems to be slight, but watch for flecainide toxicity; monitor PR and BP closely
FLECAINIDE	ANTIPSYCHOTICS – PHENOTHIAZINES, AMISULPRIDE, PIMOZIDE, SERTINDOLE	Risk of arrhythmias	Additive effect. Also, haloperidol and thioridazine inhibit CYP2D6-mediated metabolism of flecainide	Avoid co-administration
FLECAINIDE	ANTIVIRALS – PROTEASE INHIBITORS	Amprenavir, ritonavir and possibly saquinavir and tipranavir with ritonavir ↑ flecainide levels, with risk of ventricular arrhythmias	Uncertain; possibly inhibition of CYP3A4- and CYP2D6-mediated metabolism of flecainide	Manufacturers recommend avoiding co-administration of flecainide with amprenavir, ritonavir and saquinavir

FLECAINIDE	BETA-BLOCKERS	Risk of bradycardia (occasionally severe), ↓ BP and heart failure. Note, a single case report has described bradycardia when timolol eye drops given to a patient on flecainide	Additive negative inotropic and chronotropic effects	Monitor PR, BP and ECG closely; watch for development of heart failure
FLECAINIDE	CALCIUM CHANNEL BLOCKERS	Risk of heart block and ↓ BP when flecainide is co-administered with verapamil. A single case of asystole has been reported	Additive negative inotropic and chronotropic effect	Monitor PR, BP and ECG at least weekly until stable; watch for heart failure
FLECAINIDE	DIURETICS – CARBONIC ANHYDRASE INHIBITORS, LOOP DIURETICS, THIAZIDES	Risk of arrhythmias	Cardiac toxicity directly related to hypokalaemia	Monitor potassium levels closely; watch for hypokalaemia
FLECAINIDE	DRUG DEPENDENCE THERAPIES – BUPROPION	↑ levels of flecainide	Bupropion may inhibit CYP2D6-mediated metabolism of flecainide	Monitor PR and BP closely; start flecainide at the lowest dose for patients taking bupropion
FLECAINIDE	H2 RECEPTOR BLOCKERS	Cimetidine may ↑ flecainide levels	Cimetidine inhibits CYP2D6-mediated metabolism of flecainide. Ranitidine is a much weaker CYP2D6 inhibitor	Monitor PR and BP at least weekly until stable. Warn patients to report symptoms of hypotension (light-headedness, dizziness on standing, etc.). Consider alternative acid suppression therapy
FLECAINIDE	SODIUM BICARBONATE	Urinary alkalinization ↑ flecainide levels	Flecainide excretion is ↓ in the presence of an alkaline urine; flecainide exists in predominantly non-ionic form, which is more readily reabsorbed from the renal tubules	Monitor PR and BP closely

CARDIOVASCULAR DRUGS ANTIARRHYTHMICS

Primary drug	Secondary drug	Effect	Mechanism	Precautions
FLECAINIDE	TOBACCO SMOKE	Flecainide levels lower in smokers	Uncertain; postulated that hepatic metabolism ↑ by a component of tobacco smoke	Watch for poor response to flecainide and ↑ the dose accordingly (studies have suggested that smokers need up to 20% higher doses)
MEXILETINE				
MEXILETINE	**ANAESTHETICS – LOCAL**			
MEXILETINE	BUPIVACAINE, LEVOBUPIVACAINE	Risk of ↓ BP	Additive myocardial depression	Particular care should be taken to avoid inadvertent intravenous administration during bupivacaine infiltration; monitor PR, BP and ECG during epidural administration of bupivacaine
MEXILETINE	LIDOCAINE	Mexiletine ↑ lidocaine levels (with cases of toxicity when lidocaine is given intravenously)	Mexiletine displaces lidocaine from its tissue-binding sites; it also seems to ↓ its clearance but the exact mechanism is uncertain at present	Watch for the early symptoms and signs of lidocaine toxicity (perioral paraesthesia, ↑ muscle tone)
MEXILETINE	ANALGESICS – OPIOIDS	1. Absorption of oral mexiletine is ↓ by co-administration with morphine or diamorphine 2. Methadone may ↑ mexiletine levels	1. Uncertain, but thought to be due to opioid-induced delay in gastric emptying 2. Methadone inhibits CYP2D6-mediated metabolism of mexiletine	1. Watch for a poor response to mexiletine; consider starting at a higher dose or using the intravenous route 2. Monitor PR, BP and ECG closely; watch for mexiletine toxicity
MEXILETINE	**ANTIARRHYTHMICS**			
MEXILETINE	ANTIARRHYTHMICS	Risk of bradycardia and ↓ BP; however, mexiletine ↓ the Q–T prolongation of other antiarrhythmics so is often beneficial	Additive effect; antiarrhythmics are all myocardial depressants	Monitor PR, BP and ECG closely

MEXILETINE	PROPAFENONE	↑ serum levels of mexiletine	Propafenone inhibits CYP2D6-mediated metabolism of mexiletine; no case reports of adverse clinical effects but is potential for proarrhythmias	Monitor ECG closely
MEXILETINE	ANTIBIOTICS	Rifampicin ↓ mexiletine levels	Uncertain; postulated that rifampicin ↑ mexiletine metabolism	Watch for poor response to mexiletine
MEXILETINE	ANTICANCER AND IMMUNOMODULATING DRUGS – IMATINIB	Imatinib may cause an ↑ in plasma concentrations of mexiletine and a risk of toxic effects, e.g. nausea, vomiting, constipation, taste disturbances, dizziness and confusion	Imatinib is a potent inhibitor of CYP2D6 isoenzymes, which metabolize mexiletine	Mexiletine is used for life-threatening ventricular arrhythmias. Close monitoring of BP and ECG is mandatory, and watch for signs and symptoms of heart failure
MEXILETINE	**ANTIDEPRESSANTS**			
MEXILETINE	SSRIs	SSRIs may ↑ mexiletine levels	SSRIs inhibit CYP2D6-mediated metabolism of mexiletine	Monitor PR and BP closely; watch for mexiletine toxicity
MEXILETINE	TCAs	Risk of arrhythmias	Additive effect; both drugs may be proarrhythmogenic. In addition, amitriptyline and clomipramine may inhibit CYP2D6-mediated metabolism of mexiletine, while mexiletine inhibits CYP1A2-mediated metabolism of amitriptyline, clomipramine and imipramine	Monitor PR, BP and ECG closely
MEXILETINE	ANTIEMETICS – 5-HT3-ANTAGONISTS	Risk of arrhythmias with dolasetron	Additive effect	Manufacturers recommend avoiding co-administration. Also caution with tropisetron; monitor ECG closely

Primary drug	Secondary drug	Effect	Mechanism	Precautions
MEXILETINE	ANTIEPILEPTICS	Phenytoin levels are ↓ by mexiletine	Phenytoin induces CYP1A2-mediated metabolism of mexiletine	Watch for poor response to mexiletine
MEXILETINE	ANTIHISTAMINES – MIZOLASTINE	Risk of arrhythmias	Additive effect	Avoid co-administration
MEXILETINE	ANTIMALARIALS – QUININE	Quinine may ↑ mexiletine levels	Quinine inhibits CYP2D6-mediated metabolism of mexiletine	Monitor PR and BP closely
MEXILETINE	ANTIMUSCARINICS – ATROPINE	Delayed absorption of mexiletine	Anticholinergic effects delay gastric emptying and absorption	May slow the onset of action of the first dose of mexiletine, but this is not of clinical significance for regular dosing (atropine does not ↓ the total dose absorbed)
MEXILETINE	ANTIVIRALS	Mexiletine levels may be ↑ by ritonavir	Inhibition of metabolism via CYP2D6, particularly in rapid metabolizers (90% of the population)	Monitor PR, BP and ECG closely
MEXILETINE	BETA-BLOCKERS	Risk of bradycardia (occasionally severe), ↓ BP and heart failure	Additive negative inotropic and chronotropic effects. Also, mexiletine is known to inhibit CYP1A2-mediated metabolism of propanolol	Monitor PR, BP and ECG closely; watch for development of heart failure
MEXILETINE	BRONCHODILATORS – THEOPHYLLINE	Theophylline levels may be ↑ by mexiletine; cases of theophylline toxicity have been reported	Mexiletine inhibits CYP1A2-mediated metabolism of theophylline	↓ the theophylline dose (by up to 50%). Monitor theophylline levels and watch for toxicity
MEXILETINE	CNS STIMULANTS – MODAFINIL	May cause ↓ mexiletine levels if CYP1A2 is the predominant metabolic pathway and alternative metabolic pathways are either genetically deficient or affected	Modafinil is a moderate inducer of CYP1A2 in a concentration-dependent manner	Be aware

MEXILETINE	DIURETICS – CARBONIC ANHYDRASE INHIBITORS, LOOP DIURETICS, THIAZIDES	Effect of mexiletine ↓ by hypokalaemia	Uncertain	Normalize potassium levels before starting mexiletine
MEXILETINE	H2 RECEPTOR BLOCKERS	Cimetidine may ↑ plasma concentrations of mexiletine	Cimetidine inhibits CYP2D6-mediated metabolism of mexiletine. Ranitidine is a much weaker CYP2D6 inhibitor	Monitor PR and BP at least weekly until stable. Warn patients to report symptoms of hypotension (light-headedness, dizziness on standing, etc.). Consider alternative acid-suppression therapy
MORACIZINE				
MORACIZINE	BRONCHODILATORS – THEOPHYLLINE	↓ plasma concentrations of theophylline and risk of therapeutic failure	Due to induction of microsomal enzyme activity	May need to ↑ dose of theophylline by 25%
MORACIZINE	CALCIUM CHANNEL BLOCKERS	Co-administration is associated with ↑ bioavailability of moracizine and ↓ availability of diltiazem	Postulated that diltiazem inhibits metabolism of moracizine, while moracizine ↑ metabolism of diltiazem; the precise mechanism of interaction is uncertain at present	Monitor PR, BP and ECG; adjust doses of each drug accordingly
MORACIZINE	CARDIAC GLYCOSIDES – DIGOXIN	Case reports of heart block when moracizine is co-administered with digoxin	Uncertain at present	Monitor PR and ECG closely

Primary drug	Secondary drug	Effect	Mechanism	Precautions
PROCAINAMIDE				
PROCAINAMIDE	DRUGS THAT PROLONG THE Q–T INTERVAL			
PROCAINAMIDE	1. ANTIARRHYTHMICS – amiodarone, disopyramide, propafenone 2. ANTIBIOTICS – macrolides (especially azithromycin, clarithromycin, parenteral erythromycin, telithromycin), quinolones (especially moxifloxacin), quinupristin/dalfopristin 3. ANTICANCER AND IMMUNOMODULATING DRUGS – arsenic trioxide 4. ANTIDEPRESSANTS – TCAs, venlafaxine 5. ANTIEMETICS – dolasetron 6. ANTIFUNGALS – fluconazole, posaconazole, voriconazole 7. ANTIHISTAMINES – terfenadine, hydroxyzine, mizolastine 8. ANTIMALARIALS – artemether with lumefantrine, chloroquine, hydroxychloroquine, mefloquine, quinine 9. ANTIPROTOZOALS – pentamidine isetionate 10. ANTIPSYCHOTICS – atypicals, phenothiazines, pimozide 11. BETA-BLOCKERS – sotalol 12. BRONCHODILATORS – parenteral bronchodilators. 13. CNS STIMULANTS – atomoxetine	Risk of ventricular arrhythmias, particularly torsades de pointes	Additive effect; these drugs prolong the Q–T interval. In addition, procainamide levels may be ↑ by amiodarone (uncertain mechanism). Also, amitriptyline, clomipramine and quinine inhibit CYP2D6-mediated metabolism of procainamide	Avoid co-administration

PROCAINAMIDE	ANAESTHETICS – LOCAL			
PROCAINAMIDE	BUPIVICAINE, LEVOBUPIVACAINE	Risk of ↓ BP	Additive myocardial depression	Particular care should be taken to avoid inadvertent intravenous administration during bupivacaine infiltration; monitor PR, BP and ECG during epidural administration of bupivacaine
PROCAINAMIDE	LIDOCAINE	Case report of neurotoxicity when intravenous lidocaine is administered with procainamide. No significant interaction is expected when lidocaine is used for local anaesthetic infiltration	Likely to be an additive effect; both may cause neurotoxicity in overdose	Care should be taken when administering lidocaine as an infusion for patients taking procainamide
PROCAINAMIDE	ANALGESICS – OPIOIDS	Methadone may ↑ flecainide levels	Methadone inhibits CYP2D6-mediated metabolism of flecainide	Monitor PR and BP closely
PROCAINAMIDE	ANTIARRHYTHMICS	Risk of bradycardia and ↓ BP	Additive effect; antiarrhythmics are all myocardial depressants	Monitor PR, BP and ECG closely
PROCAINAMIDE	ANTIBIOTICS – TRIMETHOPRIM	Procainamide levels are ↑ by trimethoprim	Trimethoprim is a potent inhibitor of organic cation transport in the kidney, and elimination of procainamide is impaired	Watch for signs of procainamide toxicity; ↓ the dose of procainamide, particularly in the elderly
PROCAINAMIDE	ANTIDEPRESSANTS – SSRIs	SSRIs may ↑ procainamide levels	SSRIs inhibit CYP2D6-mediated metabolism of procainamide	Monitor PR and BP closely; watch for procainamide toxicity
PROCAINAMIDE	ANTIHYPERTENSIVES AND HEART FAILURE DRUGS – ACE INHIBITORS	Possible ↑ risk of leukopenia	Uncertain at present	Monitor FBC before starting treatment, 2-weekly for 3 months after initiation of therapy, then periodically thereafter

Primary drug	Secondary drug	Effect	Mechanism	Precautions
PROCAINAMIDE	BETA-BLOCKERS	Risk of bradycardia (occasionally severe), ↓ BP and heart failure	Additive negative inotropic and chronotropic effects	Monitor PR, BP and ECG closely; watch for development of heart failure
PROCAINAMIDE	CARDIAC GLYCOSIDES – DIGITOXIN	Single case report of toxicity in a patient taking both digitoxin and procainamide	Uncertain at present	Watch for digitoxin toxicity
PROCAINAMIDE	H2 RECEPTOR BLOCKERS	Cimetidine may ↑ plasma concentrations of procainamide	Cimetidine is a potent inhibitor of organic cation transport in the kidney, and elimination of procainamide is impaired. Cimetidine also inhibits CYP2D6-mediated metabolism of procainamide. Ranitidine is a much weaker CYP2D6 inhibitor	Monitor PR and BP at least weekly until stable. Warn patients to report symptoms of hypotension (light-headedness, dizziness on standing, etc.). Consider alternative acid-suppression therapy
PROCAINAMIDE	MUSCLE RELAXANTS – DEPOLARISING	Possibility of ↑ neuromuscular blockade	Uncertain; procainamide may ↓ plasma cholinesterase levels	Be aware of the possibility of a prolonged effect of suxamethonium when administered to patients taking procainamide

PROPAFENONE				
PROPAFENONE	DRUGS THAT PROLONG THE Q–T INTERVAL			
PROPAFENONE	1. ANTIARRHYTHMICS – disopyramide, procainamide 2. ANTIBIOTICS – macrolides (especially azithromycin, clarithromycin, parenteral erythromycin, telithromycin), quinolones (especially moxifloxacin), quinupristin/dalfopristin 3. ANTICANCER AND IMMUNOMODULATING DRUGS – arsenic trioxide 4. ANTIDEPRESSANTS – TCAs, venlafaxine 5. ANTIEMETICS – dolasetron 6. ANTIFUNGALS – fluconazole, posaconazole, voriconazole 7. ANTIHISTAMINES – terfenadine, hydroxyzine, mizolastine 8. ANTIMALARIALS – artemether with lumefantrine, chloroquine, hydroxychloroquine, mefloquine, quinine 9. ANTIPROTOZOALS – pentamidine isetionate 10. ANTIPSYCHOTICS – atypicals, phenothiazines, pimozide 11. BETA-BLOCKERS – sotalol 12. BRONCHODILATORS – parenteral bronchodilators 13. CNS STIMULANTS – atomoxetine	Risk of ventricular arrhythmias, particularly torsades de pointes	Additive effect; these drugs prolong the Q–T interval. Also, amitriptyline, clomipramine and desipramine levels may be ↑ by propafenone. Amitriptyline and clomipramine may ↑ propafenone levels. Propafenone and these TCAs inhibit CYP2D6-mediated metabolism of each other	Avoid co-administration

Primary drug	Secondary drug	Effect	Mechanism	Precautions
PROPAFENONE	DRUGS WITH ANTIMUSCARINIC EFFECTS			
PROPAFENONE	1. ANALGESICS – nefopam 2. ANTIARRHYTHMICS – disopyramide 3. ANTIDEPRESSANTS – TCAs 4. ANTIEMETICS – cyclizine 5. ANTIHISTAMINES – chlorphenamine, cyproheptadine, hydroxyzine 6. ANTIMUSCARINICS – atropine, benzatropine, cyclopentolate, dicycloverine, flavoxate, homatropine, hyoscine, orphenadrine, oxybutynin, procyclidine, propantheline, tolterodine, trihexyphenidyl, tropicamide 7. ANTIPARKINSON'S DRUGS – dopaminergics 8. ANTIPSYCHOTICS – phenothiazines, clozapine, pimozide 9. MUSCLE RELAXANTS – baclofen 10. NITRATES – isosorbide dinitrate	↑ risk of antimuscarinic side-effects. **NB ↓ efficacy of sublingual nitrate tablets**	Additive effect; both drugs cause antimuscarinic side-effects. **Antimuscarinic effects ↓ salivary production, which ↓ dissolution of the tablet**	Warn patient of this additive effect. **Consider changing the formulation to a sublingual nitrate spray**

PROPAFENONE	ANAESTHETICS – LOCAL	Risk of ↓ BP	Additive myocardial depression	Particular care should be taken to avoid inadvertent intravenous administration during bupivacaine infiltration; monitor PR, BP and ECG during epidural administration of bupivacaine
PROPAFENONE	**ANALGESICS**			
PROPAFENONE	NSAIDs	Serum levels of propafenone may be ↑ by parecoxib	Parecoxib is a weak inhibitor of CYP2D6-mediated metabolism of propafenone	Monitor PR and BP closely. If possible, use only short courses of NSAID
PROPAFENONE	OPIOIDS	Methadone may ↑ propafenone levels	Methadone inhibits CYP2D6-mediated metabolism of propafenone	Monitor PR and BP closely
PROPAFENONE	PARACETAMOL	Propafenone may slow the onset of action of intermittent-dose paracetamol	Anticholinergic effects delay gastric emptying and absorption	Warn patients that the action of paracetamol may be delayed. This will not be the case when paracetamol is taken regularly
PROPAFENONE	**ANTIARRHYTHMICS**			
PROPAFENONE	ANTIARRHYTHMICS	Risk of bradycardia and ↓ BP with all antiarrhythmics	Additive myocardial depression	Monitor PR and BP closely
PROPAFENONE	MEXILETINE	↑ serum levels of mexiletine	Propafenone inhibits CYP2D6-mediated metabolism of mexiletine; no case reports of adverse clinical effects, but is a potential for proarrhythmias	Monitor ECG closely
PROPAFENONE	ANTIBIOTICS – RIFAMPICIN	Rifampicin may ↓ propafenone levels	Rifampicin may inhibit CYP3A4- and CYP1A2-mediated metabolism of propafenone	Watch for poor response to propafenone

Primary drug	Secondary drug	Effect	Mechanism	Precautions
PROPAFENONE	ANTICANCER AND IMMUNOMODULATING DRUGS – CICLOSPORIN	Possible ↑ ciclosporin levels	Uncertain	Watch for signs of ciclosporin toxicity
PROPAFENONE	ANTICOAGULANTS – ORAL	Warfarin levels may be ↑ by propafenone	Propafenone seems to inhibit warfarin metabolism	Monitor INR at least weekly until stable
PROPAFENONE	**ANTIDEPRESSANTS**			
PROPAFENONE	DULOXETINE	Duloxetine may ↑ propafenone levels	Duloxetine moderately inhibits CYP2D6, which metabolizes propafenone	Monitor PR and BP closely
PROPAFENONE	SSRIs	Levels of both may be ↑	Both SSRIs and propafenone are substrates for and inhibitors of CYP2D6	Monitor PR and BP closely
PROPAFENONE	ANTIEPILEPTICS	↓ serum levels of propafenone with barbiturates	Barbiturates stimulate hepatic metabolism of propafenone	Watch for poor response to propafenone
PROPAFENONE	ANTIVIRALS – PROTEASE INHIBITORS	Amprenavir, ritonavir and possibly saquinavir and tipranavir with ritonavir ↑ propafenone levels, with risk of ventricular arrhythmias	Uncertain	Manufacturers recommend avoiding co-administration of propafenone and amprenavir, ritonavir or tipranavir
PROPAFENONE	**BETA-BLOCKERS**			
PROPAFENONE	BETA-BLOCKERS	Risk of bradycardia (occasionally severe), ↓ BP and heart failure	Additive negative inotropic and chronotropic effects	Monitor PR, BP and ECG closely; watch for development of heart failure
PROPAFENONE	METOPROLOL, PROPANOLOL	↑ plasma levels of propranolol and metoprolol	Propafenone is extensively metabolized by CYP2D6 enzymes and interferes with the metabolism of propranolol and metoprolol	Watch for propranolol and metoprolol toxicity; ↓ doses accordingly

PROPAFENONE	BRONCHODILATORS – THEOPHYLLINE	Cases of ↑ theophylline levels with toxicity when propafenone added	Uncertain at present	Watch for signs of theophylline toxicity
PROPAFENONE	CARDIAC GLYCOSIDES	Digoxin concentrations may be ↑ by propafenone	Uncertain at present	Watch for digoxin toxicity; check digoxin levels if indicated and ↓ digoxin dose as necessary (15–75% suggested by studies)
PROPAFENONE	DRUG DEPENDENCE THERAPIES – BUPROPION	Bupropion may ↑ propafenone levels	Bupropion may inhibit CYP2D6-mediated metabolism of propafenone	Monitor PR and BP closely; start propafenone at the lowest dose for patients taking bupropion
PROPAFENONE	GRAPEFRUIT JUICE	Possibly ↓ effect of propafenone	Unclear. Metabolism may be altered to CYP3A4 and CYP1A2 in patients with low CYP2D6 activity	Monitor ECG and side-effects more closely
PROPAFENONE	H2 RECEPTOR BLOCKERS	Cimetidine may ↑ propafenone levels	Cimetidine inhibits CYP2D6-mediated metabolism of propafenone. Ranitidine is a weak CYP2D6 inhibitor	Monitor PR and BP at least weekly until stable. Warn patients to report symptoms of hypotension (light-headedness, dizziness on standing, etc.). Consider alternative acid-suppression therapy
PROPAFENONE	PARASYMPATHOMIMETICS	↓ efficacy of neostigmine and pyridostigmine	Uncertain; propafenone has a degree of antinicotinic action that may oppose the action of parasympathomimetic therapy for myasthenia gravis	Watch for poor response to these parasympathomimetics and ↑ dose accordingly
SOTALOL ➢ *Beta-blockers, below*				

Primary drug	Secondary drug	Effect	Mechanism	Precautions
ANTIHYPERTENSIVES AND HEART FAILURE DRUGS				
ACE INHIBITORS, ADRENERGIC NEURONE BLOCKERS, ALPHA-BLOCKERS, ANGIOTENSIN II RECEPTOR ANTAGONISTS, CENTRALLY ACTING AND VASODILATOR ANTIHYPERTENSIVES				
ANTIHYPERTENSIVES AND HEART FAILURE DRUGS	ALBUMIN-CONTAINING SOLUTIONS	Acute ↓ BP following *rapid* infusion with captopril or enalapril	Uncertain at present	Use alternative colloids; monitor BP closely while on infusion
ANTIHYPERTENSIVES AND HEART FAILURE DRUGS	**ALCOHOL**			
ANTIHYPERTENSIVES AND HEART FAILURE DRUGS	ALCOHOL	1. Acute alcohol ingestion may ↑ hypotensive effects 2. Chronic moderate/ heavy drinking ↓ hypotensive effect	1. Additive hypotensive effect. 2. Chronic alcohol excess is associated with hypertension	Monitor BP closely as unpredictable responses can occur. Advise patients to drink only in moderation and avoid large variations in the amount of alcohol drunk
ALPHA-BLOCKERS	ALCOHOL	↑ levels of both alcohol and indoramin occurs with concurrent use	Uncertain	Warn the patient about the risk of ↑ sedation
CENTRALLY ACTING ANTIHYPERTENSIVES	ALCOHOL	Clonidine and moxonidine may exacerbate the sedative effects of alcohol, particularly during initiation of therapy	Uncertain	Warn patients of this effect and advise them to avoid driving or operating machinery if they suffer from sedation
ANGIOTENSIN II RECEPTOR ANTAGONISTS	ALISKIREN	Aliskiren levels possibly ↓ by irbesartan	Uncertain	Monitor BP at least weekly until stable
ANTIHYPERTENSIVES AND HEART FAILURE DRUGS	ANAESTHETICS – GENERAL	Risk of severe hypotensive episodes during induction of anaesthesia	Most general anaesthetics are myocardial depressants and vasodilators. Additive hypotensive effect	Monitor BP closely, especially during induction of anaesthesia

ANTIHYPERTENSIVES AND HEART FAILURE DRUGS	ANAESTHETICS – LOCAL			
ACE INHIBITORS	BUPIVICAINE	Risk of profound ↓ BP with epidural bupivacaine in patients on captopril	Additive hypotensive effect; epidural bupivacaine causes vasodilatation in the lower limbs	Monitor BP closely. Ensure that the patient is preloaded with fluids
ADRENERGIC NEURONE BLOCKERS – GUANETHIDINE	LOCAL ANAESTHETICS	↓ clinical efficacy of guanethidine when used in the treatment of complex regional pain syndrome-type I	The local anaesthetic ↓ the reuptake of guanethidine	Be aware. Consider use of a local anaesthetic that minimally inhibits reuptake, e.g. lidocaine when possible
ANTIHYPERTENSIVES AND HEART FAILURE DRUGS	**ANALGESICS**			
ANTIHYPERTENSIVES AND HEART FAILURE DRUGS	NSAIDs	↓ hypotensive effect, especially with indometacin. The effect is variable amongst different ACE inhibitors and NSAIDs, but is most notable between captopril and indometacin	NSAIDs cause sodium and water retention and raise BP by inhibiting vasodilating renal prostaglandins. ACE inhibitors metabolize tissue kinins (e.g. bradykinin) and this may be the basis for indometacin attenuating hypotensive effect of captopril	Monitor BP at least weekly until stable. Avoid co-administering indometacin with captopril
ACE INHIBITORS, ANGIOTENSIN II RECEPTOR ANTAGONISTS	NSAIDs	1. ↑ risk of renal impairment with NSAIDs and ACE inhibitors 2. ↑ risk of hyperkalaemia with ketorolac	1. Additive effect 2. Ketorolac causes hyperkalaemia, and ACE inhibitors can ↓ renal function	1. Monitor renal function and BP closely. Benefits often outweigh risks for short-term NSAID use 2. Ketorolac is only licensed for short-term control of perioperative pain. Monitor serum potassium daily
VASODILATOR ANTIHYPERTENSIVES	NSAIDs	Etoricoxib may ↑ minoxidil levels	Etoricoxib inhibits sulphotransferase activity	Monitor BP closely

Primary drug	Secondary drug	Effect	Mechanism	Precautions
ACE INHIBITORS	ANTACIDS	↓ effect, particularly of captopril, fosinopril and enalapril	↓ absorption due to ↑ in gastric pH	Watch for poor response to ACE inhibitors
ACE INHIBITORS	ANTIARRHYTHMICS – PROCAINAMIDE	Possible ↑ risk of leukopenia	Uncertain at present	Monitor FBC before starting treatment, 2-weekly for 3 months after initiation of therapy, then periodically thereafter
ANTIHYPERTENSIVES AND HEART FAILURE DRUGS	**ANTIBIOTICS**			
ACE INHIBITORS	RIFAMPICIN	↓ plasma concentrations and efficacy of imidapril and enalapril	Uncertain. ↓ production of active metabolites noted despite rifampicin being an enzyme inducer	Monitor BP at least weekly until stable
ACE INHIBITORS	TETRACYCLINES	↓ plasma concentrations and efficacy of tetracyclines with quinapril. The absorption of tetracyclines may be reduced when taken concurrently with quinapril, due to the presence of magnesium carbonate as an excipient in quinapril's pharmaceutical formulation	Magnesium carbonate (found in a formulation of quinapril) chelates with tetracyclines in the gut to form a less soluble substance that ↓ absorption of tetracycline	For short-term antibiotic use, consider stopping quinapril for duration of the course. For long-term use, consider an alternative ACE inhibitor
ACE INHIBITORS	TRIMETHOPRIM	Risk of hyperkalaemia when trimethoprim is co-administered with ACE inhibitors *in the presence of renal failure*	Uncertain at present	Avoid concurrent use in the presence of severe renal failure
ANGIOTENSIN II RECEPTOR ANTAGONISTS – LOSARTAN	RIFAMPICIN	↓ antihypertensive effect of losartan	Rifampicin induces CYP2C9	Monitor BP at least weekly until stable
VASODILATOR ANTIHYPERTENSIVES	RIFAMPICIN	↓ bosentan levels	Induction of metabolism	Avoid co-administration

ANTIHYPERTENSIVES AND HEART FAILURE DRUGS	ANTICANCER AND IMMUNOMODULATING DRUGS			
ANTIHYPERTENSIVES AND HEART FAILURE DRUGS	**CYTOTOXICS**			
ACE INHIBITORS	PORFIMER	↑ risk of photosensitivity reactions when porfimer is administered with enalapril	Attributed to additive effects	Avoid exposure of skin and eyes to direct sunlight for 30 days after porfimer therapy
ANGIOTENSIN II RECEPTOR ANTAGONISTS	IMATINIB	↑ plasma concentrations of losartan, irbesartan and valsartan	Imatinib is a potent inhibitor of CYP2C9 isoenzymes, which metabolize these angiotensin II receptor blockers	Monitor for toxic effects of losartan, e.g. hypotension, hyperkalaemia, diarrhoea, cough, vertigo and liver toxicity
ANTIHYPERTENSIVES AND HEART FAILURE DRUGS	**IMMUNOMODULATING DRUGS**			
ACE INHIBITORS	AZATHIOPRINE	Risk of anaemia with captopril and enalapril and leukopenia with captopril	The exact mechanism is uncertain. Azathioprine-induced impairment of haematopoiesis and ACE inhibitor-induced ↓ in erythropoietin may cause additive effects. Enalapril has been used to treat post-renal transplant erythrocytosis	Monitor blood counts regularly
ACE INHIBITORS, ANGIOTENSIN II RECEPTOR ANTAGONISTS	CICLOSPORIN	↑ risk of hyperkalaemia and renal failure	Ciclosporin causes a dose-dependent ↑ in serum creatinine, urea and potassium, especially in renal dysfunction	Monitor renal function and serum potassium weekly until stable, then at least every 3–6 months
VASODILATOR ANTIHYPERTENSIVES	CICLOSPORIN	1. Co-administration of bosentan and ciclosporin leads to ↑ bosentan and ↓ ciclosporin levels 2. Risk of hypertrichosis when minoxidil given with ciclosporin 3. ↑ sitaxentan levels	1. Additive effect; both drugs inhibit the bile sodium export pump, which is associated with hepatotoxicity 2. Additive effect 3. Uncertain	1. Avoid co-administration of bosentan and ciclosporin 2. Warn patients of the potential interaction 3. Avoid co-administration

Primary drug	Secondary drug	Effect	Mechanism	Precautions
ANTIHYPERTENSIVES AND HEART FAILURE DRUGS	CORTICOSTEROIDS	↓ hypotensive effect	Corticosteroids cause sodium and water retention leading to ↑ BP	Monitor BP at least weekly until stable
VASODILATOR ANTIHYPERTENSIVES	CORTICOSTEROIDS	Risk of hyperglycaemia when diazoxide is co-administered with corticosteroids	Additive effect; both drugs have a hyperglycaemic effect	Monitor blood glucose closely, particularly with diabetes
ANTIHYPERTENSIVES AND HEART FAILURE DRUGS	IL-2 (ALDESLEUKIN)	↑ hypotensive effect	Additive hypotensive effect; may be used therapeutically. Aldesleukin causes ↓ vascular resistance and ↑ capillary permeability	Monitor BP at least weekly until stable. Warn patients to report symptoms of hypotension (light-headedness, dizziness on standing, etc.).
ANGIOTENSIN II RECEPTOR ANTAGONISTS	TACROLIMUS	↑ risk of hyperkalaemia	Uncertain	Monitor serum potassium weekly until stable, then every 6 months
ANTIHYPERTENSIVES AND HEART FAILURE DRUGS	**ANTICOAGULANTS**			
ACE INHIBITORS, ANGIOTENSIN II RECEPTOR ANTAGONISTS	ANTICOAGULANTS – PARENTERAL	↑ risk of hyperkalaemia with heparins	Heparin inhibits aldosterone secretion, causing hyperkalaemia	Monitor potassium levels closely
VASODILATOR ANTIHYPERTENSIVES	ANTICOAGULANTS – ORAL	1. Bosentan may ↓ warfarin levels 2. Iloprost and sitaxentan may ↑ warfarin levels	1. Uncertain; postulated that bosentan induces CYP3A4 and 2C9 2. Uncertain	Monitor INR closely
VASODILATOR ANTIHYPERTENSIVES	ANTICOAGULANTS – PARENTERAL	Possible ↑ risk of bleeding with iloprost	Anticoagulant effects of heparins ↑ by a mechanism that is uncertain at present	Monitor APTT closely
ANTIHYPERTENSIVES AND HEART FAILURE DRUGS	**ANTIDEPRESSANTS**			
METHYLDOPA	ANTIDEPRESSANTS	Methyldopa may ↓ the effect of antidepressants	Methyldopa can cause depression	Methyldopa should be avoided in patients with depression

CARDIOVASCULAR DRUGS ANTIHYPERTENSIVES AND HEART FAILURE DRUGS

ANTIHYPERTENSIVES AND HEART FAILURE DRUGS	**LITHIUM**			
ACE INHIBITORS	LITHIUM	↑ efficacy of lithium	↑ plasma concentrations of lithium (up to one-third) due to ↓ renal excretion	Watch for lithium toxicity; monitor lithium levels
ANGIOTENSIN II RECEPTOR ANTAGONISTS	LITHIUM	Risk of lithium toxicity	↓ excretion of lithium possibly due to ↓ renal tubular reabsorption of sodium in proximal tubule	Watch for lithium toxicity; monitor lithium levels
CENTRALLY ACTING ANTIHYPERTENSIVES	LITHIUM	Case reports of lithium toxicity when co-ingested with methyldopa. It was noted that lithium levels were in the therapeutic range	Uncertain at present	Avoid co-administration if possible; if not, watch closely for clinical features of toxicity and do not rely on lithium levels
ANTIHYPERTENSIVES AND HEART FAILURE DRUGS	**MAOIs**			
ANTIHYPERTENSIVES AND HEART FAILURE DRUGS	MAOIs	Possible ↑ hypotensive effect	Additive hypotensive effect	Monitor BP at least weekly until stable. Warn patients to report symptoms of hypotension (light-headedness, dizziness on standing, etc.)
ADRENERGIC NEURONE BLOCKERS – GUANETHIDINE CENTRALLY ACTING ANTIHYPERTENSIVES – METHYLDOPA	MAOIs	Risk of adrenergic syndrome (see above). Reports of an enhanced hypotensive effect and hallucinations with methyldopa, which may cause depression	Due to inhibition of MAOI, which breaks down sympathomimetics	Avoid concurrent use. Onset may be 6–24 hours after ingestion

Primary drug	Secondary drug	Effect	Mechanism	Precautions
ANTIHYPERTENSIVES AND HEART FAILURE DRUGS	**TCAs**			
ADRENERGIC NEURONE BLOCKERS	TCAs	↓ hypotensive effect. There is possibly less effect with maprotiline and mianserin	TCAs compete with adrenergic neurone blockers for reuptake to nerve terminals	Monitor BP at least weekly until stable
CENTRALLY ACTING ANTIHYPERTENSIVES	TCAs	1. Possibly hypotensive effect of clonidine and moxonidine antagonized by TCAs (some cases of hypertensive crisis) 2. Conversely, clonidine and moxonidine may exacerbate the sedative effects of TCAs, particularly during initiation of therapy	Uncertain	1. Monitor BP at least weekly until stable 2. Warn patients of the risk of sedation and advise them to avoid driving or operating machinery if they suffer from sedation
ANTIHYPERTENSIVES AND HEART FAILURE DRUGS	**ANTIDIABETIC DRUGS**			
ACE INHIBITORS	INSULIN, METFORMIN, SULPHONYLUREAS, NATEGLINIDE, REPAGLINIDE	↑ risk of hypoglycaemic episodes	Mechanism uncertain. ACE inhibitors possibly ↑ insulin sensitivity and glucose utilization. Altered renal function may also be a factor. ACE inhibitors may ↑ bradykinin levels, which ↓ production of glucose by the liver. Hypoglycaemia is reported as a side-effect (rare) of ACE inhibitors. It is suggested that the occurrence of hypoglycaemia is greater with captopril than enalapril. Captopril and enalapril are used in the treatment of diabetic nephropathy	Concurrent treatment need not be avoided and is often beneficial in type II diabetes. Watch for and warn patients about symptoms of hypoglycaemia. Be aware that risk of hypoglycaemia is greater in elderly people and people with poor glycaemic control ➢ ***For signs and symptoms of hypoglycaemia, see Clinical Features of Some Adverse Drug Interactions, Hypoglycaemia***

ADRENERGIC NEURONE BLOCKERS	ANTIDIABETIC DRUGS	↑ hypoglycaemic effect	Catecholamines are diabetogenic; guanethidine blocks the release of catecholamines from nerve endings	Monitor blood glucose closely
ANGIOTENSIN II RECEPTOR ANTAGONISTS – IRBESARTAN	SULPHONYLUREAS	Possible ↑ hypotensive effect of irbesartan by tolbutamide	Tolbutamide competitively inhibits CYP2C9-mediated metabolism of irbesartan	Monitor BP at least weekly until stable. Warn patients to report symptoms of hypotension (light-headedness, dizziness on standing, etc.).
VASODILATOR ANTIHYPERTENSIVES – BOSENTAN	SULPHONYLUREAS	1. Risk of hepatotoxicity when bosentan is given with glibenclamide 2. ↑ risk of hypoglycaemic episodes when bosentan is given with glimepride or tolbutamide	1. Additive effect: both drugs inhibit the bile sodium export pump 2. Bosentan may inhibit CYP2C9-mediated metabolism of these sulphonylureas	1. Avoid co-administration 2. Monitor blood glucose levels closely. Warn patients about the signs and symptoms of hypoglycaemia. ➢ ***For signs and symptoms of hypoglycaemia, see Clinical Features of Some Adverse Drug Interactions, Hypoglycaemia***
DIAZOXIDE	ANTIDIABETIC DRUGS	May ↑ antidiabetic requirements	Diazoxide causes hyperglycaemia by inhibiting insulin release and probably by a catecholamine-induced extrahepatic effect. Used in the treatment of hypoglycaemia due to insulinomas	Larger doses of antidiabetic are often required; need to monitor blood sugar until adequate control of blood sugar is achieved
VASODILATOR ANTIHYPERTENSIVES	ANTIEPILEPTICS	Co-administration of diazoxide and phenytoin ↓ phenytoin levels and possibly ↓ efficacy of diazoxide	Uncertain at present	Monitor phenytoin levels and BP closely
VASODILATOR ANTIHYPERTENSIVES	ANTIFUNGALS – AZOLES	↑ bosentan levels	Azoles inhibit CYP3A4 and CYP2C9	Monitor LFTs closely

Primary drug	Secondary drug	Effect	Mechanism	Precautions
ANTIHYPERTENSIVES AND HEART FAILURE DRUGS	**ANTIGOUT DRUGS**			
ACE INHIBITORS	ALLOPURINOL	Risk of serious hypersensitivity with captopril and enalapril	Uncertain. Both drugs can cause hypersensitivity reactions	Warn patients to look for clinical features of hypersensitivity and Stevens-Johnson syndrome
ACE INHIBITORS	PROBENECID	↑ plasma concentrations of captopril and enalapril; uncertain clinical significance	Renal excretion of captopril and enalapril ↓ by probenecid	Monitor BP closely
ANTIHYPERTENSIVES AND HEART FAILURE DRUGS	**ANTIHYPERTENSIVES AND HEART FAILURE DRUGS**			
ANTIHYPERTENSIVES AND HEART FAILURE DRUGS	ANTIHYPERTENSIVES AND HEART FAILURE DRUGS	↑ hypotensive effect. Episodes of severe first dose ↓ BP when alpha-blockers are added to ACE inhibitors	Additive hypotensive effect; may be used therapeutically	Monitor BP at least weekly until stable, particularly on initiation of therapy. Consider starting therapy at night
ANGIOTENSIN II RECEPTOR ANTAGONISTS	ACE INHIBITORS	Risk of hyperkalaemia	Additive retention of potassium	Monitor renal function and serum potassium every 4–6 weeks until stable and then at least annually
CENTRALLY ACTING ANTIHYPERTENSIVES	ACE INHIBITORS	Some evidence that when switching from clonidine to captopril, there may be a delayed onset of action of captopril	Sudden cessation of clonidine causes rebound ↑ BP, and this may be the reason for the delay in onset of captopril	Monitor BP at least weekly until stable
CENTRALLY ACTING ANTIHYPERTENSIVES – CLONIDINE	ALPHA-BLOCKERS – PRAZOSIN	Small case series indicate that prazosin may ↓ the antihypertensive effect of clonidine	Uncertain at present	Monitor BP at least weekly until stable
VASODILATOR ANTIHYPERTENSIVES	VASODILATOR ANTIHYPERTENSIVES	Profound, refractory ↓ BP may occur when diazoxide is co-administered with hydralazine	Additive effect; uncertain why the effect is so refractory to treatment	Avoid co-administration of diazoxide with hydralazine

ANTIHYPERTENSIVES AND HEART FAILURE DRUGS	ANTIPARKINSON'S DRUGS			
CENTRALLY ACTING ANTIHYPERTENSIVES	ANTIPARKINSON'S DRUGS – AMANTADINE	↓ efficacy of amantadine with methyldopa	Antagonism of antiparkinsonian effect; these drugs have extrapyramidal side-effects	Use with caution; avoid in patients aged under 20 years
ANTIHYPERTENSIVES AND HEART FAILURE DRUGS	LEVODOPA	↑ hypotensive effect	Additive effect	Monitor BP at least weekly until stable. Warn patients to report symptoms of hypotension (light-headedness, dizziness on standing, etc.)
CENTRALLY ACTING ANTIHYPERTENSIVES	LEVODOPA	1. Clonidine may oppose the effect of levodopa/ carbidopa 2. Methyldopa may ↓ levodopa requirements, although there are case reports of deteriorating dyskinesias in some patients	1. Uncertain at present 2. Uncertain at present	1. Watch for deterioration in control of symptoms of Parkinson's disease 2. Levodopa needs may ↓; in cases of worsening Parkinson's control, use an alternative antihypertensive
ACE INHIBITORS	PERGOLIDE	Possible ↑ hypotensive effect	Additive effect; a single case of severe ↓ BP with lisinopril and pergolide has been reported	Monitor BP at least weekly until stable. Warn patients to report symptoms of hypotension (light-headedness, dizziness on standing, etc.)
ANTIHYPERTENSIVES AND HEART FAILURE DRUGS	**ANTIPLATELET AGENTS**			
ACE INHIBITORS, ANGIOTENSIN II RECEPTOR ANTAGONISTS	ASPIRIN	↑ risk of renal impairment. ↓ efficacy of captopril and enalapril with high-dose (>100 mg/day) aspirin	Aspirin and NSAIDs can cause elevation of BP. Prostaglandin inhibition leads to sodium and water retention and poor renal function in those with impaired renal blood flow	Monitor renal function every 3–6 months; watch for poor response to ACE inhibitors when >100 mg/day aspirin is given

CARDIOVASCULAR DRUGS ANTIHYPERTENSIVES AND HEART FAILURE DRUGS

Primary drug	Secondary drug	Effect	Mechanism	Precautions
ADRENERGIC NEURONE BLOCKERS, ALPHA-BLOCKERS, CENTRALLY ACTING ANTIHYPERTENSIVES, VASODILATOR ANTIHYPERTENSIVES	ASPIRIN	↓ hypotensive effect; not noted with low-dose aspirin	Aspirin may cause sodium retention and vasoconstriction at possibly both renal and endothelial sites	Monitor BP at least weekly until stable when high-dose aspirin is prescribed
ANGIOTENSIN II RECEPTOR BLOCKERS	ASPIRIN	Risk of renal impairment when olmesartan is administered with high-dose aspirin (>3 g daily). Effect not noted with low-dose aspirin	Additive effect on reducing glomerular filtration rate	Monitor renal function regularly until stable
VASODILATOR ANTIHYPERTENSIVES	ASPIRIN	↑ risk of bleeding when aspirin is co-administered with iloprost	Uncertain at present	Closely monitor the effects; watch for signs of excess bleeding
VASODILATOR ANTIHYPERTENSIVES	CLOPIDOGREL	↑ risk of bleeding when clopidogrel is co-administered with iloprost	Uncertain at present	Closely monitor the effects; watch for signs of excess bleeding
VASODILATOR ANTIHYPERTENSIVES	GLYCOPROTEIN IIb/IIIa INHIBITORS	↑ risk of bleeding when eptifibatide or tirofiban is co-administered with iloprost	Uncertain at present	Closely monitor the effects; watch for signs of excess bleeding
ANTIHYPERTENSIVES AND HEART FAILURE DRUGS	**ANTIPSYCHOTICS**			
ANTIHYPERTENSIVES AND HEART FAILURE DRUGS	ANTIPSYCHOTICS	↑ hypotensive effect	Dose-related ↓ BP (due to vasodilatation) is a side-effect of most antipsychotics, particularly phenothiazines	Monitor BP closely, especially during initiation of treatment. Warn patients to report symptoms of hypotension (light-headedness, dizziness on standing, etc.)
ADRENERGIC NEURONE BLOCKERS	HALOPERIDOL	↓ hypotensive effect	Haloperidol blocks the uptake of guanethidine into adrenergic neurones	Monitor BP at least weekly until stable

ADRENERGIC NEURONE BLOCKERS	PHENOTHIAZINES	Variable effect: some cases of ↑ hypotensive effect; other cases where hypotensive effects ↓ by higher doses (>100 mg) of chlorpromazine	Additive hypotensive effect. Phenothiazines cause vasodilatation; however, chlorpromazine blocks uptake of guanethidine into adrenergic neurones	Monitor BP at least weekly until stable. Warn patients to report symptoms of hypotension (light-headedness, dizziness on standing, etc.)
CENTRALLY ACTING ANTIHYPERTENSIVES	HALOPERIDOL	Case reports of sedation or confusion on initiating co-administration of haloperidol and methyldopa	Uncertain; possible additive effect	Watch for excess sedation when starting therapy
VASODILATOR ANTIHYPERTENSIVES	ANTIPSYCHOTICS	Risk of hyperglycaemia when diazoxide is co-administered with chlorpromazine	Additive effect; both drugs have a hyperglycaemic effect	Monitor blood glucose closely, particularly with diabetes
ANTIHYPERTENSIVES AND HEART FAILURE DRUGS	**ANTIVIRALS**			
ALPHA-BLOCKERS	PROTEASE INHIBITORS	Possible ↑ alfuzosin levels with ritonavir	Uncertain	Avoid co-administration
VASODILATOR ANTIHYPERTENSIVES	NNRTIs	Risk of peripheral neuropathy when hydralazine is co-administered with didanosine, stavudine or zalcitabine	Additive effect; both drugs can cause peripheral neuropathy	Warn patient to report early features of peripheral neuropathy; if it occurs, the NNRTI should be stopped
VASODILATOR ANTIHYPERTENSIVES	PROTEASE INHIBITORS	↑ adverse effects of bosentan by ritonavir	Inhibition of CYP3A4-mediated metabolism of bosentan	Co-administration is not recommended
ANTIHYPERTENSIVES AND HEART FAILURE DRUGS	**ANXIOLYTICS AND HYPNOTICS**			
ANTIHYPERTENSIVES AND HEART FAILURE DRUGS	ANXIOLYTICS AND HYPNOTICS	↑ hypotensive effect	Additive hypotensive effect	Monitor BP at least weekly until stable. Warn patients to report symptoms of hypotension (light-headedness, dizziness on standing, etc.)

Primary drug	Secondary drug	Effect	Mechanism	Precautions
CENTRALLY ACTING ANTIHYPERTENSIVES	ANXIOLYTICS AND HYPNOTICS	Clonidine and moxonidine may exacerbate the sedative effects of BZDs, particularly during initiation of therapy	Uncertain	Warn patients of this effect and advise them to avoid driving or operating machinery if they suffer from sedation
ANTIHYPERTENSIVES AND HEART FAILURE DRUGS	**BETA-BLOCKERS**			
ACE INHIBITORS, ANGIOTENSIN II RECEPTOR ANTAGONISTS, CENTRALLY ACTING ANTIHYPERTENSIVES, VASODILATOR ANTIHYPERTENSIVES	BETA-BLOCKERS	↑ hypotensive effect	Additive hypotensive effect; may be used therapeutically	Monitor BP at least weekly until stable. Warn patients to report symptoms of hypotension (light-headedness, dizziness on standing, etc.)
ALPHA-BLOCKERS	BETA-BLOCKERS	↑ efficacy of alpha-blockers; ↑ risk of first-dose ↓ BP when alfuzosin, prazosin or terazosin is started in patients already taking beta-blockers	Additive hypotensive effect; may be used therapeutically	Monitor BP at least weekly until stable. Warn patients to report symptoms of hypotension (light-headedness, dizziness on standing, etc.). Watch for first-dose ↓ BP
CENTRALLY ACTING ANTIHYPERTENSIVES	BETA-BLOCKERS	Risk of withdrawal ↑ BP (rebound ↑ BP) with clonidine and possibly moxonidine	Withdrawal of clonidine, and possibly moxonidine, is associated with ↑ circulating catecholamines; beta-blockers, especially non-cardioselective ones, will allow the catecholamines to exert an unopposed alpha action (vasoconstriction)	Do not withdraw clonidine or moxonidine while a patient is taking beta-blockers. Withdraw beta-blockers several days before slowly withdrawing clonidine and moxonidine

CARDIOVASCULAR DRUGS ANTIHYPERTENSIVES AND HEART FAILURE DRUGS

VASODILATOR ANTIHYPERTENSIVES	BETA-BLOCKERS	↑ hypotensive effect	Additive hypotensive effect with diazoxide, hydralazine, minoxidil and sodium nitroprusside. In addition, hydralazine may ↑ the bioavailability of beta-blockers with a high first-pass metabolism (e.g. propanolol and metoprolol), possibly due to alterations in hepatic blood flow or inhibited hepatic metabolism	Monitor BP closely
CENTRALLY ACTING ANTIHYPERTENSIVES	BRONCHODILATORS – BETA-2 AGONISTS	Cases of ↓ BP when intravenous salbutamol is given with methyldopa	Uncertain at present	Monitor BP closely
ANTIHYPERTENSIVES AND HEART FAILURE DRUGS	**CALCIUM CHANNEL BLOCKERS**			
ANTIHYPERTENSIVES AND HEART FAILURE DRUGS	CALCIUM CHANNEL BLOCKERS	↑ hypotensive effect	Additive hypotensive effect; may be used therapeutically	Monitor BP at least weekly until stable. Warn patients to report symptoms of hypotension (light-headedness, dizziness on standing, etc.)
ALPHA-BLOCKERS	CALCIUM CHANNEL BLOCKERS	↑ efficacy of alpha-blockers; ↑ risk of first-dose ↓ BP with alfuzosin, prazosin and terazosin	Additive hypotensive effect; may be used therapeutically	Watch for first-dose ↓ BP when starting either drug when the patient is already established on the other; consider reducing the dose of the established drug and starting the new agent at the lowest dose and titrating up
CENTRALLY ACTING ANTIHYPERTENSIVES	VERAPAMIL	Two cases of complete heart block when clonidine was added to a patient on verapamil	Additive effect; both drugs are known rarely to cause AV dysfunction	Monitor ECG closely when co-administering

Primary drug	Secondary drug	Effect	Mechanism	Precautions
ANTIHYPERTENSIVES AND HEART FAILURE DRUGS	**CARDIAC GLYCOSIDES**			
ACE INHIBITORS	DIGOXIN	↑ plasma concentrations of digoxin when captopril is co-administered in the presence of heart failure (class II or more severe) or renal insufficiency. No other ACE inhibitors seem to interact in the same way	Uncertain; postulated to be due to ↓ renal excretion of digoxin	Monitor digoxin levels; watch for digoxin toxicity
ALPHA-BLOCKERS	CARDIAC GLYCOSIDES	Possibility of ↑ plasma concentrations of digoxin; no cases of toxicity have been reported with doxazosin or prazosin	Doxazosin inhibits P-gp-mediated elimination of digoxin; mechanism with prazosin is uncertain at present	Monitor digoxin levels
ANGIOTENSIN II RECEPTOR ANTAGONISTS	DIGOXIN	Telmisartan may ↑ plasma levels of digoxin	Uncertain; telmisartan thought to ↑ the rate of absorption of digoxin	Watch for digoxin toxicity, monitor digoxin levels
ANTIHYPERTENSIVES AND HEART FAILURE DRUGS	**DIURETICS**			
ANTIHYPERTENSIVES AND HEART FAILURE DRUGS	LOOP DIURETICS	↑ hypotensive effect. Risk of first-dose ↓ BP greater when ACE inhibitors or angiotensin II receptor antagonists are added to high-dose diuretics. ↑ risk of first-dose ↓ BP also with alfuzosin, prazosin and terazosin	Additive hypotensive effect; may be used therapeutically	Monitor BP at least weekly until stable. Warn patients to report symptoms of hypotension (light-headedness, dizziness on standing, etc.). Benefits often outweigh risks. Patients with congestive cardiac failure on diuretics should be started on a low dose of alpha-blocker
ACE INHIBITORS, ANGIOTENSIN II RECEPTOR ANTAGONISTS	POTASSIUM-SPARING DIURETICS, ALDOSTERONE ANTAGONISTS	↑ risk of hyperkalaemia	Additive retention of potassium	Monitor serum potassium every week until stable, then every 3–6 months

ANTIHYPERTENSIVES AND HEART FAILURE DRUGS	THIAZIDES	↑ hypotensive effect. Risk of first-dose ↓ BP greater when ACE inhibitors are added to high-dose diuretics. ↑ risk of first-dose ↓ BP also with alfuzosin, prazosin and terazosin	Additive hypotensive effect; may be used therapeutically	Monitor BP at least weekly until stable. Warn patients to report symptoms of hypotension (light-headedness, dizziness on standing, etc.). Benefits often outweigh risks. Patients with congestive cardiac failure on diuretics should be started on a low dose of alpha-blocker
VASODILATOR ANTIHYPERTENSIVES	THIAZIDES	Risk of hyperglycaemia when diazoxide is co-administered with thiazides	Additive effect; both drugs have a hyperglycaemic effect	Monitor blood glucose closely, particularly with diabetes
ANTIHYPERTENSIVES AND HEART FAILURE DRUGS	**EPOETIN**			
ACE INHIBITORS	EPOETIN	↓ haematopoietic effects of epoetin. ↓ efficacy of ACE inhibitors	Angiotensin II is believed to be responsible for sustaining secretion of erythropoietin and for stimulating the bone marrow to produce erythrocytes. Epoetin has direct contractile effects on vessels (causing ↑ BP)	Watch for poor response to erythropoietin and to ACE inhibitors. These effects may be delayed so monitor for the duration of co-administration
ANGIOTENSIN II RECEPTOR ANTAGONISTS	EPOETIN	↓ efficacy of angiotensin II receptor antagonists and possible ↑ risk of hyperkalaemia	Angiotensin II is believed to sustain the secretion of erythropoietin and to stimulate the bone marrow to produce erythrocytes. Epoetin has a direct contractile effects on vessels	Monitor BP at least weekly until stable. Monitor serum potassium every week until stable, then every 3–6 months

Primary drug	Secondary drug	Effect	Mechanism	Precautions
ACE INHIBITORS	GOLD (SODIUM AUROTHIOMALATE)	Cases of ↓ BP	Additive vasodilating effects	Monitor BP at least weekly until stable. Warn patients to report symptoms of hypotension (light-headedness, dizziness on standing, etc.). If reaction occurs, consider changing to alternative gold formulation or stopping ACE inhibitor
ALPHA-BLOCKERS	H2 RECEPTOR BLOCKERS	↓ efficacy of tolazoline	Uncertain; possibly ↓ absorption	Watch for poor response to tolazoline
ACE INHIBITORS	INTERFERON ALFA	Risk of severe granulocytopenia	Possibly due to synergistic haematological toxicity	Monitor blood counts frequently; warn patients to report promptly any symptoms of infection
CENTRALLY ACTING ANTIHYPERTENSIVES	IRON COMPOUNDS	↓ antihypertensive effect of methyldopa	Ferrous sulphate and possibly ferrous gluconate may chelate methyldopa in the intestine and ↓ its absorption	Monitor BP at least weekly until stable
VASODILATOR ANTIHYPERTENSIVES	LIPID-LOWERING DRUGS	Bosentan lowers simvastatin levels	Uncertain; bosentan moderately inhibits CYP3A4	Monitor lipid profile closely; look for poor response to simvastatin
ANTIHYPERTENSIVES AND HEART FAILURE DRUGS	MUSCLE RELAXANTS – SKELETAL	↑ hypotensive effect with tizanidine and baclofen	Additive hypotensive effect	Monitor BP at least weekly until stable. Warn patients to report symptoms of hypotension (light-headedness, dizziness on standing, etc.)
ANTIHYPERTENSIVES AND HEART FAILURE DRUGS	NITRATES	↑ hypotensive effect	Additive hypotensive effect; may be used therapeutically	Monitor BP at least weekly until stable. Warn patients to report symptoms of hypotension (light-headedness, dizziness on standing, etc.)

ANTIHYPERTENSIVES AND HEART FAILURE DRUGS	**OESTROGENS**			
ANTIHYPERTENSIVES AND HEART FAILURE DRUGS	OESTROGENS	↓ hypotensive effect	Oestrogens cause sodium and fluid retention	Monitor BP at least weekly until stable; routine prescription of oestrogens in patients with ↑ BP is not advisable
VASODILATOR ANTIHYPERTENSIVES	OESTROGENS	Risk of hyperglycaemia when diazoxide is co-administered with combined oral contraceptives	Additive effect; both drugs have a hyperglycaemic effect	Monitor blood glucose closely, particularly with diabetics
ANTIHYPERTENSIVES AND HEART FAILURE DRUGS	**ORLISTAT**			
ACE INHIBITORS	ORLISTAT	↓ hypotensive effect found with enalapril	Uncertain at present	Monitor BP at least weekly until stable
ANGIOTENSIN II RECEPTOR ANTAGONISTS	ORLISTAT	Cases of ↓ efficacy of losartan	Uncertain at present	Monitor BP at least weekly until stable
ANTIHYPERTENSIVES AND HEART FAILURE DRUGS	PERIPHERAL VASODILATORS – MOXISYLYTE (THYMOXAMINE)	↑ hypotensive effect	Additive hypotensive effect	Monitor BP at least weekly until stable. Warn patients to report symptoms of hypotension (light-headedness, dizziness on standing, etc.)
ANTIHYPERTENSIVES AND HEART FAILURE DRUGS	**PHOSPHODIESTERASE TYPE 5 INHIBITORS**			
ALPHA-BLOCKERS	PHOSPHODIESTERASE TYPE 5 INHIBITORS	Risk of marked ↓ BP	Additive hypotensive effect	Avoid co-administration. Avoid alpha-blockers for 4 hours after intake of sildenafil (6 hours after vardenafil)
VASODILATOR ANTIHYPERTENSIVES – BOSENTAN	SILDENAFIL	↓ sildenafil levels	Probable induction of metabolism	Watch for poor response

Primary drug	Secondary drug	Effect	Mechanism	Precautions
ADRENERGIC NEURONE BLOCKERS	PIZOTIFEN	↓ hypotensive effect	Pizotifen competes with adrenergic neurone blockers for reuptake to nerve terminals	Monitor BP at least weekly until stable
ACE INHIBITORS, ANGIOTENSIN II RECEPTOR ANTAGONISTS	POTASSIUM	↑ risk of hyperkalaemia	Retention of potassium by ACE inhibitors and additional intake of potassium	Monitor serum potassium daily
VASODILATOR ANTIHYPERTENSIVES	POTASSIUM CHANNEL ACTIVATORS	↑ hypotensive effect	Additive effect	Monitor BP closely
ANTIHYPERTENSIVES AND HEART FAILURE DRUGS	**PROGESTOGENS**			
ACE INHIBITORS, ANGIOTENSIN II RECEPTOR ANTAGONISTS	PROGESTOGENS	↑ risk of hyperkalaemia	Drospirenone (component of the Yasmin brand of combined contraceptive pill) is a progestogen derived from spironolactone that can cause potassium retention	Monitor serum potassium weekly until stable, then every 6 months
VASODILATOR ANTIHYPERTENSIVES – BOSENTAN	PROGESTOGENS	↓ progesterone levels, which may lead to failure of contraception or poor response to treatment of menorrhagia	Possibly induction of metabolism of progestogens	Advise patients to use additional contraception for the period of intake and for 1 month after stopping co-administration with these drugs
ANTIHYPERTENSIVES AND HEART FAILURE DRUGS	PROSTAGLANDINS – ALPROSTADIL	↑ hypotensive effect	Additive hypotensive effect	Monitor BP at least weekly until stable. Warn patients to report symptoms of hypotension (light-headedness, dizziness on standing, etc.)

ANTIHYPERTENSIVES AND HEART FAILURE DRUGS	SYMPATHOMIMETICS			
ACE INHIBITORS, ADRENERGIC NEURONE BLOCKERS	SYMPATHOMIMETICS	↓ hypotensive effect. Note there is a risk of interactions even with topical sympathomimetics (eye and nose drops)	Adrenergic neurone blockers act mainly by preventing the release of norepinephrine. Sympathomimetics stimulate adrenergic receptors, which causes a rise in BP	Monitor BP at least weekly until stable
ADRENERGIC NEURONE BLOCKERS	SYMPATHOMIMETICS – DIRECT	For patients on guanethidine, ↑ pressor effects have been reported with the administration of norepinephrine and metaraminol, and a lower threshold for arrhythmias with norepinephrine. Prolonged mydriasis reported when eye drops are given to patients on guanethidine	Guanethidine blocks the release of norepinephrine from adrenergic neurones; this causes a hypersensitivity of the receptors that are normally stimulated by norepinephrine and leads to the ↑ response when they are stimulated by directly acting sympathomimetics	Start alpha- and beta-1 agonists at a lower dose; monitor BP and cardiac rhythm closely
CENTRALLY ACTING ANTIHYPERTENSIVES	SYMPATHOMIMETICS – DIRECT	Risk of ↑ BP when clonidine is given with epinephrine or norepinephrine	Additive effect; clonidine use associated with ↑ circulating catecholamines	Monitor BP at least weekly until stable
CENTRALLY ACTING ANTIHYPERTENSIVES	SYMPATHOMIMETICS – INDIRECT	1. Indirect sympathomimetics may ↓ the hypotensive effect of methyldopa 2. Methyldopa may ↓ the mydriatic effect of ephedrine eye drops	1. Uncertain 2. Uncertain	1. Monitor BP at least weekly until stable 2. Watch for a poor response to ephedrine eye drops
VASODILATOR ANTIHYPERTENSIVES	SYMPATHOMIMETICS – DIRECT	Cases of ↑ tachycardia when epinephrine is given for perioperative ↓ BP in patients on hydralazine	Additive effect	Avoid co-administration

Primary drug	Secondary drug	Effect	Mechanism	Precautions
ANTIPLATELET DRUGS				
ASPIRIN				
ASPIRIN	ANAESTHETICS – GENERAL	↓ requirements of thiopentone when aspirin (1 g) used as premedication	Uncertain at present	Be aware of possible ↓ dose requirements for thiopentone
ASPIRIN	ANALGESICS – NSAIDs	1. Risk of gastrointestinal bleeding when aspirin, even a low dose, is co-administered with NSAIDs 2. Ibuprofen ↓ antiplatelet effect of aspirin	1. Additive effect 2. Ibuprofen competitively inhibits binding of aspirin to platelets	1. Avoid co-administration 2. Avoid co-administration
ASPIRIN	**ANTICANCER AND IMMUNOMODULATING DRUGS**			
ASPIRIN	CYTOTOXICS – METHOTREXATE	Risk of methotrexate toxicity when co-administered with high-dose aspirin. There is a risk of toxic effects of methotrexate, e.g. liver cirrhosis, blood dyscrasias that may be fatal, pulmonary toxicity and stomatitis. Haematopoietic suppression can occur abruptly. Other adverse effects include anorexia, dyspepsia, gastrointestinal ulceration and bleeding, and pulmonary oedema	Aspirin ↓ plasma protein binding of methotrexate (a relatively minor contribution to the interaction) and the renal excretion of high doses of methotrexate. Salicylates compete with methotrexate for renal elimination	Check FBC, U&Es and LFTs before starting treatment and repeat weekly until stabilized, then every 2–3 months. Patients should be advised to report symptoms such as sore throat, fever or gastrointestinal discomfort immediately. Stop methotrexate and initiate supportive therapy if the white cell or platelet counts drop. Do not administer aspirin within 10 days of high-dose methotrexate treatment
ASPIRIN	IMMUNOMODULATING DRUGS – CORTICOSTEROIDS	Corticosteroids ↓ aspirin levels, and therefore there is a risk of salicylate toxicity when withdrawing corticosteroids. Risk of gastric ulceration when aspirin is co-administered with corticosteroids	Uncertain	Watch for features of salicylate toxicity when withdrawing corticosteroids. Use aspirin in the lowest dose. Remember that corticosteroids may mask the features of peptic ulceration

ASPIRIN	ANTICOAGULANTS	Risk of bleeding when high-dose aspirin is co-administered with anticoagulants; less risk with low-dose aspirin	Additive effect on the clotting mechanism; aspirin also irritates the gastric mucosa	Avoid co-administration of anticoagulants and high-dose aspirin. Patients on warfarin should be warned that many OTC and some herbal remedies contain aspirin
ASPIRIN	**ANTIDEPRESSANTS**			
ASPIRIN	SSRIs	Possible ↑ risk of bleeding with SSRIs	Uncertain. Possible additive effects including inhibition of serotonin release by platelets, SSRI-induced thrombocytopenia, and ↓ platelet aggregation	Avoid co-administration with high-dose aspirin
ASPIRIN	VENLAFAXINE	Possible ↑ risk of bleeding with venlafaxine	Uncertain	Avoid co-administration with high-dose aspirin
ASPIRIN	ANTIDIABETIC DRUGS	Risk of hypoglycaemia when high-dose aspirin (3.5–7.5 g/day) is given with antidiabetic agents	Additive effect; aspirin has a hypoglycaemic effect	Avoid high-dose aspirin
ASPIRIN	ANTIEMETICS	↑ aspirin levels with metoclopramide	↑ absorption of aspirin	Watch for early features of salicylate toxicity
ASPIRIN	ANTIEPILEPTICS	Possible ↑ levels of phenytoin and valproate	Possibly ↑ unbound phenytoin or valproate fraction in the blood	Monitor phenytoin or valproate levels when co-administering high-dose aspirin
ASPIRIN	**ANTIGOUT DRUGS**			
ASPIRIN	PROBENICID	Aspirin possibly ↓ the efficacy of probenicid	Uncertain	Watch for poor response to probenicid
ASPIRIN	SULFINPYRAZONE	High-dose aspirin antagonizes the urate-lowering effect of sulfinpyrazone	Salicylates block sulfinpyrazone-induced inhibition of renal tubular reabsorption of urate	Avoid long-term co-administration of high-dose aspirin with sulfinpyrazone. Low-dose aspirin does not seem to have this effect

Primary drug	Secondary drug	Effect	Mechanism	Precautions
ASPIRIN	ACE INHIBITORS	↑ risk of renal impairment. ↓ efficacy of captopril and enalapril with high-dose (>100 mg/day) aspirin	Aspirin and NSAIDs can cause elevation of BP. Prostaglandin inhibition leads to sodium and water retention and poor renal function in those with impaired renal blood flow	Monitor renal function every 3–6 months, watch for poor response to ACE inhibitors when >100 mg/day aspirin is given
ASPIRIN	ADRENERGIC NEURONE BLOCKERS, ALPHA-BLOCKERS, CENTRALLY ACTING ANTIHYPERTENSIVES, VASODILATOR ANTIHYPERTENSIVES	↓ antihypertensive effect with aspirin; effect not noted with low-dose aspirin	Aspirin may cause sodium retention and vasoconstriction at possibly both renal and endothelial sites	Monitor BP at least weekly until stable when high-dose is aspirin prescribed
ASPIRIN	ANGIOTENSIN II RECEPTOR BLOCKERS	Risk of renal impairment when olmesartan is administered with high-dose (>3 g daily) aspirin. Effect not noted with low-dose aspirin	Additive effect on reducing glomerular filtration rate	Monitor renal function regularly until stable
ASPIRIN	VASODILATOR ANTIHYPERTENSIVES	↑ risk of bleeding when aspirin is co-administered with iloprost	Uncertain at present	Closely monitor effects; watch for signs of excess bleeding
ASPIRIN	ANTIOBESITY DRUGS – SIBUTRAMINE	Risk of bleeding	Additive effect; sibutramine may cause thrombocytopenia	Warn the patient to report any signs of ↑ bleeding
ASPIRIN	ANTIPLATELET AGENTS	Risk of bleeding when aspirin is co-administered with other antiplatelet agents. The addition of dipyridamole to low-dose aspirin does not seem to confer an ↑ risk of bleeding	Additive effect	Closely monitor effects; watch for signs of excess bleeding
ASPIRIN	ANXIOLYTICS AND HYPNOTICS	↓ requirements of midazolam when aspirin (1 g) is co-administered	Uncertain at present	Be aware of possible ↓ dose requirements for midazolam

ASPIRIN	CALCIUM CHANNEL BLOCKERS	↓ antihypertensive effect with aspirin; effect not noted with low-dose aspirin	Aspirin may cause sodium retention and vasoconstriction at possibly both renal and endothelial sites	Monitor BP at least weekly until stable when high-dose is aspirin prescribed
ASPIRIN	**DIURETICS**			
ASPIRIN	CARBONIC ANHYDRASE INHIBITORS	↑ risk of salicylate toxicity with high-dose aspirin	Uncertain at present	Use low-dose aspirin
ASPIRIN	POTASSIUM-SPARING DIURETICS	↓ efficacy of spironolactone	Uncertain	Watch for poor response to spironolactone
ASPIRIN	DROTRECOGIN ALFA	↑ risk of bleeding	Additive effect on clotting mechanism; drotrecogin alfa has antithrombotic and fibrinolytic effects	Careful risk–benefit analysis should be undertaken if drotrecogin alfa is given within 7 days of aspirin
ASPIRIN	LEUKOTRIENE ANTAGONISTS	↑ levels of zafirlukast	Uncertain	Watch for early features of zafirlukast toxicity. Monitor FBC and liver function closely
ASPIRIN	MIFEPRISTONE	↓ efficacy of mifepristone	Antiprostaglandin effect of aspirin antagonizes action of mifepristone	Avoid co-administration
ASPIRIN	NITRATES	↓ antihypertensive effect with aspirin; effect not noted with low-dose aspirin	Aspirin may cause sodium retention and vasoconstriction at possibly both renal and endothelial sites	Monitor BP at least weekly until stable when high-dose is aspirin prescribed
ASPIRIN	PERIPHERAL VASODILATORS	Possible ↑ risk of bleeding with cilostazol. Low-dose aspirin (<80 mg) appears to be safe	Additive effect; cilostazol has antiplatelet activity	Warn the patient to report any signs of ↑ bleeding
ASPIRIN	THROMBOLYTICS	↑ risk of intracerebral bleeding when streptokinase is co-administered with higher dose (300 mg) aspirin	Additive effect	Avoid co-ingestion when streptokinase is given for cerebral infarction; use low-dose aspirin when co-administered for myocardial infarction

Primary drug	Secondary drug	Effect	Mechanism	Precautions
CLOPIDOGREL				
CLOPIDOGREL	ANALGESICS	1. Risk of gastrointestinal bleeding when clopidogrel is co-administered with NSAIDs. 2. Case of intracerebral haemorrhage when clopidogrel given with celecoxib	1. NSAIDs may cause gastric mucosal irritation/ulceration; clopidogrel inhibits platelet aggregation 2. Uncertain; possible that celecoxib inhibits CYP2D6-mediated metabolism of clopidogrel	1. Warn patients to report immediately any gastrointestinal symptoms; use NSAIDs for as short a course as possible 2. Avoid co-ingestion of clopidogrel and celecoxib
CLOPIDOGREL	ANTICOAGULANTS	Risk of bleeding when clopidogrel is co-administered with anticoagulants	Additive effect on different parts of the clotting mechanism	Closely monitor effects; watch for signs of excess bleeding
CLOPIDOGREL	ANTIHYPERTENSIVES AND HEART FAILURE DRUGS – VASODILATOR ANTIHYPERTENSIVES	↑ risk of bleeding when clopidogrel is co-administered with iloprost	Uncertain at present	Closely monitor effects; watch for signs of excess bleeding
CLOPIDOGREL	ANTIPLATELET AGENTS	Risk of bleeding when clopidogrel is co-administered with other antiplatelet agents	Additive effect	Closely monitor effects; watch for signs of excess bleeding
CLOPIDOGREL	CNS STIMULANTS – MODAFINIL	May cause moderate ↑ in plasma concentrations of these substrates	Modafinil is a reversible inhibitor of CYP2C19 when used in therapeutic doses	Be aware
CLOPIDOGREL	LIPID-LOWERING DRUGS	Atorvastatin and possibly simvastatin ↓ the antiplatelet effect of clopidogrel in a dose-dependent manner. The clinical significance of this effect is uncertain	Atorvastatin and simvastatin inhibit CYP3A4-mediated activation of clopidogrel	Use these statins at the lowest possible dose; otherwise consider using an alternative statin

CLOPIDOGREL	PERIPHERAL VASODILATORS	Possible ↑ risk of bleeding with cilostazol	Additive effect; cilostazol has antiplatelet activity. Clopidogrel ↑ the levels of a metabolite of cilostazol that has high anti-platelet activity, by a mechanism that is uncertain at present	Warn the patient to report any signs of ↑ bleeding
DIPYRIDAMOLE				
DIPYRIDAMOLE	ANTACIDS	Possible ↓ bioavailability of dipyridamole	Dipyridamole tablets require an acidic environment for adequate dissolution; ↑ in pH of the stomach impairs dissolution and therefore may ↓ absorption of the drug	↑ the dose of dipyridamole or consider using an alternative antiplatelet drug
DIPYRIDAMOLE	ANTIARRHYTHMICS	↑ effect of adenosine; ↓ doses needed to terminate supraventricular tachycardias; case report of profound bradycardia when adenosine infusion was given for myocardial stress testing	Dipyridamole inhibits adenosine uptake into cells	↓ bolus doses of adenosine by up to fourfold when administering it to treat supraventricular tachycardias. Some recommend avoiding adenosine for patients taking dipyridamole. Advise patients to stop dipyridamole for 24 hours before using adenosine infusions
DIPYRIDAMOLE	ANTICANCER AND IMMUNOMODULATING DRUGS	Possible ↓ efficacy of fludarabine	Uncertain	Consider using an alternative antiplatelet drug
DIPYRIDAMOLE	ANTICOAGULANTS	Cases of mild bleeding when dipyridamole is added to anticoagulants	Antiplatelet effects of dipyridamole add to the anticoagulant effects	Warn patients to report early signs of bleeding

Primary drug	Secondary drug	Effect	Mechanism	Precautions
DIPYRIDAMOLE	ANTIPLATELET AGENTS	Risk of bleeding when dipyridamole is co-administered with other antiplatelet drugs. The addition of dipyridamole to low-dose aspirin does not seem to confer an ↑ risk of bleeding	Additive effect	Closely monitor effects; watch for signs of excess bleeding
DIPYRIDAMOLE	H2 RECEPTOR BLOCKERS	Possible ↓ bioavailability of dipyridamole	Dipyridamole tablets require an acidic environment for adequate dissolution; an ↑ in pH of the stomach impairs dissolution and therefore may ↓ absorption of the drug	↑ the dose of dipyridamole or consider using an alternative antiplatelet drug
DIPYRIDAMOLE	PERIPHERAL VASODILATORS	Possible ↑ risk of bleeding with cilostazol.	Additive effect; cilostazol has antiplatelet activity	Warn the patient to report any signs of ↑ bleeding.
DIPYRIDAMOLE	PROTON PUMP INHIBITORS	Possible ↓ bioavailability of dipyridamole	Dipyridamole tablets require an acidic environment for adequate dissolution; an ↑ in pH of the stomach impairs dissolution and therefore may ↓ absorption of the drug	↑ the dose of dipyridamole or consider using an alternative antiplatelet drug

GLYCOPROTEIN IIb/IIIa INHIBITORS				
GLYCOPROTEIN IIb/IIIa INHIBITORS	ANTICOAGULANTS	Risk of bleeding when glycoprotein IIb/IIIa inhibitors are co-administered with anticoagulants	Additive effect on different parts of the clotting mechanism	Closely monitor APTT or INR as appropriate; watch for signs of excess bleeding
GLYCOPROTEIN IIb/IIIa INHIBITORS	ANTIHYPERTENSIVES AND HEART FAILURE DRUGS – VASODILATOR ANTIHYPERTENSIVES	↑ risk of bleeding when eptifibatide or tirofiban is co-administered with iloprost	Uncertain at present	Closely monitor effects; watch for signs of excess bleeding
GLYCOPROTEIN IIb/IIIa INHIBITORS	ANTIPLATELET AGENTS	Risk of bleeding when abciximab is co-administered with other antiplatelet agents	Additive effect	Closely monitor effects; watch for signs of excess bleeding
GLYCOPROTEIN IIb/IIIa INHIBITORS	PERIPHERAL VASODILATORS	Possible ↑ risk of bleeding with cilostazol	Additive effect; cilostazol has antiplatelet activity	Warn the patient to report any signs of ↑ bleeding
GLYCOPROTEIN IIb/IIIa INHIBITORS	THROMBOLYTICS	1. ↑ risk of major haemorrhage when co-administered with alteplase 2. Possible ↑ risk of bleeding complications when streptokinase is co-administered with eptifibatide	1. Uncertain; other thrombolytics do not seem to interact 2. Additive effect	1. Avoid co-administration 2. Watch for bleeding complications. Risk–benefit analysis is needed before co-administering; this will involve the availability of alternative therapies such as primary angioplasty

Primary drug **BETA-BLOCKERS**	Secondary drug	Effect	Mechanism	Precautions
SOTALOL	DRUGS THAT PROLONG THE Q–T INTERVAL			
SOTALOL	1. ANTIARRHYTHMICS – amiodarone, disopyramide, procainamide, propafenone 2. ANTIBIOTICS – macrolides (especially azithromycin, clarithromycin, parenteral erythromycin, telithromycin), quinolones (especially moxifloxacin), quinupristin/dalfopristin 3. ANTICANCER AND IMMUNOMODULATING DRUGS – arsenic trioxide 4. ANTIDEPRESSANTS – TCAs, venlafaxine 5. ANTIEMETICS – dolasetron 6. ANTIFUNGALS – fluconazole, posaconazole, voriconazole 7. ANTIHISTAMINES – terfenadine, hydroxyzine, mizolastine 8. ANTIMALARIALS – artemether with lumefantrine, chloroquine, hydroxychloroquine, mefloquine, quinine 9. ANTIPROTOZOALS – pentamidine isetionate 10. ANTIPSYCHOTICS – atypicals, phenothiazines, pimozide 11. BRONCHODILATORS – parenteral bronchodilators. 12. CNS STIMULANTS – atomoxetine	Risk of ventricular arrhythmias, particularly torsades de pointes	Additive effect; these drugs cause prolongation of the Q–T interval	Avoid co-administration

SOTALOL	DIURETICS – CARBONIC ANHYDRASE INHIBITORS, LOOP DIURETICS, THIAZIDES	↑ risk of ventricular arrhythmias, particularly torsades de pointes ventricular tachycardia, caused by sotalol	Hypokalaemia, a side-effect of these diuretics, predisposes to arrhythmias during sotalol therapy	Normalize potassium levels before starting sotalol in patients already taking these diuretics. When starting these diuretics in patients already taking sotalol, monitor potassium levels every 4–6 weeks until stable
BETA-BLOCKERS – SOTALOL	IVABRADINE	Risk of arrhythmias	Additive effect; ivabradine slows the sinus node	Monitor ECG closely
BETA-BLOCKERS				
BETA-BLOCKERS	ALCOHOL	Acute alcohol ingestion may ↑ hypotensive effect. Chronic moderate/heavy drinking ↓ hypotensive effect	Additive hypotensive effect. Mechanism of opposite effect with chronic intake is uncertain	Monitor BP closely as unpredictable responses can occur. Advise patients to drink only in moderation and to avoid large variations in the amount of alcohol drunk
BETA-BLOCKERS	ANAESTHETICS – GENERAL	Risk of severe hypotensive episodes during induction of anaesthesia (including patients using timolol eye drops)	Most general anaesthetics are myocardial depressants and vasodilators, so additive ↓ BP may occur	Monitor BP closely, especially during induction of anaesthesia
BETA-BLOCKERS	**ANAESTHETICS – LOCAL**			
Remember that ↑ BP can occur when epinephrine-containing local anaesthetics are used with patients on beta-blockers ➢ *Sympathomimetics, below*				
BETA-BLOCKERS	BUPIVACAINE	Risk of bupivacaine toxicity	Beta-blockers, particularly propranolol, inhibit hepatic microsomal metabolism of bupivacaine	Watch for bupivacaine toxicity – monitor ECG and BP

Primary drug	Secondary drug	Effect	Mechanism	Precautions
BETA-BLOCKERS	LIDOCAINE	1. Risk of bradycardia (occasionally severe), ↓ BP and heart failure with intravenous lidocaine 2. Risk of lidocaine toxicity due to ↑ plasma concentrations of lidocaine, particularly with propranolol and nadolol 3. ↑ plasma concentrations of propranolol and possibly some other beta-blockers	1. Additive negative inotropic and chronotropic effects 2. Uncertain, but possibly a combination of beta-blocker-induced reduction in hepatic blood flow (due to ↓ cardiac output) and inhibition of metabolism of lidocaine 3. Attributed to inhibition of metabolism by lidocaine	1. Monitor PR, BP and ECG closely; watch for development of heart failure when intravenous lidocaine is administered to patients on beta-blockers 2. Watch for lidocaine toxicity 3. Be aware. Regional anaesthetics should be used cautiously in patients with bradycardia. Beta-blockers could cause dangerous hypertension due to stimulation of alpha-receptors if epinephrine is used with local anaesthetic
BETA-BLOCKERS	**ANALGESICS**			
BETA-BLOCKERS	NSAIDS – INDOMETACIN, PIROXICAM, POSSIBLY IBUPROFEN, NAPROXEN	↓ hypotensive efficacy of beta-blockers. There does not seem to be this effect with other NSAIDs	Additive toxic effects on kidney, and sodium and water, retention by NSAIDs. NSAIDs can raise BP by inhibiting renal synthesis of vasodilating prostaglandins. It is uncertain why this effect is specific to these NSAIDs	Watch for ↓ response to beta-blockers
METOPROLOL	VALDECOXIB	Risk of ↑ hypotensive efficacy of metoprolol	Metoprolol is metabolized by CYP2D6, which is inhibited by valdecoxib	Monitor BP at least weekly until stable. Warn patients to report symptoms of hypotension (light-headedness, dizziness on standing, etc.)

BETA-BLOCKERS	OPIOIDS	1. Risk of ↑ plasma concentrations and effects of labetalol, metoprolol and propranolol; ↑ systemic effects of timolol eye drops 2. ↑ plasma concentrations of esmolol when morphine is added 3. ↑ plasma concentrations of metoprolol and propranolol when dextro-propoxyphene is added	1. Methadone inhibits CYP2D6, which metabolizes these beta-blockers 2. Unknown 3. ↓ hepatic clearance of metoprolol and propanolol	1. Monitor BP at least weekly until stable 2. Monitor BP closely 3. Monitor BP at least weekly until stable. Warn patients to report symptoms of hypotension (light-headedness, dizziness on standing, etc.)
BETA-BLOCKERS	ANTACIDS CONTAINING MAGNESIUM AND ALUMINIUM	↑ bioavailability of metoprolol and ↓ bioavailability of atenolol, which may produce mild variation in the response to metoprolol and atenolol	Variations in absorption of the respective beta-blockers	Clinical significance may be minimal but be aware; monitor BP at least weekly until stable when initiating antacid therapy. Warn patients to report symptoms of hypotension (light-headedness, dizziness on standing, etc.)
BETA-BLOCKERS	ANTIARRHYTHMICS – AMIODARONE, DISOPYRAMIDE, FLECAINIDE, MEXILETINE, PROCAINAMIDE, PROPAFENONE	Risk of bradycardia (occasionally severe), ↓ BP and heart failure. A single case report has described bradycardia when timolol eye drops were given to a patient on flecainide. Also, ↑ plasma levels of propranolol and metoprolol	Additive negative inotropic and chronotropic effects. In addition, high-dose amiodarone is associated with ↑ plasma levels of metoprolol due to inhibition of CYP2D. Also, mexiletine is known to inhibit CYP1A2-mediated metabolism of propanolol. Lastly, propafenone is extensively metabolized by CYP2D6 enzymes and interferes with the metabolism of propranolol and metoprolol	Monitor PR, BP and ECG closely, especially when loading patients on beta-blockers with antiarrhythmics; watch for the development of heart failure. ↓ doses of beta-blocker accordingly, especially when co-administering propafenone with metoprolol or propanolol

Primary drug	Secondary drug	Effect	Mechanism	Precautions
BETA-BLOCKERS	**ANTIBIOTICS**			
BETA-BLOCKERS	AMPICILLIN	Plasma concentrations of atenolol are halved by 1 g doses of ampicillin (but not smaller doses)	Uncertain	Monitor BP closely during initiation of therapy with ampicillin
BETA-BLOCKERS	RIFAMPICIN	↓ plasma concentrations and efficacy of bisoprolol, carvedilol, celiprolol, metoprolol and propanolol	Rifampicin induces hepatic enzymes (e.g. CYP2C19), which ↑ metabolism of the beta-blockers; in addition, it may also ↑ P-gp expression	Monitor PR and BP; watch for poor response to beta-blockers
BETA-BLOCKERS	**ANTICANCER AND IMMUNOMODULATING DRUGS**			
BETA-BLOCKERS	CYTOTOXICS	Imatinib may cause an ↑ in plasma concentrations of metoprolol, propanolol and timolol, with a risk of toxic effects	Imatinib is a potent inhibitor of CYP2D6 isoenzymes, which metabolize beta-blockers	Monitor for clinical efficacy and toxicity of beta-adrenergic blockers
BETA-BLOCKERS	**IMMUNOMODULATING DRUGS**			
ACEBUTOLOL, ATENOLOL, BETAXOLOL, BISOPROLOL, METOPROLOL, PROPANOLOL	CICLOSPORIN	↑ risk of hyperkalaemia	Beta-blockers cause an efflux of potassium from cells, and side-effect has been observed during ciclosporin therapy	Monitor serum potassium levels during co-administration ➢ ***For signs and symptoms of hyperkalaemia, see Clinical Features of Some Adverse Drug Interactions, Hyperkalaemia***
CARVEDILOL	CICLOSPORIN	Possible ↑ in plasma concentrations of ciclosporin	Carvedilol is metabolized primarily by CYP2D6 and CYP2D9, with a minor contribution from CYP3A4	Usually a dose reduction (20%) of ciclosporin is required
BETA-BLOCKERS	CORTICOSTEROIDS	↓ efficacy of beta-blockers	Mineralocorticoids cause ↑ BP as a result of sodium and water retention	Watch for poor response to beta-blockers

BETA-BLOCKERS	IL-2 (ALDESLEUKIN)	↑ hypotensive effect	Additive hypotensive effect. Aldesleukin causes ↓ vascular resistance and ↑ capillary permeability	Monitor BP at least weekly until stable
BETA-BLOCKERS	**ANTIDEPRESSANTS**			
BETA-BLOCKERS	LITHIUM	Report of episode of ↑ lithium levels in elderly patient after starting low-dose propanolol. However, propanolol is often used to treat lithium-induced tremor without problems	Mechanism uncertain at present, but propanolol seems to ↓ lithium clearance	Monitor lithium levels when starting propanolol therapy in elderly people
BETA-BLOCKERS	MAOIs	↑ hypotensive effect	Additive hypotensive effect. Postural ↓ BP is a common side-effect of MAOIs	Monitor BP at least weekly until stable. Warn patients to report symptoms of hypotension (light-headedness, dizziness on standing, etc.)
METOPROLOL	SSRIs	↑ plasma concentrations of metoprolol	SSRIs inhibit metabolism of metoprolol (paroxetine, fluoxetine, sertraline, fluvoxamine via CYP2D6, and (es)citalopram via mechanism uncertain at present)	Monitor PR and BP at least weekly; watch for metoprolol toxicity, in particular loss of its cardioselectivity
PROPANOLOL, TIMOLOL	SSRIs	↑ plasma concentrations and efficacy of propranolol and timolol	Fluvoxamine inhibits CYP1A2-, CYP2C19- and CYP2D6-mediated metabolism of propranolol. Fluoxetine inhibits CYP2C19- and CYP2D6- mediated metabolism of propanolol and timolol. Paroxetine and sertraline inhibit CYP2D6-mediated metabolism of propanolol and timolol and can impair conduction through the AV node	Monitor PR and BP at least weekly. Warn patients to report symptoms of hypotension (light-headedness, dizziness on standing, etc.). Watch for propanolol toxicity

Primary drug	Secondary drug	Effect	Mechanism	Precautions
BETA-BLOCKERS	**TCAs AND RELATED ANTIDEPRESSANTS**			
BETA-BLOCKERS	AMITRIPTYLINE, CLOMIPRAMINE	Risk of ↑ levels of beta-blockers with amitriptyline and clomipramine	These TCAs inhibit CYP2D6-mediated metabolism of beta-blockers	Monitor BP at least weekly until stable. Warn patients to report symptoms of hypotension (light-headedness, dizziness on standing, etc.)
LABETALOL, PROPANOLOL	IMIPRAMINE	↑ imipramine levels with labetalol and propanolol	Uncertain at present. Postulated that imipramine metabolism ↓ by competition at CYP2D6 and CYP2C8	Monitor plasma levels of imipramine when initiating beta-blocker therapy
PROPANOLOL	MAPROTILINE	Cases of ↑ plasma levels of maprotiline with propanolol	Uncertain at present. Postulated that maprotiline metabolism ↓ by alterations in hepatic blood flow	Monitor plasma levels of maprotiline when initiating beta-blocker therapy
BETA-BLOCKERS	**ANTIDEPRESSANTS – OTHER**			
BETA-BLOCKERS	VENLAFAXINE	↑ plasma concentrations and efficacy of metoprolol, propranolol and timolol	Venlafaxine inhibits CYP2D6-mediated metabolism of metoprolol, propanolol and timolol	Monitor PR and BP at least weekly; watch for metoprolol toxicity (in particular, loss of its cardioselectivity) and propanolol toxicity
BETA-BLOCKERS	**ANTIDIABETIC DRUGS**			
BETA-BLOCKERS	ANTIDIABETIC DRUGS	Beta-blockers may mask the symptoms and signs of hypoglycaemia. They also ↓ insulin sensitivity; however, beta-blockers that also have vasodilating properties (carvedilol, celiprolol, labetalol, nebivolol) seem to ↑ sensitivity to insulin	Beta-blockers ↓ glucose tolerance and interfere with the metabolic and autonomic responses to hypoglycaemia	Warn patients about masking of signs of hypoglycaemia. Vasodilating beta-blockers are preferred in patients with diabetes, and all beta-blockers should be avoided in those having frequent hypoglycaemic attacks. Monitor capillary blood glucose levels closely, especially during initiation of therapy ➢ ***For signs and symptoms of hypoglycaemia, see Clinical Features of Some Adverse Drug Interactions, Hypoglycaemia***

PINDOLOL, PROPRANOLOL OR TIMOLOL EYE DROPS	INSULIN	Hypoglycaemia has occurred in patients on insulin with patients taking oral propanolol and pindolol, propanolol or timolol eye drops	These beta-blockers inhibit the rebound in blood glucose that occurs as a response to a fall in blood glucose levels	Cardio-selective beta-blockers are preferred, and all beta-blockers should be avoided in those having frequent hypoglycaemic attacks. Monitor capillary blood glucose levels closely, especially during initiation of therapy ➢ ***For signs and symptoms of hypoglycaemia, see Clinical Features of Some Adverse Drug Interactions, Hypoglycaemia***
BETA-BLOCKERS	ANTIDIARRHOEALS – KAOLIN	Possibly ↓ levels of atenolol, propanolol and sotalol	↓ absorption	Separate doses by at least 2 hours
BETA-BLOCKERS	**ANTIEPILEPTICS**			
BETA-BLOCKERS	BARBITURATES	Regular barbiturate use may ↑ elimination of those beta-blockers metabolized by the liver (metoprolol, propanolol, timolol)	Barbiturates induce CYP1A2-, CYP2C9- and CYP2C19-mediated metabolism of propanolol	Monitor BP at least weekly until stable and watch for ↑ BP
BETA-BLOCKERS	PHENYTOIN	Phenytoin may ↓ propanolol levels	Phenytoin induces CYP1A2- and CYP2C19-mediated metabolism of propanolol	Monitor BP at least weekly until stable and watch for ↑ BP
BETA-BLOCKERS	ANTIGOUT DRUGS – SULFINPYRAZONE	Antihypertensive effects of oxprenolol ↓ by sulfinpyrazone	Unknown	Monitor PR and BP closely; consider starting an alternative beta-blocker
BETA-BLOCKERS	**ANTIHYPERTENSIVES AND HEART FAILURE DRUGS**			
BETA-BLOCKERS	ACE INHIBITORS, ADRENERGIC NEURONE BLOCKERS, ANGIOTENSIN II RECEPTOR ANTAGONISTS	↑ hypotensive effect	Additive hypotensive effect; may be used therapeutically	Monitor BP at least weekly until stable. Warn patients to report symptoms of hypotension (light-headedness, dizziness on standing, etc.)

Primary drug	Secondary drug	Effect	Mechanism	Precautions
BETA-BLOCKERS	ALPHA-BLOCKERS	↑ efficacy of alpha-blockers; ↑ risk of first-dose ↓ BP with alfuzosin, prazosin and terazosin	Additive hypotensive effect; may be used therapeutically. Beta-blockers prevent the ability to mount a tachycardia in response to ↓ BP; this ↑ the risk of first-dose ↓ BP when starting alpha-blockers in patients already on beta-blockers	Monitor BP at least weekly until stable; watch for first-dose ↓ BP. Warn patients to report symptoms of hypotension (light-headedness, dizziness on standing, etc.)
BETA-BLOCKERS	CENTRALLY ACTING ANTIHYPERTENSIVES	Risk of withdrawal ↑ BP (rebound ↑ BP) with clonidine and possibly moxonidine	Withdrawal of clonidine, and possibly moxonidine, is associated with ↑ circulating catecholamines; beta-blockers, especially non-cardioselective ones, allow the catecholamines to exert an unopposed alpha-receptor action (vasoconstriction)	Do not withdraw clonidine or moxonidine while a patient is taking beta-blockers. Withdraw beta-blockers several days before slowly withdrawing clonidine and moxonidine
BETA-BLOCKERS	VASODILATOR ANTIHYPERTENSIVES	↑ hypotensive effect	Additive hypotensive effect with diazoxide, hydralazine, minoxidil and sodium nitroprusside. In addition, hydralazine may ↑ the bioavailability of beta-blockers with a high first-pass metabolism (e.g. propanolol and metoprolol), possibly due to alterations in hepatic blood flow or inhibited hepatic metabolism	Monitor BP closely
BETA-BLOCKERS	**ANTIMALARIALS**			
METOPROLOL	ARTEMETHER/ LUMEFANTRINE	↑ risk of toxicity	Uncertain	Avoid co-administration

BETA-BLOCKERS	MEFLOQUINE	↑ risk of bradycardia	Mefloquine can cause cardiac conduction disorders, e.g. bradycardia. Additive bradycardic effect. Single case report of cardiac arrest with co-administration of mefloquine and propanolol, possibly caused by Q–T prolongation	Monitor PR closely
BETA-BLOCKERS	QUININE	Risk of ↑ plasma concentrations and effects of labetalol, metoprolol and propranolol; ↑ systemic effects of timolol eye drops	Quinine inhibits CYP2D6, which metabolizes these beta-blockers	Monitor BP at least weekly until stable
BETA-BLOCKERS	ANTIPARKINSON'S DRUGS – LEVODOPA	↑ hypotensive effect	Additive hypotensive effect; however, overall, adding beta-blockers to levodopa can be beneficial (e.g. by reducing the risk of dopamine-mediated risk of arrhythmias)	Monitor BP at least weekly until stable
BETA-BLOCKERS	**ANTIPSYCHOTICS**			
BETA-BLOCKERS	ANTIPSYCHOTICS	↑ hypotensive effect	Dose-related ↓ BP (due to vasodilatation) is a side-effect of most antipsychotics, particularly the phenothiazines	Monitor BP at least weekly until stable, especially during initiation of treatment. Warn patients to report symptoms of hypotension (light-headedness, dizziness on standing, etc.)
PROPANOLOL, TIMOLOL	CHLORPROMAZINE, HALOPERIDOL	↑ plasma concentrations and efficacy of both chlorpromazine and propranolol during co-administration	Propanolol and chlorpromazine mutually inhibit each other's hepatic metabolism. Haloperidol inhibits CYP2D6-mediated metabolism of propanolol and timolol	Watch for toxic effects of chlorpromazine and propranolol; ↓ doses accordingly

Primary drug	Secondary drug	Effect	Mechanism	Precautions
BETA-BLOCKERS	**ANTIVIRALS**			
BETA-BLOCKERS	RITONAVIR, TIPRANAVIR	↑ adverse effects of carvedilol, metoprolol, propanolol and timolol	Inhibition of CYP2D6-mediated metabolism of these beta-blockers and CYP2C19-mediated metabolism of propanolol	Use an alternative beta-blocker if possible; if not, monitor closely
BETA-BLOCKERS	**ANXIOLYTICS AND HYPNOTICS**			
BETA-BLOCKERS	ANXIOLYTICS AND HYPNOTICS	↑ hypotensive effect	Additive hypotensive effect; anxiolytics and hypnotics can cause postural ↓ BP	Watch for ↓ BP. Monitor BP at least weekly until stable. Warn patients to report symptoms of hypotension (light-headedness, dizziness on standing, etc.)
BETA-BLOCKERS	DIAZEPAM	May occasionally cause ↑ sedation during metoprolol and propranolol therapy	Propranolol and metoprolol inhibit the metabolism of diazepam	Warn patients about ↑ sedation
BETA-BLOCKERS	**BRONCHODILATORS**			
BETA-BLOCKERS	BETA-2 AGONISTS	Non-selective beta-blockers (e.g. propanolol) ↓ or prevents the bronchodilator effect of beta-2 agonists	Non-selective beta-blockers antagonize the effect of beta-2 agonists on bronchial smooth muscle	Avoid co-administration
BETA-BLOCKERS	THEOPHYLLINE	↑ plasma levels of theophylline with propranolol	Propranolol exerts a dose-dependent inhibitory effect on the metabolism of theophylline	Monitor theophylline levels during propranolol co-administration
BETA-BLOCKERS	**CALCIUM CHANNEL BLOCKERS**			
BETA-BLOCKERS	CALCIUM CHANNEL BLOCKERS	↑ hypotensive effect, bradycardia, conduction defects and heart failure	Additive hypotensive effect; may be used therapeutically	Monitor PR, BP and ECG at least weekly until stable. Warn patients to report symptoms of hypotension (light-headedness, dizziness on standing, etc.)

BETA-BLOCKERS	DIHYDROPYRIDINES	Rare cases of severe ↓ BP and heart failure when nifedipine and nisoldipine are given to patients on beta-blockers	It is uncertain why this severe effect occurs	Monitor PR, BP and ECG at least weekly until stable. Warn patients to report symptoms of hypotension (light-headedness, dizziness on standing, etc.)
BETA-BLOCKERS	DILTIAZEM	↑ hypotensive and bradycardic effects: cases of severe bradycardia and AV block when both drugs are administered concurrently in the presence of pre-existing heart failure or conduction abnormalities	Additive effects on conduction; diltiazem causes bradycardia, sinoatrial block and AV block. Also, diltiazem inhibits CYP1A2-mediated metabolism of propanolol	Monitor PR, BP and ECG at least weekly until stable. Warn patients to report symptoms of hypotension (light-headedness, dizziness on standing, etc.)
BETA-BLOCKERS	VERAPAMIL	1. Risk of cardiac arrest when parenteral verapamil is given to patients on beta-blockers 2. Risk of bradycardias when both are given orally	Additive effect. Also, verapamil inhibits CYP1A2-mediated metabolism of propanolol	1. Do not administer intravenous verapamil to patients taking beta-blockers 2. Monitor ECG and BP carefully when both are given orally
BETA-BLOCKERS	**CARDIAC GLYCOSIDES**			
BETA-BLOCKERS	DIGOXIN	Risk of bradycardia and AV block	Additive bradycardia	Monitor PR, BP and ECG closely
CARVEDILOL	DIGOXIN	Carvedilol may ↑ digoxin plasma concentrations, particularly in children	↓ P-gp-mediated renal clearance of digoxin	↓ the dose of digoxin by 25%; watch for signs of digoxin toxicity and monitor digoxin levels
BETA-BLOCKERS	COCAINE	Risk of hypertensive crisis	Cocaine produces both alpha- and beta-adrenergic agonist effects; selective beta-blockade leads to unopposed alpha-agonism (vasoconstriction)	Avoid concurrent use

Primary drug	Secondary drug	Effect	Mechanism	Precautions
PROPANOLOL	CNS STIMULANTS – MODAFINIL	Variable effect on propanolol levels	Modafinil is a reversible inhibitor of CYP2C19 when used in therapeutic doses, and a moderate inducer of CYP1A2 in a concentration-dependent manner	Be aware
BETA-BLOCKERS	DRUG DEPENDENCE THERAPIES – BUPROPION	↑ plasma concentrations of metoprolol, propranolol and timolol, with risk of toxic effects	Bupropion and its metabolite hydroxybupropion inhibit CYP2D6	Initiate therapy of these drugs at the lowest effective dose
BETA-BLOCKERS	DIURETICS	↑ hypotensive effect	Additive hypotensive effect; may be used therapeutically	Monitor BP at least weekly until stable. Warn patients to report symptoms of hypotension (light-headedness, dizziness on standing, etc.)
BETA-BLOCKERS	ERGOT DERIVATIVES	Three reported cases of arterial vasoconstriction and one of ↑ BP occurred when ergotamine or methysergide was added to propanolol or oxprenolol	Ergotamine can cause peripheral vasospasm, and absence of beta-adrenergic activity can ↑ the risk of vasoconstriction	Ergot derivatives and beta-blockers are often co-administered without trouble; however, monitor BP at least weekly until stable (watch for ↑ BP) and warn patients to stop the ergot derivative and seek medical attention if they develop cold, painful feet
PROPANOLOL	5-HT1 AGONISTS – RIZATRIPTAN	Plasma levels of rizatriptan almost doubled during propranolol therapy	Propanolol inhibits the metabolism of rizatriptan	Initiate therapy with 5 mg rizatriptan and do not exceed 10 mg in 24 hours. The manufacturers recommend separating doses by 2 hours, although this has not been borne out by the studies

BETA-BLOCKERS	H2 RECEPTOR BLOCKERS			
BETA-BLOCKERS	CIMETIDINE, RANITIDINE	↑ plasma concentrations and effects of labetalol, metoprolol and propranolol; ↑ systemic effects of timolol eye drops	Cimetidine inhibits CYP2D6, which metabolizes these beta-blockers, and inhibits CYP1A2- and CYP2E1-mediated metabolism of propanolol. Ranitidine is a weaker inhibitor of CYP2D6	Monitor BP at least weekly until stable
BETA-BLOCKERS	NIZATIDINE	↑ bradycardia when nizatidine is added to atenolol. Other beta-blockers have not been studied	Uncertain	Monitor PR when administering nizatidine to patients on beta-blockers
BETA-BLOCKERS	**MUSCLE RELAXANTS**			
BETA-BLOCKERS	NON-DEPOLARIZING	1. Modest ↑ in efficacy of muscle relaxants, particularly with propanolol 2. Risk of ↓ BP with atracurium and alcuronium	1 and 2. Uncertain	1. Watch for prolonged muscular paralysis after muscle relaxants 2. Monitor BP at least weekly until stable
BETA-BLOCKERS	SKELETAL – BACLOFEN, TIZANIDINE	↑ hypotensive effect with baclofen or tizanidine. Risk of bradycardia with tizanidine	Additive hypotensive effect. Tizanidine has a negative inotropic and chronotropic effect	Monitor BP at least weekly until stable. Warn patients to report symptoms of hypotension (light-headedness, dizziness on standing, etc.)
BETA-BLOCKERS	NITRATES	↑ hypotensive effect	Additive hypotensive effect; may be used therapeutically	Monitor BP at least weekly until stable
BETA-BLOCKERS	OESTROGENS	↓ hypotensive effect	Oestrogens cause sodium and fluid retention	Monitor BP at least weekly until stable; routine prescription of oestrogens in patients with ↑ BP is not advisable
BETA-BLOCKERS	ORLISTAT	Case report of severe ↑ BP when orlistat started on a patient on atenolol	Uncertain at present	Monitor BP at least weekly until stable

Primary drug	Secondary drug	Effect	Mechanism	Precautions
BETA-BLOCKERS	PARASYMPATHOMIMETICS			
BETA-BLOCKERS	NEOSTIGMINE, PYRIDOSTIGMINE	1. Cases of bradycardia and ↓ BP when neostigmine or physostigmine was given to reverse anaesthesia 2. ↓ effectiveness of neostigmine and pyridostigmine in myasthenia gravis	1. Neostigmine and pyridostigmine cause accumulation of ACh, which may cause additive bradycardia and ↓ BP 2. Beta-blockers are thought to have a depressant effect on the neuromuscular junction and thereby ↑ weakness	1. Monitor PR and BP closely when giving anticholinesterases to reverse anaesthesia to patients on beta-blockers 2. Monitor the response to neostigmine and pyridostigmine when starting beta-blockers
BETA-BLOCKERS	PILOCARPINE	↑ risk of arrhythmias	Pilocarpine is a parasympathomimetic and can cause additive bradycardia	Monitor PR and ECG closely
BETA-BLOCKERS	PERIPHERAL VASODILATORS – MOXISYLYTE (THYMOXAMINE)	↑ hypotensive effect	Additive hypotensive effect	Monitor BP at least weekly until stable
BETA-BLOCKERS	POTASSIUM CHANNEL ACTIVATORS	↑ hypotensive effect	Additive effect	Monitor BP at least weekly until stable
BETA-BLOCKERS	PROSTAGLANDINS – ALPROSTADIL	↑ hypotensive effect	Additive hypotensive effect	Monitor BP at least weekly until stable. Warn patients to report symptoms of hypotension (light-headedness, dizziness on standing, etc.)
BETA-BLOCKERS	PROTON PUMP INHIBITORS	Risk of ↑ plasma concentrations and effects of propranolol	Omeprazole inhibits CYP2D6- and CYP2C19-mediated metabolism of propanolol	Monitor BP at least weekly until stable

BETA-BLOCKERS	SYMPATHOMIMETICS			
BETA-BLOCKERS	SYMPATHOMIMETICS – INDIRECT	↓ hypotensive efficacy of beta-blockers	The hypertensive effect of sympathomimetics opposes the hypotensive actions of beta-blockers	Monitor BP at least weekly until stable; watch for poor response to beta-blockers
BETA-BLOCKERS	SYMPATHOMIMETICS – DIRECT	1. Severe ↑ BP and bradycardia with non-cardioselective beta-blockers (including reports of severe ↑ BP in patients given infiltrations of local anaesthetics containing epinephrine, and one case of a fatal reaction with phenylephrine eye drops) 2. Patients on beta-blockers may respond poorly to epinephrine when given to treat anaphylaxis	1. Unopposed alpha stimulation causes vasoconstriction, which results in a rise in BP. Beta-2 receptors, when stimulated, cause vasodilatation, which counteracts any alpha action; non-selective beta-blockers antagonize beta-2 receptors	1. Monitor BP at least weekly until stable. When using local anaesthetics with epinephrine, use small volumes of low concentrations (such as 1 in 200 000 epinephrine); avoid high concentrations (e.g. 1 in 1000 mixtures) 2. Look for failure of epinephrine therapy and consider using salbutamol or isoprenaline
BETA-BLOCKERS	X-RAY CONTRAST SOLUTIONS	Beta-blockers are associated with ↑ risk of anaphylactoid reactions to iodinated X-ray contrast materials	Uncertain, but postulated that beta-receptors have a role in suppressing the release of mediators of anaphylaxis	Consider using low-osmolality contrast media and pretreating with antihistamines and corticosteroids. Stopping beta-blockers a few days before the X-ray is associated with a risk of withdrawal ↑ BP and tachycardia; a risk–benefit assessment must therefore be made

Primary drug	Secondary drug	Effect	Mechanism	Precautions
CALCIUM CHANNEL BLOCKERS				
CALCIUM CHANNEL BLOCKERS	ALCOHOL	1. Acute alcohol ingestion may ↑ hypotensive effect. Chronic moderate/heavy drinking ↓ hypotensive effect 2. Verapamil may ↑ peak serum concentration and prolong the effects of alcohol	1. Additive hypotensive effect with acute alcohol excess. Chronic alcohol excess is associated with hypertension 2. Uncertain at present, but presumed to be due to an inhibition of hepatic metabolism of alcohol	1. Monitor BP closely as unpredictable responses can occur. Advise patients to drink only in moderation and avoid large variations in the amount of alcohol drunk 2. Warn the patient about the potentiation of the effects of alcohol, particularly the risks of driving
CALCIUM CHANNEL BLOCKERS	ANAESTHETICS – GENERAL, INHALATIONAL	↑ hypotensive effects of dihydropyridines, and hypotensive/bradycardic effects of diltiazem and verapamil	Additive hypotensive and negative inotropic effects. General anaesthetics tend to be myocardial depressants and vasodilators; they also ↓ sinus automaticity and AV conduction	Monitor BP and ECG closely
CALCIUM CHANNEL BLOCKERS	ANAESTHETICS – LOCAL	Case reports of severe ↓ BP when bupivacaine epidural was administered to patients on calcium channel blockers	Additive hypotensive effect; both bupivacaine and calcium channel blockers are cardiodepressant; in addition, epidural anaesthesia causes sympathetic block in the lower limbs, which leads to vasodilatation and ↓ BP	Monitor BP closely. Preload intravenous fluids prior to the epidural

CARDIOVASCULAR DRUGS CALCIUM CHANNEL BLOCKERS

CALCIUM CHANNEL BLOCKERS	ANALGESICS			
CALCIUM CHANNEL BLOCKERS	NSAIDs	↓ antihypertensive effect of calcium channel blockers	NSAIDs cause sodium retention and vasoconstriction at possibly both renal and endothelial sites	Monitor BP at least weekly until stable
CALCIUM CHANNEL BLOCKERS	OPIOIDS	Diltiazem prolongs the action of alfentanil	Diltiazem inhibits CYP3A4-mediated metabolism of alfentanil	Watch for the prolonged action of alfentanil in patients taking calcium channel blockers; case reports of delayed extubation in patients recovering from anaesthetics involving large doses of alfentanil in patients on diltiazem
CALCIUM CHANNEL BLOCKERS	**ANTIARRHYTHMICS**			
CALCIUM CHANNEL BLOCKERS	AMIODARONE	Risk of bradycardia, AV block and ↓ BP when amiodarone is co-administered with diltiazem or verapamil	Additive negative inotropic and chronotropic effect. Also, amiodarone inhibits intestinal P-gp, which ↑ the bioavailability of diltiazem and verapamil	Monitor PR, BP and ECG closely; watch for heart failure
CALCIUM CHANNEL BLOCKERS	DISOPYRAMIDE	Risk of myocardial depression and asystole when disopyramide is co-administered with verapamil, particularly in the presence of heart failure	Disopyramide is a myocardial depressant like verapamil and can cause ventricular tachycardia, ventricular fibrillation or torsades de pointes	Avoid co-administering verapamil with disopyramide if possible. If single-agent therapy is ineffective, monitor PR, BP and ECG closely; watch for heart failure
CALCIUM CHANNEL BLOCKERS	FLECAINIDE	Risk of heart block and ↓ BP when flecainide is co-administered with verapamil. A single case of asystole has been reported	Additive negative inotropic and chronotropic effect	Monitor PR, BP and ECG at least weekly until stable; watch for heart failure

CARDIOVASCULAR DRUGS CALCIUM CHANNEL BLOCKERS

Primary drug	Secondary drug	Effect	Mechanism	Precautions
CALCIUM CHANNEL BLOCKERS	MORACIZINE	Co-administration is associated with ↑ bioavailability of moracizine and ↓ availability of diltiazem	Postulated that diltiazem inhibits metabolism of moracizine, while moracizine ↑ metabolism of diltiazem; the precise mechanism of interaction is uncertain at present	Monitor PR, BP and ECG; adjust the doses of each drug accordingly
CALCIUM CHANNEL BLOCKERS	**ANTIBIOTICS**			
CALCIUM CHANNEL BLOCKERS	MACROLIDES	↑ plasma concentrations of felodipine when co-administered with erythromycin; cases of adverse effects of verapamil (bradycardia and ↓ BP) with both erythromycin and clarithromycin	Erythromycin inhibits CYP3A4-mediated metabolism of felodipine and verapamil. Clarithromycin and erythromycin inhibit intestinal P-gp, which may ↑ the bioavailability of verapamil	Monitor PR and BP closely; watch for bradycardia and ↓ BP. Consider reducing the dose of calcium channel blocker during macrolide therapy
CALCIUM CHANNEL BLOCKERS	RIFAMPICIN	Plasma concentrations of calcium channel blockers may be ↓ by rifampicin	Rifampicin induces CYP3A4-mediated metabolism of calcium channel blockers. It also induces CYP2C9-mediated metabolism of verapamil and induces intestinal P-gp, which may ↓ the bioavailability of verapamil	Monitor BP closely; watch for ↓ effect of calcium channel blockers
CALCIUM CHANNEL BLOCKERS	QUINUPRISTIN/ DALFOPRISTIN	Plasma levels of nifedipine may be ↑ by quinupristin–dalfopristin	Quinupristin inhibits CYP3A4-mediated metabolism of calcium channel blockers	Monitor BP closely; watch for ↓ BP

CALCIUM CHANNEL BLOCKERS	ANTICANCER AND IMMUNOMODULATING DRUGS			
CALCIUM CHANNEL BLOCKERS	CYTOTOXICS			
CALCIUM CHANNEL BLOCKERS	BUSULFAN	↑ plasma concentrations of busulfan and ↑ risk of toxicity of busulfan such as veno-occlusive disease and pulmonary fibrosis, when co-administered with diltiazem, nifedipine or verapamil	Due to inhibition of CYP3A4-mediated metabolism of busulfan by these calcium channel blockers. Busulfan clearance may be ↓ by 25%, and the AUC of busulfan may ↑ by 1500 μmol/L	Monitor clinically for veno-occlusive disease and pulmonary toxicity in transplant patients. Monitor busulfan blood levels as AUC of below 1500 μmol/L per minute tends to prevent toxicity
CALCIUM CHANNEL BLOCKERS	DOXORUBICIN	↑ serum concentrations and efficacy of doxorubicin when co-administered with verapamil, nicardipine and possibly diltiazem and nifedipine; however, no cases of doxorubicin toxicity have been reported	Uncertain; however, verapamil is known to inhibit intestinal P-gp, which may ↑ the bioavailability of doxorubicin	Watch for symptoms/signs of toxicity (tachycardia, heart failure and hand–foot syndrome)
CALCIUM CHANNEL BLOCKERS	EPIRUBICIN	Cases of ↑ bone marrow suppression when verapamil is added to epirubicin	Uncertain at present	Monitor FBC closely
CALCIUM CHANNEL BLOCKERS	ETOPOSIDE	↑ serum concentrations and risk of toxicity when verapamil is given to patients on etoposide	Verapamil inhibits CYP3A4-mediated metabolism of etoposide	Watch for symptoms/signs of toxicity (nausea, vomiting and bone marrow suppression) in patients taking calcium channel blockers
CALCIUM CHANNEL BLOCKERS	IFOSFAMIDE	↓ plasma concentrations of 4-hydroxyifosfamide, the active metabolite of ifosfamide and risk of inadequate therapeutic response when it is co-administered with diltiazem, nifedipine or verapamil	Due to inhibition of the isoenzymatic conversion to active metabolites by diltiazem	Monitor clinically the efficacy of ifosfamide and ↑ the dose accordingly

Primary drug	Secondary drug	Effect	Mechanism	Precautions
CALCIUM CHANNEL BLOCKERS	IMATINIB	↑ plasma concentrations of imatinib when is co-administered with diltiazem, nifedipine or verapamil. ↑ risk of toxicity (e.g. abdominal pain, constipation and dyspnoea) and of neurotoxicity (e.g. taste disturbances, dizziness, headache, paraesthesias and peripheral neuropathy)	Due to inhibition of hepatic metabolism of imatinib by the CYP3A4 isoenzymes by diltiazem	Monitor for clinical efficacy and for the signs of toxicity listed along with convulsions, confusion and signs of oedema (including pulmonary oedema). Monitor electrolytes and liver function, and for cardiotoxicity
CALCIUM CHANNEL BLOCKERS	IRINOTECAN	Risk of ↑ serum concentrations of irinotecan with nifedipine. No cases of toxicity reported	Inhibition of hepatic microsomal enzymes but exact mechanism uncertain at present	Watch for symptoms/signs of toxicity (especially diarrhoea, an early manifestation of acute cholinergic syndrome)
CALCIUM CHANNEL BLOCKERS	PORFIMER	↑ risk of photosensitivity reactions with diltiazem	Attributed to additive effects	Avoid exposure of skin and eyes to direct sunlight for 30 days after porfimer therapy
CALCIUM CHANNEL BLOCKERS	TRETINOIN	↓ plasma tretinoin levels and risk of ↓ anti-tumour activity when is co-administered with diltiazem, nifedipine or verapamil	Due to induction of CYP3A4-mediated metabolism of tretinoin	Avoid co-administration if possible
CALCIUM CHANNEL BLOCKERS	VINCA ALKALOIDS	1. ↑ risk of bone marrow depression, neurotoxicity and ileus due to ↑ plasma concentrations of vinblastine when is co-administered with diltiazem, nifedipine or verapamil. 2. Verapamil ↑ vincristine levels; no cases of toxicity have been reported 3. ↑ plasma concentrations of vinorelbine and ↑ risk of bone marrow and neurotoxicity when co-administered with diltiazem, nifedipine or verapamil	1. Inhibition of CYP3A4-mediated metabolism of vinblastine and ↓ efflux of vinblastine due to inhibition of renal P-gp 2. ↓ clearance, but exact mechanism not known 3. Due to inhibition of CYP3A4-mediated metabolism of vinorelbine by these calcium channel blockers	1. Avoid concurrent use of CYP3A4 inhibitors and P-gp efflux inhibitors with vinblastine. Select an alternative drug of same group with ↓ effects on enzyme inhibition and P-gp inhibition 2. Watch for symptoms/signs of toxicity 3. Monitor for clinical efficacy and monitor FBC and for neurotoxicity (pain, numbness, tingling in the fingers and toes, jaw pain, abdominal pain, constipation and ileus)

CARDIOVASCULAR DRUGS CALCIUM CHANNEL BLOCKERS

CALCIUM CHANNEL BLOCKERS	HORMONE ANTAGONISTS			
CALCIUM CHANNEL BLOCKERS	TOREMIFENE	↑ plasma concentrations of toremifene when is co-administered with diltiazem, nifedipine or verapamil	Due to inhibition of CYP3A4-mediated metabolism of toremifene	Clinical relevance is uncertain. Necessary to monitor for clinical toxicities
CALCIUM CHANNEL BLOCKERS	**IMMUNOMODULATING DRUGS**			
CALCIUM CHANNEL BLOCKERS	CICLOSPORIN	1. Plasma concentrations of ciclosporin are ↑ when co-administered with diltiazem, nicardipine, verapamil and possibly amlodipine and nisoldipine. However, calcium channel blockers seem to protect renal function 2. Ciclosporin ↑ nifedipine levels	1. Uncertain; presumed to be due to impaired hepatic metabolism. Also, diltiazem and verapamil inhibit intestinal P-gp, which may ↑ the bioavailability of ciclosporin. Uncertain mechanism of renal protection 2. Uncertain effect of ciclosporin on nifedipine	1. Monitor ciclosporin levels and ↓ dose accordingly (possibly by up to 25–50% with nicardipine) 2. Monitor BP closely and warn patients to watch for signs of nifedipine toxicity
CALCIUM CHANNEL BLOCKERS	CORTICOSTEROIDS	1. Antihypertensive effects of calcium channel blockers are antagonized by corticosteroids 2. ↑ adrenal-suppressive effects of dexamethasone, methylprednisolone and prednisolone when co-administered with diltiazem, nifedipine or verapamil. This may ↑ the risk of infections and produce an inadequate response to stress scenarios	1. Mineralocorticoids cause sodium and water retention, which antagonizes the hypotensive effects of calcium channel blockers 2. Due to inhibition of metabolism of these corticosteroids	1. Monitor BP at least weekly until stable 2. Monitor cortisol levels and warn patients to report symptoms such as fever and sore throat

CARDIOVASCULAR DRUGS CALCIUM CHANNEL BLOCKERS

Primary drug	Secondary drug	Effect	Mechanism	Precautions
CALCIUM CHANNEL BLOCKERS	IL-2 (ALDESLEUKIN)	↑ hypotensive effect	Additive hypotensive effect. Aldesleukin causes ↓ vascular resistance and ↑ capillary permeability	Monitor BP at least weekly until stable. Warn patients to report symptoms of hypotension (light-headedness, dizziness on standing, etc.)
CALCIUM CHANNEL BLOCKERS	SIROLIMUS	Plasma concentrations of sirolimus are ↑ when given with diltiazem. Plasma levels of both drugs are ↑ when verapamil and sirolimus are co-administered	Diltiazem and verapamil inhibit intestinal CYP3A4, which is the main site of sirolimus metabolism	Watch for side-effects of sirolimus when it is co-administered with diltiazem or verapamil; monitor renal and hepatic function. Monitor PR and BP closely when sirolimus is given with verapamil
CALCIUM CHANNEL BLOCKERS	TACROLIMUS	Plasma concentrations of tacrolimus are ↑ when given with diltiazem, felodipine or nifedipine; however, they appear to protect renal function	Uncertain, but presumed to be due to inhibition of CYP3A4-mediated tacrolimus metabolism	Watch for side-effects of tacrolimus; monitor ECG, blood count and renal and hepatic function
CALCIUM CHANNEL BLOCKERS	**ANTIDEPRESSANTS**			
CALCIUM CHANNEL BLOCKERS	LITHIUM	Small number of cases of neurotoxicity when co-administered with diltiazem or verapamil	Uncertain, but thought to be due to an additive effect on neurotransmission	Monitor closely for side-effects
CALCIUM CHANNEL BLOCKERS	MAOIs	↑ antihypertensive effect of calcium channel blockers when co-administered with MAOIs	Additive hypotensive effects; postural ↓ BP is a side-effect of MAOIs	Monitor BP at least weekly until stable. Warn patients to report symptoms of hypotension (light-headedness, dizziness on standing, etc.)

CALCIUM CHANNEL BLOCKERS	SSRIs	Reports of ↑ serum levels of nimodipine and episodes of adverse effects of nifedipine and verapamil (oedema, flushing and ↓ BP) attributed to ↑ levels when co-administered with fluoxetine	Fluoxetine inhibits CYP3A4-mediated metabolism of calcium channel blockers. It also inhibits intestinal P-gp, which may ↑ the bioavailability of verapamil	Monitor BP at least weekly until stable. Warn patients to report symptoms of hypotension (light-headedness, dizziness on standing, etc.). Consider reducing the dose of calcium channel blocker or using an alternative antidepressant
CALCIUM CHANNEL BLOCKERS	ST JOHN'S WORT	St John's wort is associated with ↓ verapamil levels	St John's wort induces CYP3A4, which metabolizes calcium channel blockers, and induces intestinal P-gp, which may ↓ the bioavailability of verapamil	Monitor BP regularly for at least the first 2 weeks of initiating St John's wort
CALCIUM CHANNEL BLOCKERS	TCAs	↑ plasma concentrations of TCAs when co-administered with diltiazem and verapamil. Reports of cardiotoxicity (first- and second-degree block) when imipramine is given with diltiazem or verapamil	Uncertain, but may be due to a combination of ↓ clearance of TCAs (both diltiazem and verapamil are known to inhibit CYP1A2, which has a role in the metabolism of amitriptyline, clomipramine and imipramine) and ↑ intestinal absorption (diltiazem and verapamil inhibit intestinal P-gp, which may ↑ amitriptyline bioavailability)	Monitor ECG when commencing or altering treatment
CALCIUM CHANNEL BLOCKERS	**ANTIDIABETIC DRUGS**			
CALCIUM CHANNEL BLOCKERS	INSULIN	Single case reports of impaired glucose intolerance requiring ↑ insulin requirements with diltiazem and nifedipine	Uncertain at present	Evidence suggests that calcium channel blockers are safe in diabetics; monitor blood glucose levels when starting calcium channel blockers

Primary drug	Secondary drug	Effect	Mechanism	Precautions
CALCIUM CHANNEL BLOCKERS	REPAGLINIDE	Likely to ↑ plasma concentrations of repaglinide and ↑ risk of hypoglycaemic episodes	Inhibition of CYP3A4-mediated metabolism of repaglinide	Watch for and warn patients about hypoglycaemia ➢ ***For signs and symptoms of hypoglycaemia, see Clinical Features of Some Adverse Drug Interactions, Hypoglycaemia***
CALCIUM CHANNEL BLOCKERS	**ANTIEPILEPTICS**			
CALCIUM CHANNEL BLOCKERS	BARBITURATES	↓ plasma concentrations of felodipine, nifedipine, nimodipine, nisoldipine and verapamil with phenobarbital	Phenobarbital induces CYP3A4, which metabolizes calcium channel blockers. It also induces intestinal P-gp, which may ↓ the bioavailability of verapamil	Monitor PR and BP closely; watch for ↑ BP
CALCIUM CHANNEL BLOCKERS	CARBAMAZEPINE	1. Diltiazem and verapamil ↑ plasma concentrations of carbamazepine (cases of toxicity) 2. ↓ plasma concentrations of felodipine, nifedipine and possibly nimodipine and nisoldipine	1. Diltiazem and verapamil inhibit CYP3A4-mediated metabolism of carbamazepine. They also inhibit intestinal P-gp, which may ↑ the bioavailability of carbamazepine 2. Carbamazepine, in turn, induces CYP3A4, which metabolizes calcium channel blockers	1. Monitor carbamazepine levels when initiating calcium channel blockers, particularly diltiazem and verapamil 2. Monitor PR and BP closely; watch for ↑ BP when starting carbamazepine in patients already on calcium channel blockers
CALCIUM CHANNEL BLOCKERS	PHENYTOIN	1. Phenytoin levels are ↑ by diltiazem and possibly nifedipine and isradipine 2. ↓ plasma concentrations of diltiazem, felodipine, nisoldipine, verapamil and possibly nimodipine	1. Postulated to be due to inhibition of CYP3A4-mediated metabolism of phenytoin. Diltiazem is also known to inhibit intestinal P-gp, which may ↑ the bioavailability of phenytoin 2. Phenytoin induces CYP3A4, which metabolizes calcium channel blockers	1. Monitor phenytoin levels when initiating calcium channel blockers, particularly diltiazem and verapamil 2. Monitor PR and BP closely; watch for ↑ BP when starting phenytoin in patients already on calcium channel blockers

CALCIUM CHANNEL BLOCKERS	PRIMIDONE	↓ plasma concentrations of calcium channel blockers	Primidone induces CYP3A4, which metabolizes calcium channel blockers	Monitor PR and BP closely; watch for ↑ BP
CALCIUM CHANNEL BLOCKERS	SODIUM VALPROATE	Nimodipine levels may be ↑ by valproate	Uncertain at present	Monitor BP at least weekly until stable. Warn patients to report symptoms of hypotension (light-headedness, dizziness on standing, etc.)
CALCIUM CHANNEL BLOCKERS	ANTIFUNGALS – FLUCONAZOLE, ITRACONAZOLE, KETOCONAZOLE, POSACONAZOLE	Plasma concentrations of dihydropyridine calcium channel blockers are ↑ by fluconazole, itraconazole and ketoconazole. Risk of ↑ verapamil levels with ketoconazole and itraconazole. Itraconazole and possibly posaconazole may ↑ diltiazem levels	The azoles are potent inhibitors of CYP3A4 isoenzymes, which metabolize calcium channel blockers. They also inhibit CYP2C9-mediated metabolism of verapamil. Ketoconazole and itraconazole both inhibit intestinal P-gp, which may ↑ the bioavailability of verapamil. Diltiazem is mainly a substrate of CYP3A5 and CYP3A5P1, which are inhibited by itraconazole. Around 75% of the metabolism of diltiazem occurs in the liver and the rest in the intestine. Diltiazem is a substrate of P-gp (also an inhibitor but unlikely to be significant at therapeutic doses), which is inhibited by itraconazole, resulting in ↑ bioavailability of diltiazem	Monitor PR, BP and ECG, and warn patents to watch for symptoms/signs of heart failure

CARDIOVASCULAR DRUGS CALCIUM CHANNEL BLOCKERS

CARDIOVASCULAR DRUGS CALCIUM CHANNEL BLOCKERS

Primary drug	Secondary drug	Effect	Mechanism	Precautions
CALCIUM CHANNEL BLOCKERS	ANTIGOUT DRUGS	Serum concentrations pf verapamil are significantly ↓ when co-administered with sulfinpyrazone	Uncertain, but presumed to be due to ↑ hepatic metabolism	Monitor PR and BP at least weekly until stable. Watch for poor response to verapamil
CALCIUM CHANNEL BLOCKERS	**ANTIHYPERTENSIVES AND HEART FAILURE DRUGS**			
CALCIUM CHANNEL BLOCKERS	ANTIHYPERTENSIVES AND HEART FAILURE DRUGS	↑ hypotensive effect	Additive hypotensive effect; may be used therapeutically	Monitor BP at least weekly until stable. Warn patients to report symptoms of hypotension (light-headedness, dizziness on standing, etc.)
CALCIUM CHANNEL BLOCKERS	ALPHA-BLOCKERS	↑ efficacy of alpha-blockers; ↑ risk of first-dose ↓ BP with alfuzosin, prazosin and terazosin	Additive hypotensive effect; may be used therapeutically	Watch for first-dose ↓ BP when starting either drug when the patient is already established on the other; consider reducing the dose of the established drug and starting the new agent at the lowest dose and titrating up
VERAPAMIL	CENTRALLY ACTING ANTIHYPERTENSIVES	Reports of two cases of complete heart block when clonidine was given to a patient on verapamil	Additive effect; both drugs are known to rarely cause AV dysfunction	Monitor ECG closely when co-administering
CALCIUM CHANNEL BLOCKERS	ANTIMALARIALS – MEFLOQUINE	Risk of bradycardia	Additive bradycardic effect; mefloquine can cause cardiac conduction disorders, e.g. bradycardia. Also a theoretical risk of Q–T prolongation with co-administration of mefloquine and calcium channel blockers	Monitor PR closely

VERAPAMIL	ANTIMUSCARINICS – DARIFENACIN	↑ darifenacin levels	Inhibition of CYP3A4-mediated metabolism of darifenacin	Avoid co-administration (manufacturer's recommendation)
CALCIUM CHANNEL BLOCKERS	ANTIPARKINSON'S DRUGS – LEVODOPA	↑ hypotensive effect	Additive hypotensive effect	Monitor BP at least weekly until stable. Warn patients to report symptoms of hypotension (light-headedness, dizziness on standing, etc.)
CALCIUM CHANNEL BLOCKERS	ANTIPLATELET AGENTS – ASPIRIN	↓ antihypertensive effect with aspirin; effect not noted with low-dose aspirin	Aspirin may cause sodium retention and vasoconstriction at possibly both renal and endothelial sites	Monitor BP closely when high-dose aspirin is prescribed
CALCIUM CHANNEL BLOCKERS	**ANTIPSYCHOTICS**			
CALCIUM CHANNEL BLOCKERS	ANTIPSYCHOTICS	↑ antihypertensive effect	Dose-related ↓ BP (due to vasodilatation) is a side-effect of most antipsychotics, particularly phenothiazines	Monitor BP especially during initiation of treatment. Warn patients to report symptoms of hypotension (light-headedness, dizziness on standing, etc.)
CALCIUM CHANNEL BLOCKERS	CLOZAPINE	Plasma concentrations of clozapine may be ↑ by diltiazem and verapamil	Diltiazem and verapamil inhibit CYP1A2-mediated metabolism of clozapine	Watch for side-effects of clozapine
CALCIUM CHANNEL BLOCKERS	SERTINDOLE	Plasma concentrations of sertindole are ↑ by diltiazem and verapamil	Diltiazem and verapamil inhibit CYP3A4-mediated metabolism of sertindole	Avoid co-administration; raised sertindole concentrations are associated with an ↑ risk of prolonged Q–T interval and therefore ventricular arrhythmias, particularly torsades de pointes

Primary drug	Secondary drug	Effect	Mechanism	Precautions
CALCIUM CHANNEL BLOCKERS	ANTIVIRALS – PROTEASE INHIBITORS	Plasma concentrations of calcium channel blockers are ↑ by protease inhibitors	Protease inhibitors inhibit CYP3A4-mediated metabolism of calcium channel blockers. Also, ritonavir inhibits CYP2C9-mediated metabolism of verapamil, and ritonavir and saquinavir both inhibit intestinal P-gp, which may ↑ the bioavailability of verapamil	Monitor PR, BP and ECG closely; ↓ dose of calcium channel blocker if necessary (e.g. the manufacturers of diltiazem suggest starting at 50% of the standard dose and titrating to effect)
CALCIUM CHANNEL BLOCKERS	**ANXIOLYTICS AND HYPNOTICS**			
CALCIUM CHANNEL BLOCKERS	ANXIOLYTICS AND HYPNOTICS	↑ hypotensive effect	Additive hypotensive effect; anxiolytics can cause postural ↓ BP	Monitor BP at least weekly until stable. Warn patients to report symptoms of hypotension (light-headedness, dizziness on standing, etc.). Consider reducing the dose of calcium channel blocker or using an alternative antidepressant
DILTIAZEM, VERAPAMIL	BZDs	Plasma concentrations of midazolam and triazolam are ↑ by diltiazem and verapamil	Diltiazem and verapamil inhibit CYP3A4-mediated metabolism of midazolam and triazolam	↓ the dose of BZD by 50% in patients on calcium channel blockers; warn patients not to perform skilled tasks such as driving for at least 10 hours after a dose of BZD
CALCIUM CHANNEL BLOCKERS	BUSPIRONE	Plasma concentrations of buspirone are ↑ by diltiazem and verapamil	Diltiazem and verapamil inhibit CYP3A4-mediated metabolism of buspirone	Start buspirone at a lower dose (2.5 mg twice daily suggested by the manufacturers) in patients on calcium channel blockers

CALCIUM CHANNEL BLOCKERS	BETA-BLOCKERS			
CALCIUM CHANNEL BLOCKERS	BETA-BLOCKERS	↑ hypotensive effect, bradycardia, conduction defects and heart failure	Additive hypotensive effect; may be used therapeutically	Monitor PR, BP and ECG at least weekly until stable. Warn patients to report symptoms of hypotension (light-headedness, dizziness on standing, etc.)
DIHYDROPYRIDINES	BETA-BLOCKERS	Rare cases of severe ↓ BP and heart failure when nifedipine and nisoldipine are given to patients on beta-blockers	Uncertain why this severe effect occurs	Monitor PR, BP and ECG at least weekly until stable. Warn patients to report symptoms of hypotension (light-headedness, dizziness on standing, etc.)
DILTIAZEM	BETA-BLOCKERS	↑ hypotensive and bradycardic effects: cases of severe bradycardia and AV block when both drugs are administered concurrently in the presence of pre-existing heart failure or conduction abnormalities	Additive effects on conduction; diltiazem causes bradycardia, sinoatrial block and AV block. Also, diltiazem inhibits CYP1A2-mediated metabolism of propanolol	Monitor PR, BP and ECG at least weekly until stable. Warn patients to report symptoms of hypotension (light-headedness, dizziness on standing, etc.)
VERAPAMIL	BETA-BLOCKERS	1. Risk of cardiac arrest when parenteral verapamil is given to patients on beta-blockers 2. Risk of bradycardias when both are given orally	Additive effect. Also, verapamil inhibits CYP1A2-mediated metabolism of propanolol	1. Do not administer intravenous verapamil to patients taking beta-blockers 2. Monitor ECG and BP carefully when both are given orally

CARDIOVASCULAR DRUGS CALCIUM CHANNEL BLOCKERS

CARDIOVASCULAR DRUGS CALCIUM CHANNEL BLOCKERS

Primary drug	Secondary drug	Effect	Mechanism	Precautions
CALCIUM CHANNEL BLOCKERS	**BRONCHODILATORS**			
DILTIAZEM, VERAPAMIL	THEOPHYLLINE	↑ theophylline levels with diltiazem and verapamil. Mostly not clinically significant but two cases of theophylline toxicity with verapamil have been reported	Uncertain, but thought to be due to inhibition of CYP1A2-mediated metabolism of theophylline	Be aware of the small possibility of theophylline toxicity when commencing calcium channel blockers; check levels if any problems occur, and consider either reducing the dose of theophylline or using an alternative calcium channel blocker
NIFEDIPINE	THEOPHYLLINE	Clinically non-significant ↓ theophylline levels with nifedipine, but there are case reports of theophylline toxicity after starting nifedipine	Uncertain; probably due to alterations in either metabolism or volume of distribution of theophylline	Be aware of the small possibility of theophylline toxicity when commencing calcium channel blockers; check levels if any problems occur, and consider either reducing the dose of theophylline or using an alternative calcium channel blocker
CALCIUM CHANNEL BLOCKERS	CALCIUM CHANNEL BLOCKERS	Co-administration of nifedipine and diltiazem leads to ↑ plasma concentrations of both drugs	Uncertain, but presumed mutual inhibition of CYP3A isoform-mediated metabolism	Monitor PR, BP and ECG at least weekly until stable. Warn patients to report symptoms of hypotension (light-headedness, dizziness on standing, etc.)
CALCIUM CHANNEL BLOCKERS	**CARDIAC GLYCOSIDES**			
VERAPAMIL	DIGOXIN	1. Verapamil causes an ↑ in serum digoxin levels, and there have been case reports of significant toxicity 2. ↑ AV block when digoxin is co-administered with verapamil	1. Verapamil seems to inhibit P-gp-mediated renal and biliary clearance of digoxin. Inhibition of intestinal P-gp would also ↑ the bioavailability of digoxin 2. Additive effect	1. It is recommended to ↓ digoxin doses by 33–50% when starting verapamil; monitor digoxin levels and watch for symptoms/signs of toxicity 2. Monitor ECG closely when co-administering digoxin and verapamil, especially when verapamil is being given parenterally

DILTIAZEM, NIFEDIPINE, FELODIPINE, LACIDIPINE, LERCANIDIPINE, NICARDIPINE, NISOLDIPINE	DIGOXIN	Possible ↑ plasma concentrations of digoxin	These calcium channel blockers are thought to ↓ renal excretion of digoxin	Monitor digoxin levels carefully
CALCIUM CHANNEL BLOCKERS	DIGITOXIN	Plasma concentrations of digitoxin may be ↑ by diltiazem and verapamil	Uncertain at present	Watch for digitoxin toxicity
VERAPAMIL	CNS STIMULANTS – MODAFINIL	May cause ↓ verapamil levels if CYP1A2 is the predominant metabolic pathway and alternative metabolic pathways are either genetically deficient or affected	Modafinil is a moderate inducer of CYP1A2 in a concentration-dependent manner	Be aware
CALCIUM CHANNEL BLOCKERS	**DIURETICS**			
CALCIUM CHANNEL BLOCKERS	DIURETICS	↑ hypotensive effect	Additive effect	Monitor BP at least weekly until stable. Warn patients to report symptoms of hypotension (light-headedness, dizziness on standing, etc.)
CALCIUM CHANNEL BLOCKERS	POTASSIUM-SPARING DIURETICS	↑ serum concentrations of eplerenone when given with diltiazem and verapamil	Calcium channel blockers inhibit CYP3A4-mediated metabolism of eplerenone	Restrict dose of eplerenone to 25 mg/day. Monitor serum potassium concentrations closely; watch for hyperkalaemia
CALCIUM CHANNEL BLOCKERS	DUTASTERIDE	Plasma concentrations of dutasteride may ↑ when co-administered with diltiazem or verapamil	Uncertain, but postulated that it may be due to inhibition of CYP3A4-mediated metabolism of dutasteride	Watch for side-effects of dutasteride

CARDIOVASCULAR DRUGS CALCIUM CHANNEL BLOCKERS

Primary drug	Secondary drug	Effect	Mechanism	Precautions
CALCIUM CHANNEL BLOCKERS	GRAPEFRUIT JUICE	↑ bioavailability of felodipine and nisoldipine (with reports of adverse effects), and ↑ bioavailability of isradipine, lacidipine, lercanidipine, nicardipine, nifedipine, nimodipine and verapamil (without reported adverse clinical effects)	Postulated that flavonoids in grapefruit juice (and possibly Seville oranges and limes) inhibit intestinal (but not hepatic) CYP3A4. They also inhibit intestinal P-gp, which may ↑ the bioavailability of verapamil	Avoid concurrent use of felodipine and nisoldipine and grapefruit juice
CALCIUM CHANNEL BLOCKERS	**H2 RECEPTOR BLOCKERS**			
CALCIUM CHANNEL BLOCKERS	CIMETIDINE	↑ levels of calcium channel blockers, especially diltiazem and nifedipine	Inhibition of CYP3A isoform-mediated metabolism	Monitor BP at least weekly until stable; watch for ↓ BP. Consider reducing the dose of diltiazem and nifedipine by up to 50%
CALCIUM CHANNEL BLOCKERS	FAMOTIDINE	Reports of heart failure and ↓ BP when famotidine is given with nifedipine	Additive negative inotropic effects	Caution when co-administering famotidine with calcium channel blockers, especially in elderly people
DILTIAZEM, NIFEDIPINE, VERAPAMIL	5-HT1 AGONISTS – ALMOTRIPTAN, ELETRIPTAN	↑ plasma concentrations of almotriptan and risk of toxic effects of almotriptan, e.g. flushing, sensations of tingling, heat, heaviness, pressure or tightness of any part of the body, including the throat and chest, dizziness	Almotriptan is metabolized mainly by CYP3A4 isoenzymes. Most CYP isoenzymes are inhibited by diltiazem to varying degrees, and since there is an alternative pathway of metabolism by MAO-A, toxicity responses vary between individuals	CSM has advised that if chest tightness or pressure is intense, the triptan should be discontinued immediately and the patient investigated for ischaemic heart disease by measuring cardiac enzymes and doing an ECG. Avoid concomitant use in patients with coronary artery disease and in those with severe or uncontrolled hypertension
CALCIUM CHANNEL BLOCKERS	IVABRADINE	↑ levels with diltiazem and verapamil	Uncertain	Avoid co-administration

CALCIUM CHANNEL BLOCKERS	LIPID-LOWERING DRUGS			
CALCIUM CHANNEL BLOCKERS	ANION EXCHANGE RESINS	Colestipol ↓ diltiazem levels	Colestipol binds diltiazem in the intestine	Monitor for poor response to diltiazem. Separating doses of diltiazem and colestipol does not seem to ↓ this interaction
CALCIUM CHANNEL BLOCKERS	STATINS	↑ plasma levels of atorvastatin, lovastatin and simvastatin; case reports of myopathy when atorvastatin and simvastatin are co-administered with diltiazem or verapamil	Uncertain, but postulated to be due to inhibition of CYP3A4-mediated metabolism of statins in the intestinal wall. Also, diltiazem and verapamil inhibit intestinal P-gp, which may ↑ the bioavailability of statins	Watch for side-effects of statins. It has been suggested that the dose of simvastatin should not exceed 20 mg when given with verapamil, and 40 mg when given with diltiazem
CALCIUM CHANNEL BLOCKERS	MAGNESIUM (PARENTERAL)	Cases of profound muscular weakness when nifedipine is given with parenteral magnesium	Both drugs inhibit calcium influx across cell membranes, and magnesium promotes movement of calcium into the sarcoplasmic reticulum; this results in muscular paralysis	Do not administer calcium channel blockers during parenteral magnesium therapy
CALCIUM CHANNEL BLOCKERS	**MUSCLE RELAXANTS**			
CALCIUM CHANNEL BLOCKERS	DEPOLARIZING	↑ effect of suxamethonium with parenteral, but not oral, calcium channel blockers	Uncertain; postulated that ACh release at the synapse is calcium dependent; ↓ calcium concentrations at the nerve ending may ↓ ACh release, which in turn prolongs the nerve blockade	Monitor nerve blockade carefully, particularly during short procedures

CARDIOVASCULAR DRUGS CALCIUM CHANNEL BLOCKERS

CARDIOVASCULAR DRUGS CALCIUM CHANNEL BLOCKERS

Primary drug	Secondary drug	Effect	Mechanism	Precautions
CALCIUM CHANNEL BLOCKERS	NON-DEPOLARIZING	↑ effect of non-depolarising muscle relaxants with parenteral calcium channel blockers; the effect is less certain with oral therapy. In two cohort studies, vecuronium requirements were halved in patients on diltiazem. Nimodipine does not seem to share this interaction	Uncertain; postulated that ACh release at the synapse is calcium dependent; ↓ calcium concentrations at the nerve ending may ↓ ACh release, which in turn prolongs the nerve blockade	Monitor nerve blockade carefully in patients on calcium channel blockers, particularly near to the end of surgery, when muscle relaxation may be prolonged and difficult to reverse
CALCIUM CHANNEL BLOCKERS	**SKELETAL**			
CALCIUM CHANNEL BLOCKERS	BACLOFEN AND TIZANIDINE	↑ hypotensive effect with baclofen of tizanidine. Risk of bradycardia with tizanidine	Additive hypotensive effect. Tizanidine has a negative inotropic and chronotropic effect	Monitor BP at least weekly until stable. Warn patients to report symptoms of hypotension (light-headedness, dizziness on standing, etc.)
CALCIUM CHANNEL BLOCKERS	DANTROLENE	Risk of arrhythmias when diltiazem is given with intravenous dantrolene. Risk of ↓ BP, myocardial depression and hyperkalaemia when verapamil is given with intravenous dantrolene	Uncertain at present	Extreme caution must be exercised when administering parenteral dantrolene to patients on diltiazem or verapamil. Monitor BP and cardiac rhythm closely; watch for hyperkalaemia
CALCIUM CHANNEL BLOCKERS	NITRATES	↑ hypotensive effect	Additive effect	Monitor BP at least weekly until stable. Warn patients to report symptoms of hypotension (light-headedness, dizziness on standing, etc.)

CALCIUM CHANNEL BLOCKERS	OESTROGENS	↓ hypotensive effect	Oestrogens cause sodium and fluid retention	Monitor BP at least weekly until stable; routine prescription of oestrogens in patients with ↑ BP is not advisable
CALCIUM CHANNEL BLOCKERS	ORLISTAT	Case report of ↑ BP when orlistat was started for a patient on amlodipine	Uncertain at present	Monitor BP at least weekly until stable
CALCIUM CHANNEL BLOCKERS	**PERIPHERAL VASODILATORS**			
CALCIUM CHANNEL BLOCKERS	CILOSTAZOL	↑ plasma concentrations and efficacy of cilostazol with diltiazem, verapamil and nifedipine	These calcium channel blockers inhibit CYP3A4-mediated metabolism of cilostazol	Avoid co-administration
CALCIUM CHANNEL BLOCKERS	MOXISYLYTE (THYMOXAMINE)	↑ hypotensive effect	Additive hypotensive effect	Monitor BP at least weekly until stable. Warn patients to report symptoms of hypotension (light-headedness, dizziness on standing, etc.)
CALCIUM CHANNEL BLOCKERS	PHOSPHODIESTERASE TYPE 5 INHIBITORS	↑ hypotensive action particularly with sildenafil and vardenafil	Additive effect; phosphodiesterase type 5 inhibitors cause vasodilatation	Warn patients of the small risk of postural ↓ BP
CALCIUM CHANNEL BLOCKERS	POTASSIUM CHANNEL ACTIVATORS	↑ hypotensive effect	Additive effect	Avoid co-administration of nicorandil with phosphodiesterase type 5 inhibitors. With other drugs, monitor BP closely
CALCIUM CHANNEL BLOCKERS	PROSTAGLANDINS – ALPROSTADIL	↑ hypotensive effect	Additive hypotensive effect	Monitor BP at least weekly until stable. Warn patients to report symptoms of hypotension (light-headedness, dizziness on standing, etc.)

CARDIOVASCULAR DRUGS CALCIUM CHANNEL BLOCKERS

Primary drug	Secondary drug	Effect	Mechanism	Precautions
NIFEDIPINE	PROTON PUMP INHIBITORS – OMEPRAZOLE	Possible ↑ efficacy and adverse effects	Small ↑ in bioavailability possible via ↑ intragastric pH	Unlikely to be clinically significant
CALCIUM CHANNEL BLOCKERS	X-RAY CONTRAST SOLUTIONS	↑ hypotensive effect when intravenous ionic contrast solutions are given to patients on calcium channel blockers	Additive hypotensive effect	Consider using a non-ionic X-ray contrast solution for patients on calcium channel blockers
CARDIAC GLYCOSIDES				
DIGITOXIN				
DIGITOXIN	ANTIARRHYTHMICS			
DIGITOXIN	AMIODARONE	Reports of digitoxin toxicity in two patients on digitoxin after starting amiodarone	Uncertain; thought to be due to inhibition of P-gp-mediated renal clearance of digoxin	Watch for digitoxin toxicity
DIGITOXIN	PROCAINAMIDE	Single case report of toxicity in a patient taking both digitoxin and procainamide	Uncertain at present	Watch for digitoxin toxicity
DIGITOXIN	ANTIBIOTICS – RIFAMPICIN	Plasma concentrations of digitoxin may be halved by rifampicin	Due to ↑ hepatic metabolism	Watch for poor response to digitoxin
DIGITOXIN	ANTIEPILEPTICS – BARBITURATES, CARBAMAZEPINE, PHENYTOIN	Plasma concentrations of digitoxin may be ↓ by up to half by barbiturates	Possibly ↑ hepatic metabolism	Watch for poor response to digitoxin
DIGITOXIN	CALCIUM CHANNEL BLOCKERS	Plasma concentrations of digitoxin may be ↑ by diltiazem and verapamil	Uncertain at present	Watch for digitoxin toxicity
DIGITOXIN	DIURETICS – SPIRONOLACTONE	Conflicting results from volunteer studies; some showed ↑ (up to one-third) in the half-life of digitoxin, others a ↓ (up to one-fifth)	Uncertain at present	Watch for either digitoxin toxicity or a poor response, particularly for the first month after starting spironolactone

DIGITOXIN	LIPID-REGULATING DRUGS – ANION EXCHANGE RESINS	Colestipol and colestyramine both may ↓ digitoxin levels	Both colestipol and colestyramine are ion exchange resins that bind bile sodiums and prevent reabsorption in the intestine; this breaks the enterohepatic cycle of digitoxin	Colestipol and colestyramine should be given at least 1.5 hours after digitoxin
DIGOXIN				
DIGOXIN	AMINOSALICYLATES	Sulfasalazine may ↓ digoxin levels. The manufacturers of balsalazide also warn against the possibility of this interaction in spite of a lack of case reports	Uncertain at present	Watch for poor response to digoxin; check levels if signs of ↓ effect
DIGOXIN	**ANALGESICS**			
DIGOXIN	NSAIDs	Diclofenac, indometacin and possibly fenbufen, ibuprofen and tiaprofenic acid ↑ plasma concentrations of digoxin and ↑ risk of precipitating cardiac failure and renal dysfunction	Uncertain; postulated that NSAID-induced renal impairment plays a role; however, since all NSAIDs have this effect, it is not understood why only certain NSAIDs actually influence digoxin levels	Monitor renal function closely. Monitor digoxin levels; watch for digoxin toxicity
DIGOXIN	OPIOIDS	↑ concentrations of digoxin may occur with tramadol	Uncertain at present	Watch for digoxin toxicity; check levels and ↓ the dose of digoxin as necessary
DIGOXIN	ANTACIDS	Plasma concentrations of digoxin may be ↓ by antacids	Uncertain; probably ↓ absorption of digoxin	Watch for poor response to digoxin
DIGOXIN	**ANTIARRHYTHMICS**			
DIGOXIN	AMIODARONE	Amiodarone may ↑ plasma levels of digoxin (in some cases up to fourfold)	Uncertain; thought to be due to inhibition of P-gp-mediated renal clearance of digoxin. Amiodarone is also known to inhibit intestinal P-gp, which may ↑ the bioavailability of digoxin	↓ digoxin dose by one-third to one-half when starting amiodarone. Monitor digoxin levels; watch for digoxin toxicity, especially for 4 weeks after initiating or adjusting amiodarone therapy

Primary drug	Secondary drug	Effect	Mechanism	Precautions
DIGOXIN	MORACIZINE	Case reports of heart block when moracizine is co-administered with digoxin	Uncertain at present	Monitor PR and ECG closely
DIGOXIN	PROPAFENONE	Digoxin concentrations may be ↑ by propafenone	Uncertain at present	Watch for digoxin toxicity; check digoxin levels if indicated and ↓ digoxin dose as necessary (15–70% is suggested by studies)
DIGOXIN	**ANTIBIOTICS**			
DIGOXIN	AMINOGLYCOSIDES	1. Gentamicin may ↑ plasma concentrations of digoxin 2. Neomycin may ↓ plasma concentrations of digoxin	1. Uncertain; postulated to be due to impaired renal clearance of digoxin 2. Neomycin ↓ absorption of digoxin; this may be offset in some patients by ↓ intestinal bacterial breakdown of digoxin	1. Monitor digoxin levels; watch for ↑ levels, particularly with diabetes and in the presence of renal insufficiency 2. Monitor digoxin levels; watch for poor response to digoxin
DIGOXIN	MACROLIDES	Digoxin concentrations may be ↑ by macrolides	Uncertain; postulated that macrolides inhibit P-gp in both the intestine (↑ bioavailability) and kidney (↓ clearance). It is possible that alterations in intestinal flora may also have a role	Monitor digoxin levels; watch for digoxin toxicity
DIGOXIN	RIFAMPICIN	Plasma concentrations of digoxin may be ↓ by rifampicin	Rifampicin seems to induce P-gp-mediated excretion of digoxin in the kidneys	Watch for a ↓ response to digoxin, check plasma levels and ↑ the dose as necessary
DIGOXIN	TRIMETHOPRIM, CO-TRIMOXAZOLE	Trimethoprim may ↑ plasma concentrations of digoxin, particularly in elderly people	Uncertain; postulated that trimethoprim ↓ renal clearance of digoxin	Monitor digoxin levels; watch for digoxin toxicity

DIGOXIN	**ANTICANCER AND IMMUNOMODULATING DRUGS**			
DIGOXIN	CYTOTOXICS	Cytotoxics may ↓ levels of digoxin (by up to 50%) when digoxin is given in tablet form	Cytotoxic-induced damage to the mucosa of the intestine may ↓ absorption; this does not seem to be a problem with liquid or liquid-containing capsule formulations	Watch for poor response to digoxin; check levels if signs of ↓ effect, and consider swapping to liquid digoxin or liquid-containing capsules
DIGOXIN	**IMMUNOMODULATING DRUGS**			
DIGOXIN	AMINOSALICYLATES	Sulfasalazine may ↓ digoxin levels. The manufacturers of balsalazide also warn against the possibility of this interaction in spite of a lack of case reports	Uncertain at present	Watch for poor response to digoxin; check levels if signs of ↓ effect
DIGOXIN	CICLOSPORIN	↑ plasma digoxin levels, with risk of toxicity. Digoxin may ↑ ciclosporin bioavailability (by 15–20%)	Attributed to inhibition of intestinal P-gp and renal P-gp, which ↑ bioavailability and ↑ renal elimination. Digoxin ↑ bioavailability of ciclosporin due to substrate competition for P-gp	Watch for digoxin toxicity. Monitor plasma digoxin and ciclosporin levels
DIGOXIN	CORTICOSTEROIDS	Risk of digoxin toxicity due to hypokalaemia	Corticosteroids may cause hypokalaemia	Monitor potassium levels closely. Monitor digoxin levels; watch for digoxin toxicity
DIGOXIN	INTERFERON GAMMA	Plasma concentrations of digoxin may occur with interferon gamma	Interferon gamma ↓ P-gp-mediated renal and biliary excretion of digoxin	Monitor digoxin levels; watch for digoxin toxicity
DIGOXIN	PENICILLAMINE	Plasma concentrations of digoxin may be ↓ by penicillamine	Uncertain at present	Watch for poor response to digoxin

Primary drug	Secondary drug	Effect	Mechanism	Precautions
DIGOXIN	TACROLIMUS	Digoxin toxicity (pharmacodynamic)	Possibly due to tacrolimus-induced hyperkalaemia and hypomagnesaemia	Watch for digoxin toxicity. Monitor potassium and magnesium levels
DIGOXIN	**ANTIDEPRESSANTS**			
DIGOXIN	ST JOHN'S WORT	Plasma concentrations of digoxin seem to be ↓ by St John's wort	St John's wort seems to ↓ P-gp-mediated intestinal absorption of digoxin	Watch for a ↓ response to digoxin
DIGOXIN	TRAZODONE	Reports of two cases of ↑ plasma concentrations of digoxin after starting trazodone	Uncertain at present	Watch for digoxin toxicity; check levels and ↓ the dose of digoxin as necessary
DIGOXIN	ANTIDIABETIC DRUGS – ACARBOSE	Acarbose may ↓ plasma levels of digoxin	Uncertain; possibly ↓ absorption of digoxin	Monitor digoxin levels; watch for ↓ levels
DIGOXIN	ANTIDIARRHOEALS – KAOLIN	Possibly ↓ levels of digoxin	↓ absorption	Separate doses by at least 2 hours
DIGOXIN	ANTIEPILEPTICS	Phenytoin may ↓ plasma levels of digoxin	Uncertain at present	Watch for poor response to digoxin; check levels if signs of ↓ effect
DIGOXIN	**ANTIFUNGALS**			
DIGOXIN	AMPHOTERICIN	Risk of digoxin ↑ by toxicity due to hypokalaemia	Amphotericin may cause hypokalaemia	Monitor potassium levels closely. Monitor digoxin levels; watch for digoxin toxicity
DIGOXIN	ITRACONAZOLE	Itraconazole may cause ↑ plasma levels of digoxin; cases reported of digoxin toxicity	Itraconazole inhibits P-gp-mediated renal clearance and ↑ intestinal absorption of digoxin	Monitor digoxin levels; watch for digoxin toxicity

DIGOXIN	ANTIHYPERTENSIVES AND HEART FAILURE DRUGS			
DIGOXIN	ACE INHIBITORS	↑ plasma concentrations of digoxin when captopril is co-administered in the presence of heart failure (class II or more severe) or renal insufficiency. No other ACE inhibitors seem to interact in the same way	Uncertain; postulated to be due to ↓ renal excretion of digoxin	Monitor digoxin levels; watch for digoxin toxicity
DIGOXIN	ALPHA-BLOCKERS	Possibility of ↑ plasma concentrations of digoxin; no cases of toxicity have been reported with doxazosin or prazosin	Doxazosin inhibits P-gp-mediated elimination of digoxin; mechanism with prazosin uncertain at present	Monitor digoxin levels
DIGOXIN	ANGIOTENSIN II RECEPTOR ANTAGONISTS	Telmisartan may ↑ plasma levels of digoxin	Uncertain; telmisartan thought to ↑ rate of absorption of digoxin	Monitor digoxin levels; watch for digoxin toxicity
DIGOXIN	**ANTIMALARIALS**			
DIGOXIN	CHLOROQUINE, HYDROXYCHLOROQUINE	Chloroquine may ↑ plasma concentrations of digoxin	Uncertain at present	Monitor digoxin levels; watch for digoxin toxicity
DIGOXIN	MEFLOQUINE	Risk of bradycardia	Uncertain; probably additive effect; mefloquine can cause AV block	Monitor PR and ECG closely
DIGOXIN	QUININE	Plasma concentrations of digoxin may ↑ when co-administered with quinine	Uncertain, but seems to be due to ↓ non-renal (possibly biliary) excretion of digoxin	Monitor digoxin levels; watch for digoxin toxicity
DIGOXIN	ANTIMUSCARINICS PROPANTHELINE	↑ digoxin levels (30–40%) but only with slow-release formulations	Slowed gut transit time allows more digoxin to be absorbed	Use alternative formulation of digoxin

Primary drug	Secondary drug	Effect	Mechanism	Precautions
DIGOXIN	ANTIVIRALS – RITONAVIR (WITH OR WITHOUT LOPINAVIR)	Plasma digoxin concentrations may be ↑ by ritonavir	Uncertain; probably due to inhibition of P-gp-mediated renal excretion of digoxin and ↑ intestinal absorption	Monitor digoxin levels; watch for digoxin toxicity
DIGOXIN	ANXIOLYTICS AND HYPNOTICS	Alprazolam and possibly diazepam may ↑ digoxin levels, particularly in the over-65s	Uncertain at present	Monitor digoxin levels; watch for digoxin toxicity
DIGOXIN	**BETA-BLOCKERS**			
DIGOXIN	BETA-BLOCKERS	Risk of bradycardia and AV block	Additive bradycardia	Monitor PR, BP and ECG at least weekly until stable
DIGOXIN	CARVEDILOL	Carvedilol may ↑ digoxin plasma concentrations, particularly in children	↓ P-gp-mediated renal clearance of digoxin	↓ the dose of digoxin by 25%; watch for signs of digoxin toxicity and monitor digoxin levels
DIGOXIN	BRONCHODILATORS – BETA-2 AGONISTS	1. Hypokalaemia may exacerbate digoxin toxicity 2. Salbutamol may ↓ digoxin levels (by 16–22%) after 10 days of concurrent therapy	1. Beta-2 agonists may cause hypokalaemia 2. Uncertain	1. Monitor potassium levels closely 2. Clinical significance is uncertain. Useful to monitor digoxin levels if there is a clinical indication of ↓ response to digoxin
DIGOXIN	CALCIUM	Risk of cardiac arrhythmias with large intravenous doses of calcium	Uncertain; it is known that calcium levels directly correlate with the action of digoxin; therefore, high levels, even if transient, may ↑ the chance of toxicity	It is recommended that parenteral administration of calcium should be avoided in patients taking digoxin. If this is not possible, administer calcium slowly and in small aliquots

DIGOXIN	CALCIUM CHANNEL BLOCKERS			
DIGOXIN	VERAPAMIL	1. Verapamil causes an ↑ in serum digoxin levels, and there have been case reports of significant toxicity 2. ↑ AV block when digoxin is co-administered with verapamil	1. Verapamil seems to inhibit P-gp-mediated renal and biliary clearance of digoxin. Inhibition of intestinal P-gp would also ↑ the bioavailability of digoxin 2. Additive effect	1. It is recommended to ↓ digoxin doses by 33–50% when starting verapamil; monitor digoxin levels and watch for symptoms/signs of toxicity 2. Monitor ECG closely when co-administering digoxin and verapamil, especially when verapamil is being given parenterally
DIGOXIN	DILTIAZEM, NIFEDIPINE, FELODIPINE, LACIDIPINE, LERCANIDIPINE, NICARDIPINE, NISOLDIPINE	Possible ↑ plasma concentrations of digoxin	These calcium channel blockers are thought to ↓ the renal excretion of digoxin	Monitor digoxin levels carefully
DIGOXIN	**DIURETICS**			
DIGOXIN	CARBONIC ANHYDRASE INHIBITORS, LOOP DIURETICS, THIAZIDES	Risk of digoxin toxicity ↑ due to hypokalaemia	Uncertain	Monitor potassium levels closely. Monitor digoxin levels; watch for digoxin toxicity
DIGOXIN	POTASSIUM-SPARING DIURETICS AND ALDOSTERONE ANTAGONISTS	Eplerenone and spironolactone may ↑ plasma concentrations of digoxin	Uncertain; spironolactone possibly ↓ the volume of distribution of digoxin	Monitor digoxin levels; watch for digoxin toxicity
DIGOXIN	GRAPEFRUIT JUICE	Possible ↑ efficacy and ↑ adverse effects	Possibly via altered absorption	Most patients have been unaffected; consider if unexpected bradycardia or heart block with digoxin

Primary drug	Secondary drug	Effect	Mechanism	Precautions
DIGOXIN	HERBAL MEDICINES	1. Bufalin, danshen and ginseng interfere with some of the assays for digoxin 2. Liquorice may ↑ the risk of digoxin toxicity 3. Many herbal medicines contain digoxin-like compounds, e.g. black cohosh root, cayenne pepper	1. Bufalin cross-reacts with the antibody used in some digoxin assays. The mechanism of interaction of danshen and ginseng is uncertain at present 2. Liquorice causes electrolyte imbalances, which may precipitate digoxin toxicity	Ask about Chinese herbal remedies in patients taking digoxin; inform the laboratory when monitoring digoxin levels. Watch for symptoms/signs of toxicity in patients taking liquorice-containing remedies
DIGOXIN	**LIPID-LOWERING DRUGS**			
DIGOXIN	ANION EXCHANGE RESINS	Colestipol and colestyramine both may ↓ digoxin levels	Both colestipol and colestyramine are ion exchange resins that bind bile sodiums and prevent reabsorption in the intestine; this breaks the enterohepatic cycle of digoxin	Colestipol and colestyramine should be given at least 1.5 hours after digoxin
DIGOXIN	STATINS	High-dose (80 mg) atorvastatin may ↑ digoxin levels	Atorvastatin inhibits intestinal P-gp, which ↑ absorption of digoxin	Watch for digoxin toxicity
DIGOXIN	**MUSCLE RELAXANTS**			
DIGOXIN	DEPOLARIZING	Risk of ventricular arrhythmias when suxamethonium is given to patients taking digoxin	Uncertain; postulated that the mechanism involves rapid efflux of potassium from the cells	Use caution and monitor ECG closely if suxamethonium needs to be used in patients taking digoxin
DIGOXIN	NON-DEPOLARIZING	Case reports of S–T segment/T wave changes and sinus/atrial tachycardia when pancuronium given to patients on digoxin	Uncertain	Avoid pancuronium in patients taking digoxin
DIGOXIN	SKELETAL	Risk of bradycardia when tizanidine given with digoxin	Tizanidine has a negative inotropic effect	Monitor PR closely

DIGOXIN	PARASYMPATHOMIMETICS	Cases reports of AV block and bradycardia when edrophonium was co-administered with digoxin	Uncertain at present	Avoid edrophonium in patients with atrial arrhythmias who are also taking digoxin
DIGOXIN	PROTON PUMP INHIBITORS	Plasma concentrations of digoxin are possibly ↑ by proton pump inhibitors	Small ↑ in bioavailability possible via ↑ intragastric pH or altered intestinal P-gp transport	Not thought to be clinically significant unless a poor CYP2C19 metabolizer. No specific recommendations. Different proton pump inhibitors may interaction differently – monitor if changing therapy or doses
DIGOXIN	SUCRALFATE	Plasma concentrations of digoxin may be ↓ by sucralfate	Uncertain; possibly sucralfate binds with digoxin and ↓ its absorption	Watch for poor response to digoxin
DIURETICS				
CARBONIC ANHYDRASE INHIBITORS – ACETAZOLAMIDE				
CARBONIC ANHYDRASE INHIBITORS	**ANTIARRHYTHMICS**			
CARBONIC ANHYDRASE INHIBITORS	AMIODARONE, DISOPYRAMIDE, FLECAINIDE	Risk of ↑ myocardial depression	Cardiac toxicity directly related to hypokalaemia	Monitor potassium levels closely
CARBONIC ANHYDRASE INHIBITORS	MEXILETINE	Effect of mexiletine ↓ by hypokalaemia	Uncertain	Normalize potassium levels before starting mexiletine
CARBONIC ANHYDRASE INHIBITORS	ANTIBIOTICS – METHENAMINE	↓ efficacy of methenamine	Methenamine is only effective at a low pH; raising the urinary pH ↓ its effect	Avoid co-administration
CARBONIC ANHYDRASE INHIBITORS	ANTIDEMENTIA DRUGS – MEMANTINE	Possibly ↑ memantine levels	↓ renal excretion	Watch for early features of memantine toxicity

Primary drug	Secondary drug	Effect	Mechanism	Precautions
CARBONIC ANHYDRASE INHIBITORS	ANTIDEPRESSANTS – LITHIUM	↓ plasma concentrations of lithium, with risk of inadequate therapeutic effect	↑ renal elimination of lithium	Monitor clinically and by measuring blood lithium levels to ensure adequate therapeutic efficacy
CARBONIC ANHYDRASE INHIBITORS	ANTIEPILEPTICS – BARBITURATES, PHENYTOIN	Risk of osteomalacia	Barbiturates and phenytoin have a small risk of causing osteomalacia; this may be ↑ by acetazolamide-induced urinary excretion of calcium	Be aware
CARBONIC ANHYDRASE INHIBITORS	ANTIPLATELET AGENTS – ASPIRIN	↑ risk of salicylate toxicity with high-dose aspirin	Uncertain at present	Use low-dose aspirin
CARBONIC ANHYDRASE INHIBITORS	BETA-BLOCKERS – SOTALOL	↑ risk of ventricular arrhythmias, particularly torsades de pointes, caused by sotalol	Hypokalaemia, a side-effect of these diuretics, predisposes to arrhythmias during sotalol therapy	Normalize potassium levels before starting sotalol in patients already taking these diuretics. When starting these diuretics in patients already taking sotalol, monitor potassium levels every 4–6 weeks until stable
CARBONIC ANHYDRASE INHIBITORS	BRONCHODILATORS – BETA-2 AGONISTS, THEOPHYLLINE	Risk of hypokalaemia	Additive effects	Monitor blood potassium levels prior to concomitant administration and during therapy. Administer potassium supplements to prevent hypokalaemia
CARBONIC ANHYDRASE INHIBITORS	CARDIAC GLYCOSIDES	Risk of digoxin toxicity ↑ by acetazolamide due to hypokalaemia	Uncertain	Monitor potassium levels closely. Watch for digoxin toxicity and check levels

CARDIOVASCULAR DRUGS DIURETICS

LOOP DIURETICS				
LOOP DIURETICS	**ADDITIVE HYPOTENSIVE EFFECT**			
LOOP DIURETICS	1. ANTICANCER AND IMMUNOMODULATING DRUGS – IL-2 2. ANTI-HYPERTENSIVES AND HEART FAILURE DRUGS 3. BETA-BLOCKERS 4. CALCIUM CHANNEL BLOCKERS 5. MUSCLE RELAXANTS – baclofen and tizanidine 6. NITRATES 7. PERIPHERAL VASODILATORS – moxisylyte (thymoxamine) 8. POTASSIUM CHANNEL ACTIVATORS	↑ hypotensive effect. Risk of first-dose ↓ BP greater when ACE inhibitors or angiotensin II receptor antagonists are added to high-dose diuretics. Also, ↑ risk of first-dose ↓ BP with alfuzosin, prazosin and terazosin	Additive hypotensive effect; may be used therapeutically	Monitor BP at least weekly until stable. Warn patients to report symptoms of hypotension (light-headedness, dizziness on standing, etc.). Patients with congestive cardiac failure on diuretics should be started on a low dose of alpha-blocker
LOOP DIURETICS	ALISKIREN	↓ plasma levels of furosemide	Uncertain	Watch for poor response to furosemide
LOOP DIURETICS	ANAESTHETICS – GENERAL	↑ hypotensive effect	Additive hypotensive effect	Monitor BP closely, especially during induction of anaesthesia
LOOP DIURETICS	**ANTIARRHYTHMICS**			
LOOP DIURETICS	AMIODARONE, DISOPYRAMIDE, FLECAINIDE	Risk of arrhythmias	Cardiac toxicity directly related to hypokalaemia	Monitor potassium levels every 4–6 weeks until stable, then at least annually
LOOP DIURETICS	MEXILETINE	Effect of mexiletine ↓ by hypokalaemia	Uncertain	Normalize potassium levels before starting mexiletine

Primary drug	Secondary drug	Effect	Mechanism	Precautions
LOOP DIURETICS	**ANTIBIOTICS**			
LOOP DIURETICS	AMINOGLYCOSIDES	↑ risk of ototoxicity and possible deafness as a result of concomitant use of furosemide and gentamicin	Both furosemide and gentamicin are associated with ototoxicity; this risk is ↑ if they are used together	If used concurrently patients should be monitored for any hearing impairment
LOOP DIURETICS	COLISTIN	↑ risk of ototoxicity and possible deafness as a result of concomitant use of furosemide and colistin	Additive effect	If used concurrently, patients should be monitored for any hearing impairment
LOOP DIURETICS	TETRACYCLINES	Possible risk of renal toxicity	Additive effect	Some recommend avoiding co-administration; others advise monitoring renal function closely. Doxycycline is likely to be less of a problem
LOOP DIURETICS	VANCOMYCIN	Risk of renal toxicity	Additive effect	Monitor renal function closely
LOOP DIURETICS	**ANTICANCER AND IMMUNOMODULATING DRUGS**			
LOOP DIURETICS	**CYTOTOXICS**			
LOOP DIURETICS	CISPLATIN	↑ risk of auditory toxic effects with cisplatin	Loop diuretics cause tinnitus and deafness as side-effects. Additive toxic effects on auditory system likely	Monitor hearing – test auditory function regularly, particularly if patients report symptoms such as tinnitus or impaired hearing
LOOP DIURETICS	PORFIMER	↑ risk of photosensitivity reactions when porfimer is co-administered with bumetanide or furosemide	Attributed to additive effects	Avoid exposure of skin and eyes to direct sunlight for 30 days after porfimer therapy
LOOP DIURETICS	**IMMUNOMODULATING DRUGS**			
LOOP DIURETICS	CICLOSPORIN	Risk of nephrotoxicity	Additive effect	Monitor renal function weekly

LOOP DIURETICS	ANTIDEPRESSANTS – LITHIUM	↑ plasma concentrations of lithium, with risk of toxic effects	↓ renal excretion of lithium	Monitor clinically and by measuring blood lithium levels for lithium toxicity. Loop diuretics are safer than thiazides
LOOP DIURETICS	ANTIEPILEPTICS – PHENYTOIN	↓ efficacy of furosemide	Uncertain	Be aware; watch for poor response to furosemide
LOOP DIURETICS	ANTIFUNGALS – AMPHOTERICIN	Risk of hypokalaemia	Additive effect	Monitor potassium closely
LOOP DIURETICS	ANTIPARKINSON'S DRUGS – LEVODOPA	↑ hypotensive effect	Additive effect	Monitor BP at least weekly until stable. Warn patients to report symptoms of hypotension (light-headedness, dizziness on standing, etc.)
LOOP DIURETICS	ANTIPSYCHOTICS – ATYPICALS, PHENOTHIAZINES, PIMOZIDE	Risk of arrhythmias	Cardiac toxicity directly related to hypokalaemia	Monitor potassium levels every 4–6 weeks until stable, then at least annually
LOOP DIURETICS	BETA-BLOCKERS – SOTALOL	↑ risk of ventricular arrhythmias, particularly torsades de pointes	Hypokalaemia, a side-effect of these diuretics, predisposes to arrhythmias during sotalol therapy	Normalize potassium levels before starting sotalol in patients already taking these diuretics. When starting these diuretics in patients already taking sotalol, monitor potassium levels every 4–6 weeks until stable
LOOP DIURETICS	BRONCHODILATORS – BETA-2 AGONISTS, THEOPHYLLINE	Risk of hypokalaemia	Additive effects	Monitor blood potassium levels prior to concomitant administration and during therapy. Administer potassium supplements to prevent hypokalaemia

Primary drug	Secondary drug	Effect	Mechanism	Precautions
LOOP DIURETICS	CARDIAC GLYCOSIDES	Risk of digoxin toxicity ↑ due to hypokalaemia	Uncertain	Monitor potassium levels closely. Watch for digoxin toxicity and check levels
LOOP DIURETICS	CNS STIMULANTS – ATOMOXETINE	↑ risk of arrhythmias with hypokalaemia	These diuretics may cause hypokalaemia	Monitor potassium levels closely
LOOP DIURETICS	LIPID-LOWERING DRUGS – COLESTIPOL, COLESTYRAMINE	Both colestipol and colestyramine markedly ↓ levels of loop diuretics	Colestipol and colestyramine bind diuretics in the intestine	Give the anion exchange resin 3 hours after furosemide
POTASSIUM-SPARING DIURETICS AND ALDOSTERONE ANTAGONISTS				
POTASSIUM-SPARING DIURETICS	ALISKIREN	Risk of hyperkalaemia	Additive effect	Monitor serum potassium every week until stable, then every 3–6 months
POTASSIUM-SPARING DIURETICS	ANAESTHETICS – GENERAL	↑ hypotensive effect	Additive hypotensive effect	Monitor BP closely, especially during induction of anaesthesia
POTASSIUM-SPARING DIURETICS	ANALGESICS – NSAIDs	Risk of hyperkalaemia with NSAIDs	Renal insufficiency caused by NSAIDs can exacerbate potassium retention by these diuretics	Monitor renal function and potassium closely
POTASSIUM-SPARING DIURETICS	ANTIARRHYTHMICS – AMIODARONE	Risk of ↑ levels of eplerenone with amiodarone; risk of hyperkalaemia directly related to serum levels	Amiodarone inhibits CYP3A4-mediated metabolism of eplerenone	Restrict dose of eplerenone to 25 mg/day. Monitor serum potassium concentrations closely; watch for hyperkalaemia
POTASSIUM-SPARING DIURETICS	**ANTIBIOTICS**			
POTASSIUM-SPARING DIURETICS	MACROLIDES – ERYTHROMYCIN	↑ eplerenone results in an ↑ risk of hypotension and hyperkalaemia	Eplerenone is primarily metabolized by CYP3A4; there are no active metabolites. Erythromycin moderately inhibits CYP3A4, leading to ↑ levels of eplerenone	Dosage should not exceed 25 mg daily

POTASSIUM-SPARING DIURETICS	RIFAMPICIN	↓ eplerenone levels	Induction of metabolism	Avoid co-administration
POTASSIUM-SPARING DIURETICS	TRIMETHOPRIM	Risk of hyperkalaemia when trimethoprim is co-administered with eplerenone	Additive effect	Monitor potassium levels closely
POTASSIUM-SPARING DIURETICS	**ANTICANCER AND IMMUNOMODULATING DRUGS**			
POTASSIUM-SPARING DIURETICS	CICLOSPORIN	↑ risk of hyperkalaemia	Additive effect	➢ ***For signs and symptoms of hyperkalaemia, see Clinical Features of Some Adverse Drug Interactions, Hyperkalaemia***
POTASSIUM-SPARING DIURETICS	TACROLIMUS	Risk of hyperkalaemia	Additive effect	Monitor potassium levels closely
POTASSIUM-SPARING DIURETICS	**ANTIDEPRESSANTS**			
POTASSIUM-SPARING DIURETICS	LITHIUM	↑ plasma concentrations of lithium, with risk of toxic effects	↓ renal excretion of lithium	Monitor clinically and by measuring blood lithium levels for lithium toxicity
POTASSIUM-SPARING DIURETICS	ST JOHN'S WORT	↓ eplerenone levels	Induction of metabolism	Avoid co-administration
POTASSIUM-SPARING DIURETICS	**ANTIDIABETIC DRUGS**			
AMILORIDE	METFORMIN	↑ metformin levels and risk of lactic acidosis	Metformin is not metabolized in humans and is not protein-bound. Competition for renal tubular excretion is the basis for ↑ activity or retention of metformin	Theoretical possibility. Requires reduction of metformin dose to be considered, or the avoidance of co-administration

Primary drug	Secondary drug	Effect	Mechanism	Precautions
POTASSIUM-SPARING DIURETICS	SULPHONYLUREAS – CHLORPROPAMIDE	Risk of hyponatraemia when chlorpropamide is given to a patient taking both potassium-sparing diuretics/aldosterone antagonists and thiazides	Additive effect; chlorpropamide enhances ADH secretion	Monitor serum sodium regularly
POTASSIUM-SPARING DIURETICS	REPAGLINIDE	↓ hypoglycaemic effect	Antagonistic effect	Higher doses of repaglinide needed
POTASSIUM-SPARING DIURETICS	ANTIEPILEPTICS – BARBITURATES, CARBAMAZEPINE	↓ eplerenone levels	Induction of hepatic metabolism	Be aware; watch for poor response to eplerenone
POTASSIUM-SPARING DIURETICS	ANTIFUNGALS – KETOCONAZOLE	↑ eplerenone levels	Inhibition of metabolism	Avoid co-administration
POTASSIUM-SPARING DIURETICS	ANTIHYPERTENSIVES AND HEART FAILURE DRUGS – ACE INHIBITORS, ANGIOTENSIN II RECEPTOR ANTAGONISTS	↑ risk of hyperkalaemia	Additive retention of potassium	Monitor serum potassium every week until stable, then every 3–6 months
POTASSIUM-SPARING DIURETICS	ANTIPLATELET AGENTS – ASPIRIN	↓ efficacy of spironolactone	Uncertain	Watch for poor response to spironolactone
POTASSIUM-SPARING DIURETICS	ANTIVIRALS – PROTEASE INHIBITORS	Possibly ↑ adverse effects of eplerenone with nelfinavir, ritonavir (with or without lopinavir) and saquinavir	Inhibition of CYP3A4-mediated metabolism of eplerenone	Avoid concomitant use

POTASSIUM-SPARING DIURETICS	CALCIUM CHANNEL BLOCKERS	↑ serum concentrations of eplerenone when given with diltiazem and verapamil	Calcium channel blockers inhibit CYP3A4-mediated metabolism of eplerenone	Restrict dose of eplerenone to 25 mg/day. Monitor serum potassium concentrations closely; watch for hyperkalaemia
POTASSIUM-SPARING DIURETICS	**CARDIAC GLYCOSIDES**			
POTASSIUM-SPARING DIURETICS	DIGITOXIN	Conflicting results from volunteer studies; some showed ↑ (up to one-third) in the half-life of digitoxin, others a ↓ (up to one-fifth)	Uncertain at present	Watch for either digitoxin toxicity or a poor response, particularly for the first month after starting spironolactone
POTASSIUM-SPARING DIURETICS	DIGOXIN	Eplerenone and spironolactone may ↑ plasma concentrations of digoxin	Uncertain; spironolactone possibly ↓ the volume of distribution of digoxin	Watch for digoxin toxicity; check levels
POTASSIUM-SPARING DIURETICS	POTASSIUM	Risk of hyperkalaemia	Additive effect	Monitor potassium levels closely
POTASSIUM-SPARING DIURETICS	PROGESTOGENS	↑ risk of hyperkalaemia	Drospirenone (component of the Yasmin brand of combined contraceptive pill) is a progestogen derived from spironolactone that can cause potassium retention	Monitor serum potassium weekly until stable, then every 6 months
POTASSIUM-SPARING DIURETICS	TRILOSTANE	Risk of hyperkalaemia	Additive effect	Monitor potassium levels regularly during co-administration

Primary drug	Secondary drug	Effect	Mechanism	Precautions
THIAZIDES				
THIAZIDES	**ADDITIVE HYPOTENSIVE EFFECT**			
THIAZIDES	1. IMMUNOMODULATING DRUGS – IL-2 2. ANTI-HYPERTENSIVES AND HEART FAILURE DRUGS 3. BETA-BLOCKERS 4. CALCIUM CHANNEL BLOCKERS 5. NITRATES 6. PERIPHERAL VASODILATORS – moxisylyte (thymoxamine)	↑ hypotensive effect. Risk of first-dose ↓ BP is greater when ACE inhibitors are added to high-dose diuretics. Also, ↑ risk of first-dose ↓ BP with alfuzosin, prazosin and terazosin	Additive hypotensive effect; may be used therapeutically	Monitor BP at least weekly until stable. Warn patients to report symptoms of hypotension (light-headedness, dizziness on standing, etc.). Benefits often outweigh risks. Patients with congestive cardiac failure on diuretics should be started on a low dose of alpha-blocker
THIAZIDES	ANAESTHETICS – GENERAL	↑ hypotensive effect	Additive hypotensive effect	Monitor BP closely, especially during induction of anaesthesia
THIAZIDES	**ANTIARRHYTHMICS**			
THIAZIDES	AMIODARONE, DISOPYRAMIDE, FLECAINIDE	Risk of arrhythmias	Cardiac toxicity directly related to hypokalaemia	Monitor potassium levels every 4–6 weeks until stable, then at least annually
THIAZIDES	MEXILETINE	Effect of mexiletine ↓ by hypokalaemia	Uncertain	Normalize potassium levels before starting mexiletine
THIAZIDES	ANTIBIOTICS – TETRACYCLINES	Possible risk of renal toxicity	Additive effect	Some recommend avoiding co-administration; others advise monitoring renal function closely. Doxycycline likely to be less of a problem

THIAZIDES	ANTICANCER AND IMMUNOMODULATING DRUGS			
THIAZIDES	CYTOTOXICS – PORFIMER	↑ risk of photosensitivity reactions when porfimer is co-administered with hydrochlorothiazide	Attributed to additive effects	Avoid exposure of skin and eyes to direct sunlight for 30 days after porfimer therapy
THIAZIDES	HORMONES AND HORMONE ANTAGONISTS – TOREMIFENE	Risk of hypercalcaemia	Additive effect	Monitor calcium levels closely. Warn patients about the symptoms of hypercalcaemia
THIAZIDES	IMMUNOMODULATING DRUGS – CICLOSPORIN	Risk of nephrotoxicity	Additive effect	Monitor renal function weekly
THIAZIDES	ANTIDEPRESSANTS – LITHIUM	↑ plasma concentrations of lithium, with risk of toxic effects	↓ renal excretion of lithium	Monitor clinically and by measuring blood lithium levels for lithium toxicity. Loop diuretics are safer than thiazides
THIAZIDES	**ANTIDIABETIC DRUGS**			
THIAZIDES	SULPHONYLUREAS	Hypoglycaemic efficacy is ↓	Hyperglycaemia due to antagonistic effect	Monitor blood glucose regularly until stable. Higher dose of oral antidiabetic agent often needed
THIAZIDES	CHLORPROPAMIDE	Risk of hyponatraemia when chlorpropamide is given to a patient taking both potassium-sparing diuretics/aldosterone antagonists and thiazides	Additive effect; chlorpropamide enhances ADH secretion	Monitor serum sodium regularly
THIAZIDES	ANTIFUNGALS – AMPHOTERICIN	Risk of hypokalaemia	Additive effect	Monitor potassium closely
THIAZIDES	ANTIGOUT DRUGS	Possible ↑ risk of severe allergic reactions when allopurinol is given with thiazides in the presence of renal impairment	Uncertain	Caution in co-administering allopurinol with thiazides in the presence of renal insufficiency

CARDIOVASCULAR DRUGS DIURETICS

Primary drug	Secondary drug	Effect	Mechanism	Precautions
THIAZIDES	ANTIHYPERTENSIVES AND HEART FAILURE DRUGS – VASODILATOR ANTIHYPERTENSIVES	Risk of hyperglycaemia when diazoxide is co-administered with thiazides	Additive effect; both drugs have a hyperglycaemic effect	Monitor blood glucose closely, particularly with diabetes
THIAZIDES	ANTIPARKINSON'S DRUGS – LEVODOPA	↑ hypotensive effect	Additive effect	Monitor BP at least weekly until stable. Warn patients to report symptoms of hypotension (light-headedness, dizziness on standing, etc.)
THIAZIDES	ANTIPSYCHOTICS – ATYPICAL AGENTS, PHENOTHIAZINES, PIMOZIDE	Risk of arrhythmias	Cardiac toxicity directly related to hypokalaemia	Monitor potassium levels every 4–6 weeks until stable, then at least annually
THIAZIDES	BETA-BLOCKERS – SOTALOL	↑ risk of ventricular arrhythmias, particularly torsades de pointes, caused by sotalol	Hypokalaemia, a side-effect of these diuretics, predisposes to arrhythmias during sotalol therapy	Normalize potassium levels before starting sotalol in patients already taking these diuretics. When starting these diuretics in patients already taking sotalol, monitor potassium levels every 4–6 weeks until stable
THIAZIDES	BRONCHODILATORS – BETA-2 AGONISTS, THEOPHYLLINE	Risk of hypokalaemia	Additive effects	Monitor blood potassium levels prior to concomitant administration and during therapy. Administer potassium supplements to prevent hypokalaemia
THIAZIDES	CALCIUM	Risk of hypercalcaemia with high-dose calcium	↓ renal excretion of calcium by thiazides	Monitor calcium levels closely
THIAZIDES	CARDIAC GLYCOSIDES	Risk of digoxin toxicity ↑ due to hypokalaemia	Uncertain	Monitor potassium levels closely. Watch for digoxin toxicity and check levels

THIAZIDES	CNS STIMULANTS – ATOMOXETINE	↑ risk of arrhythmias with hypokalaemia	These diuretics may cause hypokalaemia	Monitor potassium levels closely
THIAZIDES	LIPID-LOWERING DRUGS – ANION EXCHANGE RESINS	Both colestipol and colestyramine markedly ↓ levels of thiazides	Colestipol and colestyramine bind diuretics in the intestine	Give the anion exchange resin 4 hours after thiazides (although the effect of hydrochlorothiazide may still be ↓ by colestyramine)
THIAZIDES	MUSCLE RELAXANTS	↑ antihypertensive effect with baclofen and tizanidine	Additive hypotensive effect	Monitor BP at least weekly until stable. Warn patients to report symptoms of hypotension (light-headedness, dizziness on standing, etc.)
THIAZIDES	ORLISTAT	Case of ↑ BP when orlistat is started for a patient on thiazides	Uncertain at present	Monitor BP at least weekly until stable
THIAZIDES	VITAMIN D	Risk of hypercalcaemia with vitamin D	↓ renal excretion of calcium by thiazides	Monitor calcium levels closely
IVABRADINE				
IVABRADINE	ANTIARRHYTHMICS – AMIODARONE, DISOPYRAMIDE	Risk of arrhythmias	Additive effect	Monitor ECG closely
IVABRADINE	ANTIBIOTICS	1. Risk of arrhythmias with erythromycin 2. Possible ↑ levels with clarithromycin and telithromycin	1. Additive effect 2. Uncertain	Avoid co-administration
IVABRADINE	ANTIDEPRESSANTS	↓ levels with St John's wort	Uncertain	Avoid co-administration
IVABRADINE	ANTIFUNGALS	↑ levels with ketoconazole and possibly fluconazole and itraconazole	Uncertain	Avoid co-administration
IVABRADINE	ANTIMALARIALS	Risk of arrhythmias with mefloquine	Additive effect	Monitor ECG closely

Primary drug	Secondary drug	Effect	Mechanism	Precautions
IVABRADINE	ANTIPROTOZOALS	Risk of arrhythmias with pentamidine	Additive effect	Monitor ECG closely
IVABRADINE	ANTIPSYCHOTICS	Risk of arrhythmias with pimozide and sertindole	Additive effect	Monitor ECG closely
IVABRADINE	ANTIVIRALS – PROTEASE INHIBITORS	↑ levels with nelfinavir and ritonavir	Uncertain	Avoid co-administration
IVABRADINE	BETA-BLOCKERS – SOTALOL	Risk of arrhythmias	Additive effect; ivabradine slows the sinus node	Monitor ECG closely
IVABRADINE	CALCIUM CHANNEL BLOCKERS	↑ levels with diltiazem and verapamil	Uncertain	Avoid co-administration
IVABRADINE	GRAPEFRUIT JUICE	↑ levels with grapefruit juice	Uncertain	Avoid co-administration
LIPID-LOWERING DRUGS				
ANION EXCHANGE RESINS				
ANION EXCHANGE RESINS	ANALGESICS			
ANION EXCHANGE RESINS	NSAIDs	Colestyramine ↓ absorption of NSAIDs	Colestyramine binds NSAIDs in the intestine, reducing their absorption; it also binds those NSAIDs with a significant entero-hepatic recirculation (meloxicam, piroxicam, sulindac, tenoxicam)	Give the NSAID 1 hour before or 4–6 hours after colestyramine; however, meloxicam, piroxicam, sulindac and tenoxicam should not be given with colestyramine
ANION EXCHANGE RESINS	PARACETAMOL	Colestyramine ↓ paracetamol by 60% when they are given together	Colestyramine binds paracetamol in the intestine	Give colestyramine and paracetamol at least 1 hour apart

ANION EXCHANGE RESINS	ANTIARRHYTHMICS – AMIODARONE	Colestyramine ↓ amiodarone levels	Colestyramine binds amiodarone, reducing its absorption and interrupting its enterohepatic circulation	Avoid co-administration
ANION EXCHANGE RESINS	**ANTIBIOTICS**			
ANION EXCHANGE RESINS	TETRACYCLINE	↓ levels of tetracycline and possible therapeutic failure	Tetracycline binds with colestipol and colestyramine in the gut therefore reducing its absorption	Dosing should be as separate as possible
ANION EXCHANGE RESINS	VANCOMYCIN (ORAL)	↓ vancomycin levels	Inhibition of absorption	Separate doses as much as possible
ANION EXCHANGE RESINS	**ANTICANCER AND IMMUNOMODULATING DRUGS**			
ANION EXCHANGE RESINS	**CYTOTOXICS**			
ANION EXCHANGE RESINS	METHOTREXATE	Parenteral methotrexate levels may be ↓ by colestyramine	Colestyramine interrupts the enterohepatic circulation of methotrexate	Avoid co-administration
ANION EXCHANGE RESINS	MYCOPHENOLATE	↓ plasma concentrations of mycophenolate by approximately 40%. Risk of therapeutic failure	Due to interruption of enterohepatic circulation because of binding of recirculating mycophenolate with cholestyramine in the intestine	Avoid co-administration
ANION EXCHANGE RESINS	LEFLUNOMIDE	↓ levels of leflunomide	↓ absorption	Avoid co-administration
ANION EXCHANGE RESINS	ANTICOAGULANTS – ORAL	↓ anticoagulant effect with colestyramine	↓ absorption of warfarin	Give warfarin 1 hour before or 4–6 hours after colestyramine

Primary drug	Secondary drug	Effect	Mechanism	Precautions
ANION EXCHANGE RESINS	ANTIDIABETIC DRUGS			
ANION EXCHANGE RESINS	ACARBOSE	↑ hypoglycaemic effect of acarbose	Uncertain	Monitor blood glucose during and co-administration and after discontinuation of concurrent therapy
ANION EXCHANGE RESINS	SULPHONYLUREAS – GLIPIZIDE	Glipizide absorption may be ↓ by colestyramine	Colestyramine interrupts the enterohepatic circulation of glipizide	Avoid co-administration
ANION EXCHANGE RESINS	CALCIUM CHANNEL BLOCKERS	Colestipol ↓ diltiazem levels	Colestipol binds diltiazem in the intestine	Monitor for poor response to diltiazem. Separating doses of diltiazem and colestipol does not seem to ↓ this interaction
ANION EXCHANGE RESINS	CARDIAC GLYCOSIDES	Colestipol and colestyramine may ↓ digoxin and digitoxin levels	Both colestipol and colestyramine are ion exchange resins that bind bile sodiums and prevent reabsorption in the intestine; this breaks the enterohepatic cycle of digoxin and digitoxin	Colestipol and colestyramine should be given at least 1.5 hours after digoxin and digitoxin
ANION EXCHANGE RESINS	DIURETICS	Both colestipol and colestyramine markedly ↓ levels of loop diuretics and thiazides	Colestipol and colestyramine bind diuretics in the intestine	Give the anion exchange resin 3 hours after furosemide and 4 hours after thiazides (although the effect of hydrochlorothiazide may still be ↓ by colestyramine)
ANION EXCHANGE RESINS	IRON – ORAL	↓ iron levels when iron is given orally with cholestyramine	↓ absorption	Separate doses as much as possible – monitor FBC closely
ANION EXCHANGE RESINS	LIPID-LOWERING DRUGS – STATINS	Anion-binding resins ↓ the absorption of statins, but the overall lipid-lowering effect is not altered	Anion-binding resins bind statins in the intestine	Giving the statin 1 hour before or 3–6 hours after the anion exchange resin should minimize this effect

CARDIOVASCULAR DRUGS LIPID-LOWERING DRUGS

ANION EXCHANGE RESINS	RALOXIFENE	Raloxifene levels may be ↓ by colestyramine	Colestyramine interrupts the enterohepatic circulation of raloxifene	Avoid co-administration
ANION EXCHANGE RESINS	THYROID HORMONES	↓ efficacy of thyroid hormones	↓ absorption	Separate doses by at least 4–6 hours. Monitor TFTs
EZETIMIBE				
EZETIMIBE	ANTICANCER AND IMMUNOMODULATING DRUGS – CICLOSPORIN	↑ levels of both drugs when ezetimibe is co-administered with ciclosporin	Uncertain	Watch for signs of ciclosporin toxicity
EZETIMIBE	LIPID-LOWERING DRUGS	Risk of gallstones with fibrates	Uncertain	Stop co-administration if symptoms develop
FIBRATES				
FIBRATES	ANTACIDS	Gemfibrozil levels may be ↓ by antacids	Uncertain	Give gemfibrozil 1–2 hours before the antacid
FIBRATES	ANTIBIOTICS – DAPTOMYCIN	Risk of myopathy	Additive effect	Avoid co-administration
FIBRATES	**ANTICANCER AND IMMUNOMODULATING DRUGS**			
GEMFIBROZIL	CYTOTOXICS – BEXAROTENE	Gemfibrozil may ↑ bexarotene levels	Uncertain at present	Avoid co-administration
FIBRATES	IMMUNOMODULATING DRUGS – CICLOSPORIN	↑ risk with renal failure	Uncertain at present	Monitor renal function closely
FIBRATES	ANTICOAGULANTS – ORAL	↑ efficacy of warfarin and phenindione	Uncertain; postulated that fibrates displace anticoagulants from their binding sites	Monitor INR closely

Primary drug	Secondary drug	Effect	Mechanism	Precautions
FIBRATES	**ANTIDIABETIC DRUGS**			
FIBRATES	SULPHONYLUREAS – TOLBUTAMIDE	Fibrates may ↑ the efficacy of sulphonylureas	Uncertain; postulated that fibrates displace sulphonylureas from plasma proteins and ↓ their hepatic metabolism. In addition, fenofibrate may inhibit CYP2C9-mediated metabolism of tolbutamide	Monitor blood glucose levels closely
GEMFIBROZIL	REPAGLINIDE	Nearly eightfold ↑ in repaglinide levels, with risk of severe hypoglycaemia. Risk of severe and prolonged hypoglycaemia	Hepatic metabolism inhibited	The European Agency for the Evaluation of Medicinal Products contraindicated concurrent use in 2003. Bezafibrate and fenofibrate are suitable alternatives if a fibric acid derivative is required
GEMFIBROZIL	ROSIGLITAZONE	↑ in blood levels of rosiglitazone – often doubled	Gemfibrozil is a relatively selective inhibitor of CYP2C8	Watch for hypoglycaemic events and ↓ the dose of rosiglitazone after repeated blood sugar measurements. Warn patients about hypoglycaemia ➢ ***For signs and symptoms of hypoglycaemia, see Clinical Features of Some Adverse Drug Interactions, Hypoglycaemia***
FIBRATES	ANTIEPILEPTICS	Gemfibrozil may↑ carbamazepine levels	Uncertain at present	Watch for features of carbamazepine toxicity
FIBRATES	**LIPID-LOWERING DRUGS**			
FIBRATES	EZETIMIBE	Risk of gallstones with fibrates	Uncertain	Stop co-administration if symptoms develop

FIBRATES	STATINS	Gemfibrozil may ↑ atorvastatin, rosuvastatin and simvastatin levels (risk of myopathy with simvastatin)	Uncertain	Avoid co-administration of simvastatin and gemfibrozil. When using other statins, warn patients to watch for the features of myopathy
STATINS				
SIMVASTATIN	ANTIARRHYTHMICS – AMIODARONE	↑ risk of myopathy with high doses (>40 mg) of simvastatin co-administered with amiodarone	Uncertain; amiodarone inhibits intestinal P-gp, which may ↑ the bioavailability of statins	Avoid >20 mg doses of simvastatin in patients taking amiodarone; if higher doses are required, switch to an alternative statin
STATINS	**ANTIBIOTICS**			
FIBRATES	ANTIBIOTICS – DAPTOMYCIN	Risk of myopathy	Additive effect	Avoid co-administration
STATINS	FUSIDIC ACID	Cases of rhabdomyolysis reported when fusidic acid was co-administered with atorvastatin or simvastatin	Uncertain at present	Monitor LFTs and CK closely; warn patients to report any features of rhabdomyolysis
STATINS	**MACROLIDES**			
ATORVASTATIN, SIMVASTATIN	MACROLIDES	Macrolides may ↑ levels of atorvastatin and simvastatin; the risk of myopathy ↑ over 10-fold when erythromycin is co-administered with a statin	Macrolides inhibit CYP3A4-mediated metabolism of atorvastatin and simvastatin. Also, erythromycin and clarithromycin inhibit intestinal P-gp, which may ↑ the bioavailability of statins	Avoid co-administration of macrolides with atorvastatin or simvastatin (temporarily stop the statin if the patient needs macrolide therapy). Manufacturers also recommend that patients be warned to look for the early signs of rhabdomyolysis when other statins are co-ingested with macrolides

Primary drug	Secondary drug	Effect	Mechanism	Precautions
ROSUVASTATIN	ERYTHROMYCIN	↓ rosuvastatin levels with erythromycin	Uncertain	Avoid chronic co-administration
STATINS	RIFAMPICIN	Rifampicin may lower fluvastatin and simvastatin levels	Uncertain	Monitor lipid profile closely; look for poor response to fluvastatin and simvastatin
STATINS	**ANTICANCER AND IMMUNOMODULATING DRUGS**			
STATINS	**CYTOTOXICS**			
SIMVASTATIN	DASATINIB	Possible ↓ simvastatin levels	↑ metabolism of simvastatin	Monitor lipid profile closely and adjust simvastatin dose accordingly when starting and stopping co-administration
ATORVASTATIN, SIMVASTATIN	IMATINIB	Imatinib may ↑ atorvastatin and simvastatin levels	Imatinib inhibits CYP3A4-mediated metabolism of simvastatin	Monitor LFTs, U&Es and CK closely
STATINS	**IMMUNOMODULATING DRUGS**			
STATINS – ATORVASTATIN, LOVASTATIN, ROSUVASTATIN, SIMVASTATIN	CICLOSPORIN	↑ plasma concentrations of these statins, with risk of myopathy and rhabdomyolysis	Ciclosporin is a moderate inhibitor of CYP3A4, which metabolizes these statins	↓ statins to lowest possible dose (do not give simvastatin in doses >10 mg). Monitor LFTs and CK closely; warn patients to report any features of rhabdomyolysis. This interaction does not occur with pravastatin
STATINS	TACROLIMUS	Single case report of rhabdomyolysis when was simvastatin added to tacrolimus	Uncertain at present	Monitor LFTs and CK closely; warn patients to report any features of rhabdomyolysis
STATINS	ANTICOAGULANTS – ORAL	Possible ↑ anticoagulant effect with fluvastatin and simvastatin	Uncertain; possibly due to inhibition of CYP2C9-mediated metabolism of warfarin	Monitor INR closely

STATINS	ANTIDEPRESSANTS – ST JOHN'S WORT	St John's wort may lower simvastatin levels	Uncertain at present	Monitor lipid profile closely; look for poor response to simvastatin
STATINS	**ANTIDIABETIC DRUGS**			
STATINS	NATEGLINIDE, REPAGLINIDE	↑ incidence of adverse effects such as myalgia. There was an ↑ in maximum concentration of repaglinide by 25% with high variability	Uncertain. Statins are also substrates for CYP3A4, and competition for metabolism by the enzyme system may be a factor	Clinical significance is uncertain, but it is necessary to be aware of this. Warn patients about the adverse effects of statins and repaglinide
EZETIMIBE, SIMVASTATIN	REPAGLINIDE	↑ repaglinide levels, risk of hypoglycaemia	Hepatic metabolism is inhibited	Watch for and warn patients about hypoglycaemia ➢ ***For signs and symptoms of hypoglycaemia, see Clinical Features of Some Adverse Drug Interactions, Hypoglycaemia***
STATINS	ANTIFUNGALS	Azoles markedly ↑ atorvastatin, simvastatin (both with cases of myopathy reported) and possibly pravastatin. These effects are less likely with fluvastatin and rosuvastatin, although fluconazole may cause moderate rises in their levels	Itraconazole and ketoconazole inhibit CYP3A4-mediated metabolism of these statins; they also inhibit intestinal P-gp, which ↑ the bioavailability of statins; itraconazole may block the transport of atorvastatin due to inhibition of the OATP1B1 enzyme system. Some manufacturers suggest that the small ↑ in plasma levels of pravastatin may be due to ↑ absorption. Voriconazole is an inhibitor of CYP2C9. Fluconazole inhibits CYP2C9 and CYP3A4	Avoid co-administration of simvastatin and atorvastatin with azole antifungals. Care should be taken with co-administration of other statins and azoles. Although fluvastatin and rosuvastatin may be considered as alternatives, consider reducing the dose of statin and warn patients to report any features of rhabdomyolysis. Check LFTs and CK regularly

Primary drug	Secondary drug	Effect	Mechanism	Precautions
STATINS	**ANTIHYPERTENSIVES AND HEART FAILURE DRUGS**			
STATINS	VASODILATOR ANTIHYPERTENSIVES	Bosentan lowers simvastatin levels	Uncertain; bosentan moderately inhibits CYP3A4	Monitor lipid profile closely; look for poor response to simvastatin
STATINS	ANTIPLATELET AGENTS – CLOPIDOGREL	Atorvastatin and possibly simvastatin ↓ the antiplatelet effect of clopidogrel in a dose-dependent manner	Atorvastatin and simvastatin inhibit CYP3A4-mediated activation of clopidogrel	Use these statins at the lowest possible dose; otherwise consider using an alternative statin
STATINS	**ANTIVIRALS**			
STATINS	NNRTIs	↓ levels of atorvastatin, pravastatin and simvastatin with efavirenz	Uncertain; efavirenz is known to induce intestinal P-gp, which may ↓ the bioavailability of some statins (including atorvastatin)	Monitor lipid profile closely
ATORVASTATIN	PROTEASE INHIBITORS	↑ efficacy and ↑ risk of adverse effects of atorvastatin	Inhibition of CYP3A4-mediated metabolism of atorvastatin	Use with caution: monitor for atorvastatin toxicity; monitor CK. Inform patient and ↓ dose if necessary or start with 10 mg once daily. Use the lowest dose possible to attain target low-density lipoprotein reduction. Alternatives are pravastatin or fluvastatin
LOVASTATIN, SIMVASTATIN	PROTEASE INHIBITORS	↑ risk of adverse effects	Inhibition of CYP3A4-mediated metabolism of simvastatin	Avoid co-administration
STATINS	CALCIUM CHANNEL BLOCKERS	↑ plasma levels of atorvastatin, lovastatin and simvastatin; case reports of myopathy when atorvastatin and simvastatin are co-administered with diltiazem or verapamil	Uncertain, but postulated to be due to inhibition of CYP3A4-mediated metabolism of statins in the intestinal wall. Also, diltiazem and verapamil inhibit intestinal P-gp, which may ↑ the bioavailability of statins	Watch for side-effects of statins. It has been suggested that the dose of simvastatin should not exceed 20 mg when given with verapamil, and 40 mg when given with diltiazem

STATINS	CARDIAC GLYCOSIDES	High-dose (80 mg) atorvastatin may ↑ digoxin levels	Atorvastatin inhibits intestinal P-gp, which ↑ digoxin absorption	Watch for digoxin toxicity
FLUVASTATIN	CNS STIMULANTS – MODAFINIL	May cause ↑ plasma concentrations of fluvastatin if CYP2C9 is the predominant metabolic pathway and the alternative pathways are either genetically deficient or affected	Modafinil is a moderate inhibitor of CYP2C9	Be aware
STATINS	GRAPEFRUIT JUICE	↑ levels with simvastatin; slight rise with atorvastatin. ↑ risk of adverse effects such as myopathy	Constituent of grapefruit juice inhibits CYP3A4-mediated metabolism of simvastatin	Patients taking simvastatin and atorvastatin should avoid grapefruit juice
STATINS	**LIPID-LOWERING DRUGS**			
STATINS	ANION EXCHANGE RESINS	Anion-binding resins ↓ the absorption of statins, but the overall lipid-lowering effect is not altered	Anion-binding resins bind statins in the intestine	Giving the statin 1 hour before or 3–6 hours after the anion exchange resin should minimize this effect
STATINS	FIBRATES	Gemfibrozil may ↑ atorvastatin, rosuvastatin and simvastatin levels, with risk of myopathy with simvastatin	Uncertain	Avoid co-administration of simvastatin and fibrates. When using other statins, warn patients to watch for the features of myopathy
STATINS	NICOTINIC ACID	Slight risk of rhabdomyolysis	Uncertain at present	Monitor LFTs and CK closely; warn patients to report any features of rhabdomyolysis
STATINS	PROTON PUMP INHIBITORS	Possible ↑ efficacy and adverse effects of atorvastatin	Inhibition of P-gp, reducing first-pass clearance	Monitor closely

Primary drug	Secondary drug	Effect	Mechanism	Precautions
NITRATES				
NITRATES	ADDITIVE HYPOTENSIVE EFFECT			
NITRATES	1. ANAESTHETICS – GENERAL 2. ANTICANCER AND IMMUNOMODULATING DRUGS – IL-2 3. ANTIDEPRESSANTS – MAOIs 4. ANTIHYPERTENSIVES AND HEART FAILURE DRUGS 5. ANTIPSYCHOTICS 6. ANXIOLYTICS AND HYPNOTICS 7. BETA-BLOCKERS 8. CALCIUM CHANNEL BLOCKERS 9. DIURETICS 10. MUSCLE RELAXANTS – baclofen, tizanidine 11. PERIPHERAL VASODILATORS – moxisylyte (thymoxamine) 12. POTASSIUM CHANNEL ACTIVATORS	↑ hypotensive effect	Additive hypotensive effect. Aldesleukin causes ↓ vascular resistance and ↑ capillary permeability	Monitor BP at least weekly until stable. Warn patients to report symptoms of hypotension (light-headedness, dizziness on standing, etc.). During anaesthesia, monitor BP closely, especially during induction of anaesthesia
NITRATES	PHOSPHODIESTERASE TYPE 5 INHIBITORS	Risk of severe ↓ BP and precipitation of myocardial infarction	Additive effect	Avoid co-administration

CARDIOVASCULAR DRUGS NITRATES

NITRATES	ADDITIVE ANTIMUSCARINIC EFFECTS			
NITRATES	1. ANALGESICS – nefopam 2. ANTIARRHYTHMICS – disopyramide, propafenone 3. ANTIDEPRESSANTS – TCAs 4. ANTIEMETICS – cyclizine 5. ANTIHISTAMINES – chlorphenamine, cyproheptadine, hydroxyzine 6. ANTIMUSCARINICS – atropine, benzatropine, cyclopentolate, dicycloverine, flavoxate, homatropine, hyoscine, orphenadrine, oxybutynin, procyclidine, propantheline, tolterodine, trihexyphenidyl, tropicamide. 7. ANTI-PARKINSON'S DRUGS – dopaminergics 8. ANTI-PSYCHOTICS – phenothiazines, clozapine, pimozide 9. MUSCLE RELAXANTS – baclofen	1. ↑ risk of antimuscarinic side-effects when isosorbide dinitrate is co-administered with these drugs 2. ↓ efficacy of sublingual nitrate tablets	1. Additive effect; both of these drugs cause antimuscarinic side-effects 2. Antimuscarinic effects ↓ saliva production, which ↓ dissolution of the tablet	(a) Warn patients of these effects (b) Consider changing the formulation to a sublingual nitrate spray
NITRATES	ALCOHOL	↑ risk of postural ↓ BP when GTN taken with alcohol	Additive effect; both vasodilators	Warn the patient about the risk of feeling faint. Advise patients to drink only in moderation and to avoid binge drinking

CARDIOVASCULAR DRUGS NITRATES

Primary drug	Secondary drug	Effect	Mechanism	Precautions
NITRATES	ANALGESICS – NSAIDS	Hypotensive effects of hydralazine, minoxidil and nitroprusside antagonized by NSAIDs	NSAIDs cause sodium and water retention in the kidney and can raise BP due to ↓ production of vasodilating renal prostaglandins	Monitor BP at least weekly until stable
NITRATES	ANTICANCER AND IMMUNOMODULATING DRUGS – CORTICOSTEROIDS	Antihypertensive effects of calcium channel blockers are antagonized by corticosteroids	Mineralocorticoids cause sodium and water retention, which antagonizes the hypotensive effects of calcium channel blockers	Monitor BP at least weekly until stable
NITRATES	ANTICOAGULANTS – HEPARINS	Possible ↓ efficacy of heparin with GTN infusion	Uncertain	Monitor APTT closely
NITRATES	ANTIHYPERTENSIVES AND HEART FAILURE DRUGS	↑ hypotensive effect	Additive hypotensive effect; may be used therapeutically	Monitor BP at least weekly until stable. Warn patients to report symptoms of hypotension (light-headedness, dizziness on standing, etc.)
NITRATES	ANTIPARKINSON'S DRUGS – APOMORPHINE	Risk of postural ↓ BP when apomorphine is given with nitrates	Additive effect; apomorphine can cause postural ↓ BP	Monitor BP at least weekly until stable. Warn patients to report symptoms of hypotension (light-headedness, dizziness on standing, etc.)
NITRATES	ANTIPLATELET AGENTS – ASPIRIN	↓ antihypertensive effect with aspirin; effect not noted with low-dose aspirin	Aspirin may cause sodium retention and vasoconstriction at possibly both renal and endothelial sites	Monitor BP at least weekly until stable
NITRATES	OESTROGENS	↓ antihypertensive effect of nitrates	Oestrogens may cause fluid retention, and use of oestrogens with hypertension needs to be closely monitored	Monitor BP at least weekly until stable; watch for poor response to nitrates

NITRATES	PROSTAGLANDINS – ALPROSTADIL	↑ risk of ↓ BP	Additive hypotensive effect	Monitor BP at least weekly until stable. Warn patients to report symptoms of hypotension (light-headedness, dizziness on standing, etc.)
PERIPHERAL VASODILATORS				
CILOSTAZOL				
CILOSTAZOL	ANAGRELIDE	Risk of adverse effects	Additive effect; anagrelide has phosphodiesterase inhibitory activity	Avoid co-administration
CILOSTAZOL	ANTIBIOTICS	Cilostazol levels ↑ by erythromycin and possibly clarithromycin	Erythromycin and clarithromycin inhibit CYP3A4-mediated metabolism of cilostazol	Avoid co-administration
CILOSTAZOL	ANTIDEPRESSANTS – SSRIs	Fluoxetine, fluvoxamine and sertraline ↑ cilostazol levels	Fluoxetine, fluvoxamine and sertraline inhibit CYP3A4-mediated metabolism of cilostazol	Avoid co-administration
CILOSTAZOL	ANTIFUNGALS	Fluconazole, itraconazole, ketoconazole and miconazole ↑ cilostazol levels	These azoles inhibit CYP3A4-mediated metabolism of cilostazol	Avoid co-administration
CILOSTAZOL	**ANTIPLATELET DRUGS**			
CILOSTAZOL	ASPIRIN	Possible ↑ risk of bleeding. Low-dose aspirin (<80 mg) appears to be safe	Additive effect; cilostazol has antiplatelet activity	Warn the patient to report any signs of ↑ bleeding

Primary drug	Secondary drug	Effect	Mechanism	Precautions
CILOSTAZOL	CLOPIDOGREL, DIPYRIDAMOLE, GLYCOPROTEIN IIb/IIIa INHIBITORS	Possible ↑ risk of bleeding with cilostazol	Additive effect; cilostazol has antiplatelet activity. Clopidogrel ↑ the levels of a metabolite of cilostazol that has high antiplatelet activity, by an uncertain mechanism	Warn the patient to report any signs of ↑ bleeding
CILOSTAZOL	ANTIVIRALS – PROTEASE INHIBITORS	Amprenavir, indinavir, lopinavir, nelfinavir, ritonavir and saquinavir ↑ cilostazol levels	These protease inhibitors inhibit CYP3A4-mediated metabolism of cilostazol	Avoid co-administration
CILOSTAZOL	ANXIOLYTICS AND HYPNOTICS	Midazolam ↑ cilostazol levels	Midazolam inhibits CYP3A4-mediated metabolism of cilostazol	Avoid co-administration
CILOSTAZOL	CALCIUM CHANNEL BLOCKERS	↑ plasma concentrations and efficacy of cilostazol with diltiazem, verapamil and nifedipine	These calcium channel blockers inhibit CYP3A4-mediated metabolism of cilostazol	Avoid co-administration
CILOSTAZOL	FOOD	Cilostazol levels are ↑ by taking it with a high-fat meal	Uncertain	Take cilostazol at least 30 minutes before or 2 hours after a meal
CILOSTAZOL	H2 RECEPTOR BLOCKERS	Cimetidine ↑ cilostazol levels	Cimetidine inhibits CYP3A4-mediated metabolism of cilostazol	Avoid co-administration
CILOSTAZOL	PROTON PUMP INHIBITORS	Cilostazol levels are ↑ by omeprazole and possibly lansoprazole	Omeprazole inhibits CYP2C19-mediated metabolism of cilostazol	Avoid concomitant use. US manufacturer advises halving the dose of cilostazol

CARDIOVASCULAR DRUGS PERIPHERAL VASODILATORS

MOXISYLYTE (THYMOXAMINE)				
MOXISYLYTE	**ADDITIVE HYPOTENSIVE EFFECT**			
MOXISYLYTE	1. ANAESTHETICS – GENERAL 2. ANTICANCER AND IMMUNOMODULATING DRUGS – IL-2 3. ANTIDEPRESSANTS – MAOIs 4. ANTIHYPERTENSIVES AND HEART FAILURE DRUGS 5. ANTIPSYCHOTICS 6. ANXIOLYTICS AND HYPNOTICS 7. BETA-BLOCKERS 8. CALCIUM CHANNEL BLOCKERS 9. DIURETICS 10. MUSCLE RELAXANTS – baclofen, tizanidine 11. NITRATES 12. POTASSIUM CHANNEL ACTIVATORS	↑ hypotensive effect	Additive hypotensive effect	Monitor BP at least weekly until stable. Warn patients to report symptoms of hypotension (light-headedness, dizziness on standing, etc.). During anaesthesia, monitor BP closely, especially during induction of anaesthesia
MOXISYLYTE	PROSTAGLANDINS – ALPROSTADIL	Risk of priapism if intracavernous alprostadil is given with moxisylyte	Additive effect	Avoid co-administration

Primary drug	Secondary drug	Effect	Mechanism	Precautions
PENTOXIFYLLINE				
PENTOXIFYLLINE	ANALGESICS – NSAIDS	Risk of bleeding when pentoxifylline is given with ketorolac post surgery	Uncertain; possibly additive antiplatelet effect	Avoid co-administration of pentoxifylline and ketorolac
PENTOXIFYLLINE	ANTIBIOTICS	Ciprofloxacin may ↑ pentoxifylline levels	Uncertain; likely to be due to inhibition of hepatic metabolism	Warn patients of the possibility of adverse effects of pentoxifylline
PENTOXIFYLLINE	ANTICOAGULANTS – ORAL	Case reports of major haemorrhage when pentoxifylline was given with acenocoumarol	Uncertain; possibly additive effect (pentoxifylline has an antiplatelet action)	Monitor INR closely
PENTOXIFYLLINE	BRONCHODILATORS – THEOPHYLLINE	Possibly ↑ theophylline levels	Uncertain; possibly competitive inhibition of theophylline metabolism (pentoxifylline is also a xanthine derivative)	Warn patients of the possibility of adverse effects of theophylline; monitor levels if necessary
PENTOXIFYLLINE	H2 RECEPTOR BLOCKERS	Cimetidine may ↑ pentoxifylline levels	Uncertain; likely to be due to inhibition of hepatic metabolism	Avoid co-administration

CARDIOVASCULAR DRUGS PERIPHERAL VASODILATORS

POTASSIUM CHANNEL ACTIVATORS – e.g. NICORANDIL				
POTASSIUM CHANNEL ACTIVATORS	ADDITIVE HYPOTENSIVE EFFECT			
POTASSIUM CHANNEL ACTIVATORS	1. ANAESTHETICS – GENERAL 2. ANTICANCER AND IMMUNOMODULATING DRUGS – IL-2 3. ANTIDEPRESSANTS – MAOIs 4. ANTIHYPERTENSIVES AND HEART FAILURE DRUGS – VASODILATOR ANTIHYPERTENSIVES 5. ANTIPSYCHOTICS 6. ANXIOLYTICS AND HYPNOTICS 7. BETA-BLOCKERS 8. CALCIUM CHANNEL BLOCKERS 9. DIURETICS 10. MUSCLE RELAXANTS – baclofen, tizanidine 11. NITRATES 12. PERIPHERAL VASODILATORS – moxisylyte (thymoxamine) 13. PHOSPHODIESTERASE TYPE 5 INHIBITORS	↑ hypotensive effect	Additive effect	Avoid co-administration of nicorandil with phosphodiesterase type 5 inhibitors. For other drugs, monitor BP closely

CARDIOVASCULAR DRUGS POTASSIUM CHANNEL ACTIVATORS

Primary drug	Secondary drug	Effect	Mechanism	Precautions
POTASSIUM CHANNEL ACTIVATORS	ALCOHOL	Acute alcohol ingestion may ↑ hypotensive effects. Chronic moderate/heavy drinking ↓ hypotensive effect	Additive hypotensive effect. Mechanism of opposite effect with chronic intake is uncertain	Monitor BP closely as unpredictable responses can occur. Advise patients to drink only in moderation and avoid large variations in the amount of alcohol drunk
SELECTIVE PHOSPHODIESTERASE INHIBITORS				
ENOXIMONE, MILRINONE	ANAGRELIDE	Risk of adverse effects	Additive effect; anagrelide has phosphodiesterase inhibitory activity	Avoid co-administration
ENOXIMONE	BRONCHODILATORS – THEOPHYLLINE	Theophylline may ↓ efficacy of enoximone	Possibly competitive inhibition of selective phosphodiesterases	Be aware; watch for poor response to enoximone
SYMPATHOMIMETICS				
SYMPATHOMIMETICS	ANAESTHETICS – GENERAL			
DIRECT	ANAESTHETICS – GENERAL	1. Risk of arrhythmias when inhalational anaesthetics are co-administered with epinephrine or norepinephrine 2. Case report of marked ↑ BP when phenylephrine eye drops given during general anaesthesia	1. Inhalational anaesthetics seem to sensitize the myocardium to beta-adrenoceptor stimulation 2. Uncertain	1. Use epinephrine in the smallest possible dose (when using 1 in 100 000 infiltration to ↓ intraoperative bleeding, no more than 10 mL per 10 minutes and less than 30 mL/hour should be given) 2. Use alternative mydriatic drops during general anaesthesia

CARDIOVASCULAR DRUGS SYMPATHOMIMETICS

INDIRECT	ANAESTHETICS – GENERAL	1. Risk of arrhythmias when inhalational anaesthetics are co-administered with methylphenidate 2. Case report of ↓ sedative effect of midazolam and ketamine from methylphenidate	1. Uncertain; it is possible that inhalational anaesthetics sensitize the myocardium to sympathetic stimulation 2. Uncertain at present	Avoid giving methylphenidate on the day of elective surgery
INDIRECT	ANALGESICS	Dexamfetamine and methylphenidate ↑ the analgesic effects and ↓ the sedation of opioids when used for chronic pain	Uncertain; complex interaction between the sympathetic nervous system and the opioid receptors	Opioid requirements may be ↓ when patients also take indirect sympathomimetics
SYMPATHOMIMETICS	ANTACIDS – SODIUM BICARBONATE	Possibly ↑ ephedrine/ pseudoephedrine levels	Alkalinising urine ↓ excretion of these sympathomimetics	Watch for early features of toxicity
SYMPATHOMIMETICS	**ANTIBIOTICS**			
SYMPATHOMIMETICS	LINEZOLID	Risk of ↑ BP when linezolid is co-ingested with either direct or indirect sympathomimetics	Linezolid causes accumulation of norepinephrine at the nerve ends; sympathomimetics stimulate the release of these ↑ reserves of norepinephrine, which in turn causes vasoconstriction and a rise in BP	Monitor BP closely; watch for ↑ BP. Warn patients taking linezolid not to take OTC remedies containing sympathomimetics
DIRECT	VANCOMYCIN	Vancomycin levels are ↓ by dobutamine or dopamine	Uncertain at present	Monitor vancomycin levels closely

Primary drug	Secondary drug	Effect	Mechanism	Precautions
SYMPATHOMIMETICS	**ANTICANCER AND IMMUNOMODULATING DRUGS**			
SYMPATHOMIMETICS	CYTOTOXICS – PROCARBAZINE	Co-administration of ephedrine, metaraminol, methylphenidate, phenylephrine or pseudoephedrine (including nasal and ophthalmic solutions) with procarbazine may cause a prolongation and ↑ intensity of the cardiac stimulant effects and effects on BP, which may lead to headache, arrhythmias, hypertensive or hyperpyretic crisis	The metabolism of sympathomimetics is impaired due to an inhibition of MAO	It is recommended that sympathomimetics not be administered during and within 14 days of stopping procarbazine. Do not use any OTC nasal decongestants (sprays or oral preparations) or asthma relief agents without consulting the pharmacist/doctor
SYMPATHOMIMETICS	**IMMUNOMODULATING DRUGS**			
INDIRECT	CICLOSPORIN	Methylphenidate may ↑ ciclosporin levels	Uncertain at present	Watch for ciclosporin toxicity; ↓ levels as necessary and monitor levels if available
INDIRECT	CORTICOSTEROIDS	Ephedrine may ↓ dexamethasone levels	Uncertain at present	Watch for poor response to dexamethasone; uncertain at present if other corticosteroids are similarly affected
INDIRECT	ANTICOAGULANTS	Methylphenidate may ↑ efficacy of warfarin	Uncertain at present	Monitor INR closely
SYMPATHOMIMETICS	**ANTIDEPRESSANTS**			
DIRECT	MAOIs	Risk of adrenergic syndrome – see above. Unlikely to occur with moclobemide and selegiline. This is likely with some OTC medications, which may contain some of these sympathomimetics	Due to inhibition of MAOI, which breaks down sympathomimetics. Moclobemide is involved in the breakdown of serotonin, while selegiline is mainly involved in the breakdown of dopamine	Avoid concurrent use. Onset may be 6–24 hours after ingestion. Do an ECG; measure electrolytes, FBC, CK and coagulation profile. Before prescribing/dispensing, enquire about the use of MAOI antidepressants and related drugs such as linezolid

INDIRECT	SSRIs	1. Case report of serotonin syndrome when dexamfetamine was co-administered with citalopram 2. Case reports of psychiatric disturbances when methylphenidate was given with sertraline and phenylpropanolamine co-administered with phenylpropanolamine	1. Uncertain; postulated that it is an additive effect of the inhibition of serotonin reuptake by citalopram with the release of serotonin by venlafaxine 2. Uncertain	1. Avoid co-administration of dexamfetamine and citalopram 2. Warn patients to watch for early signs such as anxiety
INDIRECT	TCAs	1. Methylphenidate ↑ TCA levels, which may improve their efficacy, but cases of toxicity with imipramine have been reported 2. TCAs possibly ↓ efficacy of indirect sympathomimetics	1. Uncertain; postulated to be due to inhibition of the hepatic metabolism of TCAs 2. Indirect sympathomimetics cause release of norepinephrine from the nerve endings; this is blocked by TCAs	1. Warn patients to watch for early signs of ↑ TCA efficacy such as drowsiness and dry mouth 2. Watch for poor response to indirect sympathomimetics
DIRECT	TCAs	↑ efficacy of norepinephrine, epinephrine or phenylephrine when co-administered with TCAs; risk of ↑ BP and tachyarrhythmias	TCAs block reuptake of norepinephrine into the nerve terminals, which prolongs its activity	Monitor PR, BP and ECG closely; start inotropes at a lower dose. It would be advisable to monitor PR and BP even when using local anaesthetics containing epinephrine, although there is no evidence of significant toxicity
INDIRECT	OTHER – VENLAFAXINE	Case report of serotonin syndrome when dexamfetamine was co-administered with venlafaxine	Uncertain; postulated to be an additive effect of the inhibition of serotonin reuptake by venlafaxine and the release of serotonin by venlafaxine	Avoid co-administration

Primary drug	Secondary drug	Effect	Mechanism	Precautions
SYMPATHOMIMETICS – EPINEPHRINE	ANTIDIABETIC DRUGS	May ↑ antidiabetic therapy requirement	Epinephrine causes the release of glucose from the liver and is an important defence/homeostatic mechanism. Hyperglycaemia may occur due to an antagonistic effect	Larger doses of antidiabetic therapy may be needed during the period of epinephrine use, which is usually in the short term or in emergency situations
SYMPATHOMIMETICS	**ANTIHYPERTENSIVES AND HEART FAILURE DRUGS**			
SYMPATHOMIMETICS	ACE INHIBITORS, ADRENERGIC NEURONE BLOCKERS	↓ hypotensive effect. Note there is a risk of interactions even with topical sympathomimetics (eye and nose drops)	Adrenergic neurone blockers act mainly by preventing release of norepinephrine. Sympathomimetics ↑ cardiac output and/or cause vasoconstriction	Monitor BP at least weekly until stable
DIRECT	ADRENERGIC NEURONE BLOCKERS	For patients on guanethidine, ↑ pressor effects have been reported with the administration of norepinephrine and metaraminol, as has a lower threshold for arrhythmias with norepinephrine. Prolonged mydriasis has been reported when eye drops were given to patients on guanethidine	Guanethidine blocks the release of norepinephrine from adrenergic neurones; this causes a hypersensitivity of the receptors that are normally stimulated by norepinephrine, and leads to the ↑ response when they are stimulated by directly acting sympathomimetics	Start alpha- and beta-1 agonists at a lower dose; monitor BP and cardiac rhythm closely
DIRECT	CENTRALLY ACTING ANTIHYPERTENSIVES	Risk of ↑ BP when clonidine is given with epinephrine or norepinephrine	Additive effect; clonidine use is associated with ↑ circulating catecholamines	Monitor BP at least weekly until stable
INDIRECT	CENTRALLY ACTING ANTIHYPERTENSIVES	1. Indirect sympathomimetics may ↓ the hypotensive effect of methyldopa 2. Methyldopa may ↓ the mydriatic effect of ephedrine eye drops	1. Uncertain 2. Uncertain	Monitor BP at least weekly until stable; watch for poor response to methyldopa

DIRECT	VASODILATOR ANTIHYPERTENSIVES	Case reports of ↑ tachycardia when epinephrine was given for perioperative ↓ BP in patients on hydralazine	Additive effect	Avoid co-administration
SYMPATHOMIMETICS	ANTIMUSCARINICS – ATROPINE	Reports of hypertension when atropine was given to patients receiving 10% phenylephrine eye drops during eye surgery	Atropine abolishes the cholinergic response to phenylephrine-induced vasoconstriction	Use a lower concentration of phenylephrine
SYMPATHOMIMETICS	**ANTIPARKINSON'S DRUGS**			
INDIRECT	BROMOCRIPTINE	Case reports of severe, symptomatic ↑ BP when co-administered with indirect sympathomimetics	Likely additive effect; both can cause ↑ BP	Monitor BP closely; watch for ↑ BP
INDIRECT	ENTACAPONE	Cases of severe, symptomatic ↑ BP when co-administered with indirect sympathomimetics	Likely additive effect; both can cause ↑ BP	Monitor BP closely; watch for ↑ BP
SYMPATHOMIMETICS	RASAGILINE	Risk of adrenergic syndrome – see above	Due to inhibition of MAOI, which breaks down sympathomimetics	Avoid concurrent use. Onset may be 6–24 hours after ingestion. Do ECG; measure electrolytes, FBC, CK and coagulation profile
DIRECT	SELEGILINE	Case report of ↑ hypertensive effect of dopamine when it was given to a patient already taking selegiline	Selegiline inhibits metabolism of dopamine	Titrate dopamine carefully
SYMPATHOMIMETICS	**ANTIPSYCHOTICS**			
SYMPATHOMIMETICS	ANTIPSYCHOTICS	Hypertensive effect of sympathomimetics are antagonized by antipsychotics	Dose-related ↓ BP (due to vasodilatation) is a side-effect of most antipsychotics, particularly phenothiazines	Monitor BP closely

Primary drug	Secondary drug	Effect	Mechanism	Precautions
INDIRECT	ANTIPSYCHOTICS	1. Case reports of paralytic ileus with trifluoperazine and methylphenidate 2. Case report of acute dystonias with haloperidol and dexamfetamine 3. ↓ efficacy of chlorpromazine when dexamfetamine was added	1. Additive anticholinergic effect 2. Uncertain; possibly due to ↑ dopamine release 3. Uncertain	1. Watch for signs of altered bowel habit 2. Warn patients of this rare interaction 3. Avoid co-administration
SYMPATHOMIMETICS	ANTIVIRALS – PROTEASE INHIBITORS	1. Risk of serotonin syndrome when dexamfetamine is administered with ritonavir 2. Indinavir may ↑ phenylpropanolamine levels	1. Protease inhibitors inhibit CYP2D6-mediated metabolism 2. Likely inhibition of phenylpropanolamine metabolism	1. Avoid co-administration 2. Monitor BP closely; watch for marked ↑ BP
SYMPATHOMIMETICS	**BETA-BLOCKERS**			
DIRECT	BETA-BLOCKERS	1. Severe ↑ BP and bradycardia with non-cardioselective beta-blockers (including reports of severe ↑ BP in patients given infiltrations of local anaesthetics containing epinephrine and one case of a fatal reaction with phenylephrine eye drops) 2. Patients on beta-blockers may respond poorly to epinephrine when it is given to treat anaphylaxis	1. Unopposed alpha stimulation causes vasoconstriction, which results in a rise in BP. Beta-2 receptors, when stimulated, cause vasodilatation, which counteracts the alpha action; non-selective beta-blockers antagonize beta-2 receptors	1. Monitor BP closely. When using local anaesthetics with epinephrine, use small volumes of low concentrations (such as 1 in 200 000 epinephrine); avoid high concentrations (e.g. 1 in 1000 mixtures) 2. Look for failure of epinephrine therapy and consider using salbutamol or isoprenaline
INDIRECT	BETA-BLOCKERS	↓ hypotensive efficacy of beta-blockers	The hypertensive effect of sympathomimetics opposes the hypotensive actions of beta-blockers	Monitor BP at least weekly until stable; watch for poor response to beta-blockers

CARDIOVASCULAR DRUGS SYMPATHOMIMETICS

SYMPATHOMIMETICS	BICARBONATE	Possibly ↑ ephedrine/ pseudoephedrine levels	Alkalinizing urine ↓ the excretion of these sympathomimetics	Watch for early features of toxicity (tremor, insomnia and tachycardia)
SYMPATHOMIMETICS	**BRONCHODILATORS**			
INDIRECT	THEOPHYLLINE	↑ incidence of side-effects of theophylline (without a change in its serum concentrations) when co-administered with ephedrine	Uncertain	Warn patients to avoid OTC remedies containing ephedrine
DIRECT	THEOPHYLLINE	Case report of marked tachycardia when dobutamine was given to a patient already taking theophylline	Uncertain	Carefully titrate the dose of dobutamine in patients taking dobutamine
DIRECT	CALCIUM COMPOUNDS	Parenteral calcium administration may ↓ the positive inotropic effects of epinephrine and dobutamine	Uncertain; postulated that calcium modulates the signal transmission from the receptor	Monitor BP closely; watch for poor response to these inotropes
SYMPATHOMIMETICS	CNS STIMULANTS – MODAFINIL	May ↓ modafinil levels with dexamfetamine, methylphenidate	Due to delayed absorption	Be aware
SYMPATHOMIMETICS	DOXAPRAM	Risk of ↑ BP	Uncertain at present	Monitor BP closely
SYMPATHOMIMETICS	**DRUG DEPENDENCE THERAPIES**			
AMPHETAMINES	BUPROPION	1. ↑ plasma concentrations of these substrates, with risk of toxic effects 2. ↑ risk of seizures. This risk is marked in elderly people, patients with a history of seizures, those with an addiction to opiates/ cocaine/stimulants, and those with diabetes treated with oral hypoglycaemics or insulin	1. Bupropion and its metabolite hydroxybupropion inhibit CYP2D6 2. Bupropion is associated with a dose-related risk of seizures. These drugs that lower seizure threshold are individually epileptogenic. They have additive effects when combined	1. Initiate therapy with these drugs, particularly those with a narrow therapeutic index, at the lowest effective dose. Interaction is likely to be important with substrates for which CYP2D6 is considered the only metabolic pathway (e.g. amphetamines) 2. Extreme caution. The dose of bupropion should not exceed 450 mg/day (or 150 mg/day in those with severe hepatic cirrhosis)

CARDIOVASCULAR DRUGS SYMPATHOMIMETICS

Primary drug	Secondary drug	Effect	Mechanism	Precautions
DEXAMFETAMINE, METHYLPHENIDATE	DISULFIRAM	Risk of psychosis	Additive effects; these drugs interfere with dopamine metabolism	Caution with co-administration. Warn patients and carers to watch for early features
SYMPATHOMIMETICS	**ERGOT DERIVATIVES**			
SYMPATHOMIMETICS	ERGOT DERIVATIVES	Risk of ergot toxicity when ergotamine is co-administered with sympathomimetics	Uncertain	Watch for early features of ergotamine toxicity (vertigo and gastrointestinal disturbance)
DIRECT	ERGOT DERIVATIVES	Case report of gangrene when dopamine was given to a patient on ergotamine	Thought to be due to additive vasoconstriction	Titrate dopamine carefully
SYMPATHOMIMETICS	H2 RECEPTOR BLOCKERS	↑ efficacy and adverse effects of sympathomimetics	Unclear	↑ hypertensive response; dose reduction may be required. Monitor ECG for tachycardias
SYMPATHOMIMETICS	OXYTOCICS	Risk of ↑ BP when oxytocin co-administered with ephedrine, metaraminol, norepinephrine or pseudoephedrine	Additive vasoconstriction	Monitor PR, BP and ECG closely; start inotropes at a lower dose

Part 2 DRUGS ACTING ON THE NERVOUS SYSTEM

Antiepileptics

Antiepileptic drugs are used to prevent or treat convulsions in people with epilepsy. Long-term therapy is very often necessary. There are various classes of drug, described below.

Phenytoin is an inducer of CYP1A2, CYP2C9, CYP3A4 and UDPGT.

Barbiturates induce a wide range of CYP metabolizing enzymes, for example CYP1A2, CYP2B6, CYP2C219, CYP2C8, CYP3A4, CYP3A5, CYP3A6, CYP3A7 and CYP2C9. Secobarbital induces CYP2C9.

The antiepileptic (anticonvulsant) effect of primidone is attributed to both the parent drug and its principal metabolite, phenobarbitone.

Carbamazepine is a substrate of CYP1A2, CYP2C9, CYP3A4 and UDPGT. Carbamazepine induces CYP1A2, CYP2C9, CYP2D6, CYP3A4, glucuronyl transferases and epoxide hydrolase metabolizing enzymes. It is necessary to monitor carbamazepine blood levels weekly throughout the first 8 weeks of initiating therapy as carbamazepine can induce its own metabolism.

Oxcarbazepine is the 10-keto analogue of carbamazepine and is the prodrug for 10,11-dihydrocarbazepine. It is a weaker inducer of CYP isoenzymes than carbamazepine.

Gabapentin and *pregabalin* have very few if any significant drug interactions.

Lamotrigine cause a decreased release of glutamate and modulates the uptake of serotonin. It also tends to block the uptake of monoamines including dopamine. Lamotrigine can cause serious skin reactions (1 in 1000 in adults and 1 in 100 in children). For the first 3 months of treatment with lamotrigine, advise patients to avoid new foods, deodorants, detergents, cosmetics and fabric softeners and to avoid excessive sun exposure. They should be given advice to seek emergency treatment if a rash is accompanied by fever or discomfort in the eyes, mouth or bladder.

Tiagabine undergoes metabolism via glucuronidation and oxidation.

Serious drug interactions are uncommon with *valproate*. Approximately 25% of valproate metabolism is dependent on CYP isoenzymes. Valproic acid can cause severe liver damage during the first 6 months of treatment. Note interactions with aspirin and the need to monitor plasma free valproate levels.

Antidementia drugs

Memantine blocks NMDA receptors, inhibiting the excessive excitatory action of glutamate at the receptor, which is thought to be one mechanism which underlies Alzheimer's disease. The glutamate system is known to be involved in the formation of memory and information processing. Excessive glutamate activity masks signal transmission and possibly causes neurodegeneration. Memantine blocks both serotonin and nicotinic receptors, although this action is thought to be relatively weak.

Antidepressants

Lithium

Lithium salts have a narrow therapeutic index. Lithium levels should be monitored every 3 months. The long-term use of lithium is associated with thyroid disorders and mild cognitive and memory impairment. Thyroid and renal functions should be checked every 6–12 months.

Monoamine oxidase inhibitors

These were the first type of antidepressant used. Neurotransmitters (e.g. norepinephrine, serotonin and dopamine) are generally monoamines that, when released, are either reabsorbed into the proximal nerve and metabolized by MAO or destroyed by catechol-*O*-methyl transferase in the synaptic cleft.

There are two types of MAO: MAO-A, found mainly in the liver and gastrointestinal tract, and MAO-B, found mainly in the brain and platelets. MAO-A in the liver is involved in the elimination of ingested monoamines (e.g. tyramine) and inactivates circulating monoamines (e.g. epinephrine, norepinephrine and dopamine) when they pass through the liver. Co-ingestion of these monoamines with MAO inhibitors leads to their unopposed action, which causes severe hypertension, so the former should be avoided.

Tricyclic antidepressants

Following rapid absorption, TCAs are strongly bound to plasma albumin (90–95% at therapeutic plasma concentrations). Inactivation occurs via CYP isoenzymes by the demethylation of tertiary TCAs to secondary amine metabolites, and then glucuronidation and excretion in the urine.

- All TCAs are metabolized primarily by CYP2D6. Other pathways include CYP1A2 (e.g. amitriptyline, clomipramine, imipramine), CYP2C9 and CYP2C19 (e.g. clomipramine, imipramine).
- Amitryptiline, imipramine, clomipramine, dosulepin and doxepin are more potent CYP inhibitors, inhibiting CYP2C19 and CYP1A2.
- Desipramine and nortriptyline are the least problematic in terms of drug interaction, being weak inhibitors of CYP2D6 inhibitors.
- To varying degrees, TCAs have the ability to cause arrhythmias.

Selective serotonin reuptake inhibitors

Different SSRIs vary in their metabolism and their ability to inhibit and induce metabolising enzymes.

Fluvoxamine and *fluoxetine* are substrates of CYP1A2. Fluvoxamine is a potent inhibitor of CYP1A2, CYP2C19 and CYP2C9, a weaker inhibitor of CYP3A4 and an even weaker inhibitor of CYP1A2. Fluoxetine is a potent inhibitor of CYP2D6 and a moderate inhibitor of CYP2C19.

Paroxetine metabolism at low concentrations is dependent on CYP2D6, which is almost saturated at these concentrations. Thus, there are non-linear pharmacokinetics and an increase in the half-life of paroxetine from 10 to 20 hours when the dose is increased from 10mg to 20mg. At higher concentrations, the metabolism is mainly by CYP3A4 isoenzymes. Paroxetine inhibits the activity of CYP2D6 in the lowest usually effective antidepressant dose.

Sertraline undergoes MAO-catalysed deamination and UDGPT2B7-catalysed glucuronidation. CYP2B6 contributes most to the demethylation of sertraline, with lesser contributions from CYP2C19, CYP2C9, CYP3A4, CYP2D6 and CYP2B6. One isoform contributes more than 40% to the overall metabolism, making sertraline relatively immune to harmful interactions. Compared with fluoxetine and paroxetine, sertraline does not inhibit CYP2D6 isoenzymes in the usually lowest antidepressant dose. Sertraline is known to inhibit CYP3A4, possibly to a lesser degree than fluoxetine.

Citalopram and *escitalopram* are major substrates of CYP2C19 and CYP3A4, and weakly inhibit CYP2D6.

Other antidepressants

These include:

- *duloxetine* and *venlafaxine*, which are serotonin and norepinephrine (noradrenaline) reuptake inhibitors;
- *mirtazapine*, which blocks presynaptic alpha-adrenergic receptors;
- *reboxetine*, which is an SNRI;
- *tryptophan*, which is a precursor for several proteins, including serotonin.

St John's wort (*Hypercurium*)

Several chemicals are found in this short, yellow-flowering, wild-growing plant; they are considered to alter the balance of some neurotransmitters such as serotonin, dopamine, GABA and norepinephrine. St John's wort is an inducer of CYP3A4, CYP1A2, CYP2D6 and P-gp and is known to interact with several commonly used drugs. Topical or homeopathic preparations of St John's wort are not likely to interact with prescribed medicines.

Antiemetics

Aprepitant is a substrate for CYP3A4 and an inducer of CYP2C9 and 3A4 (it also has moderate, dose-dependent CYP3A4 inhibitory properties).

Dopamine receptor antagonists also act as antiemetics:

- *Domperidone* antagonizes D2 and D3 receptors in the chemoreceptor trigger zone. It does not cross the blood–brain barrier.
- *Metoclopramide* antagonizes D2 receptors in both the chemoreceptor trigger zone and central nervous system (as it crosses the blood–brain barrier).

5-HT3 antagonists are metabolized by various members of the CYP enzyme family; however, they neither induce nor inhibit CYP isoenzymes.

Antimigraine drugs

5-HT1 agonists – triptans

Almotriptan is principally metabolized by CYP3A4, but also MAO-A and CYP2D6.

Eletriptan is metabolized mainly by the CYP3A4 isoenzymes and is subject to activity of the P-gp efflux barrier in the brain.

Naratriptan is metabolized by the CYP isoenzymes and MAO-A enzymes, and is also subject to renal elimination.

Frovatriptan is metabolized mainly by CYP1A2 isoenzymes.

Rizatriptan and *sumatriptan* are metabolized mainly by MAO-A enzymes.

Zolmitriptan is metabolized mainly by the MAO-A enzymes and CYP1A2 isoenzymes.

Ergot alkaloids

These are used in treatment of migraine and in obstetrics (to control late uterine bleeding – postpartum haemorrhage). Their predominant action involves vasoconstriction (partial agonist effects at alpha-adrenergic receptors and 5-HT receptor-mediated effects). They are metabolized mainly via CYP3A4.

Increased plasma concentrations cause ergot poisoning (ergotism, St Anthony's fire – dementia, florid hallucinations and persistent vasospasm: gangrene may develop) and uterine muscle stimulation (it may cause abortion in pregnancy). Ergot alkaloids activates gastrointestinal serotonin receptors and central nervous system emetic centres.

Antiobesity drugs

Orlistat inhibits pancreatic lipase, thus preventing the breakdown of dietary lipids, which reduces their absorption.

Rimonabant inhibits the CB1 cannabinoid receptor. It reduces appetite. It has a high risk of precipitating depression and, at the time of writing, NICE (the UK's regulatory authority) is considering advising its withdrawal from the market.

Sibutramine inhibits the reuptake of serotonin and norepinephrine.

Antiparkinson's drugs

Parkinson's disease is caused by loss of dopamine-secreting cells in the substantia nigra. The primary aim of current therapy for Parkinson's disease is to increase the activity of dopamine in the brain.

Dopaminergic drugs act by a number of mechanisms:

- Levodopa is a precursor of dopamine.
- Dopamine receptor agonists include apomorphine, bromocriptine, cabergoline, lisuride, pergolide, pramipexole, ropinirole and rotigotine.
- Catechol-*O*-methyltransferase inhibitors (entacapone, tolcapone) reduce the peripheral breakdown of dopamine.
- Monoamine oxidase type B inhibitors (rasagiline, selegiline) reduce the metabolism of dopamine by MAO-B. They are useful to delay disease progression in the early stages of the disease and as an adjunct to levodopa.

Antimuscarinic drugs are useful for treating drug-induced, rather than primary, Parkinson's disease. They counteract the excess central cholinergic action that results from the dopamine deficiency.

Amantadine is a weak dopaminergic drug (it stimulates the release of dopamine from central nerve endings). It is considered separately from the other dopaminergic agents because it is also used as an antiviral agent.

Antipsychotic agents

Antipsychotics consist of the phenothiazines, a miscellany of non-phenothiazines and a newer class of drugs, the atypical antipsychotics.

- *Phenothiazines*: chlorpromazine, fluphenazine, levomepromazine, pericyazine, perphenazine, pipotiazine, prochlorperazine, promazine, trifluoperazine.
- *Atypical agents*: amisulpride, aripiprazole, clozapine, olanzapine, quetiapine, risperidone, sertindole, zotepine.
- *Other drugs*: benperidol, droperidol, flupentixol, haloperidol, pimozide, sulpiride, zuclopenthixol.

They act by a number of mechanisms, most notable of which is to block dopamine receptors. For example, aripiprazole has a high affinity for the serotonin type 2 (5-HT2) and dopamine types 2 (D2) and 3 (D3), moderate affinity for D4 and moderate affinity for 1- and 2-adrenergic and H1 histaminergic receptors. It also has moderate affinity for the serotonin reuptake pump.

There is also variation in the metabolic pathways involved. For example:

- *clozapine*: CYP1A2 and CYP3A4 are involved in the demethylation while CYP3A4 is involved in the *N*-oxidation. CYP2D6 may also have role in the metabolism of clozapine;

- *aripiprazole*: CYP3A4 and CYP2D6 are responsible for metabolism;
- *pimozide*: predominantly metabolized by CYP3A4.

Anxiolytics and hypnotics

Benzodiazepines

Benzodiazepines act by binding GABA receptors in the brain and potentiate other central nervous system depressants. Long-acting BZDs are oxidized in the liver and are subject to drug interactions due to the inhibition/induction of cytochrome metabolising enzymes. Clonazepam, flunitrazepam and nitrazepam are metabolized by nitro-reduction, while lorazepam and oxazepam undergo rapid conjugation with glucuronic acid and are excreted in the urine (thus being less subject to interactions associated with cytochrome, but possibly more affected by impairment of renal function).

Buspirone

Buspirone is an anxiolytic with dopaminergic, noradrenergic and antiserotonergic properties. Anxiolytic properties are attributed to effects on serotonin transmission (probably inhibiting transmission via 5-HT1A autoregulation). It may have postsynaptic 5-HT1A agonist activity and thus facilitate serotonin neurotransmission. It is metabolized by CYP3A4.

Sodium oxybate

This is a central nervous system depressant licensed for the treatment of narcolepsy with cataplexy. At recommended doses, it has been associated with confusion, depression and other neuropsychiatric effects. Sodium oxybate is related to gamma hydroxybutyrate, a known drug of abuse, which has been associated with seizures, respiratory depression, coma and death.

'Z' drugs

Zaleplon, zolpidem and zopiclone – the 'Z' drugs – are licensed only for insomnia, and NICE guidelines are available. These agents are structurally unrelated to BZDs but act at BZD receptors. They are all metabolized primarily by CYP3A4, but zopiclone (CYP2C8) and zolpidem (CYP1A2, CYP2C9, CYP2C19, and CYP2D6) have minor alternative metabolic pathways.

CNS STIMULANTS

Atomoxetine

Atomoxetine increases the brain concentrations of norepinephrine. Adverse effects (constipation, dry mouth, nausea, fatigue, decreased appetite, insomnia, chest pain, palpitations, anxiety, erectile dysfunction, mood swings, nervousness and urinary retention) are more common in poor metabolizers of CYP2D6, as atomoxetine is metabolized through the cytochrome CYP2D6 pathway.

Modafinil

Modafinil is used in patients with excessive sleepiness associated with primary disorders of sleep and wakefulness. It causes an extracellular increase in dopamine but does not increase dopamine release. Modafinil is a moderate inducer of CYP1A2, CYP2B6 and CYP3A4 in a concentration-dependent manner. It may be a moderate inhibitor of CYP2C9 and CYP2C19.

Methylphenidate

This drug is a central nervous system stimulant that is considered to prevent the reuptake of norepinephrine and dopamine into the presynaptic neurones and increase the release of these neurotransmitters to the extraneuronal space. A high-fat meal increases its absorption. Methylphenidate in animal experiments was found to inhibit CYP1A and CYP2E1 by 50%. It is metabolized by de-esterification to inactive metabolites.

Dexamphetamine sulphate

Dexamphetamine sulphate acts by stimulating the release of norepinephrine and dopamine from storage sites and may also slow down the metabolism of catecholamines by inhibiting MAO. Usually about 30% is excreted unchanged in the urine; this urinary excretion reaches 60% when the urine is acidic (pH 5.5–6). It is metabolized by cytochrome P450.

Drug-dependence therapies

Bupropion

Bupropion inhibits the reuptake of both norepinephrine and dopamine; it is used to assist smoking cessation. It is primarily metabolized by CYP2B6 isoenzymes and inhibits CYP2D6.

Disulfiram

Disulfiram inhibits the metabolism of alcohol (aldehyde dehydrogenase), leading to markedly increased levels of aldehyde. This causes a classic syndrome – the disulfiram reaction – involving facial flushing, headache, dyspnoea, copious vomiting, agitation, confusion, tachycardia and hypotension. The severity of the reaction is dose-dependent, and a severe reaction may occur resulting in cardiovascular collapse, coma, seizures and death. Disulfiram also inhibits the metabolism of dopamine beta-hydroxylase, resulting in increased dopamine levels.

Lofexidine

Lofexidine is an alpha-agonist that is used to reduce the sympathetic autonomic effects of acute opioid withdrawal symptoms.

Drugs used to treat neuromuscular diseases and movement disorders

Parasympathomimetics inhibit the enzyme cholinesterase, which is responsible for the breakdown of the neurotransmitter acetylcholine. They are a mainstay in the investigation (edrophonium) and treatment (distigmine, neostigmine, pyridostigmine) of myasthenia gravis, but they have a wide range of effects that is reflected in the different number of conditions for which they may be used therapeutically:

- reversing the effects of non-depolarizing muscle relaxants in anaesthesia (edrophonium, neostigmine);
- treating some causes of urinary retention (bethanechol, distigmine);
- increasing intestinal motility (bethanechol, distigmine, neostigmine, pyridostigmine);
- reducing raised intraocular pressure (pilocarpine).

Tetrabenazine inhibits the vesicular monoamine transporter, which results in a depletion of stores of norepinephrine (and to a lesser extent dopamine and serotonin) in the central nervous system.

Primary drug	Secondary drug	Effect	Mechanism	Precautions
ANTIDEMENTIA DRUGS				
DONEPEZIL ➢ *Drugs Used to Treat Neuromuscular Diseases and Movement Disorders, below*				
GALANTAMINE ➢ *Drugs Used to Treat Neuromuscular Diseases and Movement Disorders, below*				
MEMANTINE				
MEMANTINE	ANAESTHETICS – GENERAL – KETAMINE	↑ CNS side-effects	Additive effects on NMDA receptors	Avoid co-administration
MEMANTINE	ANALGESICS – DEXTROMETHORPHAN	↑ CNS side-effects	Additive effects on NMDA receptors	Avoid co-administration
MEMANTINE	ANTIEPILEPTICS – BARBITURATES	Possible ↓ efficacy of primidone	Uncertain	Avoid co-administration
MEMANTINE	ANTIMUSCARINICS	Possible ↑ efficacy of antimuscarinics	Additive effect; memantine has weak antimuscarinic properties	Warn patients of this effect
MEMANTINE	ANTIPARKINSON'S DRUGS – AMANTADINE	↑ CNS side-effects	Additive effects on NMDA receptors	Manufacturers recommend avoiding co-administration of amantadine and memantine
MEMANTINE	DIURETICS – CARBONIC ANHYDRASE INHIBITORS	Possible ↑ memantine levels	↓ renal excretion	Watch for early features of memantine toxicity
MEMANTINE	DOPAMINERGICS	Memantine augments the effect of dopaminergics	Memantine has some agonist activity at dopamine receptors	Be aware. May be used therapeutically
MEMANTINE	SODIUM BICARBONATE	Possible ↑ memantine levels	↓ renal excretion	Watch for early features of memantine toxicity

Primary drug	Secondary drug	Effect	Mechanism	Precautions
RIVASTIGMINE ➢ *Drugs Used to Treat Neuromuscular Diseases and Movement Disorders, below*				
ANTIDEPRESSANTS				
LITHIUM				
LITHIUM	ANALGESICS – NSAIDs	NSAIDs may ↑ lithium levels; cases of toxicity have been reported	Uncertain; NSAIDs possibly ↓ renal clearance of lithium	Monitor lithium levels closely
LITHIUM	ANTIARRHYTHMICS – AMIODARONE	1. Rare risk of ventricular arrythmias, particularly torsades de pointes 2. Risk of hypothyroidism	1. Additive effect; lithium rarely causes Q–T prolongation 2. Additive effect; both drugs can cause hypothyroidism	1. Manufacturers of amiodarone recommend avoiding co-administration 2. If co-administration thought to be necessary, watch for symptoms/ signs of hypothyroidism; check TFTs every 3–6 months
LITHIUM	ANTIBIOTICS – METRONIDAZOLE	↑ plasma concentrations of lithium with risk of toxicity	Uncertain	Monitor clinically and by measuring blood lithium levels for lithium toxicity
LITHIUM	**ANTIDEPRESSANTS**			
LITHIUM	SSRIs	Lithium may enhance the pharmacologic effects of SSRIs and potentiate the risk of serotonin syndrome. Excessive somnolence has been reported with fluvoxamine. However, there are reports of both ↑ and ↓ plasma concentrations of lithium. There are reports of lithium toxicity and of serotonergic effects	Lithium is a direct stimulant of 5-HT receptors, while SSRIs ↓ the reuptake of 5- HT; these are considered to ↑ the effects of serotonin in the brain. Seizures are a neurotoxic effect of lithium and could occur even with plasma lithium concentrations within the normal range. SSRIs and lithium may have additive effects to cause seizures	Be aware of the possibility of serotonin syndrome. Also need to monitor lithium levels with appropriate dose adjustments during co-administration ➢ ***For signs and symptoms of serotonin toxicity, see Clinical Features of Some Adverse Drug Interactions, Serotonin toxicity and serotonin syndrome***

LITHIUM	OTHER – VENLAFAXINE	Possible risk of serotonin syndrome	Additive effect	Be aware of the possibility of serotonin syndrome. Also need to monitor lithium levels with appropriate dose adjustments during co-administration ➢ ***For signs and symptoms of serotonin toxicity, see Clinical Features of Some Adverse Drug Interactions, Serotonin toxicity and serotonin syndrome***
LITHIUM	ANTIEPILEPTICS – CARBAMAZEPINE, PHENYTOIN	↑ risk of neurotoxicity	Uncertain; this may occur with normal lithium blood levels	Warn patients and carers to watch for drowsiness, ataxia and tremor
LITHIUM	**ANTIHYPERTENSIVES AND HEART FAILURE DRUGS**			
LITHIUM	ACE INHIBITORS	↑ efficacy of lithium	↑ plasma concentrations of lithium (up to one-third) due to ↓ renal excretion	Watch for lithium toxicity. Monitor lithium levels
LITHIUM	ANGIOTENSIN II RECEPTOR ANTAGONISTS	Risk of lithium toxicity	↓ excretion of lithium possibly due to ↓ renal tubular reabsorption of sodium in the proximal tubule	Watch for lithium toxicity. Monitor lithium levels
LITHIUM	CENTRALLY ACTING ANTIHYPERTENSIVES	1. Methyldopa may reduce the effect of antidepressants 2. Case reports of lithium toxicity when co-ingested with methyldopa. It was noted that lithium levels were in the therapeutic range	1. Methyldopa can cause depression 2. Uncertain at present	1. Methyldopa should be avoided in patients with depression 2. Avoid co-administration if possible; if not, watch closely for clinical features of toxicity and do not rely on lithium levels

Primary drug	Secondary drug	Effect	Mechanism	Precautions
LITHIUM	**ANTIPSYCHOTICS**			
LITHIUM	CLOZAPINE, HALOPERIDOL, PHENOTHIAZINES, SULPIRIDE	↑ risk of extra-pyramidal side-effects and of neurotoxicity	Uncertain	Watch for development of these symptoms
LITHIUM	SERTINDOLE	↑ risk of ventricular arrhythmias	Uncertain	Avoid concomitant use
LITHIUM	ANTIVIRALS – ACICLOVIR/VALACICLOVIR	↑ lithium levels with risk of toxicity	Possible ↓ renal excretion	Ensure adequate hydration, monitor lithium levels if intravenous aciclovir or $>$4 g/day valaciclovir required
LITHIUM	BETA-BLOCKERS	Report of episode of ↑ lithium levels in an elderly patient after starting low-dose propanolol. However, propanolol is often used to treat lithium-induced tremor without problems	Mechanism uncertain at present, but propanolol seems to reduce lithium clearance	Monitor lithium levels when starting propanolol therapy in elderly patients
LITHIUM	BRONCHODILATORS – THEOPHYLLINE	↓ plasma levels of lithium, with risk of therapeutic failure	Theophylline ↑ renal clearance of lithium	May need to ↑ dose of lithium by 60%
LITHIUM	CALCIUM CHANNEL BLOCKERS	Small number of cases of neurotoxicity when co-administered with diltiazem or verapamil	Uncertain, but thought to be due to additive effect on neurotransmission	Monitor closely for side-effects
LITHIUM	**DIURETICS**			
LITHIUM	ACETAZOLAMIDE	↓ plasma concentrations of lithium, with risk of inadequate therapeutic effect	↑ renal elimination of lithium	Monitor clinically and by measuring blood lithium levels to ensure adequate therapeutic efficacy
LITHIUM	LOOP DIURETICS, POTASSIUM-SPARING DIURETICS, ALDOSTERONE ANTAGONISTS, THIAZIDES	↑ plasma concentrations of lithium, with risk of toxic effects	↓ renal excretion of lithium	Monitor clinically and by measuring blood lithium levels for lithium toxicity. Loop diuretics are safer than thiazides

LITHIUM	MUSCLE RELAXANTS			
LITHIUM	NON-DEPOLARIZING	Antagonism of effects of non-depolarizing muscle relaxants	Uncertain	Monitor intraoperative muscle relaxation closely; may need ↑ doses of muscle relaxants
LITHIUM	BACLOFEN	Enhancement of hyperkinesias associated with lithium	Uncertain	Consider alternative skeletal muscle relaxant
LITHIUM	PARASYMPATHOMIMETICS	↓ efficacy of neostigmine and pyridostigmine	Uncertain	Watch for poor response to these parasympathomimetics and ↑ dose accordingly
LITHIUM	SODIUM BICARBONATE	↓ plasma concentrations of lithium with risk of lack of therapeutic effect	Due to ↑ renal excretion of lithium	Monitor clinically and by measuring blood lithium levels to ensure adequate therapeutic efficacy
MONOAMINE OXIDASE INHIBITORS				
MAOIs	ALCOHOL	Additive depression of CNS ranging from drowsiness to coma and respiratory depression.	Synergistic depressant effects on CNS function	Necessary to warn patients, particularly regards activities that require attention, e.g. driving or using machinery and equipment that could cause self-harm
MAOIs	ANAESTHETICS – GENERAL	Some cases of both ↑ and ↓ BP on induction of anaesthesia. Mostly no significant changes	Uncertain	Some recommend stopping MAOIs 2 weeks before surgery; others suggest no need for this; monitor BP closely, especially during induction of anaesthesia
MAOIs	**ANALGESICS**			
MAOIs	NEFOPAM	Risk of arrhythmias	Additive effect; both drugs have sympathomimetic effects	Avoid co-administration

NERVOUS SYSTEM DRUGS ANTIDEPRESSANTS

Primary drug	Secondary drug	Effect	Mechanism	Precautions
MAOIs	OPIOIDS	Additive depression of CNS ranging from drowsiness to coma and respiratory depression	Synergistic depressant effects on CNS function	Necessary to warn patients, particularly regards activities that require attention, e.g. driving or using machinery and equipment that could cause self-harm
MAOIs	PETHIDINE, MORPHINE, PHENOPERIDINE, DEXTROMETHORPHAN	Two types of reaction are reported: 1. Risk of serotonin syndrome with dextromethorphan, pethidine or tramadol and MAOIs 2. Depressive – respiratory depression, hypotension, coma	Type I reactions are attributed to inhibition of reuptake of serotonin – more common with pethidine, phenoperidine, dextromethorphan. Type II reactions are attributed to MAOI inhibition of metabolism of opioids – more common with morphine	Avoid co-administration; do not give dextromethorphan, pethidine or tramadol for at least 2 weeks after cessation of MAOI
PHENELZINE	ANTIBIOTICS – ERYTHROMYCIN	Report of fainting and severe hypotension on initiation of erythromycin	Attributed to ↑ absorption of phenelzine due to rapid gastric emptying caused by erythromycin	Be aware
MAOIs	ANTICANCER AND IMMUNOMODULATING DRUGS – PROCARBAZINE	Concurrent therapy ↑ risk of hypertensive crisis and severe seizures	Additive effect on inhibiting MAO	Concurrent treatment should not be started on an outpatient basis. 14 days should elapse before starting these medications after procarbazine treatment
MAOIs	**ANTIDEPRESSANTS**			
MAOIs	SSRIs	↑ risk of serotonin syndrome ➢ ***For signs and symptoms of serotonin toxicity, see Clinical Features of Some Adverse Drug Interactions, Serotonin toxicity and serotonin syndrome***	Additive inhibitory on serotonin reuptake	Avoid co-administration. MAOIs should not be started for at least 1 week after stopping SSRIs (2 weeks after sertraline, 5 weeks after fluoxetine). Conversely, SSRIs should not be started for at least 2 weeks after stopping MAOIs

MAOIs	TCAs – AMITRIPTYLINE CLOMIPRAMINE DESIPRAMINE IMIPRAMINE NORTRIPTYLINE	↑ risk of stroke, hyperpyrexia and convulsions. ↑ plasma concentrations of TCAs, with risk of toxic effects. ↑ risk of serotonin syndrome and of adrenergic syndrome with older MAOIs. Clomipramine may trigger acute confusion in Parkinson's disease when used with selegiline	TCAs are believed to also act by inhibiting the reuptake of serotonin and norepinephrine, increasing the risk of serotonin and adrenergic syndromes. The combination of TCAs and antidepressants can ↑ risk of seizures	Very hazardous interaction. Avoid concurrent use and consider the use of an alternative antidepressant. Be aware that seizures occur with overdose of TCAs just before cardiac arrest
MAOIs	**OTHER**			
MAOIs	DULOXETINE, VENLAFAXINE	Risk of severe hypertensive reactions and of serotonin syndrome ➢ ***For signs and symptoms of serotonin toxicity, see Clinical Features of Some Adverse Drug Interactions, Serotonin toxicity and serotonin syndrome.***	Duloxetine inhibits the reuptake of both serotonin and norepinephrine. Due to impaired metabolism of these amines, there is an accumulation of serotonin and norepinephrine in the brain and at peripheral sites	Do not co-administer duloxetine and venlafaxine prior to 14 days after discontinuing an MAOI, and do not co-administer MAOI for 5 days after discontinuing duloxetine, 1 week after venlafaxine
MAOIs	MIRTAZAPINE	Risk of severe hypertensive reactions and of serotonin syndrome ➢ ***For signs and symptoms of serotonin toxicity, see Clinical Features of Some Adverse Drug Interactions, Serotonin toxicity and serotonin syndrome***	Additive inhibition of both serotonin and norepinephrine reuptake	Avoid co-administration. MAOIs should not be started for at least 2 weeks after stopping mirtazapine (moclobemide can be started at least 1 week after stopping mirtazapine). Conversely, mirtazapine should not be started for at least 2 weeks after stopping MAOIs

Primary drug	Secondary drug	Effect	Mechanism	Precautions
MAOIs	REBOXETINE	Risk of severe hypertensive reactions	Additive inhibition of norepinephrine reuptake	Avoid co-administration. MAOIs should not be started for at least 1 week after stopping reboxetine. Conversely, reboxetine should not be started for at least 2 weeks after stopping MAOIs
MAOIs	TRYPTOPHAN	Risk of confusion and agitation	Tryptophan is a precursor to a number of neurotransmitters including serotonin. MAOIs inhibit the breakdown of neurotransmitters	Reduce dose of tryptophan
MAOIs	ANTIDIABETIC DRUGS – INSULIN, SULPHONAMIDES	↑ risk of hypoglycaemic episodes	Monoamine oxidase inhibitors have an intrinsic hypoglycaemic effect. MAOIs are considered to enhance the effect of hypoglycaemic drugs	Watch for and warn patients about symptoms of hypoglycaemia ➢ ***For signs and symptoms of hypoglycaemia, see Clinical Features of Some Adverse Drug Interactions, Hypoglycaemia***
MAOIs	ANTIEPILEPTICS – BARBITURATES	1. ↑ risk of seizures 2. Reports of prolonged hypnotic effects	1. MAOIs lower seizure threshold 2. Animal experiments showed that pretreatment with tranylcypromine prolonged amobarbital-induced hypnotic effects 2.5-fold. Inhibition of hepatic enzymes other than MAO has been proposed as an explanation for the exaggerated depressant effects associated with barbiturates and opioids	1. Care with co-administration. Watch for ↑ fit frequency; warn patients of this risk when starting these drugs, and take suitable precautions. Consider increasing the dose of antiepileptic 2. Be aware. Warn patients taking sleeping aids about activities requiring attention and co-ordination, e.g. driving or using machinery

MAOIs	ANTIHYPERTENSIVES AND HEART FAILURE DRUGS			
MAOIs	ANTIHYPERTENSIVES AND HEART FAILURE DRUGS	Possible ↑ hypotensive effect	Additive hypotensive effect	Monitor BP at least weekly until stable. Warn patients to report symptoms of hypotension (light-headedness, dizziness on standing, etc.)
MAOIs	ADRENERGIC NEURONE BLOCKERS – GUANETHIDINE, CENTRALLY ACTING ANTIHYPERTENSIVES – METHYLDOPA	Risk of adrenergic syndrome. Reports of an enhanced hypotensive effect and hallucinations with methyldopa, which may cause depression	Due to inhibition of MAOI, which breaks down sympathomimetics	Avoid concurrent use. Onset may be 6–24 hours after ingestion
MAOIs	**ANTIHISTAMINES**			
MAOIs	ANTIHISTAMINES	↑ occurrence of antimuscarinic effects such as blurred vision, confusion (in elderly patients), restlessness and constipation	Additive antimuscarinic effects	Warn patients and carers, particularly those managing elderly patients
MAOIs	ANTIHISTAMINES – SEDATIVE	Additive depression of CNS ranging from drowsiness to coma and respiratory depression	Synergistic depressant effects on CNS function	Necessary to warn patients, particularly regards activities that require attention, e.g. driving or using machinery and equipment that could cause self-harm
MAOIs	ANTIMUSCARINICS	↑ occurrence of antimuscarinic effects such as blurred vision, confusion (in elderly patients), restlessness and constipation	Additive antimuscarinic effects	Warn patients and carers, particularly those managing elderly patients
MAOIs	ANTIOBESITY DRUGS – SIBUTRAMINE	Risk of hypertension and agitation	Additive effect on norepinephrine transmission	Avoid co-administration. Do not start sibutramine for at least 2 weeks after stopping MAOIs

Primary drug	Secondary drug	Effect	Mechanism	Precautions
MAOIs	ANTIPARKINSON'S DRUGS – DOPAMINERGICS – levodopa, selegiline, possibly rasagiline, entacapone, tolcapone	Risk of adrenergic syndrome – hypertension, hyperthermia, arrhythmias – and dopaminergic effects with selegiline	Levodopa and related drugs are precursors of dopamine. Levodopa is predominantly metabolized to dopamine, and a smaller proportion is converted to epinephrine and norepinephrine. Due to inhibition of MAOI, which breaks down dopamine and sympathomimetics	Avoid concurrent use. Onset may be 6–24 hours after ingestion. Carbidopa and benserazide, which inhibit dopa decarboxylase that converts L-dopa to dopamine, is considered to minimize this interaction. However, MAOIs should not be used in patients with Parkinson's disease on treatment with levodopa. Imipramine and amitriptyline are considered safer by some clinicians
MAOIs	ANTIPSYCHOTICS	Additive depression of CNS ranging from drowsiness to coma and respiratory depression	Synergistic depressant effects on CNS function	Necessary to warn patients, particularly regards activities that require attention, e.g. driving and using machinery and equipment that could cause self-harm
MAOIs	**ANXIOLYTICS AND HYPNOTICS**			
MAOIs	BZDs	Additive depression of CNS ranging from drowsiness to coma and respiratory depression	Synergistic depressant effects on CNS function	Necessary to warn patients, particularly regards activities that require attention, e.g. driving and using machinery and equipment that could cause self-harm
MAOIs	BUSPIRONE	Cases of hypertension	Uncertain	Monitor BP closely
MAOIs	CHLORAL HYDRATE	Case of fatal hyperpyrexia and cases of hypertension	Uncertain	Avoid co-administration
MAOIs	BETA-BLOCKERS	↑ hypotensive effect	Additive hypotensive effect. Postural ↓ BP is a common side-effect of MAOIs	Monitor BP at least weekly until stable. Warn patients to report symptoms of hypotension (light-headedness, dizziness on standing, etc.)

MAOIs	BRONCHODILATORS			
MAOIs	IPRATROPIUM, TIOTROPIUM	↑ occurrence of antimuscarinic effects such as blurred vision, confusion (in elderly patients), restlessness and constipation	Additive antimuscarinic effects	Warn patients and carers, particularly those managing elderly patients
MAOIs	BETA-2 AGONISTS	↑ occurrence of headache, hypertensive episodes. Unlikely to occur with moclobemide and selegiline	Due to impaired metabolism of these sympathomimetic amines because of inhibition of MAO. Moclobemide is involved in the breakdown of serotonin, while selegiline is mainly involved in the breakdown of dopamine	Be aware. Monitor BP closely
MAOIs	CALCIUM CHANNEL BLOCKERS	↑ antihypertensive effect of calcium channel blockers when co-administered with MAOIs	Additive hypotensive effects; postural ↓ BP is a side-effect of MAOIs	Monitor BP at least weekly until stable. Warn patients to report symptoms of hypotension (light-headedness, dizziness on standing, etc.)
MAOIs	**CNS STIMULANTS**			
MAOIs	ATOMOXETINE	Risk of severe hypertensive reactions	Additive inhibition of norepinephrine reuptake	Avoid co-administration. MAOIs should not be started for at least 2 weeks after stopping atomoxetine; conversely, atomoxetine should not be started for at least 2 weeks after stopping MAOI
MOCLOBEMIDE	MODAFINIL	May cause moderate ↑ plasma concentrations of these substrates	Modafinil is a reversible inhibitor of CYP2C19 when used in therapeutic doses	Be aware
PHENELZINE	DRUG DEPENDENCE THERAPIES – BUPROPION	↑ acute toxicity of bupropion	Uncertain	Be aware

Primary drug	Secondary drug	Effect	Mechanism	Precautions
MAOIs	FOODS – TYRAMINE-CONTAINING – aged cheeses, aged pickles, smoked meats (e.g. salami), yeast extracts, beer (dark more than light, and tap more than bottles), red wine more than white wine, avocado, sauerkraut, marmite, banana peel, soy bean products, broad bean pods, foods containing MSG	Risk of severe tyramine reactions – hypertension, occipital headaches, vomiting, palpitations, nausea, apprehension, chills, sweating. This reaction develops 20–60 minutes after ingestion of these foods	Tyramine has both direct and indirect sympathomimetic effects, and tyramine effects of foods may be potentiated by MAOIs 10–20-fold. A mild tyramine reaction occurs with 6 mg, moderate reaction with 10 mg and severe reactions with 25 mg	Prompt treatment with phentolamine (0.5 mg intravenously) or nifedipine is effective, and death is rare (0.01–0.02%). There is a recommendation that 25 mg tablet of chlorpromazine be given to patients on MAOIs to be taken if a tyramine reaction occurs
MAOIs	H2 RECEPTOR BLOCKERS – CIMETIDINE	↑ plasma concentrations of moclobemide (by up to 40%)	Due to cimetidine inhibiting its metabolism	Reduce dose of moclobemide to one-half to one-third of original, then alter as required
MAOIs	**5-HT1 AGONISTS**			
MAOIs	RIZATRIPTAN, SUMATRIPTAN	↑ plasma concentrations of rizatriptan and sumatriptan, with risk of toxic effects, e.g. flushing, sensations of tingling, heat, heaviness, pressure or tightness of any part of body including the throat and chest, dizziness	These triptans are metabolized primarily by MAO-A	Avoid starting these triptans for at least 2 weeks after stopping MAOIs; conversely, avoid starting MAOIs for at least 2 weeks after stopping these triptans
MOCLOBEMIDE	ZOLMITRIPTAN	Risk of agitation, confusion when zolmitriptan is co-administered with moclobemide	Uncertain	Watch for these effects and consider reducing the dose of zolmitriptan

MAOIs	MUSCLE RELAXANTS – BACLOFEN, TIZANIDINE	↑ hypotensive effect	Additive hypotensive effect	Monitor BP at least weekly until stable. Warn patients to report symptoms of hypotension (light-headedness, dizziness on standing, etc.)
MAOIs	NITRATES	↑ hypotensive effect	Additive hypotensive effect. Postural ↓ BP is a common side-effect of MAOIs	Monitor BP at least weekly until stable. Warn patients to report symptoms of hypotension (light-headedness, dizziness on standing, etc.)
MAOIs	OTC MEDICATIONS – COUGH SYRUPS, SLEEP AIDS, MEDICINES FOR COLDS AND HAY FEVER, SOME PAIN RELIEVERS, SLIMMING AIDS, NASAL DECONGESTANTS	Due to the presence of sympathomimetics (amphetamines, ephedrine, ephedra, pseudoephedrine, phenylpropanolamine, etc. in nasal decongestants), opioids (pain relievers, e.g. codeine, dextromethorphan), fenfluramine (in slimming preparations), sedating antihistamines (promethazine, chlorpheniramine in hay fever and antiallergy preparations)	Patients on MAOIs cannot metabolize several of the active constituents of these OTC drugs	Mandatory that prior to dispensing these OTC medications, purchasers are questioned about use of MAOIs
MAOIs	PERIPHERAL VASODILATORS – MOXISYLYTE	↑ hypotensive effect	Additive hypotensive effect. Postural ↓ BP is a common side-effect of MAOIs	Monitor BP at least weekly until stable. Warn patients to report symptoms of hypotension (light-headedness, dizziness on standing, etc.)
MAOIs	POTASSIUM CHANNEL ACTIVATORS	↑ hypotensive effect	Additive hypotensive effect. Postural ↓ BP is a common side-effect of MAOIs	Monitor BP at least weekly until stable. Warn patients to report symptoms of hypotension (light-headedness, dizziness on standing, etc.)

NERVOUS SYSTEM DRUGS ANTIDEPRESSANTS

Primary drug	Secondary drug	Effect	Mechanism	Precautions
MOCLOBEMIDE	PROTON PUMP INHIBITORS – OMEPRAZOLE/ ESOMEPRAZOLE	Possible ↑ efficacy and adverse effects of moclobemide	Inhibition of CYP2C19	Monitor more closely; effect only seen in extensive CYP2C19 metabolizers. Dose ↓ may be required
MAOIs	SYMPATHOMIMETICS	Risk of adrenergic syndrome. Unlikely to occur with moclobemide and selegiline. This is likely with some OTC medications, which may contain some of these sympathomimetics	Due to inhibition of MAOI, which breaks down sympathomimetics. Moclobemide is involved in the breakdown of serotonin, while selegiline is mainly involved in the breakdown of dopamine	Avoid concurrent use. Onset may be 6–24 hours after ingestion. Do ECG, measure electrolytes, FBC, CK and coagulation profile. Before prescribing/dispensing, enquire about use of MAOI antidepressants and related drugs such as linezolid
MAOIs	TETRABENAZINE	Risk of confusion and agitation	Uncertain; although tetrabenazine depletes norepinephrine, if it is started on a patient who is already taking MAOIs it may stimulate the release of accumulated neurotransmitter. This would not be expected if a patient started MAOI while already taking tetrabenazine	Tetrabenazine may cause depression so should be used with caution in patients with depression. If necessary, consider using an alternative antidepressant or start an MAOI after tetrabenazine has been established
SELECTIVE SEROTONIN REUPTAKE INHIBITORS				
SSRIs	ALCOHOL	↑ risk of sedation	Additive CNS depressant effects. Acute ingestion of alcohol inhibits CYP2D6 and CYP2C19, whereas chronic use induces CYP2E1 and CYP3A4	Be aware and caution against excessive alcohol intake

FLUVOXAMINE	ANAESTHETICS – LOCAL ROPIVACAINE	↑ plasma concentrations and prolonged effects of ropivacaine – a local anaesthetic related to bupivacaine but less potent and cardiotoxic. Adverse effects include nausea, vomiting, tachycardia, headache and rigors	Fluvoxamine inhibits the metabolism of ropivacaine	Be aware of the possibility of prolonged effects and of toxicity. Take note of any numbness or tingling around the lips and mouth or slurring of speech after administration as they may be warning signs of more severe toxic effects such as seizures or loss of consciousness
SSRIs	**ANALGESICS**			
SSRIs	OPIOIDS	1. Possible ↓ analgesic effect of oxycodone and tramadol 2. ↑ serotonin effects, including possible cases of serotonin syndrome, when opioids (oxycodone, pethidine, pentazocine, tramadol) are co-administered with SSRIs (fluoxetine and sertraline) 3. SSRIs may ↑ codeine, fentanyl, methadone, pethidine and tramadol levels	1. Uncertain. Paroxetine inhibits CYP2D6, which is required to produce the active form of tramadol. 2. Uncertain 3. SSRIs inhibit CYP2D6-mediated metabolism of these opioids	1. Consider using an alternative opioid 2. Look for signs of ↑ serotonin activity, particularly on initiating therapy 3. Watch for excessive narcotization
SSRIs	NSAIDs	Slight ↑ risk of bleeding	Unknown	Warn patients to watch for early signs of bleeding
SSRIs	**ANTIARRHYTHMICS**			
SERTRALINE	AMIODARONE	Sertraline may ↑ amiodarone levels	Sertraline may inhibit CYP3A4-mediated metabolism of amiodarone	Watch for amiodarone toxicity; for those taking high doses of amiodarone, consider using an alternative SSRI with a lower affinity for CYP3A4

Primary drug	Secondary drug	Effect	Mechanism	Precautions
SSRIs	FLECAINIDE, MEXILETINE, PROCAINAMIDE	SSRIs may ↑ levels of these antiarrhythmics	SSRIs inhibit CYP2D6-mediated metabolism	Monitor PR and BP closely; watch for toxicity
SSRIs	PROPAFENONE	Levels of both may be ↑	Both SSRIs and propafenone are substrates for and inhibitors of CYP2D6	Monitor PR and BP closely
SSRIs	**ANTICANCER AND IMMUNOMODULATING DRUGS**			
SSRIs	**CYTOTOXICS**			
SSRIs	PROCARBAZINE	↑ risk of serotonin syndrome and CNS toxicity	Additive toxicity	Monitor BP closely and also CNS side-effects. Because of the long half-life of fluoxetine and its active metabolites, at least 5 weeks should elapse between discontinuation of fluoxetine and initiation of therapy with an MAOI
SERTRALINE	IMATINIB	↑ plasma concentrations with risk of toxic effects of these drugs	Imatinib is a potent inhibitor of CYP2C9 isoenzymes, which metabolize these drugs	Watch for the early toxic effects of these drugs. If necessary, consider using alternative drugs while the patient is being given imatinib
SSRIs – FLUOXETINE	IMMUNOMODULATING DRUGS – CICLOSPORIN	↑ plasma concentrations of ciclosporin with risk of nephrotoxicity, myelosuppression and neurotoxicity	Inhibition of CYP3A4-mediated metabolism of ciclosporin; these inhibitors vary in potency	Monitor plasma ciclosporin levels to prevent toxicity
SSRIs	ANTICOAGULANTS – ORAL	Possible ↑ in anticoagulant effect with citalopram, fluoxetine, fluvoxamine and paroxetine	Uncertain at present	Monitor INR at least weekly until stable

SSRIs	ANTIDEPRESSANTS			
SSRIs	LITHIUM	Lithium may enhance the pharmacological effects of SSRIs and potentiate the risk of serotonin syndrome. Excessive somnolence has been reported with fluvoxamine. However, there are reports of both ↑ and ↓ plasma concentrations of lithium. There are reports of lithium toxicity and of serotonergic effects	Lithium is a direct stimulant of 5-HT receptors, while SSRIs ↓ reuptake of 5-HT; these are considered to ↑ effects of serotonin in the brain. Seizures are a neurotoxic effect of lithium and could occur even with plasma lithium concentrations within the normal range. SSRIs and lithium may have additive effects to cause seizures	Be aware of the possibility of serotonin syndrome ➢ ***For signs and symptoms of serotonin toxicity, see Clinical Features of Some Adverse Drug Interactions, Serotonin toxicity and serotonin syndrome***. Also need to monitor lithium levels with appropriate dose adjustments during co-administration
SSRIs	MAOIs	↑ risk of serotonin syndrome ➢ ***For signs and symptoms of serotonin toxicity, see Clinical Features of Some Adverse Drug Interactions, Serotonin toxicity and serotonin syndrome***	Additive inhibitory effects on serotonin reuptake	Avoid co-administration. MAOIs should not be started for at least 1 week after stopping SSRIs (2 weeks after sertraline, 5 weeks after fluoxetine). Conversely, SSRIs should not be started for at least 2 weeks after stopping MAOIs
SSRIs	DULOXETINE, ST JOHN'S WORT, SSRIs, TCAs, TRAZODONE	↑ risk of serotonin syndrome ➢ ***For signs and symptoms of serotonin toxicity, see Clinical Features of Some Adverse Drug Interactions, Serotonin toxicity and serotonin syndrome***	Additive effect. In addition, TCAs inhibit CYP2D6-mediated metabolism of SSRIs	Caution with co-administration with TCAs or trazodone. Specialist advice should be sought and alternatives considered. Avoid co-administration of two SSRIs, and SSRIs with duloxetine or St John's wort
FLUVOXAMINE	REBOXETINE	May ↑ fluvoxamine levels	Reboxetine is a selective norepinephrine reuptake inhibitor. Reboxetine inhibits metabolism of fluvoxamine	Avoid concurrent use (manufacturers' recommendation)

Primary drug	Secondary drug	Effect	Mechanism	Precautions
SSRIs	ANTIDIABETIC DRUGS	Fluctuations in blood sugar are very likely, with both hypoglycaemic and hyperglycaemic events being reported in diabetics receiving hypoglycaemic treatment. ↑ plasma concentrations of sulphonylureas (e.g. tolbutamide) may occur	Brain serotonin and corticotropin-releasing hormone systems participate in the control of blood sugar levels. ↑ (usually acute) in brain serotonergic activity induces a hyperglycaemic response. Fluvoxamine is a potent inhibitor and fluoxetine a less potent inhibitor of CYP2C9, which metabolizes sulphonylureas	Both hyper- and hypoglycaemic responses have been reported with SSRIs; there is a need to monitor blood glucose closely prior to, during and after discontinuing SSRI treatment ➢ ***For signs and symptoms of hypoglycaemia, see Clinical Features of Some Adverse Drug Interactions, Hypoglycaemia, Hyperglycaemia***
FLUVOXAMINE	ANTIEMETICS – ONDANSETRON	Possible ↑ plasma concentrations of ondansetron	Fluvoxamine is potent inhibitor of CYP1A2, and fluoxetine is less potent as an inhibitor. Paroxetine, sertraline, escitalopram and citalopram are not currently known to cause any inhibition	Warn patients to report ↑ in side-effects of ondansetron
SSRIs	**ANTIEPILEPTICS**			
SSRIs	ANTIEPILEPTICS	↑ risk of seizures	SSRIs lower seizure threshold	Risk of seizures is high; need to warn carers
PAROXETINE	BARBITURATES	↓ paroxetine levels	Induction of hepatic metabolism	Be aware; watch for poor response to paroxetine
SSRIs	CARBAMAZEPINE	Risk of serotonin syndrome with carbamazepine	Carbamazepine ↑ serotonin concentrations in the brain	Avoid co-administration
SSRIs	PHENYTOIN	↑ plasma concentrations of phenytoin	Phenytoin is a substrate of CYP2C9 and CYP2C19. SSRIs are known to inhibit CYP2C9/10	Monitor plasma phenytoin levels

SSRIs	ANTIHISTAMINES			
SSRIs	CYPROHEPTADINE	Antidepressant effect of SSRIs are possibly antagonized by cyproheptadine	Cyproheptadine is an antihistamine with anti-serotonergic activity	Be aware
SSRIs	TERFENADINE	Possibility of ↑ plasma concentrations of these drugs and potential risk of dangerous arrhythmias	These drugs are metabolized mainly by CYP3A4. Fluvoxamine and fluoxetine are inhibitors of CYP3A4 but are relatively weak compared with ketoconazole, which is possibly 100 times more potent as an inhibitor	The interaction is unlikely to be of clinical significance but need to be aware
SSRIs	ANTIHYPERTENSIVES AND HEART FAILURE DRUGS – METHYLDOPA	Methyldopa may ↓ effect of antidepressants	Methyldopa can cause depression	Methyldopa should be avoided in patients with depression
SSRIs	ANTIMALARIALS – ARTEMETHER/ LUMEFANTRINE	This antimalarial may cause dose-related dangerous arrhythmias	A substrate, mainly of CYP3A4, which may be inhibited by high doses of fluvoxamine and to a lesser degree by fluoxetine	Manufacturers recommend avoidance of antidepressants
PAROXETINE	ANTIMUSCARINICS – DARIFENACIN, PROCYCLIDINE	↑ levels of these antimuscarinics	Inhibition of metabolism	Watch for early features of toxicity
FLUVOXAMINE	ANTIPARKINSON'S DRUGS – ROPINIROLE	↑ ropinirole levels	Inhibition of CYP1A2-mediated metabolism	Watch for early features of toxicity (nausea, drowsiness)
SSRIs	ANTIPARKINSON'S DRUGS – SELEGILINE, RASAGILINE	Risk of severe hypertensive reactions and of serotonin syndrome ➢ ***For signs and symptoms of serotonin toxicity, see Clinical Features of Some Adverse Drug Interactions, Serotonin toxicity and serotonin syndrome***	Additive inhibitory effect on serotonin reuptake with SSRIs. There is an accumulation of serotonin in the brain and at peripheral sites. These dopaminergics are MAO-B inhibitors	Avoid co-administration. Rasagiline and selegiline should not be started for at least 2 weeks after stopping SSRIs (5 weeks after fluoxetine). Conversely, SSRIs should not be started for at least 2 weeks after stopping rasagiline and selegiline

Primary drug	Secondary drug	Effect	Mechanism	Precautions
SSRIs	ANTIPLATELET AGENTS – ASPIRIN	Possible ↑ risk of bleeding with SSRIs	Uncertain. Possible additive effects including inhibition of serotonin release by platelets, SSRI-induced thrombocytopenia and ↓ platelet aggregation	Avoid co-administration with high-dose aspirin
SSRIs	**ANTIPSYCHOTICS**			
SSRIs	ARIPIPRAZOLE, CLOZAPINE, HALOPERIDOL, PERPHENAZINE, RISPERIDONE, SERTINDOLE, THIORIDAZINE	Possible ↑ plasma concentrations of these antipsychotics	Inhibition of CYP2D6-mediated metabolism of these drugs. The clinical significance of this depends upon whether alternative pathways of metabolism of these substrates are also inhibited by co-administered drugs. The risk is theoretically greater with clozapine, haloperidol and olanzapine because their CYP1A2-mediated metabolism is also inhibited by SSRIs	Warn patients to report ↑ side-effects of these drugs, and consider reducing the dose of the antipsychotic
SERTRALINE	PIMOZIDE	↑ plasma concentrations of these drugs and potential risk of dangerous arrhythmias	Sertraline inhibits metabolism of pimozide. Precise site of inhibition uncertain	Avoid co-administration
SSRIs	**ANTIVIRALS**			
SSRIs	NNRTIs – EFAVIRENZ	1. Possible ↑ efficacy and ↑ adverse effects, including serotonin syndrome, with fluoxetine 2. Possible ↓ efficacy with sertraline	1. Uncertain mechanism; possibly ↑ bioavailability 2. CYP2B6 contributed most to the demethylation of sertraline, with lesser contributions from CYP2C19, CYP2C9, CYP3A4 and CYP2D6	1. Use with caution; consider ↓ dose of fluoxetine 2. Watch for therapeutic failure, and advise patients to report persistence or lack of improvement of symptoms of depression. ↑ dose of sertraline as required; titrate to clinical response

SSRIs	PROTEASE INHIBITORS – RITONAVIR	↑ adverse effects of fluoxetine, paroxetine and sertraline when co-administered with ritonavir (with or without lopinavir). Cardiac and neurological events reported, including serotonin syndrome	Ritonavir is associated with the most significant interaction of the protease inhibitors due to potent inhibition of CYP3A, CYP2D6, CYP2C9 and CYP2C19 isoenzymes	Warn patients to watch for ↑ side-effects of SSRIs, and consider reducing the dose of SSRI
SSRIs	**ANXIOLYTICS AND HYPNOTICS**			
FLUOXETINE, FLUVOXAMINE, PAROXETINE	BZDs – ALPRAZOLAM, DIAZEPAM, MIDAZOLAM	↑ in plasma concentrations of these BZDs. Likely ↑ sedation and interference with psychomotor activity	Alprazolam, diazepam and midazolam are subject to metabolism by CYP3A4. Fluvoxamine, fluoxetine and possibly paroxetine are inhibitors of CYP3A4; sertraline is a weak inhibitor. SSRIs are relatively weak compared with ketoconazole, which is possibly 100 times more potent as an inhibitor	Warn patients about risks associated with activities that require alertness. Consider use of alternatives such as oxazepam, lorazepam and temazepam, which are metabolized by glucuronidation ➢ ***For signs and symptoms of CNS depression, see Clinical Features of Some Adverse Drug Interactions, Central nervous system depression***
SSRIs	CHLORAL HYDRATE	Case of excessive drowsiness	Uncertain; possibly additive effects, possibly displacement of chloral hydrate from protein binding sites	Warn patients to be aware of additional sedation
FLUOXETINE, PAROXETINE, SERTRALINE, VENLAFAXINE	ZOLPIDEM	Cases of agitation ± hallucinations	Uncertain	Avoid co-administration
SSRIs	**BETA-BLOCKERS**			
SSRIs	METOPROLOL	↑ plasma concentrations of metoprolol	SSRIs inhibit metabolism of metoprolol (paroxetine, fluoxetine, sertraline, fluvoxetine, and venlafaxine via CYP2D6; (es)citalopram uncertain at present)	Monitor PR and BP closely; watch for metoprolol toxicity, in particular loss of its cardioselectivity

Primary drug	Secondary drug	Effect	Mechanism	Precautions
SSRIs	PROPANOLOL AND TIMOLOL	↑ plasma concentrations and efficacy of propranolol	Fluvoxamine inhibits the CYP1A2-, CYP2C19- and CYP2D6-mediated metabolism of propranolol. Fluoxetine inhibits CYP2C19- and CYP2D6-mediated metabolism of propanolol and timolol. Paroxetine, sertraline, and venlafaxine inhibit CYP2D6-mediated metabolism of propanolol and timolol and can impair conduction through the AV node	Monitor PR and BP at least weekly. Warn patients to report symptoms of hypotension (light-headedness, dizziness on standing, etc.). Watch for propanolol toxicity
FLUVOXAMINE	BRONCHODILATORS – THEOPHYLLINE	Possible ↑ plasma concentrations of theophylline	Fluvoxamine is potent inhibitor of CYP1A2, and fluoxetine is less potent as an inhibitor. Paroxetine, sertraline, escitalopram and citalopram are not currently known to cause any inhibition	Consider an alternative antidepressant
SSRIs	CALCIUM CHANNEL BLOCKERS	Reports of ↑ serum levels of nimodipine and episodes of adverse effects of nifedipine and verapamil (oedema, flushing, ↓ BP) attributed to ↑ levels when co-administered with fluoxetine	Fluoxetine inhibits the CYP3A4-mediated metabolism of calcium channel blockers. It also inhibits intestinal P-gp, which may ↑ bioavailability of verapamil	Monitor BP at least weekly until stable. Warn patients to report symptoms of hypotension (light-headedness, dizziness on standing, etc.). Consider reducing the dose of calcium channel blocker or using an alternative antidepressant

SSRIs	CNS STIMULANTS			
SSRIs	ATOMOXETINE	↑ plasma concentrations and risk of adverse effects (abdominal pain, vomiting, nausea, fatigue, irritability)	Atomoxetine is a selective norepinephrine reuptake inhibitor. ↑ plasma concentrations due to inhibition of CYP2D6 by fluoxetine and paroxetine (potent), fluvoxamine and sertraline (less potent) and escitalopram and citalopram (weak)	Avoid concurrent use. The interaction is usually severe with fluoxetine and paroxetine
FLUVOXAMINE	MODAFINIL	May cause ↓ imipramine levels if CYP1A2 is the predominant metabolic pathway and alternative metabolic pathways are either genetically deficient or affected	Modafinil is a moderate inducer of CYP1A2 in a concentration-dependent manner	Be aware
SSRIs	**DRUG DEPENDENCE THERAPIES**			
FLUOXETINE, FLUVOXAMINE, PAROXETINE, SERTRALINE	BUPROPION	↑ plasma concentrations of bupropion and risk of adverse effects	Inhibition of CYP2B6	Warn patients about adverse effects, and use alternatives when possible
ESCITALOPRAM, FLUOXETINE, FLUVOXAMINE, PAROXETINE, SERTRALINE	BUPROPION	↑ plasma concentrations of these SSRIs, with risk of toxic effects	Bupropion and its metabolite hydroxybupropion inhibit CYP2D6	Initiate therapy of these drugs at the lowest effective dose. Interaction is likely to be important with substrates for which CYP2D6 is considered the only metabolic pathway (e.g. paroxetine)

Primary drug	Secondary drug	Effect	Mechanism	Precautions
FLUVOXAMINE	FOOD – CHARGRILLED MEAT, BROCCOLI, CABBAGE, SPROUTS	↓ plasma concentrations of fluvoxamine with loss of therapeutic efficacy	Fluvoxamine and fluoxetine are metabolized mainly by CYP1A2 isoenzymes, while the role of CYP1A2 in the metabolism of sertraline is probably not clinically significant	Monitor for lack of therapeutic effect. When inducers are withdrawn, monitor for fluvoxamine toxicity
FLUVOXAMINE, SERTRALINE	GRAPEFRUIT JUICE	Possibly ↑ efficacy and ↑ adverse effects	Possibly ↓ metabolism	Clinical significance unclear
SSRIs	H2 RECEPTOR BLOCKERS – CIMETIDINE	↑ efficacy and adverse effects, e.g. nausea, diarrhoea, dyspepsia, dizziness, sexual dysfunction	↑ bioavailability	Use with caution, monitor for ↑ side-effects. ↓ dose may be necessary
SSRIs	5-HT1 AGONISTS	↑ risk of serotonin syndrome ➢ ***For signs and symptoms of serotonin toxicity, see Clinical Features of Some Adverse Drug Interactions, Serotonin toxicity and serotonin syndrome***	Triptans cause direct stimulation of 5-HT receptors, while SSRIs ↓ uptake of 5-HT, thus leading to ↑ serotonergic activity in the brain	The US FDA (July 2006) issued a warning of possibility of occurrence of this life-threatening serotonin syndrome when SSRIs are used together with triptans. Advise patients to report immediately the onset of symptoms such as tremors, agitation, confusion, ↑ heart beat (palpitations) and fever, and either ↓ dose or discontinue SSRI
PAROXETINE	PARASYMPATHOMIMETICS – GALANTAMINE	↑ galantamine levels	Inhibition of CYP2D6-mediated metabolism of galantamine	Monitor PR and BP closely, watching for bradycardia and hypotension. Be aware that there is a theoretical risk with other SSRIs

SSRIs	PERIPHERAL VASODILATORS – CILOSTAZOL	Fluoxetine, fluvoxamine and sertraline ↑ cilostazol levels	Fluoxetine, fluvoxamine and sertraline inhibit CYP3A4-mediated metabolism of cilostazol	Avoid co-administration
FLUVOXAMINE	PROTON PUMP INHIBITORS – OMEPRAZOLE	↓ fluvoxamine levels with loss of therapeutic efficacy	Inhibition of CYP1A2-mediated metabolism	Monitor for lack of therapeutic effect. When omeprazole is withdrawn, monitor for fluvoxamine toxicity
SSRIs	SYMPATHOMIMETICS	1. Case report of serotonin syndrome when dexamfetamine was co-administered with citalopram 2. Case reports of psychiatric disturbances when methylphenidate was given with sertraline, and phenylpropanolamine was co-administered with phenylpropanolamine	1. Uncertain; postulated that there is an additive effect of inhibition of serotonin reuptake by citalopram with release of serotonin by venlafaxine 2. Uncertain	1. Avoid co-administration of dexamfetamine and citalopram 2. Warn patients to watch for early signs such as anxiety
FLUVOXAMINE	TOBACCO	↓ plasma concentrations of fluvoxamine with loss of therapeutic efficacy	Fluvoxamine and fluoxetine are metabolized mainly by CYP1A2 isoenzymes, while the role of CYP1A2 in the metabolism of sertraline is probably not clinically significant	Monitor for lack of therapeutic effect. When inducers are withdrawn, monitor for fluvoxamine toxicity

Primary drug	Secondary drug	Effect	Mechanism	Precautions
TRICYCLIC ANTIDEPRESSANTS				
TCAs	DRUGS THAT PROLONG THE Q–T INTERVAL			
TCAs	1. ANTIARRHYTHMICS – amiodarone, disopyramide, procainamide, propafenone 2. ANTIBIOTICS – macrolides (especially azithromycin, clarithromycin, parenteral erythromycin, telithromycin), quinolones (especially moxifloxacin), quinupristin/dalfopristin 3. ANTICANCER AND IMMUNOMODULATING DRUGS – arsenic trioxide 4. ANTIDEPRESSANTS – venlafaxine 5. ANTIEMETICS – dolasetron 6. ANTIFUNGALS – fluconazole, posaconazole, voriconazole 7. ANTIHISTAMINES – terfenadine, hydroxyzine, mizolastine 8. ANTIMALARIALS – artemether with lumefantrine, chloroquine, hydroxychloroquine, mefloquine, quinine 9. ANTIPROTOZOALS – pentamidine isetionate 10. ANTIPSYCHOTICS – atypicals, phenothiazines, pimozide 11. BETA-BLOCKERS – sotalol 12. BRONCHODILATORS – parenteral bronchodilators 13. CNS STIMULANTS – atomoxetine	Risk of ventricular arrhythmias, particularly torsades de pointes	Additive effect; these drugs cause prolongation of the Q–T interval. In addition, amiodarone inhibits CYP2C9 and CYP2D6, which have a role in metabolizing TCAs. Also, amitriptyline and clomipramine inhibit CYP2D6-mediated metabolism of procainamide. Propafenone and amitriptyline and clomipramine inhibit CYP2D6-mediated metabolism of each other	Avoid co-administration

TCAs	DRUGS WITH ANTIMUSCARINIC EFFECTS			
TCAs	1. ANALGESICS – nefopam 2. ANTIARRHYTHMICS – disopyramide, propafenone 3. ANTIEMETICS – cyclizine 4. ANTIHISTAMINES – chlorphenamine, cyproheptadine, hydroxyzine 5. ANTIMUSCARINICS – atropine, benzatropine, cyclopentolate, dicycloverine, flavoxate, homatropine, hyoscine, orphenadrine, oxybutynin, procyclidine, propantheline, tolterodine, trihexyphenidyl, tropicamide 6. ANTIPARKINSON'S DRUGS – dopaminergics 7. ANTIPSYCHOTICS – phenothiazines, clozapine, pimozide 8. MUSCLE RELAXANTS – baclofen 9. NITRATES – isosorbide dinitrate	↑ risk of antimuscarinic side-effects. Also, possibly ↓ levodopa levels. **NB ↓ efficacy of sublingual nitrate tablets**	Additive effect. Delayed gastric emptying may cause more levodopa to be metabolized within the wall of the gastrointestinal tract. **Antimuscarinic effects ↓ saliva production, which ↓ dissolution of the tablet**	Warn patients of this additive effect. Consider increasing the dose of levodopa. **Consider changing the formulation to a sublingual nitrate spray**

Primary drug	Secondary drug	Effect	Mechanism	Precautions
TCAs	ALCOHOL	↑ sedation	Additive effect	Warn patients about this effect
TCAs	ANAESTHETICS – GENERAL	A few cases of arrhythmia	Uncertain	Monitor ECG, PR and BP closely
TCAs	ANALGESICS			
TCAs	OPIOIDS	1. Risk of ↑ respiratory depression and sedation 2. ↑ levels of morphine 3. Case reports of seizures when tramadol was co-administered with TCAs 4. TCAs may ↑ codeine, fentanyl, pethidine and tramadol levels	1. Additive effect 2. Uncertain; likely ↑ bioavailability of morphine 3. Unknown 4. TCAs inhibit CYP2D6-mediated metabolism of these opioids	1. Warn patients of this effect. Titrate doses carefully 2. Warn patients of this effect. Titrate doses carefully 3. Consider an alternative opioid 4. Watch for excessive narcotization
TCAs	NEFOPAM	Risk of seizures with TCAs	Additive effect; both drugs lower the seizure threshold	Avoid co-administration
TCAs	PARACETAMOL	TCAs may slow the onset of action of intermittent-dose paracetamol	Anticholinergic effects delay gastric emptying and absorption	Warn patients that the action of paracetamol may be delayed. This will not be the case when paracetamol is taken regularly
TCAs	ANTIARRHYTHMICS – FLECAINIDE, MEXILETINE	Risk of arrhythmias	Additive effect; both drugs may be proarrhythmogenic. In addition, amitriptyline and clomipramine may inhibit CYP2D6-mediated metabolism of flecainide and mexiletine, while mexiletine inhibits CYP1A2-mediated metabolism of amitriptyline, clomipramine and imipramine	Monitor PR, BP and ECG closely; watch for flecainide toxicity

TCAs	ANTICANCER AND IMMUNOMODULATING DRUGS			
TCAs	FLUOROURACIL, IMATINIB, LEFLUNOMIDE	Possible ↑ plasma concentrations of these cytotoxics	Inhibition of CYP2C9-mediated metabolism. The clinical significance of this depends upon whether alternative pathways of metabolism are also inhibited by co-administered drugs	Warn patients to report ↑ side-effects and monitor blood count carefully
TCAs	VINBLASTINE	Possible ↑ plasma concentrations of vinblastine	Inhibition of CYP2D6-mediated metabolism of vinblastine. The clinical significance of this depends upon whether vinblastine's alternative pathways of metabolism are also inhibited by co-administered drugs	Warn patients to report ↑ side-effects of vinblastine and monitor blood count carefully
TCAs	ANTICOAGULANTS – ORAL	Cases of both ↑ and ↓ effect of warfarin	Uncertain at present	Monitor INR at least weekly until stable
TCAs	**ANTIDEPRESSANTS**			
TCAs – AMITRIPTYLINE CLOMIPRAMINE DESIPRAMINE IMIPRAMINE NORTRIPTYLINE	MAOIs	↑ risk of stroke, hyperpyrexia and convulsions. ↑ plasma concentrations of TCAs, with risk of toxic effects. ↑ risk of serotonin syndrome and of adrenergic syndrome with older MAOIs. Clomipramine may trigger acute confusion in Parkinson's disease when used with selegiline	TCAs are believed to act also by inhibiting the reuptake of serotonin and norepinephrine, increasing the risk of serotonin and adrenergic syndromes. A combination of TCAs and antidepressants can ↑ risk of seizures	Very hazardous interaction. Avoid concurrent use and consider use of alternative antidepressant. Be aware that seizures occur with overdose of TCAs just before cardiac arrest

Primary drug	Secondary drug	Effect	Mechanism	Precautions
TCAs	DULOXETINE, SSRIs, TRAZODONE	↑ risk of serotonin syndrome ➢ ***For signs and symptoms of serotonin toxicity, see Clinical Features of Some Adverse Drug Interactions, Serotonin toxicity and serotonin syndrome***	Additive effect; TCAs block uptake reuptake of serotonin. In addition, TCAs inhibit CYP2D6-mediated metabolism of SSRIs	Caution with co-administration. Specialist advice should be sought and alternatives considered
TCAs	ANTIDIABETIC DRUGS	Likely to impair control of diabetes.	TCAs may ↑ serum glucose levels by up to 150%, ↑ appetite (particularly carbohydrate craving) and ↓ metabolic rate	Be aware and monitor blood sugar weekly until stable. Generally considered safe unless diabetes is poorly controlled or is associated with significant cardiac or renal disease. Amitriptyline, imipramine and citalopram are also used to treat painful diabetic neuropathy
TCAs	ANTIEMETICS – ONDANSETRON, TROPISETRON	Possible ↑ plasma concentrations of these antiemetics	Inhibition of CYP2D6-mediated metabolism of these antiemetics. The clinical significance of this depends upon whether their alternative pathways of metabolism are also inhibited by co-administered drugs. The risk is theoretically higher with ondansetron because TCAs also inhibit CYP1A2-mediated metabolism	Warn patients to report ↑ side-effects of ondansetron and tropisetron
TCAs	**ANTIEPILEPTICS**			
TCAs	ANTIEPILEPTICS	Possible ↓ effect of antiepileptics	TCAs lower seizure threshold	Caution with co-administration. Consider an alternative antidepressant in patients on antiepileptics

TCAs	BARBITURATES	↓ mianserin levels	Induction of hepatic metabolism	Be aware and watch for signs of ↓ antidepressant effect of mianserin
TCAs	CARBAMAZEPINE	1. ↑ risk of bone marrow depression in patients on chemotherapy when used with TCAs 2. ↓ plasma concentrations of mianserin	1. Additive effects 2. ↑ metabolism of mianserin	1. Avoid concurrent use during chemotherapy 2. Be aware and watch for signs of ↓ antidepressant effect of mianserin
TCAs	PHENYTOIN	1. ↑ plasma concentrations of phenytoin and risk of phenytoin toxicity 2. ↓ plasma concentrations of mianserin	1. ↓ metabolism of phenytoin 2. ↑ metabolism of mianserin	1. Caution with co-administration. Consider an alternative antidepressant in patients on phenytoin 2. Be aware and watch for signs of ↓ antidepressant effect of mianserin
TCAs	VALPROATE	↑ amitriptyline and nortriptyline levels	Uncertain	Be aware; watch for clinical features of ↑ levels of these TCAs (e.g. sedation, dry mouth)
TCAs	ANTIFUNGALS – ITRACONAZOLE, KETOCONAZOLE, MICONAZOLE, GRISEOFULVIN	Possible ↑ plasma concentrations of TCAs	All TCAs are metabolized primarily by CYP2D6. Other pathways include CYP1A2 (e.g. amitriptyline, clomipramine, imipramine), CYP2C9 and CYP2C19 (e.g. clomipramine, imipramine). Ketoconazole and voriconazole are documented inhibitors of CYP2C19. Fluconazole and voriconazole are reported to inhibit CYP2C9	Warn patients to report ↑ side-effects of TCAs such as dry mouth, blurred vision and constipation, which may be an early sign of increasing TCA levels. In this case, consider reducing the dose of TCA
TCAs	**ANTIHYPERTENSIVES AND HEART FAILURE DRUGS**			
TCAs	ADRENERGIC NEURONE BLOCKERS	↓ hypotensive effect. There is possibly less effect with maprotiline and mianserin	TCAs compete with adrenergic neurone blockers for reuptake to nerve terminals	Monitor BP at least weekly until stable

Primary drug	Secondary drug	Effect	Mechanism	Precautions
TCAs	CENTRALLY ACTING ANTIHYPERTENSIVES	1. Possibly hypotensive effect of clonidine and moxonidine antagonized by TCAs (some case reports of hypertensive crisis). 2. Conversely, clonidine and moxonidine may exacerbate the sedative effects of TCAs, particularly during initiation of therapy 3. Methyldopa may ↓ effect of antidepressants	1 and 2. Uncertain 3. Methyldopa can cause depression	1. Monitor BP at least weekly until stable 2. Warn patients of the risk of sedation and advise them to avoid driving or operating machinery if they suffer from sedation. 3. Methyldopa should be avoided in patients with depression
TCAs	ANTIMALARIALS – PROGUANIL	Possible ↑ plasma concentrations of proguanil	Inhibition of CYP2C19-mediated metabolism of proguanil. The clinical significance of this depends upon whether proguanil's alternative pathways of metabolism are also inhibited by co-administered drugs	Warn patient to report any evidence of excessive side-effects such as change in bowel habit or stomatitis
TCAs	ANTIPARKINSON'S DRUGS – RASAGILINE, SELEGILINE	↑ risk of stroke, hyperpyrexia and convulsions. ↑ plasma concentrations of TCAs, with risk of toxic effects. ↑ risk of serotonin syndrome and of adrenergic syndrome with older MAOIs. Clomipramine may trigger acute confusion in Parkinson's disease when used with selegiline	TCAs are believed to act also by inhibiting the reuptake of serotonin and norepinephrine, increasing the risk of serotonin and adrenergic syndromes. The combination of TCAs and antidepressants can ↑ risk of seizures	Very hazardous interaction. Avoid concurrent use and consider the use of an alternative antidepressant. Be aware that seizures occur with overdose of TCAs just before cardiac arrest

TCAs	ANTIPSYCHOTICS ➢ *also Q–T-prolonging drugs*			
TCAs	HALOPERIDOL	Possible ↑ haloperidol levels	Inhibition of CYP2D6- and CYP1A2-mediated metabolism of thioridazine	Warn patients to report ↑ side-effects of these drugs
TCAs	**ANTIVIRALS – PROTEASE INHIBITORS**			
AMITRIPTYLINE	PROTEASE INHIBITORS	↑ adverse effects when amitriptyline is co-administered with ritonavir (with or without lopinavir) and possibly atazanavir	Inhibition of CYP3A4-mediated metabolism. Note that SSRIs are metabolized by a number of enzymes, including CYP2C9, CYP2C19, CYP2D6 as well as CYP3A4; therefore the effect of protease inhibitors is variable	Monitor closely
AMOXAPINE, CLOMIPRAMINE, DOXEPIN, IMIPRAMINE, NORTRIPTYLINE, TRIMIPRAMINE	PROTEASE INHIBITORS	Possibly ↑ adverse effects of amoxapine with atazanavir and ritonavir	Inhibition of CYP3A4-mediated metabolism of amoxapine, clomipramine and doxepin; inhibition of CYP3A4-, CYP2D6- and CYP2C9-mediated metabolism of imipramine; inhibition of CYP2D6-mediated metabolism of nortriptyline and trimipramine	Monitor closely
TACs	**ANXIOLYTICS AND HYPNOTICS**			
TCAs	ANXIOLYTICS AND HYPNOTICS – BZDs	Possible ↑ plasma concentrations of diazepam	Inhibition of CYP2C19-mediated metabolism of diazepam. The clinical significance of this depends upon whether diazepam's alternative pathways of metabolism are also inhibited by co-administered drugs	Watch for excessive sedation with diazepam

Primary drug	Secondary drug	Effect	Mechanism	Precautions
TCAs	ANXIOLYTICS AND HYPNOTICS – SODIUM OXYBATE	Risk of CNS depression – coma, respiratory depression	Additive depression of CNS	Avoid co-administration
TCAs	**BETA-BLOCKERS**			
AMITRIPTYLINE, CLOMIPRAMINE	BETA-BLOCKERS	Risk of ↑ levels of beta-blockers with amitriptyline and clomipramine	These TCAs inhibit CYP2D6-mediated metabolism of beta-blockers	Monitor BP at least weekly until stable. Warn patients to report symptoms of hypotension (light-headedness, dizziness on standing, etc.)
IMIPRAMINE	LABETALOL, PROPANOLOL	↑ imipramine with labetalol and propanolol	Uncertain at present. Postulated that imipramine metabolism ↓ by competition at CYP2D6 and CYP2C8	Monitor plasma levels of imipramine when initiating beta-blocker therapy
MAPROTILINE	PROPANOLOL	Cases of ↑ plasma levels of maprotiline with propanolol	Uncertain at present. Postulated that maprotiline metabolism ↓ by alterations in hepatic blood flow	Monitor plasma levels of maprotiline when initiating beta-blocker therapy
TCAs	**BRONCHODILATORS**			
TCAs	THEOPHYLLINE	Possible ↑ plasma concentrations of theophylline	Inhibition of CYP1A2- and CYP2D6-mediated metabolism of theophylline. The clinical significance of this depends upon whether theophylline's alternative pathways of metabolism are also inhibited by co-administered drugs	Warn patients to report ↑ side-effects of theophylline, and monitor PR and ECG carefully

TCAs	ZAFIRLUKAST	Possible ↑ plasma concentrations of zafirlukast	Inhibition of CYP2C9-mediated metabolism of zafirlukast. The clinical significance of this depends upon whether alternative pathways of metabolism are also inhibited by co-administered drugs	Warn patients to report ↑ side-effects
TCAs	CALCIUM CHANNEL BLOCKERS	↑ plasma concentrations of TCAs when co-administered with diltiazem and verapamil. Reports of cardiotoxicity (first- and second-degree block) when imipramine is given with diltiazem or verapamil	Uncertain but may be due to a combination of ↓ clearance of TCAs (both diltiazem and verapamil are known to inhibit CYP1A2, which has a role in the metabolism of amitriptyline, clomipramine and imipramine) and ↑ intestinal absorption (diltiazem and verapamil inhibit intestinal P-gp, which may ↑ amitriptyline bioavailability)	Monitor ECG when commencing/altering treatment
TRAZODONE	CARDIAC GLYCOSIDES – DIGOXIN	Two reported cases of ↑ plasma concentrations of digoxin after starting trazodone	Uncertain at present	Watch for digoxin toxicity; check levels and ↓ dose of digoxin as necessary
TCAs	**CNS STIMULANTS**			
AMITRIPTYLINE	MODAFINIL	Variable effect on amitriptyline	Modafinil inhibits CYP2C9 and induces CYP1A2	Watch for both poor response and early features of toxicity of amitriptyline
CLOMIPRAMINE	MODAFINIL	Variable effect on clomipramine	CYP2C19 provides an ancillary pathway for the metabolism of clomipramine. Modafinil inhibits CYP2C19 reversibly at pharmacologically relevant concentrations. Modafinil also induces CYP1A2	Watch for both poor response and early features of toxicity of clomipramine

Primary drug	Secondary drug	Effect	Mechanism	Precautions
IMIPRAMINE	MODAFINIL	May cause ↓ imipramine levels if CYP1A2 is the predominant metabolic pathway and alternative metabolic pathways are either genetically deficient or affected	Modafinil is a moderate inducer of CYP1A2 in a concentration-dependent manner	Be aware
DESIPRAMINE	MODAFINIL	↑ plasma concentrations of TCAs in a subset of the population (7–10% of white people) who are deficient in CYP2D6	CYP2C19 provides an ancillary pathway for the metabolism of desipramine. Modafinil inhibits CYP2C19 reversibly at pharmacologically relevant concentrations	↓ in dose of TCAs is often necessary
TCAs	DRUG DEPENDENCE THERAPIES – BUPROPION	1. ↑ risk of seizures This risk is marked in elderly people, in patients with a history of seizures, addiction to opiates/cocaine/stimulants, and in diabetics treated with oral hypoglycaemics or insulin 2. ↑ plasma concentrations of amitriptyline, clomipramine, desipramine, doxepin and imipramine, with risk of toxic effects	1. Bupropion is associated with a dose-related risk of seizures. TCAs lower the seizure threshold. Additive effects when combined 2. Bupropion and its metabolite hydroxybupropion inhibit CYP2D6	1. Extreme caution. The dose of bupropion should not exceed 450 mg/day (or 150 mg/day in those with severe hepatic cirrhosis) 2. Initiate therapy of these drugs at the lowest effective dose
TCAs	H2 RECEPTOR BLOCKERS – CIMETIDINE	↑ efficacy and adverse effects, e.g. dry mouth, urinary retention, blurred vision, constipation	↓ metabolism	Use alternative acid suppression or monitor more closely and ↓ dose. Rapid hydroxylators may be at ↑ risk
TCAs	NITRATES	1. ↑ risk of antimuscarinic side-effects when isosorbide dinitrate is co-administered with TCAs 2. ↓ efficacy of sublingual nitrate tablets with TCAs	1. Additive effect; both of these drugs cause antimuscarinic side-effects 2. Antimuscarinic effects ↓ saliva production, which ↓ dissolution of the tablet	1. Warn patients of this additive effect 2. Consider changing the formulation to a sublingual nitrate spray

TCAs	SUCRALFATE	Possible ↓ amitriptyline levels	↓ absorption of amitriptyline	Watch for poor response to amitriptyline
TCAs	**SYMPATHOMIMETICS**			
TCAs	INDIRECT	1. Methylphenidate ↑ TCA levels, which may improve their efficacy, but cases of toxicity with imipramine reported 2. TCAs possibly ↓ efficacy of indirect sympathomimetics	1. Uncertain; postulated to be due to inhibition of hepatic metabolism of TCAs 2. Indirect sympathomimetics cause release of norepinephrine from nerve endings; this is blocked by TCAs	1. Warn patients to watch for early signs of ↑ TCA efficacy such as drowsiness and dry mouth 2. Watch for poor response to indirect sympathomimetics
TCAs	DIRECT	↑ efficacy of norepinephrine, epinephrine or phenylephrine when co-administered with TCAs; risk of ↑ BP and tachyarrhythmias	TCAs block reuptake of norepinephrine into the nerve terminals, which prolongs its activity	Monitor PR, BP and ECG closely; start inotropes at a lower dose. It is advisable to monitor PR and BP even when using local anaesthetics containing epinephrine, although there is no evidence of significant toxicity
TCAs	THYROID HORMONES	Possible ↑ antidepressant effect	Uncertain	May be beneficial, but there are cases of nausea and dizziness; warn patients to report these symptoms
ST JOHN'S WORT				
ST JOHN'S WORT	ANTIBIOTICS – TELITHROMYCIN	↓ telithromycin levels	Due to induction of CYP3A4-mediated metabolism of telithromycin	Avoid co-administration for up to 2 weeks after stopping St John's wort
ST JOHN'S WORT	**ANTICANCER AND IMMUNOMODULATING DRUGS**			
ST JOHN'S WORT	IFOSFAMIDE	↑ rate of biotransformation to 4-hydroxyifosfamide, the active metabolite, but there is no change in AUC of4-hydroxyifosfamide	Due to ↑ rate of metabolism and of clearance due to induction of CYP3A4 and CYP2D6	Be aware – but clinical significance may be minimal or none

Primary drug	Secondary drug	Effect	Mechanism	Precautions
ST JOHN'S WORT	IMATINIB	↓ imatinib levels	Due to induction of CYP3A4-mediated metabolism of imatinib	Monitor for clinical efficacy and adjust dose as required. Avoid co-administration of imatinib and rifampicin
ST JOHN'S WORT	IRINOTECAN	↓ plasma concentrations of irinotecan and risk of ↓ therapeutic efficacy. The effects may last for 3 weeks after discontinuation of CYP-inducer therapy	Due to induction of CYP3A4-mediated metabolism of irinotecan	Avoid concomitant use when ever possible; if not, ↑ dose of irinotecan by 50%
ST JOHN'S WORT	PACLITAXEL	↓ plasma concentration of paclitaxel and ↓ efficacy of paclitaxel	Due to induction of hepatic metabolism of paclitaxel by the CYP isoenzymes	Monitor for clinical efficacy; need to ↑ dose if inadequate response is due to interaction
ST JOHN'S WORT	VINCA ALKALOIDS – VINBLASTINE, VINCRISTINE	↓ of plasma concentrations of vinblastine and vincristine, with risk of inadequate therapeutic response. Reports of AUC ↓ by 40%, elimination half-life ↓ by 35%, and clearance ↑ by 63% in patients with brain tumours taking vincristine	Due to induction of CYP3A4-mediated metabolism	Monitor for clinical efficacy, and ↑ dose of vinblastine and vincristine as clinically indicated; in the latter case, monitor clinically and radiologically for clinical efficacy in patients with brain tumours, and ↑ dose to obtain the desired response
ST JOHN'S WORT	**HORMONES AND HORMONE ANTAGONISTS**			
ST JOHN'S WORT	TAMOXIFEN	↓ plasma concentrations of tamoxifen and risk of inadequate therapeutic response	Due to induction of metabolism of tamoxifen by the CYP3A isoenzymes as a result of taking St John's wort	Avoid concurrent use
ST JOHN'S WORT	**IMMUNOMODULATING DRUGS**			
ST JOHN'S WORT	CICLOSPORIN	↓ plasma concentrations of ciclosporin, with risk of transplant rejection	Due to induction of metabolism of ciclosporin by these drugs. The potency of induction varies. St John's wort may produce its effects by an effect on P-gp	Avoid co-administration

ST JOHN'S WORT	CORTICOSTEROIDS	↓ plasma concentrations of corticosteroids and risk of poor or inadequate therapeutic response, which would be undesirable if used for e.g. cerebral oedema	Due to induction of the hepatic metabolism by the CYP3A4 isoenzymes	Monitor therapeutic response closely – clinically, with ophthalmoscopy and radiologically – and ↑ dose of corticosteroids for desired therapeutic effect
ST JOHN'S WORT	TACROLIMUS	↓ tacrolimus levels	Induction of CYP3A4-mediated metabolism of tacrolimus	Avoid co-administration
ST JOHN'S WORT	ANTICOAGULANTS – ORAL	↓ warfarin levels	Induction of metabolism	Avoid co-administration
ST JOHN'S WORT	**ANTIDEPRESSANTS**			
ST JOHN'S WORT	DULOXETINE	↑ risk of serotonin syndrome ➢ ***For signs and symptoms of serotonin toxicity, see Clinical Features of Some Adverse Drug Interactions, Serotonin toxicity and serotonin syndrome***	Additive effect	Avoid co-administration
ST JOHN'S WORT	SSRIs	↑ risk of serotonin syndrome ➢ ***For signs and symptoms of serotonin toxicity, see Clinical Features of Some Adverse Drug Interactions, Serotonin toxicity and serotonin syndrome***	Additive effect. In addition, TCAs inhibit CYP2D6-mediated metabolism of SSRIs	Caution with co-administration with TCAs or trazodone. Specialist advice should be sought and alternatives considered. Avoid co-administration of two SSRIs, and SSRIs with duloxetine or St John's wort
ST JOHN'S WORT	**ANTIDIABETIC DRUGS**			
ST JOHN'S WORT	REPAGLINIDE	↓ plasma concentrations of repaglinide likely	Due to inducing CYP3A4 isoenzymes, which metabolize repaglinide. However, the alternative pathway – CYP2C8 – is unaffected by these inducers	Be aware and monitor for hyperglycaemia ➢ ***For signs and symptoms of hyperglycaemia, see Clinical Features of Some Adverse Drug Interactions, Hyperglycaemia***

Primary drug	Secondary drug	Effect	Mechanism	Precautions
ST JOHN'S WORT	SULPHONYLUREAS	↓ hypoglycaemic efficacy	↓ plasma levels of sulphonylureas by induction of CYP-mediated metabolism	Watch for and warn patients about symptoms of hyperglycaemia ➢ ***For signs and symptoms of hyperglycaemia, see Clinical Features of Some Adverse Drug Interactions, Hyperglycaemia***
ST JOHN'S WORT	ANTIEMETICS – APREPITANT	↑ aprepitant levels	Inhibition of CYP3A4-mediated metabolism of aprepitant	Avoid co-administration (manufacturers' recommendation)
ST JOHN'S WORT	ANTIEPILEPTICS – BARBITURATES, CARBAMAZEPINE, PHENYTOIN LEVELS	↓ antiepileptic levels	↑ metabolism	Avoid co-administration
ST JOHN'S WORT	ANTIMALARIALS – ARTEMETHER/ LUMEFANTRINE	This antimalarial may cause dose-related dangerous arrhythmias	A substrate mainly of CYP3A4, which may be inhibited by St John's wort	Manufacturers recommend avoidance of antidepressants
ST JOHN'S WORT	ANTIMIGRAINE DRUGS – TRIPTANS	↑ risk of serotonin syndrome ➢ ***For signs and symptoms of serotonin toxicity, see Clinical Features of Some Adverse Drug Interactions, Serotonin toxicity and serotonin syndrome***	Possibly additive effect	Avoid co-administration
ST JOHN'S WORT	ANTIVIRALS – PROTEASE INHIBITORS	Markedly ↓ levels and efficacy of protease inhibitors by St John's wort	Possibly ↑ CYP3A4-mediated metabolism of the protease inhibitors	Avoid co-administration
ST JOHN'S WORT	BRONCHODILATORS – THEOPHYLLINE	↓ theophylline levels	Inhibition of CYP1A2-mediated metabolism of theophylline	Avoid co-administration

ST JOHN'S WORT	CALCIUM CHANNEL BLOCKERS	St John's wort is associated with ↓ verapamil levels	St John's wort induces CYP3A4, which metabolizes calcium channel blockers, and induces intestinal P-gp, which may ↓ bioavailability of verapamil	Monitor BP regularly for at least the first 2 weeks of initiating St John's wort
ST JOHN'S WORT	CARDIAC GLYCOSIDES – DIGOXIN	Plasma concentrations of digoxin seem to be ↓ by St John's wort	St John's wort seems to ↓ P-gp-mediated intestinal absorption of digoxin	Watch for ↓ response to digoxin
ST JOHN'S WORT	CNS STIMULANTS – MODAFINIL	May ↓ modafinil levels	Induction of CYP3A4, which has a partial role in the metabolism of modafinil	Be aware
ST JOHN'S WORT	DIURETICS – POTASSIUM-SPARING	↓ eplerenone levels	Induction of metabolism	Avoid co-administration
ST JOHN'S WORT	IVABRADINE	↓ levels with St John's wort	Uncertain	Avoid co-administration
ST JOHN'S WORT	LIPID-LOWERING DRUGS – STATINS	St John's wort may lower simvastatin levels	Uncertain at present	Monitor lipid profile closely; look for poor response to simvastatin
ST JOHN'S WORT	OESTROGENS	Marked ↓ contraceptive effect	Induction of metabolism of oestrogens	Avoid co-administration
ST JOHN'S WORT	PROGESTOGENS	↓ progesterone levels, which may lead to failure of contraception or a poor response to the treatment of menorrhagia	Possibly induction of metabolism of progestogens	Avoid co-administration

Primary drug	Secondary drug	Effect	Mechanism	Precautions
SEROTONIN NOREPINEPHRINE REUPTAKE INHIBITORS – DULOXETINE, VENLAFAXINE				
VENLAFAXINE	DRUGS THAT PROLONG THE Q–T INTERVAL			
VENLAFAXINE	1. ANTIARRHYTHMICS – amiodarone, disopyramide, procainamide, propafenone 2. ANTIBIOTICS – macrolides (especially azithromycin, clarithromycin, parenteral erythromycin, telithromycin), quinolones (especially moxifloxacin), quinupristin/ dalfopristin 3. ANTICANCER AND IMMUNOMODULATING DRUGS – arsenic trioxide 4. ANTIDEPRESSANTS – TCAs 5. ANTIEMETICS – dolasetron 6. ANTIFUNGALS – fluconazole, posaconazole, voriconazole 7. ANTIHISTAMINES – terfenadine, hydroxyzine, mizolastine 8. ANTIMALARIALS – artemether with lumefantrine, chloroquine, hydroxychloroquine, mefloquine, quinine 9. ANTIPROTOZOALS – pentamidine isetionate 10. ANTIPSYCHOTICS – atypicals, phenothiazines, pimozide 11. BETA-BLOCKERS – sotalol 12. BRONCHODILATORS – parenteral bronchodilators 13. CNS STIMULANTS – atomoxetine	Risk of ventricular arrhythmias, particularly torsades de pointes	Additive effect; these drugs cause prolongation of the Q–T interval	Avoid co-administration

SNRIs	ANALGESICS			
VENLAFAXINE	NSAIDs	Slight ↑ risk of bleeding	Unknown	Warn patients to watch for early signs of bleeding
DULOXETINE	OPIOIDS	↑ serotonin effects, including possible cases of serotonin syndrome, when opioids (oxycodone, pethidine, pentazocine, tramadol) are given	Uncertain	Look for signs of ↑ serotonin activity, particularly on initiating therapy
DULOXETINE	ANTIARRHYTHMICS – FLECAINIDE, PROPAFENONE	Possibly ↑ flecainide and propafenone levels	Duloxetine moderately inhibits CYP2D6	Monitor PR and BP weekly until stable
DULOXETINE	ANTIBIOTICS – CIPROFLOXACIN	↑ duloxetine levels with risk of side-effects, e.g. arrhythmias	Inhibition of metabolism of duloxetine	Avoid co-administration
SNRIs	**ANTIDEPRESSANTS**			
VENLAFAXINE	LITHIUM	Possible risk of serotonin syndrome	Additive effect	Be aware of the possibility of serotonin syndrome. Also need to monitor lithium levels, with appropriate dose adjustments during co-administration ➢ ***For signs and symptoms of serotonin toxicity, see Clinical Features of Some Adverse Drug Interactions, Serotonin toxicity and serotonin syndrome***

Primary drug	Secondary drug	Effect	Mechanism	Precautions
SNRIs	MAOIs	Risk of severe hypertensive reactions and of serotonin syndrome ➢ ***For signs and symptoms of serotonin toxicity, see Clinical Features of Some Adverse Drug Interactions, Serotonin toxicity and serotonin syndrome***	Duloxetine and venlafaxine inhibits the reuptake of both serotonin and norepinephrine. Due to impaired metabolism of these amines, there is an accumulation of serotonin and norepinephrine in the brain and at peripheral sites	Do not co-administer duloxetine and venlafaxine prior to 14 days after discontinuing an MAOI, and do not co-administer an MAOI for 5 days after discontinuing duloxetine, 1 week after venlafaxine
DULOXETINE	ST JOHN'S WORT, SSRIs, TCAs	↑ risk of serotonin syndrome ➢ ***For signs and symptoms of serotonin toxicity, see Clinical Features of Some Adverse Drug Interactions, Serotonin toxicity and serotonin syndrome***	Additive effect	Avoid co-administration
SNRIs	ANTIHYPERTENSIVES AND HEART FAILURE DRUGS – CENTRALLY ACTING ANTIHYPERTENSIVES – methyldopa	Methyldopa may ↓ effect of antidepressants	Methyldopa can cause depression	Methyldopa should be avoided in patients with depression
SNRIs	ANTIMALARIALS – ARTEMETHER/ LUMEFANTRINE	↑ artemether/lumefantrine levels with risk of toxicity, including arrhythmias	Venlafaxine inhibits CYP3A4, which is partly responsible for the metabolism of artemether	Avoid co-administration with venlafaxine and caution with duloxetine
VENLAFAXINE	ANTIPARKINSON'S DRUGS – SELEGILINE, POSSIBLY RASAGILINE	Risk of severe hypertensive reactions and of serotonin syndrome ➢ ***For signs and symptoms of serotonin toxicity, see Clinical Features of Some Adverse Drug Interactions, Serotonin toxicity and serotonin syndrome***	Venlafaxine inhibits the reuptake of both serotonin and norepinephrine. Due to impaired metabolism of these amines, there is an accumulation of serotonin and norepinephrine in the brain and at peripheral sites. These dopaminergics are MAO-B inhibitors	Do not start selegiline or rasagiline for at least 1 week after stopping venlafaxine; conversely, do not start venlafaxine for at least 2 weeks after stopping selegiline or rasagiline

VENLAFAXINE	ANTIPLATELET AGENTS – ASPIRIN	Possible ↑ risk of bleeding with venlafaxine	Uncertain	Avoid co-administration with high-dose aspirin
VENLAFAXINE	**ANTIPSYCHOTICS** ➢ ***also Q-T-prolonging drugs, above***			
VENLAFAXINE	HALOPERIDOL	↑ haloperidol levels	Inhibited metabolism	Avoid co-administration
DULOXETINE	ANTIMIGRAINE DRUGS – 5-HT1 AGONISTS	Possible ↑ risk of serotonin syndrome ➢ ***For signs and symptoms of serotonin toxicity, see Clinical Features of Some Adverse Drug Interactions, Serotonin toxicity and serotonin syndrome***	Triptans cause direct stimulation of 5-HT receptors, while SSRIs ↓ uptake of 5-HT, thus leading to ↑ serotonergic activity in the brain	The US FDA (July 2006) warned of the possibility of life-threatening serotonin syndrome when SNRIs are used together with triptans (5-HT receptor agonists). Avoid concomitant use, or ↓ dose of SNRI
VENLAFAXINE	BETA-BLOCKERS	↑ plasma concentrations and efficacy of metoprolol, propranolol and timolol	Venlafaxine inhibits CYP2D6-mediated metabolism of metoprolol, propanolol and timolol	Monitor PR and BP at least weekly; watch for metoprolol toxicity (in particular, loss of its cardioselectivity) and propanolol toxicity
VENLAFAXINE	H2 RECEPTOR BLOCKERS – CIMETIDINE	↑ efficacy and adverse effects	Inhibition of metabolism	Not thought to be clinically significant, but take care in elderly people and in patients with hepatic impairment
VENLAFAXINE	SYMPATHOMIMETICS – INDIRECT	Case of serotonin syndrome when dexamfetamine is co-administered with venlafaxine	Uncertain; postulated that there is an additive effect of inhibition of serotonin reuptake by venlafaxine, with a release of serotonin by venlafaxine	Avoid co-administration
MIRTAZAPINE				
MIRTAZAPINE	ALCOHOL	↑ sedation	Additive effect	Warn patients about this effect
MIRTAZAPINE	ANTICOAGULANTS – ORAL	↑ anticoagulant effect of warfarin	Inhibition of metabolism of warfarin	Monitor INR at least weekly until stable

Primary drug	Secondary drug	Effect	Mechanism	Precautions
MIRTAZAPINE	ANTIDEPRESSANTS – MAOIs	Risk of severe hypertensive reactions and of serotonin syndrome ➢ ***For signs and symptoms of serotonin toxicity, see Clinical Features of Some Adverse Drug Interactions, Serotonin toxicity and serotonin syndrome***	Additive inhibition of both serotonin and norepinephrine reuptake	Avoid co-administration. MAOIs should not be started for at least 2 weeks after stopping mirtazapine (moclobemide can be started at least 1 week after stopping mirtazapine). Conversely, mirtazapine should not be started for at least 2 weeks after stopping MAOIs
MIRTAZAPINE	ANTIEPILEPTICS	↓ mirtazapine levels with carbamazepine and phenytoin	Induction of metabolism of mirtazapine, possibly by CYP2D6	Watch for poor response to mirtazapine
MIRTAZAPINE	ANTIFUNGALS – KETOCONAZOLE	↑ mirtazapine levels	Inhibition of metabolism via CYP1A2, CYP2D6 and CYP3A4	Consider alternative antifungals
MIRTAZAPINE	ANTIHYPERTENSIVES AND HEART FAILURE DRUGS – CENTRALLY ACTING ANTIHYPERTENSIVES – METHYLDOPA	Methyldopa may ↓ effect of antidepressants	Methyldopa can cause depression	Methyldopa should be avoided in patients with depression
MIRTAZAPINE	ANTIOBESITY DRUGS – SIBUTRAMINE	Risk of hypertension and agitation	Additive effect on norepinephrine transmission	Avoid co-administration
MIRTAZAPINE	ANXIOLYTICS AND HYPNOTICS	↑ sedation	Additive effect	Warn patients about this effect
MIRTAZAPINE	H2 RECEPTOR BLOCKERS – CIMETIDINE	↑ mirtazapine levels	Inhibition of metabolism via CYP1A2, CYP2D6 and CYPA4	Consider alternative acid suppression, e.g. H2 antagonist (proton pump inhibitors will interact in poor CYP2D6 metabolizers) or monitor more closely for side-effects; ↓ dose as necessary

REBOXETINE				
REBOXETINE	ANTIBIOTICS – MACROLIDES	Risk of ↑ reboxetine levels	Possibly inhibition of CYP3A4-mediated metabolism of reboxetine	Avoid co-administration
REBOXETINE	**ANTIDEPRESSANTS**			
REBOXETINE	MAOIs	Risk of severe hypertensive reactions	Additive inhibition of norepinephrine reuptake	Avoid co-administration. MAOIs should not be started for at least 1 week after stopping reboxetine. Conversely, reboxetine should not be started for at least 2 weeks after stopping MAOIs
REBOXETINE	FLUVOXAMINE	May ↑ fluvoxamine levels	Reboxetine is a selective norepinephrine reuptake inhibitor. Reboxetine inhibits metabolism of fluvoxamine	Avoid concurrent use (manufacturers' recommendation)
REBOXETINE	ANTIFUNGALS – AZOLES	Risk of ↑ reboxetine levels	Possibly inhibition of CYP3A4-mediated metabolism of reboxetine	Avoid co-administration
REBOXETINE	ANTIHYPERTENSIVES AND HEART FAILURE DRUGS – CENTRALLY ACTING ANTIHYPERTENSIVES – methyldopa	Methyldopa may ↓ effect of antidepressants	Methyldopa can cause depression	Methyldopa should be avoided in patients with depression
REBOXETINE	ANTIMALARIALS – ARTEMETHER/ LUMEFANTRINE	↑ artemether/lumefantrine levels, with risk of toxicity, including arrhythmias	Uncertain	Avoid co-administration
REBOXETINE	ANTIMIGRAINE DRUGS – ERGOT DERIVATIVES	Risk of hypertension	Additive effect	Monitor BP closely
REBOXETINE	ANTIOBESITY DRUGS – SIBUTRAMINE	Risk of hypertension and agitation	Additive inhibition of norepinephrine reuptake	Avoid co-administration

Primary drug	Secondary drug	Effect	Mechanism	Precautions
TRYPTOPHAN				
TRYPTOPHAN	ANTICANCER AND IMMUNOMODULATING DRUGS – PROCARBAZINE	Risk of hyperreflexia, shivering, hyperventilation, hyperthermia, mania or hypomania, disorientation/confusion	Tryptophan is a precursor of a number of neurotransmitters, including serotonin. Procarbazine has MAOI activity, which inhibits the breakdown of neurotransmitters	Tryptophan should be started under specialist supervision. Recommended to start with low doses and titrate the dose upwards with close monitoring of mental status and BP
TRYPTOPHAN	ANTIDEPRESSANTS – MAOIs	Risk of confusion and agitation	Tryptophan is a precursor of a number of neurotransmitters, including serotonin. MAOIs inhibit the breakdown of neurotransmitters	↓ dose of tryptophan
TRYPTOPHAN	ANTIHYPERTENSIVES AND HEART FAILURE DRUGS – CENTRALLY ACTING ANTIHYPERTENSIVES – methyldopa	Methyldopa may ↓ effect of antidepressants	Methyldopa can cause depression	Methyldopa should be avoided in patients with depression
TRYPTOPHAN	ANTIMALARIALS – ARTEMETHER/LUMEFANTRINE	↑ artemether/lumefantrine levels, with risk of toxicity, including arrhythmias	Uncertain	Avoid co-administration
TRYPTOPHAN	ANTIOBESITY DRUGS – SIBUTRAMINE	Risk of hypertension and agitation	Additive effect. Tryptophan is a precursor of neurotransmitters such as serotonin; sibutramine inhibits serotonin and norepinephrine reuptake	Avoid co-administration

ANTIEMETICS

APREPITANT

APREPITANT	ANTIBIOTICS			
APREPITANT	MACROLIDES	↑ aprepitant levels	Inhibition of CYP3A4-mediated metabolism of aprepitant	Use with caution; clinical significance unclear so monitor closely
APREPITANT	RIFAMPICIN	↓ aprepitant levels	Induction of CYP3A4-mediated metabolism of aprepitant	Watch for poor response to aprepitant
APREPITANT	ANTICANCER AND IMMUNOMODULATING DRUGS – CORTICOSTEROIDS	↑ dexamethasone and methylprednisolone levels	Inhibition of CYP3A4-mediated metabolism of these corticosteroids	Be aware
APREPITANT	ANTICOAGULANTS – ORAL	Possible ↓ INR when aprepitant is added to warfarin	Aprepitant ↑ CYP2C9-mediated metabolism of warfarin	Monitor INR carefully for 2 weeks after completing each course of aprepitant
APREPITANT	ANTIDEPRESSANTS – ST JOHN'S WORT	↑ aprepitant levels	Inhibition of CYP3A4-mediated metabolism of aprepitant	Avoid co-administration (manufacturers' recommendation)
APREPITANT	ANTIDIABETIC DRUGS – TOLBUTAMIDE	↓ tolbutamide levels	Aprepitant ↑ CYP2C9-mediated metabolism of tolbutamide	Monitor blood glucose closely
APREPITANT	ANTIEPILEPTICS – CARBAMAZEPINE, PHENOBARBITAL, PHENYTOIN	↓ aprepitant levels	Induction of CYP3A4-mediated metabolism of aprepitant	Watch for poor response to aprepitant
APREPITANT	ANTIFUNGALS – KETOCONAZOLE	↑ aprepitant levels	Inhibition of CYP3A4-mediated metabolism of aprepitant	Use with caution; clinical significance unclear; monitor closely
APREPITANT	ANTIPSYCHOTICS – PIMOZIDE	↑ aprepitant levels	Inhibition of metabolism	Avoid co-administration (manufacturers' recommendation)

Primary drug	Secondary drug	Effect	Mechanism	Precautions
APREPITANT	ANTIVIRALS – PROTEASE INHIBITORS	↑ aprepitant levels with nelfinavir and ritonavir (with or without lopinavir)	Inhibition of CYP3A4-mediated metabolism of aprepitant	Use with caution; clinical significance unclear; monitor closely
APREPITANT	OESTROGENS	↓ oestrogen levels with risk of contraceptive failure	Uncertain	Clinical significance uncertain. It would seem wise to advise patients to use an alternative form of contraception during and for 1 month after stopping co-administration with these drugs
APREPITANT	PROGESTOGENS	↓ progestogen levels with risk of contraceptive failure	Uncertain	Advise patients to use an alternative form of contraception during and for 1 month after completing the course of aprepitant
ANTIHISTAMINES – CINNARIZINE, CYCLIZINE, PROMETHAZINE ➢ *Respiratory Drugs, Antihistamines*				
DOPAMINE RECEPTOR ANTAGONISTS – DOMPERIDONE, METOCLOPRAMIDE				
DOPAMINE RECEPTOR ANTAGONISTS	ANALGESICS			
DOMPERIDONE, METOCLOPRAMIDE	OPIOIDS	1. ↓ efficacy of domperidone on gut motility by opioids 2. Metoclopramide ↑ speed of onset and effect of oral morphine	1. Antagonist effect 2. Uncertain; metoclopramide may promote the absorption of morphine by increasing gastric emptying	1. Caution with co-administration 2. Be aware that the effects of oral morphine are ↑

METOCLOPRAMIDE	NSAIDs	1. Metoclopramide speeds up the onset of action of tolfenamic acid 2. Metoclopramide ↓ efficacy of ketoprofen	Metoclopramide promotes gastric emptying 1. Tolfenamic acid reaches its main site of absorption in the small intestine more rapidly 2. Ketoprofen has low solubility and has less time to dissolve in the stomach; therefore less ketoprofen is absorbed	1. This interaction can be used beneficially to hasten the onset of analgesia 2. Take ketoprofen at least 2 hours before metoclopramide
METOCLOPRAMIDE	ANTIMALARIALS – ATOVAQUONE	↓ atovaquone levels	Uncertain	Avoid; consider an alternative antiemetic
DOMPERIDONE, METOCLOPRAMIDE	ANTIMUSCARINICS	↓ efficacy of domperidone on gut motility by antimuscarinics	Some effects of metoclopramide are considered to be due to ↑ release of ACh and ↑ sensitivity of the cholinergic receptors to ACh. Antimuscarinics prevent the effects on muscarinic receptors	The gastrointestinal effects of metoclopramide will be impaired, while the antiemetic effects may not be. Thus, concurrent use with antimuscarinics is not advised because of effects on the gastrointestinal system
DOPAMINE RECEPTOR ANTAGONISTS	**ANTIPARKINSON'S DRUGS**			
DOMPERIDONE, METOCLOPRAMIDE	AMANTADINE	↓ efficacy of amantadine	Antagonism of antiparkinson's effect; these drugs have extrapyramidal side-effects	Use with caution; avoid in patients <20 years

Primary drug	Secondary drug	Effect	Mechanism	Precautions
DOMPERIDONE, METOCLOPRAMIDE	BROMOCRIPTINE, CABERGOLINE	↓ efficacy of bromocriptine and cabergoline for reducing prolactin levels	Domperidone and metoclopramide are associated with prolactin secretion	Use alternative antiemetics when bromocriptine and cabergoline are being used to treat prolactinomas. Domperidone has minimal central antidopaminergic effect and may therefore be used when bromocriptine and cabergoline are administered as treatments for Parkinson's disease
METOCLOPRAMIDE	DOPAMINERGICS	↓ efficacy of dopaminergics	Metoclopramide is a centrally acting antidopaminergic	Use with caution; avoid in patients <20 years. Manufacturers recommend avoiding the co-administration of metoclopramide with ropinirole or rotigotine
METOCLOPRAMIDE	ANTIPLATELET AGENTS – ASPIRIN	↑ aspirin levels with metoclopramide	↑ absorption of aspirin	Watch for early features of salicylate toxicity
METOCLOPRAMIDE	ANTIPSYCHOTICS	↑ risk of extrapyramidal effects	Additive effect	Consider using an alternative antiemetic
METOCLOPRAMIDE	DRUG DEPENDENCE THERAPIES – BUPROPION	↑ plasma concentrations of these substrates, with risk of toxic effects	Bupropion and its metabolite hydroxybupropion inhibit CYP2D6	Initiate therapy of these drugs at the lowest effective dose.
METOCLOPRAMIDE	MUSCLE RELAXANTS – DANTROLENE	Possibly ↑ dantrolene levels	Uncertain	Be aware; monitor BP and LFTs closely
METOCLOPRAMIDE	SUXAMETHONIUM	Possible ↑ efficacy of suxamethonium	Uncertain	Be aware and monitor effects of suxamethonium closely
METOCLOPRAMIDE	TETRABENAZINE	Risk of extrapyramidal symptoms	Additive effect	Avoid co-administration

5-HT3 ANTAGONISTS				
5-HT3 ANTAGONISTS	**DRUGS THAT PROLONG THE Q–T INTERVAL**			
5-HT3 ANTAGONISTS	1. ANTIARRHYTHMICS – amiodarone, disopyramide, procainamide, propafenone 2. ANTIBIOTICS – macrolides (especially azithromycin, clarithromycin, parenteral erythromycin, telithromycin), quinolones (especially moxifloxacin), quinupristin/dalfopristin 3. ANTI-CANCER AND IMMUNOMODULATING DRUGS – arsenic trioxide 4. ANTIDEPRESSANTS – TCAs, venlafaxine 5. ANTIFUNGALS – fluconazole, posaconazole, voriconazole 6. ANTIHISTAMINES – terfenadine, hydroxyzine, mizolastine 7. ANTIMALARIALS – artemether with lumefantrine, chloroquine, hydroxychloroquine, mefloquine, quinine 8. ANTIPROTOZOALS – pentamidine isetionate 9. ANTIPSYCHOTICS – atypicals, phenothiazines, pimozide 10. BETA-BLOCKERS – sotalol 11. BRONCHODILATORS – parenteral bronchodilators 12. CNS STIMULANTS – atomoxetine	Risk of ventricular arrhythmias, particularly torsades de pointes	Additive effect; these drugs cause prolongation of the Q–T interval	Avoid co-administration with dolasetron. Caution with other 5-HT3 antagonists; monitor ECG carefully

Primary drug	Secondary drug	Effect	Mechanism	Precautions
ONDANSETRON	ANALGESICS – OPIOIDS	Ondansetron seems to ↓ analgesic effect of tramadol	Uncertain; tramadol exerts its analgesic properties via serotoninergic pathways in addition to stimulation of opioid receptors. Ondansetron is a serotonin receptor antagonist	Avoid co-administration. Although increasing tramadol restored the analgesic effect, it also caused a significant ↑ in vomiting that was poorly responsive to antiemetic
ONDANSETRON, TROPISETRON	ANTIBIOTICS – RIFAMPICIN	↓ levels of these drugs	Induction of metabolism	Watch for poor response to ondansetron and tropisetron; consider using an alternative antiemetic
5-HT3 ANTAGONISTS	ANTIDEPRESSANTS			
ONDANSETRON	FLUVOXAMINE	Possible ↑ plasma concentrations of ondansetron	Fluvoxamine is potent inhibitor of CYP1A2, and fluoxetine is less potent as an inhibitor. Paroxetine, sertraline, escitalopram and citalopram are not currently known to cause any inhibition	Warn patients to report ↑ side-effects of ondansetron
ONDANSETRON, TROPISETRON	TCAs	Possible ↑ plasma concentrations of these antiemetics	Inhibition of CYP2D6-mediated metabolism of these antiemetics. The clinical significance of this depends upon whether their alternative pathways of metabolism are also inhibited by co-administered drugs. The risk is theoretically higher with ondansetron because TCAs also inhibit CYP1A2-mediated metabolism	Warn patients to report ↑ side-effects of ondansetron and tropisetron
5-HT3 ANTAGONISTS	ANTIEPILEPTICS			
ONDANSETRON	CARBAMAZEPINE, PHENYTOIN	Reports of ↓ ondansetron levels	Induction of metabolism of ondansetron	Watch for poor response to ondansetron; care with other 5-HT3 antagonists
TROPISETRON	PRIMIDONE	Reports of ↓ tropisetron levels	Induction of metabolism of tropisetron	Watch for poor response to ondansetron; care with other 5-HT3 antagonists

ONDANSETRON	CNS STIMULANTS – MODAFINIL	May cause ↓ ondansetron levels if CYP1A2 is the predominant metabolic pathway and alternative metabolic pathways are either genetically deficient or affected	Modafinil is moderate inducer of CYP1A2 in a concentration-dependent manner	Be aware
HYOSCINE ➢ *Antiparkinson's drugs, below*				
PHENOTHIAZINES – CHLORPROMAZINE, PERPHENAZINE, PROCHLORPERAZINE, TRIFLUOPERAZINE ➢ *Antipsychotics, below*				
ANTIEPILEPTICS				
INTERACTIONS BETWEEN ANTIEPILEPTICS				
BARBITURATES	1. CARBAMAZEPINE 2. LAMOTRIGINE 3. TIAGABINE 4. VALPROATE 5. ZONISAMIDE	↓ levels of these antiepileptics	Induction of metabolism	Watch for poor response to these antiepileptics
BARBITURATES	PHENYTOIN	Variable effect on phenytoin levels. ↑ phenobarbital levels	Phenobarbital induces metabolism of phenytoin but at high levels may competitively inhibit it. Uncertain why ↑ phenobarbital level occurs	Be aware and monitor levels. Watch for early features of phenytoin toxicity
CARBAMAZEPINE	1. ?ETHOSUXIMIDE 2. LAMOTRIGINE 3. TIAGABINE 4. TOPIRAMATE 5. VALPROATE 6. ZONISAMIDE	↓ levels of these antiepileptics	Induction of metabolism	Watch for poor response to these antiepileptics
CARBAMAZEPINE	PHENYTOIN	Variable effect on phenytoin levels. ↓ carbamazepine levels	Mutual induction of metabolism; uncertain why cases of ↑ phenytoin levels	Be aware and monitor levels. Watch for early features of phenytoin toxicity
ETHOSUXIMIDE	PHENYTOIN	Cases of ↑ phenytoin levels	Uncertain	Watch for early features of phenytoin toxicity

Primary drug	Secondary drug	Effect	Mechanism	Precautions
LAMOTRIGINE	1. CARBAMAZEPINE 2. OXCARBAZEPINE	1. Cases of ↑ levels of an active metabolite of carbamazepine with toxicity 2. Case of toxicity with oxcarbazepine	Uncertain	Be aware; watch for early features of toxicity of carbamazepine and oxcarbazepine
OXCARBAZEPINE	1. BARBITURATES – phenobarbital 2. PHENYTOIN	↑ levels of these antiepileptics	Uncertain	Watch for early features of toxicity
OXCARBAZEPINE	CARBAMAZEPINE	Variable effect on carbamazepine levels	Uncertain	Be aware; monitor carbamazepine levels
PHENYTOIN	1. LAMOTRIGINE 2. TIAGABINE 3. TOPIRAMATE 4. VALPROATE 5. ZONISAMIDE	↓ levels of these antiepileptics. Topiramate sometimes ↑ phenytoin levels	Induction of metabolism. Uncertain why phenytoin alters topiramate levels	Watch for poor response to these antiepileptics
VALPROATE	1. BARBITURATES – phenobarbital, primidone 2. ?ETHOSUXIMIDE 3. LAMOTRIGINE	↑ levels of these antiepileptics	Uncertain	Watch for early features of toxicity. Measure levels where possible
VALPROATE	PHENYTOIN	Variable effect on phenytoin levels	Uncertain	Be aware and monitor levels. Watch for early features of phenytoin toxicity
VIGABATRIN	1. BARBITURATES – phenobarbital, primidone 2. PHENYTOIN	↓ levels of these antiepileptics	Possibly induction of metabolism	Watch for poor response to these antiepileptics
INTERACTIONS WITH DRUGS THAT LOWER SEIZURE THRESHOLD				
ANTIEPILEPTICS	1. ANTIMALARIALS – chloroquine, mefloquine 2. ANTIDEPRESSANTS – MAOIs, SSRIs, TCAs 3. ANTIPSYCHOTICS	↑ risk of seizures	These drugs lower seizure threshold	Care with co-administration. Watch for ↑ fit frequency; warn patient of this risk when starting these drugs and take suitable precautions. Consider increasing dose of antiepileptic

BARBITURATES				
BARBITURATES	**INTERACTIONS DUE TO ENZYME INDUCTION BY BARBITURATES**			
BARBITURATES	1. ANTIARRHYTHMICS – disopyramide, propafenone 2. ANTIBIOTICS – chloramphenicol, doxycycline, metronidazole, rifampicin, telithromycin 3. ANTICANCER AND IMMUNOMODULATING DRUGS – carmustine, ciclosporin, corticosteroids, doxorubicin, etoposide, imatinib, lomustine, paclitaxel, tacrolimus, tamoxifen, toremifene, vinca alkaloids 4. ANTICOAGULANTS – ORAL 5. ANTIDEPRESSANTS – mianserin, paroxetine 6. ANTIDIABETIC DRUGS – repaglinide, sulphonylureas 7. ANTIEMETICS – aprepitant 5-HT3-antagonists 8. ANTIFUNGALS – fluconazole, itraconazole, ketoconazole, voriconazole 9. ANTIPSYCHOTICS – apiprazole, chlorpromazine, haloperidol 10. BETA-BLOCKERS – metoprolol, propanolol, timolol 11. BRONCHODILATORS – montelukast, theophylline 12. CARDIAC GLYCOSIDES – digitoxin 13. CALCIUM CHANNEL BLOCKERS – felodipine, nifedipine, nimodipine, nisoldipine, verapamil 14. DIURETICS – eplerenone 15. 5-HT1 AGONISTS – almotriptan, eletriptan 16. GESTRINONE 17. OESTROGENS 18. PROGESTOGENS 19. THYROID HORMONES – levothyroxine	↓ levels of these drugs with risk of therapeutic failure. The ↓ anticoagulant effect of warfarin reaches a maximum after 3 weeks and can last up to 6 weeks after stopping barbiturates	Induction of hepatic metabolism	1. Avoid co-administration of barbiturates with carmustine, eplerenone, etoposide, griseofulvin, imatinib, lomustine, tacrolimus, tamoxifen; consider alternative non-enzyme-inducing antiepileptics. Avoid co-administration of telithromycin for up to 2 weeks after stopping phenobarbital 2. With the other drugs, monitor for ↓ clinical efficacy and ↑ their dose as required (a) Monitor ciclosporin levels (b) With anticoagulants, monitor INR carefully. Dose of anticoagulant may need to be ↑ by up to 60% (c) With antidiabetic drugs, monitor capillary blood glucose and warn patients about symptoms of hyperglycaemia (d) Beta-blockers, calcium channel blockers and digitoxin – monitor PR and BP weekly until stable and watch for ↑ BP (e) Levothyroxine – monitor TFTs regularly (f) May need to ↑ dose of theophylline by 25% (g) With oestrogens and progestogens, advise patients to use additional contraception for period of intake and for 1 month after stopping co-administration with these drugs ➢ ***For signs and symptoms of hyperglycaemia, see Clinical Features of Some Adverse Drug Interactions, Hyperglycaemia***

Primary drug	Secondary drug	Effect	Mechanism	Precautions
BARBITURATES	ALCOHOL	↑ sedation	Additive sedative effect	Warn patients about this effect
BARBITURATES	ANAESTHETICS – LOCAL – PROCAINE SOLUTIONS	Precipitation of drugs, which may not be immediately apparent	Pharmaceutical interaction	Do not mix in the same infusion or syringe
BARBITURATES	ANALGESICS – OPIOIDS	1. Barbiturates ↑ sedative effects of opioids 2. ↓ efficacy of fentanyl and methadone with phenobarbital and primidone	1. Additive sedative effect. 2. ↑ hepatic metabolism of fentanyl and methadone	1. Monitor respiratory rate and conscious levels 2. Be aware that the dose of fentanyl and methadone may need to ↑
BARBITURATES	**ANTICANCER AND IMMUNOMODULATING DRUGS**			
BARBITURATES	IFOSFAMIDE	↑ rate of biotransformation to 4-hydroxyifosfamide, the active metabolite, but no change in AUC of 4-hydroxyifosfamide	Due to ↑ rate of metabolism and of clearance resulting from induction of CYP3A4 and CYP2D6	Be aware – clinical significance may be minimal or none
BARBITURATES	PROCARBAZINE	↑ risk of hypersensitivity reactions in patients with brain tumours	Strong correlation between therapeutic antiepileptic level and hypersensitivity reactions	Consider using non-enzyme-inducing agents
BARBITURATES	ANTIDEMENTIA DRUGS – MEMANTINE	Possible ↓ efficacy of primidone	Uncertain	Avoid co-administration
BARBITURATES	**ANTIDEPRESSANTS**			
BARBITURATES	MAOIs – PHENELZINE	Reports of prolonged hypnotic effects	Animal experiments showed that pretreatment with tranylcypromine prolonged amobarbital-induced hypnotic effects 2.5-fold. Inhibition of hepatic enzymes other than MAO has been proposed as an explanation for the exaggerated depressant effects associated with barbiturates and opioids	Be aware. Warn patients taking sleeping aids about activities requiring attention and co-ordination (e.g. driving or using machinery)
BARBITURATES	ST JOHN'S WORT	↓ barbiturate levels	↑ metabolism	Avoid co-administration

BARBITURATES	ANTIFUNGALS			
BARBITURATES	AZOLES			
BARBITURATES	FLUCONAZOLE, ITRACONAZOLE, KETOCONAZOLE, VORICONAZOLE	↓ azole levels with risk of therapeutic failure	Barbiturates induce CYP3A4, which metabolizes itraconazole and the active metabolite of itraconazole. Primidone is metabolized to phenobarbitone	Watch for inadequate therapeutic effects and ↑ dose of azole if effect due to interaction
BARBITURATES	MICONAZOLE	↑ phenobarbital levels	Inhibition of metabolism	Be aware; watch for early features of toxicity (e.g. ↑ sedation)
BARBITURATES	OTHER ANTIFUNGALS – GRISEOFULVIN	↓ griseofulvin levels	↓ absorption	Although the effect of ↓ plasma concentrations on therapeutic effect has not been established, concurrent use is preferably avoided
BARBITURATES	ANXIOLYTICS AND HYPNOTICS			
BARBITURATES	BZDs – clonazepam	↓ barbiturate levels	Induction of metabolism	Watch for poor response to barbiturates
BARBITURATES	SODIUM OXYBATE	Risk of CNS depression – coma, respiratory depression	Additive depression of CNS	Avoid co-administration. Caution even with relatively non-sedating antihistamines (cetrizine, desloratidine, fexofenadine, levocetirizine, loratidine, mizolastine) as they can impair performance of skilled tasks

Primary drug	Secondary drug	Effect	Mechanism	Precautions
BARBITURATES	BETA-BLOCKERS	↑ hypotensive effect	Additive hypotensive effect; anxiolytics and hypnotics can cause postural ↓ BP	Watch for ↓ BP; monitor BP at least weekly until stable. Warn patients to report symptoms of hypotension (light-headedness, dizziness on standing, etc.)
PHENOBARBITONE	CNS STIMULANTS – MODAFINIL	1. ↓ plasma concentrations of modafinil with possibility of ↓ therapeutic effect 2. May cause moderate ↑ in plasma concentrations of phenobarbitone and primidone	1. Induction of CYP3A4, which has a partial role in the metabolism of modafinil 2. Modafinil is a reversible inhibitor of CYP2C19 when used in therapeutic doses	1 and 2. Be aware
BARBITURATES	DIURETICS – CARBONIC ANHYDRASE INHIBITORS	Risk of osteomalacia	Barbiturates have a small risk of causing osteomalacia; this may be ↑ by acetazolamide-induced urinary excretion of calcium	Be aware
BARBITURATES	FOLIC ACID	↓ levels of these antiepileptics	Uncertain; postulated that induction of CYP enzymes by these antiepileptics depletes folate reserves. Replacement of these reserves ↑ formation of CYP further, which ↑ metabolism of the antiepileptics	Watch for poor response to these antiepileptics and ↑ doses as necessary
BARBITURATES	LOFEXIDINE	↑ sedation	Additive effect	Warn patients of risk of excessive sedation
BARBITURATES	TIBOLONE	↓ tibolone levels	Induction of metabolism of tibolone	Watch for poor response to tibolone; consider increasing its dose
BARBITURATES	VITAMIN B6	↓ plasma concentrations of these antiepileptics	Uncertain	Watch for poor response to these antiepileptics if large doses of vitamin B6 are given

BENZODIAZEPINES ➢ *Anxiolytics and hypnotics, below*

CARBAMAZEPINE

CARBAMAZEPINE	INTERACTIONS DUE TO ENZYME INDUCTION BY CARBAMAZEPINE			
CARBAMAZEPINE	1. ANALGESICS – parecoxib, fentanyl, methadone, tramadol 2. ANTIBIOTICS – doxycycline, telithromycin 3. ANTICANCER AND IMMUNOMODULATING DRUGS – ciclosporin, corticosteroids, imatinib, irinotecan, paclitaxel, tamoxifen, toremifene, vinca alkaloids 4. ANTICOAGULANTS – ORAL 5. ANTIDEPRESSANTS – mirtazapine 6. ANTIDIABETIC DRUGS – glipizide, repaglinide 7. ANTIEMETICS – aprepitant, ondansetron 8. ANTIFUNGALS – itraconazole, ketoconazole, posaconazole, voriconazole, caspofungin 9. ANTIPROTOZOALS – mebendazole 10. ANTIPSYCHOTICS – apiprazole, clozapine, haloperidol, olanzapine, quetiapine, risperidone, sertindole 11. ANXIOLYTICS AND HYPNOTICS – zaleplon, zolpidem, zopiclone 12. BRONCHODILATORS – theophylline 13. CALCIUM CHANNEL BLOCKERS – felodipine, nifedipine, and possibly nimodipine and nisoldipine 14. CARDIAC GLYCOSIDES – digitoxin 15. DIURETICS – eplerenone 16. 5-HT1 AGONISTS almotriptan, eletriptan 17. GESTRINONE 18. OESTROGENS 19. PROGESTOGENS 20. THYROID HORMONES – levothyroxine	1. ↓ levels of these drugs with risk of therapeutic failure 2. Azoles also ↑ carbamazepine levels 3. Risk of serotonin syndrome with almotriptan and eletriptan	1. Induction of hepatic metabolism 2. Inhibition of P-gp ↑ bioavailability of carbamazepine 3. Triptans and carbamazepine are both stimulants of 5-HT receptors, and carbamazepine also prevents reuptake of 5-HT	1. Avoid co-administration of carbamazepine with azoles (consider using fluconazole), eplerenone, irinotecan (if not able to avoid, ↑ dose of irinotecan by 50%) or tamoxifen. Avoid co-administration of telithromycin for up to 2 weeks after stopping carbamazepine 2. With the other drugs, monitor for ↓ clinical efficacy and ↑ their dose as required (a) Monitor ciclosporin levels (b) With anticoagulants, monitor INR at least weekly until stable; dose of anticoagulant may need to be ↑ (c) With antidiabetic drugs, monitor capillary blood glucose and warn patients about symptoms of hyperglycaemia (d) Calcium channel blockers and digitoxin – monitor PR and BP weekly until stable and watch for ↑ BP (e) Levothyroxine – monitor TFTs regularly (f) ↑ dose of caspofungin to 70 mg daily (g) Be aware of the possibility of the occurrence of serotonin syndrome with 5-HT1 agonists (h) May need to ↑ dose of theophylline by 25% (i) With oestrogens and progestogens, advise patients to use additional contraception for period of intake and for 1 month after stopping co-administration with these drugs ➢ ***For signs and symptoms of hyperglycaemia, see Clinical Features of Some Adverse Drug Interactions, Hyperglycaemia***

Primary drug	Secondary drug	Effect	Mechanism	Precautions
CARBAMAZEPINE	ANALGESICS – OPIOIDS	1. ↓ efficacy of fentanyl and methadone 2. ↓ tramadol levels	1. ↑ hepatic metabolism of fentanyl and methadone, and possibly an effect at the opioid receptor 2. ↑ metabolism of tramadol	1. Be aware that the dose of fentanyl and methadone may need to be ↑ 2. Watch for poor effect of tramadol. Consider using an alternative opioid
CARBAMAZEPINE	ANTIBIOTICS			
CARBAMAZEPINE	ISONIAZID	↑ carbamazepine levels	Inhibition of metabolism	Monitor carbamazepine levels
CARBAMAZEPINE	MACROLIDES – CLARITHROMYCIN, ERYTHROMYCIN, TELITHROMYCIN, ISONIAZID	↑ carbamazepine levels	Inhibition of metabolism	Monitor carbamazepine levels
CARBAMAZEPINE	RIFABUTIN	↓ carbamazepine levels	Induction of metabolism	Monitor carbamazepine levels
CARBAMAZEPINE	ANTICANCER AND IMMUNOMODULATING DRUGS			
CARBAMAZEPINE	PLATINUM COMPOUNDS	↓ plasma concentrations of antiepileptic, which ↑ risk of seizures	Due to impaired absorption of antiepileptic	Monitor closely for seizure activity, and warn patient and carers. Need to adjust dosage using parameters such as blood levels to ensure therapeutic levels
CARBAMAZEPINE	PROCARBAZINE	↑ risk of hypersensitivity reactions in patients with brain tumours	Strong correlation between therapeutic antiepileptic level and hypersensitivity reactions	Consider using non-enzyme-inducing agents
CARBAMAZEPINE	ANTIDEPRESSANTS			
CARBAMAZEPINE	LITHIUM	↑ risk of neurotoxicity	Uncertain; this may occur with normal lithium blood levels	Warn patient and carers to watch for drowsiness, ataxia and tremor
CARBAMAZEPINE	ST JOHN'S WORT	↓ carbamazepine levels	Induction of metabolism	Avoid co-administration
CARBAMAZEPINE	SSRIs	Risk of serotonin syndrome with carbamazepine	Carbamazepine ↑ serotonin concentrations in the brain	Avoid co-administration

CARBAMAZEPINE	TCAs	1. ↑ risk of bone marrow depression in patients on chemotherapy when used with TCAs 2. ↓ plasma concentrations of mianserin	1. Additive effects 2. ↑ metabolism of mianserin	1. Avoid concurrent use during chemotherapy 2. Be aware and watch for signs of ↓ antidepressant effect of mianserin
CARBAMAZEPINE	ANTIFUNGALS – ITRACONAZOLE, KETOCONAZOLE, MICONAZOLE, POSACONAZOLE, VORICONAZOLE	↓ plasma concentrations of itraconazole and of its active metabolite, ketoconazole, posaconazole and voriconazole, with risk of therapeutic failure. ↑ carbamazepine plasma concentrations	These azoles are highly lipophilic, and clearance is heavily dependent upon metabolism by CYP isoenzymes. Carbamazepine is a powerful inducer of CYP3A4 and other CYP isoenzymes (CYP2C18/19, CYP1A2), and the result is very low or undetectable plasma levels. Inhibition of P-gp ↑ bioavailability of carbamazepine	Avoid co-administration of posaconazole or voriconazole with carbamazepine. Watch for inadequate therapeutic effects, and ↑ dose of itraconazole. Higher doses of itraconazole may not overcome this interaction. Consider use of the less lipophilic fluconazole, which is less dependent on CYP metabolism. Necessary to monitor carbamazepine levels
CARBAMAZEPINE	ANTIGOUT DRUGS – ALLOPURINOL	High-dose allopurinol (600 mg/day) may ↑ carbamazepine levels over a period of several weeks. 300 mg/day allopurinol does not seem to have this effect	Uncertain	Monitor carbamazepine levels in patients taking long-term, high-dose allopurinol
CARBAMAZEPINE	**ANTIVIRALS**			
CARBAMAZEPINE	NNRTIs	Possible ↓ efficacy of carbamazepine	Uncertain	Monitor carbamazepine levels and side-effects when initiating or changing treatment
CARBAMAZEPINE	PROTEASE INHIBITORS	Possibly ↑ adverse effects of carbamazepine with protease inhibitors	Inhibition of CYP3A4-mediated metabolism of carbamazepine	Use with caution. Monitor carbamazepine levels and side-effects when initiating or changing treatment

Primary drug	Secondary drug	Effect	Mechanism	Precautions
CARBAMAZEPINE	ANXIOLYTICS AND HYPNOTICS – BZDs – clonazepam	↓ carbamazepine levels	Induction of metabolism	Watch for poor response to carbamazepine
CARBAMAZEPINE	CALCIUM CHANNEL BLOCKERS	Diltiazem and verapamil ↑ plasma concentrations of carbamazepine (have been cases of toxicity)	Diltiazem and verapamil inhibit CYP3A4-mediated metabolism of carbamazepine. They also inhibit intestinal P-gp, which may ↑ bioavailability of carbamazepine	Monitor carbamazepine levels when initiating calcium channel blockers, particularly diltiazem/verapamil
CARBAMAZEPINE	CNS STIMULANTS – MODAFINIL	↓ plasma concentrations of modafinil, with possibility of ↓ therapeutic effect	Induction of CYP3A4, which has a partial role in the metabolism of modafinil	Be aware
CARBAMAZEPINE	DANAZOL	↑ plasma concentrations of carbamazepine, with risk of toxic effects	Inhibition of carbamazepine metabolism	Watch for toxic effects of carbamazepine
CARBAMAZEPINE	GRAPEFRUIT JUICE	↑ efficacy and ↑ adverse effects	Grapefruit juice irreversibly inhibits intestinal CYP3A4. Transport via P-gp and the MRP-2 efflux pumps is also inhibited	Monitor for ↑ side-effects/toxicity and check carbamazepine levels. If levels or control of fits are variable remove grapefruit juice and grapefruit from the diet
CARBAMAZEPINE	H2 RECEPTOR BLOCKERS – CIMETIDINE, FAMOTIDINE, RANITIDINE	↑ plasma concentrations of phenytoin and risk of adverse effects including phenytoin toxicity, bone marrow depression and skin reactions	Inhibition of metabolism via CYP2C9 and CYP2C19	Use alternative acid suppression (e.g. ranitidine) or warn patients that effects last about 1 week. Consider monitoring carbamazepine levels, and adjust dose as necessary
CARBAMAZEPINE	LIPID-LOWERING DRUGS – FIBRATES	Gemfibrozil may ↑ carbamazepine levels	Uncertain at present	Watch for features of carbamazepine toxicity

CARBAMAZEPINE	PROTON PUMP INHIBITORS	Possible altered efficacy of carbamazepine	Unclear; possibly via ↓ clearance	Use with caution. Monitor carbamazepine levels when starting or stopping and use proton pump inhibitor regularly not PRN. Not reported with pantoprazole or rabeprazole
CARBAMAZEPINE	TIBOLONE	↓ tibolone levels	Induction of metabolism of tibolone	Watch for poor response to tibolone; consider increasing its dose
ETHOSUXIMIDE				
ETHOSUXIMIDE	ANTIBIOTICS – ISONIAZID	Case of ↑ ethosuximide levels with toxicity	Inhibition of metabolism	Watch for early features of ethosuximide toxicity
GABAPENTIN				
GABAPENTIN	ANTACIDS	↓ gabapentin levels	↓ absorption	Separate doses by at least 3 hours
LAMOTRIGINE				
LAMOTRIGINE	1. ANTIBIOTICS – rifampicin 2. OESTROGENS 3. PROGESTOGENS	↓ lamotrigine levels	↑ metabolism	Monitor levels
OXCARBAZEPINE				
OXCARBAZEPINE	OESTROGENS	Marked ↓ contraceptive effect	Induction of metabolism of oestrogens	Advise patients to use additional contraception for period of intake and for 1 month after stopping co-administration
OXCARBAZEPINE	PROGESTOGENS	↓ progesterone levels, which may lead to failure of contraception or poor response to treatment of menorrhagia	Possibly induction of metabolism of progestogens	Advise patients to use additional contraception for period of intake and for 1 month after stopping co-administration

Primary drug	Secondary drug	Effect	Mechanism	Precautions
PHENYTOIN/FOSPHENYTOIN				
PHENYTOIN	INTERACTIONS DUE TO ENZYME INDUCTION BY PHENYTOIN			
PHENYTOIN	1. ANALGESICS – parecoxib, fentanyl, methadone 2. ANTIARRHYTHMICS – amiodarone, disopyramide, mexiletine 3. ANTIBIOTICS – doxycycline, telithromycin 4. ANTICANCER AND IMMUNOMODULATING DRUGS – busulfan, ciclosporin, corticosteroids, etoposide, ifosfamide, imatinib, irinotecan, paclitaxel, tacrolimus, tamoxifen, topotecan, toremifene, vinca alkaloids 5. ANTICOAGULANTS – ORAL 6. ANTIDEPRESSANTS – mirtazapine, TCAs 7. ANTIDIABETIC DRUGS – repaglinide 8. ANTIEMETICS – aprepitant, ondansetron 9. ANTIFUNGALS – itraconazole, ketoconazole, posaconazole, voriconazole, caspofungin 10. ANTIPROTOZOALS – mebendazole 11. ANTIPSYCHOTICS – apiprazole, clozapine, quetiapine, sertindole 12. ANXIOLYTICS AND HYPNOTICS – zaleplon, zolpidem, zopiclone 13. BETA-BLOCKERS – propanolol 14. BRONCHODILATORS – theophylline 15. CALCIUM CHANNEL BLOCKERS – diltiazem, felodipine, nisoldipine, verapamil, possibly nimodipine 16. CARDIAC GLYCOSIDES – digitoxin, digoxin 17. 5-HT1 AGONISTS – almotriptan, eletriptan 18. GESTRINONE 19. OESTROGENS 20. PROGESTOGENS	1. ↓ levels of these drugs, with risk of therapeutic failure 2. Report of ↑ phenytoin levels with celecoxib, mianserin, diltiazem and possibly nifedipine and isradipine 3. Phenytoin levels may be ↓ by amiodarone and theophylline	1. Induction of hepatic metabolism 2. Inhibition of phenytoin metabolism (parecoxib – CYP2C9; calcium channel blockers – CYP3A4; mianserin – unknown) 3. Uncertain; amiodarone inhibits CYP2C9, which plays a role in phenytoin metabolism and inhibits intestinal P-gp, which may ↑ bioavailability of phenytoin. Theophylline ↓ absorption of phenytoin	1. Avoid co-administration of phenytoin with azoles (consider using fluconazole), etoposide, irinotecan (if not able to avoid, ↑ dose of irinotecan by 50%), tacrolimus, tamoxifen. Avoid co-administration of telithromycin for up to 2 weeks after stopping phenytoin 2. With the other drugs, monitor for ↓ clinical efficacy and ↑ their dose as required (a) Monitor ciclosporin levels (b) With anticoagulants, monitor INR at least weekly until stable; dose of anticoagulant may need to be ↑ (c) With antidiabetic drugs, monitor capillary blood glucose and warn patients about symptoms of hyperglycaemia (d) Antiarrhythmics, beta-blockers, calcium channel blockers and cardiac glycosides – monitor PR and BP weekly until stable, and watch for ↑ BP (e) ↑ dose of caspofungin to 70 mg daily (f) May need to ↑ dose of theophylline by 25% (g) With oestrogens and progestogens, advise patients to use additional contraception for period of intake and for 1 month after stopping co-administration with these drugs 3. Monitor phenytoin levels when co-administered with amiodarone, diltiazem, isradipine, mianserin, nifedipine, parecoxib or theophylline ➢ ***For signs and symptoms of hyperglycaemia, see Clinical Features of Some Adverse Drug Interactions, Hyperglycaemia***

PHENYTOIN	ANAESTHETICS – LOCAL – LIDOCAINE AND PROCAINE SOLUTIONS	Precipitation of drugs, which may not be immediately apparent	A pharmaceutical interaction	Do not mix in the same infusion or syringe
PHENYTOIN	ANALGESICS – OPIOIDS	1. ↓ efficacy of fentanyl and methadone 2. Risk of pethidine toxicity	1. ↑ hepatic metabolism of fentanyl and methadone, and possibly an effect at the opioid receptor 2. Phenytoin induces metabolism of pethidine, which causes ↑ levels of a neurotoxic metabolite	1. Be aware that the dose of fentanyl and methadone may need to be ↑ 2. Co-administer with caution; the effect may be ↓ by administering pethidine intravenously
PHENYTOIN	ANTACIDS	↓ phenytoin levels	↓ absorption	Separate doses by at least 3 hours
PHENYTOIN	ANTIARRHYTHMICS – AMIODARONE	Phenytoin levels may be ↑ by amiodarone; conversely, amiodarone levels may be ↓ by phenytoin	Uncertain; amiodarone inhibits CYP2C9, which plays a role in phenytoin metabolism, while phenytoin is a known hepatic enzyme inducer. Also, amiodarone inhibits intestinal P-gp, which may ↑ bioavailability of phenytoin	↓ phenytoin dose by 25–30% and monitor levels; watch for amiodarone toxicity. Note that phenytoin and amiodarone share similar features of toxicity, such as arrhythmias and ataxia
PHENYTOIN	**ANTIBIOTICS**			
PHENYTOIN	CHLORAMPHENICOL, CLARITHROMYCIN, ISONIAZID, METRONIDAZOLE, SULPHONAMIDES, TRIMETHOPRIM	↑ phenytoin levels	Inhibited metabolism	Monitor phenytoin levels
PHENYTOIN	CIPROFLOXACIN	Variable effect on phenytoin levels	Unknown	Monitor phenytoin levels
PHENYTOIN	RIFAMPICIN, RIFABUTIN	↓ phenytoin levels	Induced metabolism	Monitor phenytoin levels

Primary drug	Secondary drug	Effect	Mechanism	Precautions
PHENYTOIN	**ANTICANCER AND IMMUNOMODULATING DRUGS**			
PHENYTOIN	METHOTREXATE	↑ risk of hepatotoxicity, especially with high-dose and long-term use of methotrexate. Likely ↓ in phenytoin levels and ↑ risk of folic acid deficiency. High-dose and long-term therapy with methotrexate ↑ risk of liver injury with other potentially hepatotoxic drugs. Additive antifolate effects. Cytotoxics in general ↓ absorption of phenytoin	High doses of methotrexate ↓ elimination of phenytoin and risk of folic acid deficiency	Monitor phenytoin levels and clinically watch for signs and symptoms of phenytoin toxicity, e.g. nausea, vomiting, insomnia, tremor, acne and hirsutism
PHENYTOIN	PLATINUM COMPOUNDS	↓ phenytoin levels with risk of seizures	Impaired absorption of antiepileptic	Monitor closely for seizure activity, and warn patients and carers. Need to adjust dosage using parameters such as blood levels to ensure therapeutic levels
PHENYTOIN	PROCARBAZINE	↑ risk of hypersensitivity reactions in patients with brain tumours	Strong correlation between therapeutic antiepileptic level and hypersensitivity reactions	Consider using non-enzyme-inducing agents
PHENYTOIN	**ANTIDEPRESSANTS**			
PHENYTOIN	LITHIUM	↑ risk of neurotoxicity	Uncertain; this may occur with normal lithium blood levels	Warn patients and carers to watch for drowsiness, ataxia and tremor
CARBAMAZEPINE	ST JOHN'S WORT	↓ phenytoin levels	Induction of metabolism	Avoid co-administration
PHENYTOIN	SSRIs	↑ phenytoin levels	Phenytoin is a substrate of CYP2C9 and CYP2C19. SSRIs are known to inhibit CYP2C9/10	Monitor plasma phenytoin levels
PHENYTOIN	ANTIDIABETIC DRUGS – METFORMIN, SULPHONYLUREAS	↓ hypoglycaemic efficacy	Hydantoins are considered to ↓ release of insulin	Monitor capillary blood glucose closely; higher doses of antidiabetic drugs needed

PHENYTOIN	ANTIFUNGALS – FLUCONAZOLE, MICONAZOLE	↓ plasma concentrations of itraconazole and of its active metabolite, ketoconazole, posaconazole and voriconazole, with risk of therapeutic failure. ↑ phenytoin levels but clinical significance uncertain	These azoles are highly lipophilic, and clearance is heavily dependent upon metabolism by CYP isoenzymes. Phenytoin is a powerful inducer of CYP3A4 and other CYP isoenzymes (CYP2C18/19, CYP1A2), and the result is very low or undetectable plasma levels. Phenytoin extensively ↓ AUC of itraconazole by more than 90%	Watch for inadequate therapeutic effects and ↑ dose of itraconazole. Higher doses of itraconazole may not overcome this interaction. Consider use of the less lipophilic fluconazole, which is less dependent on CYP metabolism. Necessary to monitor phenytoin levels
PHENYTOIN	ANTIGOUT DRUGS – ALLOPURINOL, SULFINPYRAZONE	Phenytoin levels may be ↑ in some patients	Uncertain	Monitor phenytoin levels
PHENYTOIN	ANTIMALARIALS – PYRIMETHAMINE	1. ↓ efficacy of phenytoin 2. ↑ antifolate effect	1. Uncertain 2. Additive effect	1. Care with co-administration; ↑ dose of antiepileptic if ↑ incidence of fits 2. Monitor FBC closely; the effect may take a number of weeks to occur
PHENYTOIN	ANTIPARKINSON'S DRUGS – LEVODOPA	Possibly ↓ levodopa levels	Uncertain	Watch for poor response to levodopa and consider increasing its dose
PHENYTOIN	ANTIPLATELET AGENTS – ASPIRIN	Possible ↑ phenytoin levels	Possibly ↑ unbound phenytoin fraction in the blood	Monitor phenytoin levels when co-administering high- dose aspirin
PHENYTOIN	ANTIPROTOZOALS – LEVAMISOLE	Possible ↑ phenytoin levels	Uncertain; case report of this interaction when levamisole and fluorouracil were co-administered with phenytoin	Monitor phenytoin levels and ↓ phenytoin dose as necessary

Primary drug	Secondary drug	Effect	Mechanism	Precautions
PHENYTOIN	ANTIVIRALS			
PHENYTOIN	NUCLEOSIDE REVERSE TRANSCRIPASE INHIBITORS – DIDANOSINE, STAVUDINE, ZIDOVUDINE	Possibly ↑ adverse effects (e.g. peripheral neuropathy) with didanosine, stavudine and zidovudine	Additive effect	Monitor closely for peripheral neuropathy during prolonged combination
PHENYTOIN	PROTEASE INHIBITORS	Possibly ↓ efficacy of phenytoin, with a risk of fits when co-administered with indinavir, nelfinavir and ritonavir (with or without lopinavir)	Uncertain; ↓ plasma levels of phenytoin	Use with caution. Monitor phenytoin levels weekly. Adjust doses at 7–10-day intervals. Maximum suggested dose adjustment each time is 25 mg
PHENYTOIN	ACICLOVIR/VALACICLOVIR	↓ efficacy of phenytoin	Unclear	Warn patients and monitor seizure frequency
PHENYTOIN	ANXIOLYTICS AND HYPNOTICS – BZDs – clonazepam	↓ phenytoin levels	Induction of metabolism	Watch for poor response to phenytoin
PHENYTOIN	CNS STIMULANTS – MODAFINIL	May ↓ modafinil levels	Induction of CYP3A4, which has a partial role in the metabolism of modafinil	Be aware
PHENYTOIN	DIURETICS			
PHENYTOIN	CARBONIC ANHYDRASE INHIBITORS	Risk of osteomalacia	Phenytoin is associated with a small risk of causing osteomalacia; this may be ↑ by acetazolamide-induced urinary excretion of calcium	Be aware
PHENYTOIN	LOOP DIURETICS – FUROSEMIDE	↓ efficacy of furosemide	Uncertain	Be aware; watch for poor response to furosemide
PHENYTOIN	DRUG DEPENDENCE THERAPIES – DISULFIRAM	↑ phenytoin levels	Inhibited metabolism	Monitor phenytoin levels closely

PHENYTOIN	FOLIC ACID	↓ phenytoin levels	Uncertain; postulated that induction of CYP enzymes by these antiepileptics depletes folate reserves. Replacement of these reserves ↑ formation of CYP further, which ↑ metabolism of the antiepileptics	Watch for poor response to phenytoin and ↑ dose as necessary
PHENYTOIN	H2 RECEPTOR BLOCKERS – CIMETIDINE, FAMOTIDINE, RANITIDINE	↑ phenytoin levels with risk of adverse effects	Inhibition of metabolism via CYP2C9 and CYP2C19	Use alternative acid suppression (e.g. ranitidine) or warn patients that effects last about 1 week
PHENYTOIN	PROTON PUMP INHIBITORS	Possible ↑ efficacy and adverse effects of phenytoin	Unclear; possible altered metabolism via CYP2C19	↓ dose may be required. Use the proton pump inhibitor regularly, not PRN; monitor phenytoin levels when starting or stopping treatment. Patients have received omeprazole for 3 weeks without altered phenytoin levels. Effect not reported with pantoprazole or rabeprazole
PHENYTOIN	SUCRALFATE	↓ phenytoin levels	↓ absorption of phenytoin	Give phenytoin at least 2 hours after sucralfate
PHENYTOIN	TIBOLONE	↓ tibolone levels	Induction of metabolism of tibolone	Watch for poor response to tibolone; consider ↑ its dose
PHENYTOIN	VASODILATOR ANTIHYPERTENSIVES	Co-administration of diazoxide and phenytoin ↓ phenytoin levels and possibly ↓ efficacy of diazoxide	Uncertain at present	Monitor phenytoin levels and BP closely
PHENYTOIN	VITAMIN B6	↓ phenytoin levels	Uncertain	Watch for poor response to phenytoin if large doses of vitamin B6 are given
PHENYTOIN	VITAMIN D	↓ efficacy of vitamin D	Uncertain	Be aware; consider increasing dose of vitamin D

Primary drug	Secondary drug	Effect	Mechanism	Precautions
TOPIRAMATE				
TOPIRAMATE	ALCOHOL	↑ sedation	Additive sedative effect	Warn patients about this effect
TOPIRAMATE	ANTICANCER AND IMMUNOMODULATING DRUGS – IMATINIB	↑ topiramate levels	Imatinib is a potent inhibitor of CYP2C9-mediated metabolism of topiramate	Watch for the early features of toxicity. If necessary, consider using alternative drugs while the patient is being given imatinib
TOPIRAMATE	ANTIDIABETIC DRUGS – METFORMIN	↑ metformin levels	Unknown mechanism	Watch for and warn patients about hypoglycaemia ➢ ***For signs and symptoms of hypoglycaemia, see Clinical Features of Some Adverse Drug Interactions, Hypoglycaemia***
TOPIRAMATE	OESTROGENS	Marked ↓ contraceptive effect	Induction of metabolism of oestrogens	Advise patients to use additional contraception for period of intake and for 1 month after stopping co-administration with topiramate
TOPIRAMATE	PROGESTOGENS	↓ progesterone levels, which may lead to failure of contraception or poor response to treatment of menorrhagia	Possibly induction of metabolism of progestogens	Advise patients to use additional contraception for period of intake and for 1 month after stopping co-administration with topiramate
VALPROATE				
VALPROATE	ANTIBIOTICS			
VALPROATE	ERTAPENEM, MEROPENEM	↓ valproate levels	Induced metabolism	Monitor levels
VALPROATE	ERYTHROMYCIN	↑ valproate levels	Inhibited metabolism	Monitor levels

NERVOUS SYSTEM DRUGS ANTIEPILEPTICS

VALPROATE	ANTICANCER AND IMMUNOMODULATING DRUGS			
VALPROATE	PLATINUM COMPOUNDS	↓ plasma concentrations of antiepileptic, which ↑ risk of seizures	Impaired absorption of valproate	Monitor for seizure activity closely, and warn patients and carers. Monitor valproate levels
VALPROATE	PROCARBAZINE	↑ risk of hypersensitivity reactions in patients with brain tumours	Strong correlation between therapeutic antiepileptic level and hypersensitivity reactions	Consider using non-enzyme-inducing agents
VALPROATE	ANTIDEPRESSANTS – TCAs	↑ amitriptyline and nortriptyline levels	Uncertain	Be aware; watch for clinical features of ↑ levels of these TCAs (e.g. sedation, dry mouth, etc.)
VALPROATE	ANTIDIABETIC DRUGS – ACARBOSE	Case of ↓ valproate levels	Uncertain	Monitor valproate levels
VALPROATE	ANTIPLATELET AGENTS – ASPIRIN	Possible ↑ levels of phenytoin and valproate	Possibly ↑ unbound phenytoin or valproate fraction in the blood	Monitor phenytoin or valproate levels when co-administering high-dose aspirin
VALPROATE	ANTIPSYCHOTICS – OLANZAPINE	Risk of bone marrow toxicity	Additive effect	Monitor FBC closely; warn patients to report sore throat, fever, etc.
VALPROATE	ANTIVIRALS – ZIDOVUDINE	↑ zidovudine levels	Inhibition of metabolism	Watch for early features of toxicity of zidovudine
VALPROATE	CALCIUM CHANNEL BLOCKERS	Nimodipine levels may be ↑ by valproate	Uncertain at present	Monitor BP at least weekly until stable. Warn patients to report symptoms of hypotension (light-headedness, dizziness on standing, etc.)
VALPROATE	SODIUM PHENYLBUTYRATE	Possibly ↓ efficacy of sodium phenylbutyrate	These drugs are associated with ↑ ammonia levels	Avoid co-administration

Primary drug	Secondary drug	Effect	Mechanism	Precautions
ANTIMIGRAINE DRUGS				
ERGOT DERIVATIVES (INCLUDING METHYSERGIDE)				
ERGOT DERIVATIVES	ANAESTHETICS – GENERAL – HALOTHANE	↓ efficacy of ergometrine on the uterus	Uncertain	Use alternative form of anaesthesia for surgery requiring use of ergotamine
ERGOT DERIVATIVES	ANTIBIOTICS			
ERGOT DERIVATIVES	MACROLIDES, QUINUPRISTIN/DALFOPRISTIN,	↑ ergotamine/methysergide levels with risk of toxicity	Inhibition of CYP3A4-mediated metabolism of the ergot derivatives	Avoid co-administration
ERGOT DERIVATIVES	TETRACYCLINES	Cases of ergotism with tetracyclines and ergotamine	Uncertain	Avoid co-administration. If absolutely necessary, advise patients to discontinue treatment immediately if numbness and tingling of the extremities are felt
ERGOT DERIVATIVES	ANTIDEPRESSANTS – REBOXETINE	Risk of hypertension	Additive effect	Monitor BP closely
ERGOT DERIVATIVES	ANTIFUNGALS – VORICONAZOLE	↑ ergotamine/methysergide levels with risk of toxicity	Inhibition of metabolism of the ergot derivatives	Avoid co-administration. If absolutely necessary, advise patients to discontinue treatment immediately if numbness and tingling of the extremities are felt
ERGOT DERIVATIVES	ANTIVIRALS – PROTEASE INHIBITORS, EFAVIRENZ	↑ ergotamine/methysergide levels with risk of toxicity	↓ CYP3A4-mediated metabolism of ergot derivatives	Avoid co-administration
ERGOT DERIVATIVES	BETA-BLOCKERS	Three cases of arterial vasoconstriction and one of ↑ BP occurred when ergotamine or methysergide was added to propanolol or oxprenolol	Ergotamine can cause peripheral vasospasm, and absence of beta-adrenergic activity can ↑ risk of vasoconstriction	Ergot derivatives and beta-blockers are often co-administered without trouble; however, monitor BP at least weekly until stable (watch for ↑ BP) and warn patients to stop the ergot derivative and seek medical attention if they develop cold, painful feet

NERVOUS SYSTEM DRUGS ANTIMIGRAINE DRUGS

ERGOTAMINE	GRAPEFRUIT JUICE	Possibly ↑ efficacy and ↑ adverse effects, e.g. vasospasm, ergotism, peripheral vasoconstriction, gangrene	Possibly ↑ bioavailability by ↓ presystemic metabolism. Constituents of grapefruit juice irreversibly inhibit intestinal cytochrome CYP3A4	Monitor for ↑ side-effects and stop intake of grapefruit preparations if side-effects occur
ERGOT DERIVATIVES	H2 RECEPTOR BLOCKERS – CIMETIDINE	↑ ergotamine/methysergide levels with risk of toxicity	Inhibition of metabolism via CYP3A4	Avoid co-administration
ERGOTAMINE, METHYSERGIDE	5-HT1 AGONISTS – TRIPTANS	↑ risk of vasospasm	Additive effect	1. Do not administer ergotamine and almotriptan, rizatriptan, sumatriptan or zolmitriptan within 6 hours of each other 2. Do not administer methy-sergide and almotriptan, rizatriptan, sumatriptan or zolmitriptan within 24 hours of each other 3. Do not administer an ergot derivative and eletriptan or frovatriptan within 24 hours of each other
ERGOT DERIVATIVES	**SYMPATHOMIMETICS**			
ERGOT DERIVATIVES	SYMPATHOMIMETICS	Risk of ergot toxicity when ergotamine is co-administered with sympathomimetics	Uncertain	Watch for early features of ergotamine toxicity (vertigo and gastrointestinal disturbance)
ERGOT DERIVATIVES	DIRECT	Case report of gangrene when dopamine was given to a patient on ergotamine	Thought to be due to additive vasoconstriction	Titrate dopamine carefully

Primary drug	Secondary drug	Effect	Mechanism	Precautions
5-HT1 AGONISTS – TRIPTANS				
TRIPTANS	**ANTIBIOTICS**			
ALMOTRIPTAN, ELETRIPTAN	MACROLIDES – CLARITHROMYCIN, ERYTHROMYCIN, TELITHROMYCIN	↑ plasma concentrations of almotriptan and eletriptan, with risk of toxic effects, e.g. flushing, sensations of tingling, heat, heaviness, pressure or tightness of any part of body including the throat and chest, dizziness	Almotriptan is metabolized mainly by CYP3A4 isoenzymes. Most CYP isoenzymes are inhibited by clarithromycin to varying degrees, and since there is an alternative pathway of metabolism by MAO-A, toxicity responses will vary between individuals	Avoid co-administration
ALMOTRIPTAN	RIFAMPICIN	Possible ↓ plasma concentrations of almotriptan, with risk of inadequate therapeutic efficacy	One of the major metabolizing enzymes of almotriptan – CYP3A4 isoenzymes – are induced by rifampicin. As there are alternative metabolic pathways, the effect may not be significant and can vary from individual to individual	Be aware of the possibility of ↓ response to triptan, and consider ↑ of dose if considered to be due to interaction
ZOLMITRIPTAN	QUINOLONES	Possible ↓ plasma concentrations of zolmitriptan, with risk of inadequate therapeutic efficacy	Possibly induced metabolism of zolmitriptan	Be aware of possibility of ↓ response to triptan, and consider ↑ of dose if considered to be due to interaction.
ALMOTRIPTAN	**ANTICANCER AND IMMUNOMODULATING DRUGS**			
ALMOTRIPTAN, ELETRIPTAN	CYTOTOXICS – IMATINIB	↑ plasma concentrations of almotriptan and risk of toxic effects of almotriptan, e.g. flushing, sensations of tingling, heat, heaviness, pressure or tightness of any part of body including the throat and chest, dizziness	Almotriptan is metabolized mainly by CYP3A4 isoenzymes. Most CYP isoenzymes are inhibited by imatinib mesylate to varying degrees, and since there is an alternative pathway of metabolism by MAO-A, toxicity responses will vary between individuals	The CSM has advised, particularly for sumatriptan, that if chest tightness or pressure is intense, the triptan should be discontinued immediately and the patient investigated for ischaemic heart disease by measuring cardiac enzymes and doing an ECG. Avoid concomitant use in patients with coronary artery disease and in those with severe or uncontrolled hypertension

NERVOUS SYSTEM DRUGS ANTIMIGRAINE DRUGS

ALMOTRIPTAN, ELETRIPTAN	IMMUNOMODULATING DRUGS – CORTICOSTEROIDS – DEXAMETHASONE	Possible ↓ plasma concentrations of almotriptan and risk of inadequate therapeutic efficacy	One of the major metabolizing enzymes of almotriptan – CYP3A4 isoenzymes – are induced by rifampicin. As there are alternative metabolic pathways, the effect may not be significant and can vary from individual to individual	Be aware of possibility of ↓ response to triptan, and consider ↑ dose if considered to be due to interaction
TRIPTANS	**ANTIDEPRESSANTS**			
TRIPTANS	SSRIs	↑ risk of serotonin syndrome ➢ ***For signs and symptoms of serotonin toxicity, see Clinical Features of Some Adverse Drug Interactions, Serotonin toxicity and serotonin syndrome***	Triptans cause direct stimulation of 5-HT receptors, while SSRIs ↓ uptake of 5-HT, thus leading to ↑ serotonergic activity in the brain	The US FDA (July 2006) issued a warning of the possibility of this life-threatening serotonin syndrome when SSRIs are used together with triptans. Advise patients to report immediately the onset of symptoms such as tremors, agitation, confusion, ↑ heart beat (palpitations) and fever, and either ↓ dose or discontinue the SSRI
TRIPTANS	**MAOIs**			
RIZATRIPTAN, SUMATRIPTAN	MAOIs	↑ plasma concentrations of rizatriptan and sumatriptan, with risk of toxic effects, e.g. flushing, sensations of tingling, heat, heaviness, pressure or tightness of any part of body including the throat and chest, dizziness	These triptans are metabolized primarily by MAOI-A	Avoid starting these triptans for at least 2 weeks after stopping MAOIs; conversely, avoid starting MAOIs for at least 2 weeks after stopping these triptans
ZOLMITRIPTAN	MOCLOBEMIDE	Risk of agitation and confusion when zolmitriptan is co-administered with moclobemide	Uncertain	Watch for these effects and consider reducing the dose of zolmitriptan

Primary drug	Secondary drug	Effect	Mechanism	Precautions
TRIPTANS	DULOXETINE	Possible ↑ risk of serotonin syndrome ➢ ***For signs and symptoms of serotonin toxicity, see Clinical Features of Some Adverse Drug Interactions, Serotonin toxicity and serotonin syndrome***	Triptans cause direct stimulation of 5-HT receptors, while SSRIs ↓ uptake of 5-HT, thus leading to ↑ serotonergic activity in the brain	The US FDA (July 2006) issued a warning of the possibility of this life-threatening serotonin syndrome when SSRIs are used together with triptans (5-HT receptor agonists). Avoid concomitant use or ↓ dose of the SSRI
TRIPTANS	ST JOHN'S WORT	↑ risk of serotonin syndrome ➢ ***For signs and symptoms of serotonin toxicity, see Clinical Features of Some Adverse Drug Interactions, Serotonin toxicity and serotonin syndrome***	Possibly additive effect	Avoid co-administration
ALMOTRIPTAN	**ANTIEPILEPTICS**			
ALMOTRIPTAN, ELETRIPTAN	CARBAMAZEPINE	Possible ↓ plasma concentrations of almotriptan and risk of inadequate therapeutic efficacy. Risk of serotonin syndrome	One of the major metabolizing enzymes of almotriptan – CYP3A4 isoenzymes – is induced by rifampicin. As there are alternative metabolic pathways, the effect may not be significant and can vary from individual to individual. Triptans and carbamazepine are both stimulants of 5-HT receptors, and carbamazepine in addition prevents the reuptake of 5-HT	Be aware of possibility of ↓ response to triptan, and consider ↑ dose if considered to be due to interaction. Be aware of the possibility of the occurrence of serotonin syndrome ➢ ***For signs and symptoms of serotonin toxicity, see Clinical Features of Some Adverse Drug Interactions, Serotonin toxicity and serotonin syndrome***

ALMOTRIPTAN, ELETRIPTAN	PHENOBARBITAL	Possible ↓ plasma concentrations of almotriptan and risk of inadequate therapeutic efficacy	One of the major metabolizing enzymes of almotriptan – CYP3A4 isoenzymes – is induced by rifampicin. As there are alternative metabolic pathways, the effect may not be significant and can vary from individual to individual	Be aware of possibility of ↓ response to triptan, and consider ↑ dose if considered to be due to interaction
ALMOTRIPTAN, ELETRIPTAN	PHENYTOIN	Possible ↓ plasma concentrations of almotriptan and risk of inadequate therapeutic efficacy	One of the major metabolizing enzymes of almotriptan – CYP3A4 isoenzymes – is induced by rifampicin. As there are alternative metabolic pathways, the effect may not be significant and can vary from individual to individual	Be aware of possibility of ↓ response to triptan, and consider ↑ dose if considered to be due to interaction
ANTIMIGRAINE DRUGS – 5-HT1 AGONISTS	ANTIFUNGALS – AZOLES	↑ levels of almotriptan and eletriptan	Inhibited metabolism	Avoid co-administration
ALMOTRIPTAN, ELETRIPTAN	**ANTIVIRALS**			
ALMOTRIPTAN, ELETRIPTAN	NON-NUCLEOSIDE REVERSE TRANSCRIPTASE INHIBITORS – EFAVIRENZ	↑ plasma concentrations of almotriptan and eletriptan and risk of toxic effects, e.g. flushing, sensations of tingling, heat, heaviness, pressure or tightness of any part of body including the throat and chest, dizziness	Almotriptan and eletriptan are metabolized by CYP3A4 isoenzymes, which may be inhibited by efavirenz. However, since there is an alternative pathway of metabolism by MAO-A, toxicity responses would vary between individuals	The CSM has advised that if chest tightness or pressure is intense, the triptan should be discontinued immediately and the patient investigated for ischaemic heart disease by measuring cardiac enzymes and doing an ECG. Avoid concomitant use in patients with coronary artery disease and in those with severe or uncontrolled hypertension

Primary drug	Secondary drug	Effect	Mechanism	Precautions
ALMOTRIPTAN, ELETRIPTAN	PROTEASE INHIBITORS – INDINAVIR, NELFINAVIR, RITONAVIR	Possibly ↑ adverse effects when almotriptan or eletriptan is co-administered with indinavir, ritonavir (with or without lopinavir), or nelfinavir	Inhibition of CYP3A4- and possibly CYP2D6-mediated metabolism of eletriptan, and CYP3A4-mediated metabolism of almotriptan	Avoid co-administration
RIZATRIPTAN	BETA-BLOCKERS – PROPRANOLOL	Plasma levels of rizatriptan almost doubled during propranolol therapy	Propanolol inhibits the metabolism of rizatriptan	Initiate therapy with 5 mg rizatriptan and do not exceed 10 mg in 24 hours. The manufacturers recommend separating doses by 2 hours, although this has not been borne out by studies
ALMOTRIPTAN, ELETRIPTAN	CALCIUM CHANNEL BLOCKERS – DILTIAZEM, NIFEDIPINE, VERAPAMIL	↑ plasma concentrations of almotriptan and risk of toxic effects of almotriptan, e.g. flushing, sensations of tingling, heat, heaviness, pressure or tightness of any part of body including the throat and chest, dizziness	Almotriptan is metabolized mainly by CYP3A4 isoenzymes. Most CYP isoenzymes are inhibited by diltiazem to varying degrees, and since there is an alternative pathway of metabolism by MAO-A, toxicity responses vary between individuals	The CSM has advised that if chest tightness or pressure is intense, the triptan should be discontinued immediately and the patient investigated for ischaemic heart disease by measuring cardiac enzymes and doing an ECG. Avoid concomitant use in patients with coronary artery disease and in those with severe or uncontrolled hypertension
ZOLMITRIPTAN	CNS STIMULANTS – MODAFINIL	May cause ↓ zolmitriptan levels if CYP1A2 is the predominant metabolic pathway and alternative metabolic pathways are either genetically deficient or affected	Modafinil is a moderate inducer of CYP1A2 in a concentration-dependent manner	Be aware

TRIPTANS	ERGOT ALKALOIDS – ERGOTAMINE, METHYSERGIDE	↑ risk of vasospasm	Additive effect	1. Do not administer ergotamine and almotriptan, rizatriptan, sumatriptan or zolmitriptan within 6 hours of each other 2. Do not administer methysergide and almotriptan, rizatriptan, sumatriptan or zolmitriptan within 24 hours of each other 3. Do not administer an ergot derivative and eletriptan or frovatriptan within 24 hours of each other
ALMOTRIPTAN, ELETRIPTAN	GRAPEFRUIT JUICE	↑ plasma concentrations of almotriptan and eletriptan, with risk of toxic effects, e.g. flushing, sensations of tingling, heat, heaviness, pressure or tightness of any part of body including the throat and chest, dizziness	Almotriptan and eletriptan are metabolized mainly by CYP3A4 isoenzymes. Most CYP isoenzymes are inhibited by grapefruit juice to varying degrees, and since there is an alternative pathway of metabolism by MAO-A, toxicity responses will vary between individuals	The CSM has advised that if chest tightness or pressure is intense, the triptan should be discontinued immediately and the patient investigated for ischaemic heart disease by measuring cardiac enzymes and doing an ECG. Avoid concomitant use in patients with coronary artery disease and in those with severe or uncontrolled hypertension
ALMOTRIPTAN, ELETRIPTAN, ZOLMITRIPTAN	H2-RECEPTOR BLOCKERS – CIMETIDINE	↑ efficacy and adverse effects of zolmitriptan, e.g. flushing, sensations of tingling, heat, heaviness, pressure or tightness of any part of body including the throat and chest, dizziness	Inhibition of metabolism via CYP1A2	Consider alternative acid suppression, e.g. H2 antagonist or proton pump inhibitors (not omeprazole or lansoprazole), or monitor more closely and ↓ maximum dose of zolmitriptan to 5 mg/24 hours

Primary drug	Secondary drug	Effect	Mechanism	Precautions
PIZOTIFEN				
PIZOTIFEN	ADRENERGIC NEURONE BLOCKERS	↓ hypotensive effect	Pizotifen competes with adrenergic neurone blockers for reuptake to nerve terminals	Monitor BP at least weekly until stable
ANTIOBESITY DRUGS				
ORLISTAT				
ORLISTAT	ANTIARRHYTHMICS – AMIODARONE	Possible ↓ amiodarone levels	↓ absorption of amiodarone	Watch for poor response to amiodarone
ORLISTAT	ANTICANCER DRUGS – CICLOSPORIN	↓ plasma concentrations of ciclosporin and risk of transplant rejection	↓ absorption of ciclosporin	Avoid co-administration
ORLISTAT	ANTICOAGULANTS – ORAL	↓ anticoagulant effect	Probably ↓ absorption of coumarins	Monitor INR closely until stable
ORLISTAT	ANTIDIABETIC DRUGS – ACARBOSE, INSULIN, NATEGLINIDE, REPAGLINIDE, SULPHONYLUREAS	Tendency for blood glucose levels to fluctuate	Antiobesity drugs change the dietary intake of carbohydrates and other foods, and the risk of such fluctuations is greater if there is a concurrent dietary regimen. A side-effect of orlistat is hypoglycaemia	These agents are used often in patients with type II diabetes who are on hypoglycaemic therapy. Need to monitor blood sugars twice weekly until stable. Advise self-monitoring and warn about symptoms of hypoglycaemia. Watch for and warn patients about symptoms of hypoglycaemia. Avoid co-administration of acarbose and orlistat ➢ ***For signs and symptoms of hypoglycaemia, see Clinical Features of Some Adverse Drug Interactions, Hypoglycaemia***

NERVOUS SYSTEM DRUGS ANTIOBESITY DRUGS

ORLISTAT	ANTIHYPERTENSIVES AND HEART FAILURE DRUGS			
ORLISTAT	ACE INHIBITORS	↓ hypotensive effect found with enalapril	Uncertain at present	Monitor BP at least weekly until stable
ORLISTAT	ANGIOTENSIN II RECEPTOR ANTAGONISTS	Cases of ↓ efficacy of losartan	Uncertain at present	Monitor BP at least weekly until stable
ORLISTAT	BETA-BLOCKERS	Case of severe ↑ BP when orlistat is started in a patient on atenolol	Uncertain at present	Monitor BP at least weekly until stable
ORLISTAT	CALCIUM CHANNEL BLOCKERS	Case report of ↑ BP when orlistat was started in a patient on amlodipine	Uncertain at present	Monitor BP at least weekly until stable
ORLISTAT	THIAZIDES	Case report of ↑ BP when orlistat was started in a patient on thiazides	Uncertain at present	Monitor BP at least weekly until stable
RIMONABANT				
RIMONABANT	ANTIDIABETIC DRUGS – ACARBOSE, INSULIN, NATEGLINIDE, REPAGLINIDE, SULPHONYLUREAS	Tendency for blood glucose levels to fluctuate	Antiobesity drugs change the dietary intake of carbohydrates and other foods, and the risk of such fluctuations is greater if there is a concurrent dietary regimen. A side-effect of orlistat is hypoglycaemia	These agents are used often in patients with type II diabetes who are on hypoglycaemic therapy. Need to monitor blood sugars twice weekly until stable. Advise self-monitoring and warn about symptoms of hypoglycaemia. Watch for and warn patients about symptoms of hypoglycaemia ➣ ***For signs and symptoms of hypoglycaemia, see Clinical Features of Some Adverse Drug Interactions, Hypoglycaemia***

Primary drug	Secondary drug	Effect	Mechanism	Precautions
RIMONABANT	ANTIFUNGALS – KETOCONAZOLE	↑ rimonabant levels	Ketoconazole inhibits CYP3A4-mediated metabolism of rimonabant	Avoid co-administration
SIBUTRAMINE				
SIBUTRAMINE	ANALGESICS – NSAIDs	↑ risk of bleeding	Additive effect	Avoid co-administration
SIBUTRAMINE	ANTICOAGULANTS – HEPARINS	Possible ↑ risk of bleeding	Uncertain	Monitor APTT closely
SIBUTRAMINE	ANTIDIABETIC DRUGS – ACARBOSE, INSULIN, NATEGLINIDE, REPAGLINIDE, SULPHONYL UREAS	Tendency for blood glucose levels to fluctuate	Antiobesity drugs change the dietary intake of carbohydrates and other foods, and the risk of such fluctuations is greater if there is a concurrent dietary regimen. A side-effect of orlistat is hypoglycaemia	These agents are used often in patients with type II diabetes who are on hypoglycaemic therapy. Need to monitor blood sugars twice weekly until stable. Advise self-monitoring and warn about symptoms of hypoglycaemia. Watch for and warn patients about symptoms of hypoglycaemia ➢ ***For signs and symptoms of hypoglycaemia, see Clinical Features of Some Adverse Drug Interactions, Hypoglycaemia***
SIBUTRAMINE	ANTIPLATELET AGENTS – ASPIRIN	Risk of bleeding	Additive effect; sibutramine may cause thrombocytopenia	Warn the patient to report any signs of ↑ bleeding
SIBUTRAMINE	**ANTIDEPRESSANTS**			
SIBUTRAMINE	MAOIs	Risk of hypertension and agitation	Additive effect on norepinephrine transmission	Avoid co-administration. Do not start sibutramine for at least 2 weeks after stopping MAOIs

SIBUTRAMINE	TCAs, MIRTAZAPINE, REBOXETINE, TRYPTOPHAN	Risk of hypertension and agitation	Additive effect on norepinephrine transmission. In addition, tryptophan is a precursor of neurotransmitters such as serotonin; sibutramine inhibits serotonin and norepinephrine reuptake	Avoid co-administration
SIBUTRAMINE	ANTIPSYCHOTICS	Risk of headache, agitation and fits	Additive effect	Avoid co-administration
SIBUTRAMINE	GRAPEFRUIT JUICE	Possibly ↑ efficacy and ↑ adverse effects, e.g. higher BP and raised heart rate	Unclear	Monitor PR and BP
ANTIPARKINSON'S DRUGS				
AMANTADINE				
AMANTADINE	ANTIMUSCARINICS	↑ risk of antimuscarinic side-effects	Additive effect; both drugs cause antimuscarinic side-effects	Warn patient of this additive effect
AMANTADINE	1. ANTIEMETICS – metoclopramide 2. ANTIPSYCHOTICS 3. CENTRALLY ACTING ANTIHYPERTENSIVES – methyldopa 4. TETRABENAZINE	↓ efficacy of amantadine	Antagonism of antiparkinson's effect; these drugs have extrapyramidal side-effects	Use with caution; avoid in patients <20 years
AMANTADINE	1. ANTIPARKINSON'S DRUGS – dopaminergics 2. ANTIDEMENTIA DRUGS – memantine 3. DRUG DEPENDENCE THERAPIES – bupropion	↑ CNS side-effects	Additive effects	Monitor more closely for confusion and gastrointestinal side-effects. Initiate therapy with bupropion at the lowest dose and ↑ it gradually. Manufacturers recommend avoiding co-administration of amantadine and memantine

Primary drug	Secondary drug	Effect	Mechanism	Precautions
AMANTADINE	1. ANTIMALARIALS – quinine 2. ANTIPARKINSON'S DRUGS – pramipexole	↑ side-effects	↓ renal excretion	Monitor closely for confusion, disorientation, headache, dizziness and nausea
ANTIMUSCARINICS				
ANTIMUSCARINICS	ADDITIVE ANTICHOLINERGIC EFFECTS			
ANTIMUSCARINICS	1. ANALGESICS – nefopam 2. ANTIARRHYTHMICS – disopyramide, propafenone 3. ANTIDEPRESSANTS – TCAs 4. ANTIEMETICS – cyclizine 5. ANTIHISTAMINES – chlorphenamine, cyproheptadine, hydroxyzine 6. ANTIPARKINSON'S DRUGS – dopaminergics 7. ANTIPSYCHOTICS – phenothiazines, clozapine, pimozide 8. MUSCLE RELAXANTS – baclofen 9. NITRATES – isosorbide dinitrate	↑ risk of antimuscarinic side-effects. **NB ↓ efficacy of sublingual nitrate tablets**	Additive effect; both drugs cause antimuscarinic side-effects. **Antimuscarinic effects ↓ saliva production, which ↓ dissolution of the tablet**	Warn patient of this additive effect. **Consider changing the formulation to a sublingual nitrate spray**
ATROPINE, GLYCOPYRRONIUM	ALCOHOL	↑ sedation	Additive effect	Warn patients about this effect and advise them not to drink while taking these antimuscarinics
ANTIMUSCARINICS	ANALGESICS – PARACETAMOL	Atropine, benzatropine, orphenadrine, procyclidine and trihexyphenidyl may slow the onset of action of intermittent-dose paracetamol	Anticholinergic effects delay gastric emptying and absorption	Warn patients that the action of paracetamol may be delayed. This will not be the case when paracetamol is taken regularly

ATROPINE	ANTIARRHYTHMICS – MEXILETINE	Delayed absorption of mexiletine	Anticholinergic effects delay gastric emptying and absorption	May slow the onset of action of the first dose of mexiletine, but is not of clinical significance for regular dosing (atropine does not ↓ total dose absorbed)
TOLTERODINE	ANTIBIOTICS – CLARITHROMYCIN, ERYTHROMYCIN	↑ tolterodine levels	Inhibition of CYP3A4-mediated metabolism	Avoid co-administration (manufacturers' recommendation)
DARIFENACIN	ANTICANCER AND IMMUNOMODULATING DRUGS – CICLOSPORIN	↑ levels of darifenacin	Ciclosporin inhibits P-gp and CYP3A4, which results in ↓ clearance of darifenacin	Avoid co-administration
ANTIMUSCARINICS	ANTIDEMENTIA DRUGS – MEMANTINE	Possible ↑ efficacy of antimuscarinics	Additive effect; memantine has weak antimuscarinic properties	Warn patients of this effect
ANTIMUSCARINICS	**ANTIDEPRESSANTS**			
DARIFENACIN, PROCYCLIDINE	PAROXETINE	↑ levels of these antimuscarinics	Inhibition of metabolism	Watch for early features of toxicity
IPRATROPIUM, TIOTROPIUM	MAOIs	↑ occurrence of antimuscarinic effects such as blurred vision, confusion (in elderly people), restlessness and constipation	Additive antimuscarinic effects	Warn patients and carers, particularly those managing elderly patients
ANTIMUSCARINICS	ANTIDEPRESSANTS – MAOIs	↑ occurrence of antimuscarinic effects such as blurred vision, confusion (in elderly people), restlessness and constipation	Additive antimuscarinic effects	Warn patients and carers, particularly those managing elderly patients
ANTIMUSCARINICS	ANTIEMETICS – DOMPERIDONE, METOCLOPRAMIDE	↓ efficacy of domperidone on gut motility by antimuscarinics	Some effects of metoclopramide are considered to be due to ↑ release of ACh and ↑ sensitivity of the cholinergic receptors to ACh. Antimuscarinics prevent the effects on muscarinic receptors	The gastrointestinal effects of metoclopramide will be impaired, while the antiemetic effects may not be. Thus, concurrent use with antimuscarinics is not advised because of effects on the gastrointestinal system

Primary drug	Secondary drug	Effect	Mechanism	Precautions
ANTIMUSCARINICS	ANTIFUNGALS – ITRACONAZOLE, KETOCONAZOLE	1. ↓ ketoconazole levels. 2. ↑ darifenacin, solifenacin and tolterodine levels	1. ↓ absorption 2. Inhibited metabolism	1. Watch for poor response to ketoconazole 2. Avoid co-administration of itraconazole, ketoconazole and these antimuscarinics. The US manufacturer of darifenacin recommends that its dose should not exceed 7.5 mg/day
PROTEASE INHIBITORS	**ANTIVIRALS**			
SOLIFENACIN	PROTEASE INHIBITORS	↑ adverse effects with nelfinavir and ritonavir (with or without lopinavir)	Inhibition of CYP3A4-mediated metabolism of solifenacin	Limit maximum dose of solifenacin to 5 mg daily
TOLTERODINE	PROTEASE INHIBITORS	Possibly ↑ adverse effects, including arrythmias, with protease inhibitors	Inhibition of CYP2D6- and 3A4-mediated metabolism of tolterodine	Avoid co-administration
ANTIMUSCARINICS	ANTIPARKINSON'S – AMANTADINE	↑ risk of antimuscarinic side-effects	Additive effect; both drugs cause antimuscarinic side-effects	Warn patients of this additive effect
IPRATROPIUM	BRONCHODILATORS – SALBUTAMOL	A few reports of acute angle closure glaucoma when nebulized ipratropium and salbutamol were co-administered	Ipratropium dilates the pupil, which ↓ drainage of aqueous humour, while salbutamol ↑ production of aqueous humour	Warn patients to prevent the solution to mist or enter the eye. Extreme caution in co-administering these bronchodilators by the nebulized route in patients with a history of acute closed-angle glaucoma
DARIFENACIN	CALCIUM CHANNEL BLOCKERS – VERAPAMIL	↑ darifenacin levels	Inhibition of CYP3A4-mediated metabolism of darifenacin	Avoid co-administration (manufacturers' recommendation)
PROPANTHELINE	CARDIAC GLYCOSIDES – DIGOXIN	↑ digoxin levels (30–40%) but only with slow-release formulations	Slowed gut transit time allows more digoxin to be absorbed	Use alternative formulation of digoxin
ANTIMUSCARINICS	PARASYMPATHOMIMETICS	↓ efficacy of parasympathomimetics	Parasympathomimetics and antimuscarinics have opposing effects	Avoid co-administration where possible

ATROPINE	SYMPATHOMIMETICS	Reports of hypertension when atropine was given to patients receiving 10% phenylephrine eye drops during eye surgery	Atropine abolishes the cholinergic response to phenylephrine-induced vasoconstriction	Use a lower concentration of phenylephrine
DOPAMINERGICS				
DOPAMINERGICS	DRUGS WITH ANTIMUSCARINIC EFFECTS			
DOPAMINERGICS	1. ANALGESICS – nefopam 2. ANTIARRHYTHMICS – disopyramide, propafenone 3. ANTIDEPRESSANTS – TCAs 4. ANTIEMETICS – cyclizine 5. ANTIHISTAMINES – chlorphenamine, cyproheptadine, hydroxyzine 6. ANTIMUSCARINICS – atropine, benzatropine, cyclopentolate, dicycloverine, flavoxate, homatropine, hyoscine, orphenadrine, oxybutynin, procyclidine, propantheline, tolterodine, trihexyphenidyl, tropicamide 7. ANTIPSYCHOTICS – phenothiazines, clozapine, pimozide 8. MUSCLE RELAXANTS – baclofen 9. NITRATES – isosorbide dinitrate	↑ risk of antimuscarinic side-effects. Also, possibly ↓ levodopa levels. **NB ↓ efficacy of sublingual nitrate tablets**	Additive effect. Delayed gastric emptying may cause more levodopa to be metabolized within the wall of the gastrointestinal tract. **Antimuscarinic effects ↓ saliva production, which ↓ dissolution of the tablet**	Warn patients of this additive effect. Consider increasing the dose of levodopa. **Consider changing the formulation to a sublingual nitrate spray**

Primary drug	Secondary drug	Effect	Mechanism	Precautions
LEVODOPA	ANAESTHETICS – GENERAL – VOLATILE AGENTS	Possible risk of arrhythmias	Uncertain	Monitor EGC and BP closely. Consider using intravenous agents for maintenance of anaesthesia
DOPAMINERGICS	**ANALGESICS**			
DOPAMINERGICS	NEFOPAM	↑ anticholinergic effects	Additive effects	Warn patients about these effects
RASAGILINE, SELEGILINE	OPIOIDS – PETHIDINE, TRAMADOL	1. Risk of neurological toxicity when pethidine is co-administered with rasagiline 2. Risk of hyperpyrexia when pethidine and possibly tramadol is co-administered with selegiline	Unknown	1. Avoid co-administration; do not use pethidine for at least 2 weeks after stopping rasagiline 2. Avoid co-administration
DOPAMINERGICS	PARACETAMOL	Amantadine, bromocriptine, levodopa, pergolide, pramipexole and selegiline may slow the onset of action of intermittent-dose paracetamol	Anticholinergic effects delay gastric emptying and absorption	Warn patients that the action of paracetamol may be delayed. This will not be the case when paracetamol is taken regularly
DOPAMINERGICS	**ANTIBIOTICS**			
BROMOCRIPTINE, CABERGOLINE	ERYTHROMYCIN	↑ bromocriptine and cabergoline levels	Inhibition of metabolism	Monitor BP closely and watch for early features of toxicity (nausea, headache, drowsiness)
ROPINIROLE	CIPROFLOXACIN	↑ ropinirole levels	Inhibition of CYP1A2-mediated metabolism	Watch for early features of toxicity (nausea, drowsiness)
DOPAMINERGICS	**ANTICANCER AND IMMUNOMODULATING DRUGS**			
BROMOCRIPTINE	CYTOTOXICS – PROCARBAZINE	May cause ↑ serum prolactin levels and interfere with the effects of bromocriptine	Uncertain	Watch for ↓ effect of bromocriptine
BROMOCRIPTINE	HORMONE ANTAGONISTS – OCTREOTIDE	↑ bromocriptine levels	Uncertain	Be aware

ENTACAPONE	ANTICOAGULANTS – ORAL	↑ anticoagulant effect	Uncertain at present	Monitor INR at least weekly until stable
DOPAMINERGICS	ANTIDEMENTIA DRUGS – MEMANTINE	Memantine augments the effect of dopaminergics	Memantine has some agonist activity at dopamine receptors	Be aware. May be used therapeutically
DOPAMINERGICS	**ANTIDEPRESSANTS**			
LEVODOPA, SELEGILINE, POSSIBLY RASAGILINE, ENTACAPONE, TOLCAPONE	MAOIs	Risk of adrenergic syndrome – hypertension, hyperthermia, arrhythmias – and dopaminergic effects with selegiline	Levodopa and related drugs are precursors of dopamine. Levodopa is predominantly metabolized to dopamine, and a smaller proportion is converted to epinephrine and norepinephrine. Effects are due to inhibition of MAOI, which breaks down dopamine and sympathomimetics	Avoid concurrent use. Onset may be 6–24 hours after ingestion. Carbidopa and benserazide, which inhibit dopa decarboxylase that converts L-dopa to dopamine, is considered to minimize this interaction. However, MAOIs should not be used in patients with Parkinson's disease on treatment with levodopa. Imipramine and amitriptyline are considered safer by some clinicians
RASAGILINE, SELEGILINE	SSRIs, VENLAFAXINE	Risk of severe hypertensive reactions and of serotonin syndrome ➢ ***For signs and symptoms of serotonin toxicity, see Clinical Features of Some Adverse Drug Interactions, Serotonin toxicity and serotonin syndrome***	Additive inhibitory effect on serotonin the reuptake with SSRIs. Venlafaxine inhibits the reuptake of both serotonin and norepinephrine. Due to impaired metabolism of these amines, there is an accumulation of serotonin and norepinephrine in the brain and at peripheral sites. These dopaminergics are MAO-B inhibitors	Avoid co-administration. Rasagiline and selegiline should not be started for at least 2 weeks after stopping SSRIs (5 weeks after fluoxetine). Do not start selegiline or rasagiline for at least 1 week after stopping venlafaxine. Conversely, SSRIs and venlafaxine should not be started for at least 2 weeks after stopping rasagiline and selegiline

Primary drug	Secondary drug	Effect	Mechanism	Precautions
RASAGILINE, SELEGILINE	TCAs	↑ risk of stroke, hyperpyrexia and convulsions. ↑ plasma concentrations of TCAs, with risk of toxic effects. ↑ risk of serotonin syndrome and of adrenergic syndrome with older MAOIs. Clomipramine may trigger acute confusion in Parkinson's disease when used with selegiline	TCAs are believed to also act by inhibiting the reuptake of serotonin and norepinephrine, increasing the risk of serotonin and adrenergic syndromes. The combination of TCAs and antidepressants can ↑ risk of seizures	Very hazardous interaction. Avoid concurrent use and consider the use of an alternative antidepressant. Be aware that seizures occur with overdose of TCAs just before cardiac arrest
ROPINIROLE	SSRI – FLUVOXAMINE	↑ ropinirole levels	Inhibition of CYP1A2-mediated metabolism	Watch for early features of toxicity (nausea, drowsiness)
RASAGILINE, SELEGILINE	ANTIDIABETIC DRUGS – INSULIN, SULPHONYLUREAS	↑ risk of hypoglycaemic episodes	These drugs are MAO-B inhibitors. MAOIs have an intrinsic hypoglycaemic effect and are considered to enhance the effect of hypoglycaemic drugs	Watch for and warn patients about symptoms of hypoglycaemia ➢ ***For signs and symptoms of hypoglycaemia, see Clinical Features of Some Adverse Drug Interactions, Hypoglycaemia***
DOPAMINERGICS	**ANTIEMETICS**			
DOPAMINERGICS	METOCLOPRAMIDE	↓ efficacy of dopaminergics	Metoclopramide is a centrally acting antidopaminergic	Use with caution, avoid in patients <20 years. Manufacturers recommend avoiding co-administration of metoclopramide with ropinirole or rotigotine

BROMOCRIPTINE, CABERGOLINE	DOMPERIDONE, METOCLOPRAMIDE	↓ efficacy of bromocriptine and cabergoline at reducing prolactin levels	Domperidone and metoclopramide are associated with prolactin secretion	Use alternative antiemetics when bromocriptine and cabergoline are being used to treat prolactinomas. Domperidone has minimal central antidopaminergic effect and may therefore be used when bromocriptine and cabergoline are administered as treatments for Parkinson's disease
LEVODOPA	ANTIEPILEPTICS – PHENYTOIN	Possibly ↓ levodopa levels	Uncertain	Watch for poor response to levodopa and consider increasing its dose
DOPAMINERGICS	**ANTIHYPERTENSIVES AND HEART FAILURE DRUGS**			
LEVODOPA	ANTIHYPERTENSIVES AND HEART FAILURE DRUGS	↑ hypotensive effect	Additive effect	Monitor BP at least weekly until stable. Warn patients to report symptoms of hypotension (light-headedness, dizziness on standing, etc.)
LEVODOPA	CENTRALLY ACTING ANTIHYPERTENSIVES	1. Clonidine may oppose the effect of levodopa/carbidopa 2. Methyldopa may ↓ levodopa requirements, although there are case reports of deteriorating dyskinesias in some patients	1. Uncertain at present 2. Uncertain at present	1. Watch for deterioration in control of symptoms of Parkinson's disease 2. Levodopa needs may ↓; in cases of worsening Parkinson's control, use an alternative antihypertensive
PERGOLIDE	ACE INHIBITORS	Possible ↑ hypotensive effect	Additive effect; a single case of severe ↓ BP with lisinopril and pergolide has been reported	Monitor BP at least weekly until stable. Warn patients to report symptoms of hypotension (light-headedness, dizziness on standing, etc.)

Primary drug	Secondary drug	Effect	Mechanism	Precautions
DOPAMINERGICS	ANTIPARKINSON'S DRUGS			
DOPAMINERGICS	AMANTADINE	↑ CNS side-effects	Additive effects	Monitor more closely for confusion, gastrointestinal side-effects. Initiate therapy with bupropion at the lowest dose and ↑ gradually. Manufacturers recommend avoiding co-administration of amantadine and memantine
PRAMIPEXOLE	AMANTADINE	↑ side-effects	↓ renal excretion	Monitor closely for confusion, disorientation, headache, dizziness and nausea
DOPAMINERGICS	ANTIPSYCHOTICS	↓ efficacy of dopaminergics	Antipsychotics may cause extrapyramidal side-effects, which oppose the effect of antiparkinson's drugs. The atypical antipsychotics cause less effect than the older drugs	Caution with co-administration; consider using atypical antipsychotics, and use antimuscarinic drugs if extrapyramidal symptoms occur. Manufacturers recommend avoiding co-administration of amisulpride with levodopa, and co-administration of antipsychotics with pramipexole, ropinirole and rotigotine. Clozapine can be co-administered with Sinemet and pergolide
LEVODOPA	ANXIOLYTICS AND HYPNOTICS – BZDs	Risk of ↓ effect of levodopa	Uncertain	Watch for poor response to levodopa and consider increasing its dose. If there is severe antagonism of effect, stop the BZD
LEVODOPA	BETA-BLOCKERS	↑ hypotensive effect	Additive hypotensive effect; however, overall, adding beta-blockers to levodopa can be beneficial (e.g. by reducing the risk of a dopamine-mediated risk of arrhythmias)	Monitor BP at least weekly until stable
LEVODOPA	CALCIUM CHANNEL BLOCKERS	↑ hypotensive effect	Additive hypotensive effect	Monitor BP at least weekly until stable. Warn patients to report symptoms of hypotension (light-headedness, dizziness on standing, etc.)

LEVODOPA	DIURETICS	↑ hypotensive effect	Additive effect	Monitor BP at least weekly until stable. Warn patients to report symptoms of hypotension (light-headedness, dizziness on standing, etc.)
DOPAMINERGICS – ENTACAPONE, TOLCAPONE	DOPAMINERGICS – SELEGILINE	Possible risk of severe hypertensive reactions	Theoretical risk due to additive inhibitory effect on dopamine metabolism	Manufacturers recommend limiting the dose of selegiline to a maximum of 10 mg
LEVODOPA	DRUG DEPENDENCE THERAPIES – BUPROPION	↑ CNS side-effects	Additive effects	Initiate therapy with bupropion at the lowest dose and ↑ gradually
PRAMIPEXOLE, ROPINIROLE	H2-RECEPTOR BLOCKER – CIMETIDINE	↑ efficacy and adverse effects of pramipexole	↓ renal excretion of pramipexole by inhibition of cation transport system. Inhibition of CYP1A2-mediated metabolism of ropinirole	Monitor closely; ↓ dose of pramipexole may be required. Adjust dose of ropinirole as necessary or use alternative acid suppression, e.g. H2 antagonist proton pump inhibitor (not omeprazole or lansoprazole)
ENTACAPONE, LEVODOPA	IRON – ORAL	↓ entacapone levels	Iron chelates with entacapone and levodopa, which ↓ their absorption	Separate doses as much as possible. Consider increasing the dose of antiparkinson's therapy
LEVODOPA	MUSCLE RELAXANTS – BACLOFEN	Reports of CNS agitation and ↓ efficacy of levodopa	Uncertain	Avoid co-administration
APOMORPHINE	NITRATES	Risk of postural ↓ BP when apomorphine is given with nitrates	Additive effect; apomorphine can cause postural ↓ BP	Monitor BP at least weekly until stable. Warn patients to report symptoms of hypotension (light-headedness, dizziness on standing, etc.)
ROPINIROLE, SELEGILINE	OESTROGENS	↑ levels of ropinirole and selegiline	Inhibition of metabolism (possibly *N*-demethylation)	Watch for early features of toxicity (nausea, drowsiness) when starting oestrogens in a patient stabilized on these dopaminergics. Conversely, watch for poor response to them if oestrogens are stopped

NERVOUS SYSTEM DRUGS ANTIPARKINSON'S DRUGS

Primary drug	Secondary drug	Effect	Mechanism	Precautions
APOMORPHINE	PERIPHERAL VASODILATORS – MOXISYLYTE	↑ hypotensive effect	Additive hypotensive effect	Monitor BP at least weekly until stable. Warn patients to report symptoms of hypotension (light-headedness, dizziness on standing, etc.)
SELEGILINE	PROGESTOGENS	↑ selegiline levels	Inhibition of metabolism	Watch for early features of toxicity (nausea, drowsiness) when starting progestogens in a patient stabilized on these dopaminergics. Conversely, watch for poor response to them if progestogens are stopped
DOPAMINERGICS	**SYMPATHOMIMETICS**			
BROMOCRIPTINE	INDIRECT	Cases of severe, symptomatic ↑ BP when co-administered with indirect sympathomimetics	Likely additive effect; both can cause ↑ BP	Monitor BP closely; watch for ↑ BP
ENTACAPONE	INDIRECT	Cases of severe, symptomatic ↑ BP when co-administered with indirect sympathomimetics	Likely additive effect; both can cause ↑ BP	Monitor BP closely; watch for ↑ BP
RASAGILINE	SYMPATHOMIMETICS	Risk of adrenergic syndrome	Due to inhibition of MAOI, which breaks down sympathomimetics	Avoid concurrent use. Onset may be 6–24 hours after ingestion. Do ECG and measure electrolytes, FBC, CK and coagulation profile
SELEGILINE	DOPAMINE	Case report of ↑ hypertensive effect of dopamine when it was given to a patient already taking selegiline	Selegiline inhibits metabolism of dopamine	Titrate dopamine carefully
LEVODOPA	VITAMIN B6	↓ efficacy of levodopa (in the absence of a dopa decarboxylase inhibitor)	A derivative of vitamin B6 is a co-factor in the peripheral conversion of levodopa to dopamine, which ↓ the amount available for conversion in the CNS. Dopa decarboxylase inhibitors inhibit this peripheral reaction	Avoid co-administration of levodopa with vitamin B6; co-administration of vitamin B6 with co-beneldopa or co-careldopa is acceptable

ANTIPSYCHOTICS

ANTIPSYCHOTICS	DRUGS THAT PROLONG THE Q–T INTERVAL			
ATYPICALS, PHENOTHIAZINE, PIMOZIDE	1. ANTIARRHYTHMICS – amiodarone, disopyramide, procainamide, propafenone 2. ANTIBIOTICS – macrolides (especially azithromycin, clarithromycin, parenteral erythromycin, telithromycin), quinolones (especially moxifloxacin), quinupristin/dalfopristin 3. ANTI-DEPRESSANTS – TCAs, venlafaxine 4. ANTIEMETICS – dolasetron 5. ANTIFUNGALS – fluconazole, posaconazole, voriconazole 6. ANTI-HISTAMINES – terfenadine, hydroxyzine, mizolastine 7. ANTIMALARIALS – artemether with lumefantrine, chloroquine, hydroxy-chloroquine, mefloquine, quinine 8. ANTIPROTOZOALS – pentamidine isetionate 9. BETA-BLOCKERS – sotalol 10. BRONCHODILATORS – parenteral bronchodilators 11. CNS STIMULANTS – atomoxetine	Risk of ventricular arrhythmias, particularly torsades de pointes	Additive effect; these drugs cause prolongation of the Q–T interval	Avoid co-administration

NERVOUS SYSTEM DRUGS ANTIPSYCHOTICS

Primary drug	Secondary drug	Effect	Mechanism	Precautions
ANTIPSYCHOTICS	**DRUGS WITH ANTIMUSCARINIC EFFECTS**			
ANTIPSYCHOTICS – PHENOTHIAZINES, CLOZAPINE, PIMOZIDE	1. ANALGESICS – nefopam 2. ANTIARRHYTHMICS – disopyramide, propafenone 3. ANTIDEPRESSANTS – TCAs 4. ANTIEMETICS – cyclizine 5. ANTIHISTAMINES – chlorphenamine, cyproheptadine, hydroxyzine 6. ANTIMUSCARINICS – atropine, benzatropine, cyclopentolate, dicycloverine, flavoxate, homatropine, hyoscine, orphenadrine, oxybutynin, procyclidine, propantheline, tolterodine, trihexyphenidyl or tropicamide 7. ANTIPSYCHOTICS – phenothiazines, clozapine, pimozide 8. MUSCLE RELAXANTS – baclofen 9. NITRATES – isosorbide dinitrate	↑ risk of antimuscarinic side-effects. Also, possibly ↓ levodopa levels. **NB ↓ efficacy of sublingual nitrate tablets**	Additive effect. Delayed gastric emptying may cause more levodopa to be metabolized within the wall of the gastrointestinal tract. **Antimuscarinic effects ↓ saliva production, which ↓ dissolution of the tablet**	Warn patients of this additive effect. Consider increasing the dose of levodopa. **Consider changing the formulation to a sublingual nitrate spray**
ANTIPSYCHOTICS	ALCOHOL	Risk of excessive sedation	Additive effect	Warn patients of this effect, and advise them to drink alcohol only in moderation
ANTIPSYCHOTICS	ANAESTHETICS – GENERAL	Risk of hypotension	Additive effect	Monitor BP closely, especially during induction of anaesthesia

ANTIPSYCHOTICS	ANALGESICS			
ANTIPSYCHOTICS	NSAIDs	1. Reports of ↑ sedation when indometacin is added to haloperidol 2. Risk of agranulocytosis when azapropazone given with clozapine	1. Unknown 2. Unknown	1. Avoid co-administration 2. Avoid co-administration
ANTIPSYCHOTICS	OPIOIDS	Risk of ↑ respiratory depression, sedation and ↓ BP. This effect seems to be particularly marked with clozapine	Additive effects	Warn patients of these effects. Monitor BP closely. Titrate doses carefully
ANTIPSYCHOTICS	TRAMADOL	↑ risk of fits	Additive effects	Consider using an alternative analgesic
PHENOTHIAZINES, SULPIRIDE	ANTACIDS	↓ levels of these antipsychotics	↓ absorption	Separate doses by 2 hours (in the case of sulpiride, give sulpiride 2 hours after but not before the antacid)
ANTIPSYCHOTICS	**ANTIARRHYTHMICS**			
ANTIPSYCHOTICS	ADENOSINE	Risk of ventricular arrhythmias, particularly torsades de pointes, with phenothiazines and pimozide. There is also a theoretical risk of Q–T prolongation with atypical antipsychotics	All of these drugs prolong the Q–T interval	Avoid co-administration of phenothiazines, amisulpride, pimozide or sertindole with adenosine. Monitor the ECG closely when adenosine is co-administered with atypical antipsychotics
AMISULPRIDE, PHENOTHIAZINES, PIMOZIDE, SERTINDOLE	FLECAINIDE	Risk of arrhythmias	Additive effect. Also, haloperidol and thioridazine inhibit CYP2D6-mediated metabolism of flecainide	Avoid co-administration
ANTIPSYCHOTICS	**ANTIBIOTICS** ➢ *Q–T-prolonging drugs, above*			
ARIPIPRAZOLE, CLOZAPINE, HALOPERIDOL	RIFABUTIN, RIFAMPICIN	↓ levels of these antipsychotics	↑ metabolism	Watch for poor response to these antipsychotics; consider increasing the dose

Primary drug	Secondary drug	Effect	Mechanism	Precautions
CLOZAPINE	CHLORAMPHENICOL, SULPHONAMIDES	↑ risk of bone marrow toxicity	Additive effect	Avoid co-administration
CLOZAPINE, OLANZAPINE	CIPROFLOXACIN	↑ clozapine levels and possibly ↑ olanzapine levels	Ciprofloxacin inhibits CYP1A2; clozapine is primarily metabolized by CYP1A2, while olanzapine is partly metabolized by it	Watch for the early features of toxicity to these antipsychotics. A ↓ in dose of clozapine and olanzapine may be required
CLOZAPINE	MACROLIDES – ERYTHROMYCIN	↑ clozapine levels with risk of clozapine toxicity	Clozapine is metabolized by CYPIA2, which is moderately inhibited by erythromycin. Erythromycin is a potent inhibitor of CYP3A4, which has a minor role in the metabolism of clozapine. This may lead to ↓ clearance and therefore ↑ levels of clozapine	Cautious use advised
ANTIPSYCHOTICS	**ANTICANCER AND IMMUNOMODULATING DRUGS**			
CLOZAPINE	CYTOTOXICS	↑ risk of bone marrow toxicity	Additive effect	Avoid co-administration
CLOZAPINE, HALOPERIDOL, PERPHENAZINE, RISPERIDONE	IMATINIB	Imatinib may cause ↑ plasma concentrations of these drugs with a risk of toxic effects	Inhibition of CYP2D6-mediated metabolism of these drugs	Watch for early features of toxicity of these drugs
CHLORPROMAZINE, FLUPHENAZINE	PORFIMER	↑ risk of photosensitivity reactions	Attributed to additive effects	Avoid exposure of skin and eyes to direct sunlight for 30 days after porfimer therapy
CLOZAPINE	PROCARBAZINE, PENICILLAMINE	↑ risk of bone marrow toxicity	Additive effect	Avoid co-administration
FLUPENTIXOL, PIMOZIDE, ZUCLOPENTHIXOL	PROCARBAZINE	Prolongation or greater intensity of sedative, hypotensive and anticholinergic effects	Additive effect	Avoid co-administration

NERVOUS SYSTEM DRUGS ANTIPSYCHOTICS

ANTIPSYCHOTICS	ANTIDEPRESSANTS			
CLOZAPINE, HALOPERIDOL, PHENOTHIAZINE, SULPIRIDE	LITHIUM	↑ risk of extrapyramidal side-effects and neurotoxicity	Uncertain	Watch for development of these symptoms
SERTINDOLE	LITHIUM	↑ risk of ventricular arrhythmias	Uncertain	Avoid concomitant use
ANTIPSYCHOTICS	MAOIs	Additive depression of CNS ranging from drowsiness to coma and respiratory depression	Synergistic depressant effects on CNS function	Necessary to warn patients, particularly regards activities that require attention, e.g. driving or using machinery and equipment that could cause self-harm
ARIPIPRAZOLE, CLOZAPINE, HALOPERIDOL, PERPHENAZINE, RISPERIDONE, SERTINDOLE	SSRIs	Possible ↑ plasma concentrations of these antipsychotics	Inhibition of CYP2D6-mediated metabolism of these drugs. The clinical significance of this depends upon whether alternative pathways of metabolism of these substrates are also inhibited by co-administered drugs. The risk is theoretically greater with clozapine, haloperidol and olanzapine because their CYP1A2-mediated metabolism is also inhibited by SSRIs	Warn patients to report ↑ side-effects of these drugs, and consider reducing the dose of the antipsychotic
PIMOZIDE	SERTRALINE	↑ plasma concentrations of these drugs and potential risk of dangerous arrhythmias	Sertraline inhibits metabolism of pimozide. The precise site of inhibition is uncertain	Avoid co-administration
HALOPERIDOL	TCAs	Possible ↑ haloperidol levels	Inhibition of CYP2D6- and CYP1A2-mediated metabolism of thioridazine	Warn patients to report ↑ side-effects of these drugs
HALOPERIDOL	VENLAFAXINE	↑ haloperidol levels	Inhibited metabolism	Avoid co-administration

Primary drug	Secondary drug	Effect	Mechanism	Precautions
ANTIPSYCHOTICS	ANTIDIABETIC DRUGS			
CLOZAPINE	ANTIDIABETIC DRUGS	May cause ↑ blood sugar and loss of control of blood sugar	Clozapine can cause resistance to the action of insulin	Watch for diabetes mellitus in patients on long-term clozapine treatment
OLANZAPINE, PHENOTHIAZINES	REPAGLINIDE	↓ hypoglycaemic effect	Antagonistic effect	Higher doses of repaglinide needed
PHENOTHIAZINES	METFORMIN	May ↑ blood sugar-lowering effect and risk of hypoglycaemic episodes. Likely to occur with doses exceeding 100 mg/day	Phenothiazines such as chlorpromazine inhibit the release of epinephrine and ↑ risk of hypoglycaemia. May inhibit the release of insulin	Chlorpromazine is nearly always used in the long term. Watch for and warn patients about symptoms of hypoglycaemia ➢ ***For signs and symptoms of hypoglycaemia, see Clinical Features of Some Adverse Drug Interactions, Hypoglycaemia***
PHENOTHIAZINES	SULPHONYLUREAS	May ↑ blood sugar-lowering effect and risk of hypoglycaemic episodes. Likely to occur with doses exceeding 100 mg/day	Phenothiazines such as chlorpromazine inhibit the release of epinephrine and ↑ risk of hypoglycaemia. May inhibit the release of insulin, which is the mechanism by which sulphonylureas act	Chlorpromazine is nearly always used in the long term. Watch for and warn patients about symptoms of hypoglycaemia ➢ ***For signs and symptoms of hypoglycaemia, see Clinical Features of Some Adverse Drug Interactions, Hypoglycaemia***
RISPERIDONE	NATEGLINIDE, REPAGLINIDE	↑ risk of hypoglycaemic episodes	Attributed to a synergistic effect	Watch for and warn patients about symptoms of hypoglycaemia ➢ ***For signs and symptoms of hypoglycaemia, see Clinical Features of Some Adverse Drug Interactions, Hypoglycaemia***
PIMOZIDE	ANTIEMETICS – APREPITANT	↑ aprepitant levels	Inhibition of metabolism	Avoid co-administration (manufacturers' recommendation)

ANTIPSYCHOTICS	**ANTIEPILEPTICS**			
ANTIPSYCHOTICS	ANTIEPILEPTICS	↓ efficacy of antiepileptics	Antipsychotics lower seizure threshold	Watch for ↑ fit frequency; warn patients of this risk when starting antipsychotics, and take suitable precautions. Consider increasing the dose of antiepileptic
ANTIPSYCHOTICS	CARBAMAZEPINE, PHENYTOIN, PHENOBARBITAL, PRIMIDONE	↓ levels of apiprazole (all), haloperidol (carbamazepine, phenobarbital), clozapine, quetiapine, sertindole (carbamazepine, phenytoin), risperidone and olanzapine (carbamazepine)	Induction of metabolism	Watch for poor response to these antipsychotics, and consider increasing the dose
OLANZAPINE	VALPROATE	Risk of bone marrow toxicity	Additive effect	Monitor FBC closely; warn patients to report sore throat, fevers, etc.
CHLORPROMAZINE	PHENOBARBITAL	↓ levels of both drugs	Induction of metabolism	Watch for poor response to these drugs, and consider increasing the dose
ANTIPSYCHOTICS	**ANTIFUNGALS ➢ *Q–T-prolonging drugs, above***			
ARIPIPRAZOLE	ITRACONAZOLE, KETOCONAZOLE	↑ aripiprazole levels	Inhibition of metabolism	↓ dose of aripiprazole
ANTIPSYCHOTICS	**ANTIHYPERTENSIVES AND HEART FAILURE DRUGS**			
ANTIPSYCHOTICS	ANTIHYPERTENSIVES AND HEART FAILURE DRUGS	↑ hypotensive effect	Dose-related ↓ BP (due to vasodilatation) is a side-effect of most antipsychotics, particularly phenothiazines	Monitor BP closely, especially during initiation of treatment. Warn patients to report symptoms of hypotension (light-headedness, dizziness on standing, etc.)

NERVOUS SYSTEM DRUGS ANTIPSYCHOTICS

NERVOUS SYSTEM DRUGS ANTIPSYCHOTICS

Primary drug	Secondary drug	Effect	Mechanism	Precautions
ANTIPSYCHOTICS	VASODILATOR ANTIHYPERTENSIVES	Risk of hyperglycaemia when diazoxide is co-administered with chlorpromazine	Additive effect; both drugs have a hyperglycaemic effect	Monitor blood glucose closely, particularly with diabetes
HALOPERIDOL	ADRENERGIC NEURONE BLOCKERS	↓ hypotensive effect	Haloperidol blocks the uptake of guanethidine into adrenergic neurones	Monitor BP at least weekly until stable
HALOPERIDOL	CENTRALLY ACTING ANTIHYPERTENSIVES	Case reports of sedation or confusion on initiating co-administration of haloperidol and methyldopa	Uncertain; possible additive effect	Watch for excess sedation when starting therapy
PHENOTHIAZINES	ADRENERGIC NEURONE BLOCKERS	Variable effect: some cases of ↑ hypotensive effect; other cases where hypotensive effects ↓ by higher doses (>100 mg) of chlorpromazine	Additive hypotensive effect. Phenothiazines cause vasodilatation; however, chlorpromazine blocks the uptake of guanethidine into adrenergic neurones	Monitor BP at least weekly until stable. Warn patients to report symptoms of hypotension (light-headedness, dizziness on standing, etc.)
ANTIPSYCHOTICS	ANTIOBESITY – SIBUTRAMINE	Risk of headache, agitation, fits	Additive effect	Avoid co-administration
ANTIPSYCHOTICS	**ANTIPARKINSON'S DRUGS**			
ANTIPSYCHOTICS	AMANTADINE	↑ extrapyramidal side-effects	Additive effects	Use with caution, avoid in patients <20 years
ANTIPSYCHOTICS	DOPAMINERGICS	↓ efficacy of dopaminergics	Antipsychotics may cause extrapyramidal side-effects, which oppose the effect of antiparkinson's drugs. The atypical antipsychotics cause less effect than the older drugs	Caution with co-administration; consider using atypical antipsychotics, and use antimuscarinic drugs if extrapyramidal symptoms occur. Manufacturers recommend avoiding co-administration of amisulpride with levodopa, and co-administration of antipsychotics with pramipexole, ropinirole and rotigotine. Clozapine can be co-administered with co-careldopa and pergolide

ANTIPSYCHOTICS	ANTIPSYCHOTICS ➢ *Q-T-prolonging drugs, above*			
CLOZAPINE	DEPOT ANTIPSYCHOTICS	Risk of prolonged bone marrow toxicity	Additive effect	Avoid co-administration
ANTIPSYCHOTICS	**ANTIVIRALS**			
ARIPIPRAZOLE	NNRTIs	↓ efficacy of aripiprazole	↑ CYP3A4-mediated metabolism of aripiprazole	Monitor patient closely, and ↑ dose of aripiprazole as necessary
PIMOZIDE	NNRTIs	Possible ↑ efficacy and ↑ adverse effects, e.g. ventricular arrhythmias of pimozide	↓ CYP3A4-mediated metabolism of pimozide	Avoid co-administration
ARIPIPRAZOLE, HALOPERIDOL, CLOZAPINE, PIMOZIDE, RISPERIDONE, SERTINDOLE	PROTEASE INHIBITORS	Possibly ↑ levels of antipsychotic	Inhibition of CYP3A4- and/or CYP2D6-mediated metabolism	Avoid co-administration of clozapine with ritonavir, and pimozide or sertindole with protease inhibitors. Use other antipsychotics with caution as ↓ dose may be required; with risperidone, watch closely for extrapyramidal side-effects and neuroepileptic malignant syndrome
OLANZAPINE	PROTEASE INHIBITORS	Possibly ↓ efficacy of olanzapine when co-ingested with ritonavir (with or without lopinavir)	Possibly ↑ metabolism via CYP1A2 and glucuronyl transferases	Monitor clinical response; ↑ dose as necessary
ANTIPSYCHOTICS	**ANXIOLYTICS AND HYPNOTICS**			
ANTIPSYCHOTICS	BZDs	Risk of excessive sedation. This effect seems to be particularly marked with clozapine	Additive effect	Warn patients and carers of this effect. Particular care should be exercised when parenteral doses are given, e.g. for emergency sedation
ANTIPSYCHOTICS	SODIUM OXYBATE	Risk CNS depression – coma, respiratory depression of	Additive depression of CNS	Avoid co-administration
CHLORPROMAZINE	ZOLPIDEM, ZOPICLONE	Risk of sedation	Additive effect; uncertain why this occurs more with chlorpromazine	Warn patients of this effect

NERVOUS SYSTEM DRUGS ANTIPSYCHOTICS

Primary drug	Secondary drug	Effect	Mechanism	Precautions
ANTIPSYCHOTICS	BETA-BLOCKERS			
ANTIPSYCHOTICS	BETA-BLOCKERS	↑ hypotensive effect	Dose-related ↓ BP (due to vasodilatation) is a side-effect of most antipsychotics, particularly phenothiazines	Monitor BP at least weekly until stable, especially during initiation of treatment. Warn patients to report symptoms of hypotension (light-headedness, dizziness on standing, etc.)
CHLORPROMAZINE, HALOPERIDOL	PROPANOLOL, TIMOLOL	↑ plasma concentrations and efficacy of both chlorpromazine and propranolol during co-administration	Propanolol and chlorpromazine mutually inhibit each other's hepatic metabolism. Haloperidol inhibits CYP2D6-mediated metabolism of propanolol and timolol	Watch for toxic effects of chlorpromazine and propranolol; ↓ doses accordingly
CLOZAPINE	CAFFEINE	↑ clozapine levels	Possibly ↑ metabolism via CYP1A2	Warn patients to avoid wide variations in caffeine intake once established on clozapine
ANTIPSYCHOTICS	CALCIUM CHANNEL BLOCKERS			
ANTIPSYCHOTICS	CALCIUM CHANNEL BLOCKERS	↑ antihypertensive effect	Dose-related ↓ BP (due to vasodilatation) is a side-effect of most antipsychotics, particularly phenothiazines	Monitor BP, especially during initiation of treatment. Warn patients to report symptoms of hypotension (light-headedness, dizziness on standing, etc.)
CLOZAPINE	CALCIUM CHANNEL BLOCKERS	Plasma concentrations of clozapine may be ↑ by diltiazem and verapamil	Diltiazem and verapamil inhibit CYP1A2-mediated metabolism of clozapine	Watch for side-effects of clozapine
SERTINDOLE	CALCIUM CHANNEL BLOCKERS	Plasma concentrations of sertindole are ↑ by diltiazem and verapamil	Diltiazem and verapamil inhibit CYP3A4-mediated metabolism of sertindole	Avoid co-administration; raised sertindole concentrations are associated with ↑ risk of prolonged Q–T interval and therefore ventricular arrhythmias, particularly torsades de pointes

CLOZAPINE, HALOPERIDOL, OLANZAPINE	CNS STIMULANTS – MODAFINIL	May cause ↓ plasma concentrations of these substrates if CYP1A2 is the predominant metabolic pathway and alternative metabolic pathways are either genetically deficient or affected	Modafinil is a moderate inducer of CYP1A2 in a concentration-dependent manner	Be aware. Patients who are using oestrogen-containing contraceptives should be warned to use alternative forms of contraception during and for at least 1 month after cessation of modafinil
PROCHLORPERAZINE	DESFERRIOXAMINE	Reports of coma when prochlorperazine is given with desferrioxamine	Uncertain	Avoid co-administration
ATYPICALS, PHENOTHIAZINES PIMOZIDE	DIURETICS – LOOP AND THIAZIDES	Risk of arrhythmias	Cardiac toxicity directly related to hypokalaemia	Monitor potassium levels every 4–6 weeks until stable, then at least annually
ANTIPSYCHOTICS	**DRUG DEPENDENCE THERAPIES**			
ANTIPSYCHOTICS	BUPROPION	↑ risk of seizures. This risk is marked in elderly people, in patients with a history of seizures, with addiction to opiates/cocaine/stimulants, and in diabetics treated with oral hypoglycaemics or insulin	Bupropion is associated with a dose-related risk of seizures. These drugs, which lower seizure threshold, are individually epileptogenic. Additive effects occur when they are combined	Extreme caution. The dose of bupropion should not exceed 450 mg/day (or 150 mg/day in patients with severe hepatic cirrhosis)
CHLORPROMAZINE, PERPHENAZINE, RISPERIDONE	BUPROPION	↑ plasma concentrations of these substrates with risk of toxic effects	Bupropion and its metabolite hydroxybupropion inhibit CYP2D6	Initiate therapy of these drugs at the lowest effective dose
CHLORPROMAZINE, CLOZAPINE, HALOPERIDOL, OLANZAPINE	BUPROPION	↑ plasma concentrations of these drugs with risk of toxic/adverse effects	Smoking induces mainly CYP1A2 and CYP2E1. Thus de-induction takes place following cessation of smoking	Be aware and watch for early features of toxicity. Consider reducing the dose
ANTIPSYCHOTICS – PIMOZIDE	GRAPEFRUIT JUICE	Possibly ↑ efficacy and ↑ adverse effects	Not evaluated	Avoid concomitant use

Primary drug	Secondary drug	Effect	Mechanism	Precautions
ANTIPSYCHOTICS – CHLORPROMAZINE, CLOZAPINE, HALOPERIDOL, OLANZAPINE, PERPHENAZINE, RISPERIDONE, SERTINDOLE, THIORIDAZINE, ZUCLOPENTHIXOL	H2 RECEPTOR BLOCKERS – CIMETIDINE	↑ plasma concentrations of these antipsychotics, with risk of associated adverse effects	Cimetidine is an inhibitor of CYP3A4 (sertindole, haloperidol, risperidone), CYP2D6 (chlorpromazine, risperidone, zuclopenthixol, thioridazine, perphenazine) and CYP1A2 (clozapine, olanzapine, sertindole, haloperidol)	Avoid concomitant use. Choose an alternative acid suppression, e.g. H2 antagonist
ANTIPSYCHOTICS	IVABRADINE	Risk of arrhythmias with pimozide and sertindole	Additive effect	Monitor ECG closely
ANTIPSYCHOTICS	**NITRATES**			
ANTIPSYCHOTICS	NITRATES	↑ hypotensive effect	Additive hypotensive effect. Aldesleukin causes ↓ vascular resistance and ↑ capillary permeability	Monitor BP at least weekly until stable. Warn patients to report symptoms of hypotension (light-headedness, dizziness on standing, etc.)
ANTIPSYCHOTICS – PHENOTHIAZINE, CLOZAPINE, PIMOZIDE	NITRATES	1. ↑ risk of antimuscarinic side-effects when isosorbide dinitrate is co-administered with these drugs. 2. ↓ efficacy of sublingual nitrate tablets	1. Additive effect; both of these drugs cause antimuscarinic side-effects 2. Antimuscarinic effects ↓ saliva production, which ↓ dissolution of the tablet	1. Warn patient of these effects 2. Consider changing the formulation to a sublingual nitrate spray
ANTIPSYCHOTICS	POTASSIUM CHANNEL ACTIVATORS	↑ hypotensive effect	Additive effect	Avoid co-administration of nicorandil with phosphodiesterase type 5 inhibitors. For other drugs, monitor BP closely
ANTIPSYCHOTICS – CLOZAPINE	PROTON PUMP INHIBITORS – OMEPRAZOLE	Possible ↓ efficacy of clozapine	↑ metabolism via CYP1A2	Clinical significance unclear; monitor more closely
HALOPERIDOL	SODIUM PHENYLBUTYRATE	Possibly ↓ efficacy of sodium phenylbutyrate	These drugs are associated with ↑ ammonia levels	Avoid co-administration

NERVOUS SYSTEM DRUGS ANTIPSYCHOTICS

SULPIRIDE	SUCRALFATE	↓ sulpiride levels	↓ absorption of sulpiride	Give sulpiride at least 2 hours after sucralfate
ANTIPSYCHOTICS	**SYMPATHOMIMETICS**			
ANTIPSYCHOTICS	SYMPATHOMIMETICS	Hypertensive effect of sympathomimetics are antagonized by antipsychotics	Dose-related ↓ BP (due to vasodilatation) is a side-effect of most antipsychotics, particularly phenothiazines	Monitor BP closely
ANTIPSYCHOTICS	INDIRECT	1. Case reports paralytic ileus with trifluoperazine and methylphenidate 2. Case report of acute dystonias with haloperidol and dexamfetamine 3. ↓ efficacy of chlorpromazine when dexamfetamine is added	1. Additive anticholinergic effect 2. Uncertain; possibly due to ↑ dopamine release 3. Uncertain	1. Watch for signs of altered bowel habit 2. Warn patients of this rare interaction 3. Avoid co-administration
ANTIPSYCHOTICS	TETRABENAZINE	Case report of extrapyramidal symptoms when tetrabenazine is given with chlorpromazine	Uncertain	Warn patients to report any extrapyramidal symptoms
ANXIOLYTICS AND HYPNOTICS				
ALL	CNS DEPRESSANTS – INCLUDING ALCOHOL	↑ sedation	Additive effect	Warn patients to be aware of this added effect
ALL	DRUGS WITH HYPOTENSIVE EFFECTS	↑ hypotensive effect	Additive hypotensive effect	Monitor BP at least weekly until stable. Warn patients to report symptoms of hypotension (light-headedness, dizziness on standing, etc.)
BARBITURATES ➢ *Antiepileptics, above*				

Primary drug	Secondary drug	Effect	Mechanism	Precautions
BENZODIAZEPINES				
BZDs	ANALGESICS			
BZDs	NSAIDs	Parenteral diclofenac may ↓ dose of midazolam needed to produce sedation	Unknown	Titrate the dose of midazolam carefully
BZDs	OPIOIDS	1. ↑ sedation with BZDs 2. Respiratory depressant effect of morphine is antagonized by lorazepam.	1. Additive effect; both drugs are sedatives 2. Uncertain	1. Closely monitor vital signs during co-administration 2. Although this effect may be considered to be beneficial, it should be borne in mind if the combination of an opioid and BZD is used for sedation for painful procedures
BZDs	ANTIBIOTICS			
DIAZEPAM	ISONIAZID	↑ diazepam levels	Inhibited metabolism	Watch for excessive sedation; consider reducing the dose of diazepam
MIDAZOLAM, TRIAZOLAM, POSSIBLY ALPRAZOLAM	MACROLIDES – ERYTHROMYCIN, CLARITHROMYCIN, TELITHROMYCIN	↑ BZD levels	Inhibition of CYP3A4-mediated metabolism	↓ dose of BZD by 50%; warn patients not to perform skilled tasks such as driving for at least 10 hours after the dose of BZD
MIDAZOLAM	QUINUPRISTIN/ DALFOPRISTIN	↑ midazolam levels	Inhibited metabolism	Watch for excessive sedation; consider reducing the dose of midazolam
BZDs, NOT LORAZEPAM, OXAZEPAM, TEMAZEPAM	RIFAMPICIN	↓ BZD levels	Induction of CYP3A4-mediated metabolism	Watch for poor response to these BZDs; consider increasing the dose, e.g. diazepam or nitrazepam 2–3-fold

NERVOUS SYSTEM DRUGS ANXIOLYTICS AND HYPNOTICS

ALPRAZOLAM, MIDAZOLAM, DIAZEPAM	ANTICANCER AND IMMUNOMODULATING DRUGS – CICLOSPORIN	Likely ↑ plasma concentrations and risk of ↑ sedation	These BZDs are metabolized primarily by CYP3A4, which is inhibited moderately by ciclosporin	Warn patients about ↑ sedation. Consider using alternative drugs, e.g. flurazepam. Warn about activities requiring attention ➢ ***For signs and symptoms of CNS depression, see Clinical Features of Some Adverse Drug Interactions, Central nervous system depression***
BZDs	**ANTIDEPRESSANTS**			
BZDs	MAOIs	Additive depression of CNS ranging from drowsiness to coma and respiratory depression	Synergistic depressant effects on CNS function	Necessary to warn patients, particularly regards activities that require attention, e.g. driving or using machinery and equipment that could cause self-harm
BZDs	MIRTAZAPINE	↑ sedation	Additive effect	Warn patients about this effect
BZDs	TCAs	Possible ↑ plasma concentrations of diazepam	Inhibition of CYP2C19-mediated metabolism of diazepam. The clinical significance of this depends upon whether diazepam's alternative pathways of metabolism are also inhibited by co-administered drugs	Watch for excessive sedation with diazepam
ALPRAZOLAM, DIAZEPAM, MIDAZOLAM	SSRIs – FLUOXETINE, FLUVOXAMINE, PAROXETINE	↑ in plasma concentrations of these BZDs. Likely ↑ sedation and interference with psychomotor activity	Alprazolam, diazepam and midazolam are subject to metabolism by CYP3A4. Fluvoxamine, fluoxetine and possibly paroxetine are inhibitors of CYP3A4; sertraline is a weak inhibitor	Warn patients about risks associated with activities that require alertness. Consider use of alternatives such as oxazepam, lorazepam and temazepam, which are metabolized by glucuronidation ➢ ***For signs and symptoms of CNS depression, see Clinical Features of Some Adverse Drug Interactions, Central nervous system depression***

Primary drug	Secondary drug	Effect	Mechanism	Precautions
CLONAZEPAM	ANTIEPILEPTICS – BARBITURATES, CARBAMAZEPINE, PHENYTOIN	↓ levels of these antiepileptics	Induction of metabolism	Watch for poor response to these antiepileptics
ALPRAZOLAM, CHLORDIAZEPOXIDE, DIAZEPAM, LORAZEPAM, MIDAZOLAM, OXAZEPAM, TEMAZEPAM	ANTIFUNGALS – ITRACONAZOLE, KETOCONAZOLE, VORICONAZOLE	↑ plasma concentrations of these BZDs with ↑ risk of adverse effects. These risks are greater following intravenous administration of midazolam compared with oral midazolam	Itraconazole and ketoconazole are potent inhibitors of phase I metabolism (oxidation and functionalization) of these BZDs by CYP3A4. In addition, the more significant ↑ in plasma concentrations following oral midazolam – 15 times compared with 5 times following intravenous use – indicates that the inhibition of P-gp by ketoconazole is important following oral administration	Aim to avoid co-administration. If co-administration is necessary, always start with ↓ dose and monitor the effects closely. Consider the use of alternative BZDs, which predominantly undergo phase II metabolism by glucuronidation, e.g. flurazepam, quazepam. Fluconazole and posaconazole are unlikely to cause this interaction
BZDs	ANTIHYPERTENSIVES AND HEART FAILURE DRUGS – CLONIDINE AND MOXONIDINE	Clonidine and moxonidine may exacerbate the sedative effects of BZDs, particularly during initiation of therapy	Uncertain	Warn patients of this effect and advise them to avoid driving or operating machinery if they suffer from sedation
BZDs	ANTIPARKINSON'S DRUGS – LEVODOPA	Risk of ↓ effect of levodopa	Uncertain	Watch for poor response to levodopa and consider increasing its dose. If severe antagonism of effect, stop the BZD
BZDs	ANTIPLATELET AGENTS – ASPIRIN	↓ requirements of midazolam when aspirin (1 g) is co-administered	Uncertain at present	Be aware of possible ↓ dose requirements for midazolam

NERVOUS SYSTEM DRUGS ANXIOLYTICS AND HYPNOTICS

BZDs	ANTIPSYCHOTICS	Risk of excessive sedation. This effect seems to be particularly marked with clozapine	Additive effect	Warn patients and carers of this effect. Particular care should be exercised when parenteral doses are given, e.g. for emergency sedation
BZDs	**ANTIVIRALS**			
DIAZEPAM, MIDAZOLAM	NNRTIs – EFAVIRENZ	↑ efficacy and ↑ adverse effects, e.g. prolonged sedation	↓ CYP3A4-mediated metabolism of diazepam and midazolam	1. Monitor more closely, especially sedation levels. May need ↓ dose of diazepam or alteration of timing of dose 2. Avoid co-administration with midazolam
BZDs	NUCLEOSIDE REVERSE TRANSCRIPTASE INHIBITORS – ZIDOVUDINE	↑ adverse effects including ↑ incidence of headaches when oxazepam is co-administered with zidovudine	Uncertain	Monitor closely
BZDs	PROTEASE INHIBITORS	↑ adverse effects, e.g. prolonged sedation	Inhibition of CYP3A4-mediated metabolism of BZDs and buspirone	Watch closely for ↑ sedation; ↓ dose of sedative as necessary. Some recommend considering substituting long-acting for shorter-acting BZDs with less active metabolites (e.g. lorazepam for diazepam)
BZDs	ANXIOLYTICS AND HYPNOTICS – SODIUM OXYBATE	Risk of CNS depression – coma, respiratory depression	Additive depression of CNS	Avoid co-administration. Caution even with relatively non-sedating antihistamines (cetrizine, desloratidine, fexofenadine, levocetirizine, loratidine, mizolastine) as they can impair the performance of skilled tasks

Primary drug	Secondary drug	Effect	Mechanism	Precautions
BZDs	**BETA-BLOCKERS**			
BZDs	BETA-BLOCKERS	↑ hypotensive effect	Additive hypotensive effect; anxiolytics and hypnotics can cause postural ↓ BP	Watch for ↓ BP. Monitor BP at least weekly until stable. Warn patients to report symptoms of hypotension (light-headedness, dizziness on standing, etc.)
DIAZEPAM	BETA-BLOCKERS	May occasionally cause ↑ sedation during metoprolol and propranolol therapy	Propranolol and metoprolol inhibit the metabolism of diazepam	Warn patients about ↑ sedation
BZDs	BRONCHODILATORS – THEOPHYLLINE	↓ therapeutic effect of BZDs	BZDs ↑ CNS concentrations of adenosine, a potent CNS depressant, while theophylline blocks adenosine receptors	Larger doses of diazepam are required to produce the desired therapeutic effects such as sedation. Discontinuation of theophylline without ↓ dose of BZD ↑ risk of sedation and of respiratory depression
BZDs	CALCIUM CHANNEL BLOCKERS – DILTIAZEM, VERAPAMIL	Plasma concentrations of midazolam and triazolam are ↑ by diltiazem and verapamil	Diltiazem and verapamil inhibit CYP3A4-mediated metabolism of midazolam and triazolam	↓ dose of BZD by 50% in patients on calcium channel blockers; warn patients not to perform skilled tasks such as driving for at least 10 hours after the dose of BZD
ALPRAZOLAM, DIAZEPAM	CARDIAC GLYCOSIDES – DIGOXIN	Alprazolam and possibly diazepam may ↑ digoxin levels, particularly in the over-65s	Uncertain at present; possibly ↓ renal excretion of digoxin	Monitor digoxin levels; watch for digoxin toxicity
BZDs	**CNS STIMULANTS**			
DIAZEPAM	MODAFINIL	May cause moderate ↑ plasma concentrations of diazepam	Modafinil is a reversible inhibitor of CYP2C19 when used in therapeutic doses	Be aware
TRIAZOLAM	MODAFINIL	May ↓ triazolam levels	Uncertain	Be aware

BZDs	DRUG DEPENDENCE THERAPIES			
BZDs	DISULFIRAM	↑ BZDs levels	Inhibited metabolism	Warn patients of risk of excessive sedation
BZDs	LOFEXIDINE	↑ sedation	Additive effect	Warn patients of risk of excessive sedation
ALPRAZOLAM, DIAZEPAM, MIDAZOLAM – ORAL	GRAPEFRUIT JUICE	Possibly ↑ efficacy and ↑ adverse effects, e.g. sedation, CNS depression	Possibly ↑ bioavailability, ↓ presystemic metabolism. Constituents of grapefruit juice irreversibly inhibit intestinal CYP3A4. Transport via P-gp and MRP-2 efflux pumps is also inhibited	Avoid concomitant use. Be particularly vigilant in elderly patients or those with impaired liver function. Consider alternative, e.g. temazepam
BZDs (NOT LORAZEPAM OR TEMAZEPAM)	H2 RECEPTOR BLOCKERS – CIMETIDINE, RANITIDINE	↑ efficacy and adverse effects of BZD, e.g. sedation	Cimetidine is an inhibitor of CYP3A4, CYP2D6, CYP2C19 and CYP1A2	Not clinically significant for most patients. Conflicting information for some BZDs. Monitor more closely, and ↓ dose if necessary
BZDs	**MUSCLE RELAXANTS**			
BZDs	BACLOFEN, TIZANIDINE	↑ hypotensive effect	Additive hypotensive effect	Monitor BP at least weekly until stable. Warn patients to report symptoms of hypotension (light-headedness, dizziness on standing, etc.)
BZDs	BACLOFEN, METHOCARBAMOL, TIZANIDINE	↑ sedation	Additive effect	Warn patients
BZDs	NITRATES	↑ hypotensive effect	Additive hypotensive effect	Monitor BP at least weekly until stable. Warn patients to report symptoms of hypotension (light-headedness, dizziness on standing, etc.)

Primary drug	Secondary drug	Effect	Mechanism	Precautions
BZDs	OESTROGENS, PROGESTERONES	Reports of breakthrough bleeding when BZDs are co-administered with oral contraceptives	Uncertain	The clinical significance is uncertain. It would seem to be wise to advise patients to use an alternative form of contraception during and for 1 month after stopping BZDs
BZDs	**PERIPHERAL VASODILATORS**			
BZDs	CILOSTAZOL	Midazolam ↑ cilostazol levels	Midazolam inhibits CYP3A4-mediated metabolism of cilastazol	Avoid co-administration
BZDs	MOXISYLYTE	↑ hypotensive effect	Additive hypotensive effect	Monitor BP at least weekly until stable. Warn patients to report symptoms of hypotension (light-headedness, dizziness on standing, etc.)
BZDs	POTASSIUM CHANNEL ACTIVATORS	↑ hypotensive effect	Additive effect	Avoid co-administration of nicorandil with phosphodiesterase type 5 inhibitors. For other drugs, monitor BP closely
BZDs	PROTON PUMP INHIBITORS – OMEPRAZOLE/ ESOMEPRAZOLE	↑ efficacy and adverse effects, e.g. prolonged sedation	Inhibition of metabolism via CYP450 (some show competitive inhibition via CYP2C19)	Monitor for ↑ side-effects, and ↓ dose as necessary. Likely to delay recovery after procedures for which BZDs have been used. Consider alternative proton pump inhibitor, e.g. lansoprazole or pantoprazole
BUSPIRONE				
BUSPIRONE	**ANTIBIOTICS**			
BUSPIRONE	MACROLIDES	↑ buspirone levels	Inhibition of CYP3A4-mediated metabolism	Warn patients to be aware of additional sedation

BUSPIRONE	RIFAMPICIN	↓ buspirone levels	Induction of CYP3A4-mediated metabolism	Watch for poor response to buspirone; consider increasing the dose
BUSPIRONE	ANTICANCER AND IMMUNOMODULATING DRUGS – PROCARBAZINE	Risk of elevation of blood pressure	Additive effect; buspirone acts at serotonin receptors; procarbazine inhibits the breakdown of sympathomimetics	Avoid concurrent use
BUSPIRONE	ANTIDEPRESSANTS – MAOIs	Cases of hypertension	Uncertain	Monitor BP closely
BUSPIRONE	ANTIFUNGALS – ITRACONAZOLE, KETOCONAZOLE	↑ buspirone levels	Inhibition of CYP3A4-mediated metabolism	Warn patients to be aware of additional sedation
BUSPIRONE	ANTIVIRALS – PROTEASE INHIBITORS	↑ adverse effects, e.g. prolonged sedation	Inhibition of CYP3A4-mediated metabolism of BZDs and buspirone	Watch closely for ↑ sedation; ↓ dose of sedative as necessary. Some recommend considering substituting long-acting for shorter-acting BZDs with less active metabolites (e.g. lorazepam for diazepam)
BUSPIRONE	ANXIOLYTICS AND HYPNOTICS – SODIUM OXYBATE	Risk of CNS depression – coma, respiratory depression	Additive depression of CNS	Avoid co-administration
BUSPIRONE	CALCIUM CHANNEL BLOCKERS	Plasma concentrations of buspirone are ↑ by diltiazem and verapamil	Diltiazem and verapamil inhibit CYP3A4-mediated metabolism of buspirone	Start buspirone at a lower dose (2.5 mg twice a day is suggested by the manufacturers) in patients on calcium channel blockers

Primary drug	Secondary drug	Effect	Mechanism	Precautions
BUSPIRONE – ORAL	GRAPEFRUIT JUICE	Possibly ↑ efficacy and ↑ adverse effects, e.g. sedation, CNS depression	Possibly ↑ bioavailability, ↓ presystemic metabolism. Constituents of grapefruit juice irreversibly inhibit intestinal CYP3A4. Transport via P-gp and MRP-2 efflux pumps is also inhibited	Avoid concomitant use. Be particularly vigilant in elderly patients or those with impaired liver function. Consider an alternative, e.g. temazepam
CHLORAL HYDRATE				
CHLORAL HYDRATE	ANTIDEPRESSANTS			
CHLORAL HYDRATE	MAOIs	Case report of fatal hyperpyrexia and cases of hypertension	Uncertain	Avoid co-administration
CHLORAL HYDRATE	SSRIs	Case of excessive drowsiness	Uncertain; possibly additive effects, possibly displacement of chloral hydrate from protein-binding sites	Warn patients to be aware of additional sedation
CHLORMETHIAZOLE				
CHLORMETHIAZOLE	H2 RECEPTOR BLOCKERS – CIMETIDINE	↑ efficacy and adverse effects, e.g. sedation, 'hangover' effect	Inhibition of metabolism	Monitor closely; ↓ dose may be required
MEPROBAMATE				
MEPROBAMATE	OESTROGENS, PROGESTERONES	Reports of breakthrough bleeding when meprobamate is co-administered with oral contraceptives	Uncertain	The clinical significance is uncertain. It would seem to be wise to advise patients to use an alternative form of contraception during and for 1 month after stopping meprobamate

SODIUM OXYBATE				
SODIUM OXYBATE	1. ALCOHOL 2. ANALGESICS – opioids 3. ANTIDEPRESSANTS – TCAs 4. ANTIEPILEPTICS – barbiturates 5. ANTIHISTAMINES 6. ANTIPSYCHOTICS 7. ANXIOLYTICS AND HYPNOTICS – BZDs, buspirone	Risk of CNS depression – coma, respiratory depression	Additive depression of CNS	Avoid co-administration. Caution even with relatively non-sedating antihistamines (cetrizine, desloratidine, fexofenadine, levocetirizine, loratidine, mizolastine) as they can impair the performance of skilled tasks
ZALEPLON, ZOLPIDEM, ZOPICLONE				
ZALEPLON, ZOLPIDEM, ZOPICLONE	ANTIBIOTICS – RIFAMPICIN	↓ levels of these hypnotics	Induction of CYP3A4-mediated metabolism	Watch for poor response to these agents
ZOLPIDEM	ANTIDEPRESSANTS – FLUOXETINE, PAROXETINE, SERTRALINE, VENLAFAXINE	Cases of agitation ± hallucinations	Uncertain	Avoid co-administration
ZALEPLON, ZOLPIDEM, ZOPICLONE	ANTIEPILEPTICS – CARBAMAZEPINE, RIFAMPICIN	↓ levels of these hypnotics	Induction of CYP3A4-mediated metabolism	Watch for poor response to these agents
ZALEPLON, ZOLPIDEM, ZOPICLONE	ANTIFUNGALS – KETOCONAZOLE	↑ zolpidem levels reported; likely to occur with zaleplon and zopiclone	Inhibition of CYP3A4-mediated metabolism	Warn patients of the risk of ↑ sedation
ZOLPIDEM, ZOPICLONE	ANTIPSYCHOTICS – CHLORPROMAZINE	Risk of sedation	Additive effect; uncertain why this occurs more with chlorpromazine	Warn patients of this effect
ZOLPIDEM	DRUG DEPENDENCE THERAPIES – BUPROPION	Cases of agitation ± hallucinations	Uncertain	Avoid co-administration

Primary drug	Secondary drug	Effect	Mechanism	Precautions
CNS STIMULANTS				
ATOMOXETINE				
ATOMOXETINE	DRUGS THAT PROLONG THE Q–T INTERVAL			
ATOMOXETINE	1. ANTIARRHYTHMICS – amiodarone, disopyramide, procainamide, propafenone 2. ANTIBIOTICS – macrolides (especially azithromycin, clarithromycin, parenteral erythromycin, telithromycin), quinolones (especially moxifloxacin), quinupristin/dalfopristin 3. ANTICANCER AND IMMUNOMODULATING DRUGS – arsenic trioxide 4. ANTIDEPRESSANTS – TCAs, venlafaxine 5. ANTIEMETICS – dolasetron 6. ANTIFUNGALS – fluconazole, posaconazole, voriconazole 7. ANTIHISTAMINES – terfenadine, hydroxyzine, mizolastine 8. ANTIMALARIALS – artemether with lumefantrine, chloroquine, hydroxychloroquine, mefloquine, quinine 9. ANTIPROTOZOALS – pentamidine isetionate 10. ANTIPSYCHOTICS – atypicals, phenothiazines, pimozide 11. BETA-BLOCKERS – sotalol 12. BRONCHODILATORS – parenteral bronchodilators	Risk of ventricular arrhythmias, particularly torsades de pointes	Additive effect; these drugs cause prolongation of the Q–T interval	Avoid co-administration

ATOMOXETINE	ANALGESICS – METHADONE, TRAMADOL	Risk of arrhythmias with methadone and possible risk of fits with tramadol	Uncertain	Avoid co-administration of atomoxetine with methadone or tramadol
ATOMOXETINE	**ANTIDEPRESSANTS**			
ATOMOXETINE	MAOIs	Risk of severe hypertensive reactions	Additive inhibition of norepinephrine reuptake	Avoid co-administration. MAOIs should not be started for at least 2 weeks after stopping atomoxetine; conversely, atomoxetine should not be started for at least 2 weeks after stopping MAOI
ATOMOXETINE	SSRIs	↑ plasma concentrations and risk of adverse effects (abdominal pain, vomiting, nausea, fatigue, irritability)	Atomoxetine is a selective norepinephrine reuptake inhibitor. ↑ plasma concentrations are due to inhibition of CYP2D6 – it is inhibited by fluoxetine and paroxetine (potent), fluvoxamine and sertraline (less potent) and escitalopram and citalopram (weak)	Avoid co-administration. The interaction is usually severe with fluoxetine and paroxetine
ATOMOXETINE	BRONCHODILATORS – SALBUTAMOL	↑ risk of arrhythmias with parenteral salbutamol	Additive effect	Avoid co-administration of atomoxetine with parenteral salbutamol
ATOMOXETINE	DRUG DEPENDENCE THERAPIES – BUPROPION	1. ↑ plasma concentrations of atomoxetine with risk of toxic effects 2. ↑ risk of seizures. This risk is marked in elderly people, in patients with a history of seizures, with addiction to opiates/cocaine/stimulants, and in diabetics treated with oral hypoglycaemics or insulin	1. Bupropion and its metabolite hydroxybupropion inhibit CYP2D6 2. Bupropion is associated with a dose-related risk of seizures. These drugs, which lower seizure threshold, are individually epileptogenic. Additive effects when combined	1. Initiate therapy of these drugs, particularly those with a narrow therapeutic index at the lowest effective dose 2. Extreme caution. The dose of bupropion should not exceed 450 mg/day (or 150 mg/day in patients with severe hepatic cirrhosis)

Primary drug	Secondary drug	Effect	Mechanism	Precautions
ATOMOXETINE	DIURETICS – LOOP AND THIAZIDES	↑ risk of arrhythmias with hypokalaemia	These diuretics may cause hypokalaemia	Monitor potassium levels closely
DEXAMFETAMINE ➢ *Cardiovascular Drugs, Sympathomimetics*				
METHYLPHENIDATE ➢ *Cardiovascular Drugs, Sympathomimetics*				
MODAFINIL				
MODAFINIL	POTENT INDUCERS OF CYP3A4			
MODAFINIL	CARBAMAZEPINE, PHENOBARBITONE, RIFAMPICIN	↓ plasma concentrations of modafinil with possibility of ↓ therapeutic effect	Induction of CYP3A4, which has a partial role in the metabolism of modafinil	Be aware
MODAFINIL	OTHER INDUCERS OF CYP3A4			
MODAFINIL	1. ANTIBIOTICS – rifabutin 2. ANTICANCER AND IMMUNOMODULATING DRUGS – corticosteroids 3. ANTIDEPRESSANTS – St John's wort 4. ANTIEPILEPTICS – phenytoin 5. ANTIDIABETIC DRUGS – pioglitazone 6. ANTIVIRALS – efavirenz, nevirapine	May ↓ modafinil levels	Induction of CYP3A4, which has a partial role in the metabolism of modafinil	Be aware
MODAFINIL	POTENT INHIBITORS OF CYP3A4			
MODAFINIL	1. ANTIBIOTICS – clarithromycin, telithromycin 2. ANTIFUNGALS – itraconazole, ketoconazole 3. ANTIVIRALS – indinavir, nelfinavir, ritonavir, saquinavir	↑ plasma concentrations of modafinil, with risk of adverse effects	Due to inhibition of CYP3A4, which has a partial role in the metabolism of modafinil	Be aware. Warn patients to report dose-related adverse effects, e.g. headache, anxiety

MODAFINIL	CYP2C19 SUBSTRATES			
MODAFINIL	1. ANALGESICS – indometacin 2. ANTIBIOTICS – chloramphenicol 3. ANTICANCER AND IMMUNO-MODULATING DRUGS – cyclophosphamide 4. ANTICOAGULANTS – warfarin 5. ANTIDEPRESSANTS – moclobemide 6. ANTIEPILEPTICS – phenobarbitone, primidone 7. ANTIMALARIALS – proguanil 8. ANTIPLATELET AGENTS – clopidogrel 9. ANTIVIRALS – nelfinavir 10. ANXIOLYTICS AND HYPNOTICS – diazepam 11. BETA-BLOCKERS – propanolol 12. MUSCLE RELAXANTS – carisoprodol 13. PROTON PUMP INHIBITORS	May cause moderate ↑ plasma concentrations of these substrates	Modafinil is a reversible inhibitor of CYP2C19 when used in therapeutic doses	Be aware
MODAFINIL	**CYP2C9 SUBSTRATES**			
MODAFINIL	1. ANALGESICS – NSAIDs 2. ANTICANCER AND IMMUNOMODULATING DRUGS – tamoxifen 3. ANTICOAGULANTS – warfarin 4. ANTIDEPRESSANTS – amitriptyline 5. ANTIDIABETIC DRUGS – nateglinide, rosiglitazone, sulphonylureas 6. LIPID-LOWERING DRUGS – fluvastatin	May cause ↑ plasma concentrations of these substrates if CYP2C9 is the predominant metabolic pathway and the alternative pathways are either genetically deficient or affected	Modafinil is a moderate inhibitor of CYP2C9	Be aware

Primary drug	Secondary drug	Effect	Mechanism	Precautions
MODAFINIL	CYP1A2 SUBSTRATES			
MODAFINIL	1. ANALGESICS – naproxen, paracetamol 2. ANAESTHETICS, LOCAL – ropivacaine 3. ANTIARRHYTHMICS – mexiletine 4. ANTIDEPRESSANTS – amitriptyline, clomipramine, fluvoxamine, imipramine 5. ANTIEMETICS – ondansetron 6. ANTIMIGRAINE DRUGS – zolmitriptan 7. ANTIPSYCHOTICS – clozapine, haloperidol, olanzapine 8. BETA-BLOCKERS – propanolol 9. BRONCHODILATORS – theophylline 10. CALCIUM CHANNEL BLOCKERS – verapamil 11. MUSCLE RELAXANTS – tizanidine 12. OESTROGENS 13. RILUZOLE	May cause ↓ plasma concentrations of these substrates if CYP1A2 is the predominant metabolic pathway and alternative metabolic pathways are either genetically deficient or affected	Modafinil is moderate inducer of CYP1A2 in a concentration-dependent manner	Be aware. Patients who are using oestrogen-containing contraceptives should be warned to use alternative forms of contraception during and for at least 1 month after cessation of modafinil
MODAFINIL	ANTICANCER AND IMMUNOMODULATING DRUGS – ciclosporin	↓ ciclosporin levels up to 50%, with risk of lack of therapeutic effect	↑ metabolism of ciclosporin. Modafinil is a moderate inducer of CYP3A4	Monitor ciclosporin levels
MODAFINIL	ANTIDEPRESSANTS – clomipramine, desipramine ➢ ***CYP1A2 substrates, CYP2C9 substrates, above***	↑ of plasma concentrations of TCAs in a subset of the population (7–10% of Caucasians) who are deficient in CYP2D6	CYP2C19 provides an ancillary pathway for the metabolism of clomipramine and desipramine. Modafinil inhibited CYP2C19 reversibly at pharmacologically relevant concentrations	↓ dose of TCAs is often necessary
MODAFINIL	ANXIOLYTICS AND HYPNOTICS – triazolam	May ↓ triazolam levels	Uncertain	Be aware
MODAFINIL	DRUG DEPENDENCE THERAPIES – Bupropion	↑ risk of seizures. This risk is marked in elderly people, in patients with a history of seizures, with addiction to opiates/cocaine/stimulants, and in diabetics treated with oral hypoglycaemics or insulin	Bupropion is associated with a dose-related risk of seizures. These drugs, which lower seizure threshold, are individually epileptogenic. Additive effects when combined	Extreme caution. The dose of bupropion should not exceed 450 mg/day (or 150 mg/day in patients with severe hepatic cirrhosis)

MODAFINIL	SYMPATHOMIMETICS – DEXAMFETAMINE, METHYLPHENIDATE	May ↓ modafinil levels	Due to delayed absorption	Be aware
DRUG DEPENDENCE THERAPIES				
BUPRENORPHINE ➢ *Analgesics, Opioids*				
BUPROPION				
BUPROPION	ALCOHOL	Rare reports of adverse neuropsychiatric events and ↓ alcohol tolerance	Uncertain	Warn patients to avoid or minimize alcohol intake during bupropion treatment
BUPROPION	ANTIDEPRESSANTS – PHENELZINE	↑ acute toxicity of bupropion	Uncertain	Be aware
BUPROPION	ANTIPARKINSON'S DRUGS – amantadine, levodopa	↑ CNS side-effects	Additive effects	Initiate therapy with bupropion at the lowest dose and ↑ gradually
BUPROPION	**INHIBITORS OF CYP2B6**			
BUPROPION	1. ANTICANCER DRUGS – thiotepa 2. ANTIDEPRESSANTS – fluoxetine, fluvoxamine, paroxetine, sertraline 3. ANTIVIRALS – efavirenz, protease inhibitors	↑ plasma concentrations of bupropion and risk of adverse effects	Inhibition of CYP2B6	Warn patients about adverse effects and use alternatives when possible. Avoid co-administration of bupropion with protease inhibitors. Co-administer efavirenz and bupropion with caution. A retrospective study showed that two patients received a combination without reported adverse effects. Potential ↑ risk of seizures

NERVOUS SYSTEM DRUGS DRUG DEPENDENCE THERAPIES

Primary drug	Secondary drug	Effect	Mechanism	Precautions
BUPROPION	**INDUCERS OF CYP2B6**			
BUPROPION	RIFAMPICIN	↓ plasma concentrations of bupropion and lack of therapeutic effect	Induction of CYP2B6	↑ dose of bupropion cautiously
BUPROPION	**DRUGS METABOLIZED BY CYP2D6**			
BUPROPION	1. ANALGESICS – celecoxib, opioids 2. ANTIARRHYTHMICS – amiodarone, flecainide, propafenone 3. ANTICANCER DRUGS – doxorubicin 4. ANTIDEPRESSANTS – duloxetine, moclobemide, SSRIs – escitalopram, fluoxetine, fluvoxamine, paroxetine, sertraline, TCAs – amitriptyline, clomipramine, desipramine, doxepin, imipramine 5. ANTIEMETICS – metoclopramide 6. ANTIHISTAMINES – chlorphenamine, clemastine, hydroxyzine 7. ANTIPSYCHOTICS – chlorpromazine, perphenazine, risperidone, thioridazine 8. BETA-BLOCKERS – metoprolol, propranolol, timolol 9. CINACALCET 10. CNS STIMULANTS – amphetamines, atomoxetine 11. H2 RECEPTOR BLOCKERS – cimetidine, ranitidine	↑ plasma concentrations of these substrates with risk of toxic effects	Bupropion and its metabolite hydroxybupropion inhibit CYP2D6	Initiate therapy of these drugs, particularly those with a narrow therapeutic index, at the lowest effective dose. Interaction is likely to be important with substrates for which CYP2D6 is considered the only metabolic pathway (e.g. hydrocodone, oxycodone, desipramine, paroxetine, chlorpheniramine, mesoridazine, alprenolol, amphetamines, atomoxetine)

BUPROPION	**DRUGS THAT LOWER THRESHOLD FOR SEIZURES**			
BUPROPION	1. ANTIBIOTICS – fluoroquinolones 2. ANTICANCER AND IMMUNO-MODULATING DRUGS – corticosteroids, interferons 3. ANTIDEPRESSANTS – TCAs 4. ANTIMALARIALS – chloroquine, mefloquine 5. ANTIPSYCHOTICS 6. BRONCHODILATORS – theophylline 7. CNS STIMULANTS 8. PARASYMPATHOMIMETICS	↑ risk of seizures. This risk is marked in elderly people, in patients with a history of seizures, with addiction to opiates/cocaine/stimulants, and in diabetics treated with oral hypoglycaemics or insulin	Bupropion is associated with a dose-related risk of seizures. These drugs, which lower seizure threshold, are individually epileptogenic. Additive effects occur when combined	Extreme caution. The dose of bupropion should not exceed 450 mg/day (or 150 mg/day in patients with severe hepatic cirrhosis)
BUPROPION	**DRUGS WHOSE METABOLISM WOULD ALTER AFTER CESSATION OF SMOKING**			
BUPROPION	1. ANTIARRHYTHMICS – flecainide, mexiletine 2. ANTICOAGULANTS – warfarin 3. ANTIDEPRESSANTS – fluvoxamine 4. ANTIPSYCHOTICS – chlorpromazine, clozapine, haloperidol, olanzapine 5. BETA-BLOCKERS – propanolol 6. BRONCHODILATORS – theophylline	↑ plasma concentrations of these drugs, with risk of toxic/adverse effects	Smoking induces mainly CYP1A2 and CYP2E1. Thus de-induction takes place following cessation of smoking	Be aware, particularly with drugs with a narrow therapeutic index. Monitor clinically and biochemically (e.g. INR, plasma theophylline levels)
BUPROPION	ANXIOLYTICS AND HYPNOTICS – ZOLPIDEM	Cases of agitation ± hallucinations	Uncertain	Avoid co-administration
BUPROPION	DRUG DEPENDENCE THERAPIES – DISULFIRAM	Risk of psychosis	Additive effects; these drugs interfere with dopamine metabolism	Caution with co-administration. Warn patients and carers to watch for early features

Primary drug	Secondary drug	Effect	Mechanism	Precautions
CLONIDINE ➢ *Cardiovascular Drugs, Antihypertensives and heart failure drugs*				
DISULFIRAM				
DISULFIRAM	ALCOHOL	Disulfiram reaction	See above	Do not co-administer. Disulfiram must not be given within 12 hours of ingestion of alcohol
DISULFIRAM	ANTIBIOTICS – METRONIDAZOLE	Report of psychosis	Additive effect; both drugs may cause neurological/psychiatric side-effects (disulfiram by inhibiting the metabolism of dopamine, metronodazole by an unknown mechanism)	Caution with co-administration. Warn patients and carers to watch for early features
DISULFIRAM	ANTICOAGULANTS – WARFARIN	↑ anticoagulant effect	Uncertain at present	Monitor INR at least weekly until stable
DISULFIRAM	ANTIEPILEPTICS – PHENYTOIN	↑ phenytoin levels	Inhibited metabolism	Monitor phenytoin levels closely
DISULFIRAM	ANTIVIRALS – PROTEASE INHIBITORS	↑ risk of disulfiram reaction with ritonavir (with or without lopinavir)	Ritonavir and lopinavir/ritonavir oral solutions contain 43% alcohol	Warn patients. Consider using capsule preparations as an alternative
DISULFIRAM	ANXIOLYTICS AND HYPNOTICS	↑ BZD levels	Inhibited metabolism	Warn patients of risk of excessive sedation
DISULFIRAM	BRONCHODILATORS – THEOPHYLLINE	↑ theophylline levels	Disulfiram ↓ theophylline clearance by inhibiting hydroxylation and demethylation	Monitor theophylline levels before, during and after co-administration
DISULFIRAM	DRUG DEPENDENCE THERAPIES – BUPROPION	Risk of psychosis	Additive effects; these drugs interfere with dopamine metabolism	Caution with co-administration. Warn patients and carers to watch for early features
DISULFIRAM	PROTON PUMP INHIBITORS – OMEPRAZOLE	Possible ↑ adverse effects of disulfiram	Accumulation of metabolites	Monitor closely for ↑ side-effects, although patients have received combinations without reported problems

DISULFIRAM	SYMPATHOMIMETICS – DEXAMFETAMINE, METHYLPHENIDATE	Risk of psychosis	Additive effects; these drugs interfere with dopamine metabolism	Caution with co-administration. Warn patients and carers to watch for early features
LOFEXIDINE				
LOFEXIDINE	ALCOHOL, BZDs, BARBITURATES	↑ sedation	Additive effect	Warn patients of risk of excessive sedation
METHADONE ➢ *Analgesics, Opioids*				
DRUGS USED TO TREAT NEUROMUSCULAR DISEASES AND MOVEMENT DISORDERS				
HALOPERIDOL ➢ *Antipsychotics, above*				
PARASYMPATHOMIMETICS				
PARASYMPATHOMIMETICS	ANTIARRHYTHMICS – PROPAFENONE	↓ efficacy of neostigmine and pyridostigmine	Uncertain; propafenone has a degree of antinicotinic action that may oppose the action of parasympathomimetic therapy for myasthenia gravis	Watch for poor response to these parasympathomimetics and ↑ dose accordingly
PARASYMPATHOMIMETICS	ANTIBIOTICS			
GALANTAMINE	ERYTHROMYCIN	↑ galantamine levels	Inhibition of CYP3A4-mediated metabolism of galantamine	Be aware; watch for ↑ side-effects from galantamine
NEOSTIGMINE, PYRIDOSTIGMINE	AMINOGLYCOSIDES, CLINDAMYCIN, COLISTIN	↓ efficacy of neostigmine and pyridostigmine	Uncertain	Watch for poor response to these parasympathomimetics and ↑ dose accordingly
PARASYMPATHOMIMETICS	ANTIDEPRESSANTS			
GALANTAMINE	PAROXETINE	↑ galantamine levels	Inhibition of CYP2D6-mediated metabolism of galantamine	Monitor PR and BP closely, watching for bradycardia and hypotension. Be aware that there is a theoretical risk with other SSRIs

NERVOUS SYSTEM DRUGS NEUROMUSCULAR AND MOVEMENT DISORDERS

Primary drug	Secondary drug	Effect	Mechanism	Precautions
PARASYMPATHOMIMETICS	LITHIUM	↓ efficacy of neostigmine and pyridostigmine	Uncertain	Watch for poor response to these parasympathomimetics and ↑ dose accordingly
GALANTAMINE	ANTIFUNGALS – KETOCONAZOLE	↑ galantamine levels	Inhibition of 3A4-mediated metabolism of galantamine	Monitor PR and BP closely, watching for bradycardia and hypotension
PARASYMPATHOMIMETICS	ANTIMALARIALS – CHLOROQUINE, QUININE	↓ efficacy of parasympathomimetics	These antimalarials occasionally cause muscle weakness, which may exacerbate the symptoms of myasthenia gravis	Watch for poor response to these parasympathomimetics and ↑ dose accordingly
PARASYMPATHOMIMETICS	ANTIMUSCARINICS	↓ efficacy of parasympathomimetics	Parasympathomimetics and antimuscarinics have opposing effects	Avoid co-administration where possible
PARASYMPATHOMIMETICS	**BETA-BLOCKERS**			
NEOSTIGMINE, PYRIDOSTIGMINE	BETA-BLOCKERS	1. Cases of bradycardia and ↓ BP when neostigmine or physostigmine is given to reverse anaesthesia. This is a potential risk with all parasympathomimetics 2. ↓ effectiveness of neostigmine and pyridostigmine in myasthenia gravis	1. Neostigmine and pyridostigmine causes an accumulation of ACh, which may cause additive bradycardia and ↓ BP 2. Beta-blockers are thought to have a depressant effect on the neuromuscular junction and thereby ↑ weakness	1. Monitor PR and BP closely when giving anticholinesterases to reverse anaesthesia to patients on beta-blockers 2. Monitor the response to neostigmine and pyridostigmine when starting beta-blockers
PILOCARPINE	BETA-BLOCKERS	↑ risk of arrhythmias	Additive bradycardia	Monitor PR and ECG closely
PARASYMPATHOMIMETICS	CARDIAC GLYCOSIDES – DIGOXIN	Cases of AV block and bradycardia have been reported when edrophonium was co-administered with digoxin	Uncertain at present	Avoid edrophonium in patients with atrial arrhythmias who are also taking digoxin

PARASYMPATHOMIMETICS	DRUG DEPENDENCE THERAPIES – BUPROPION	↑ risk of seizures. This risk is marked in elderly people, in patients with a history of seizures, with addiction to opiates/cocaine/stimulants, and in diabetics treated with oral hypoglycaemics or insulin	Bupropion is associated with a dose-related risk of seizures. These drugs, which lower seizure threshold, are individually epileptogenic. Additive effects occur when combined	Extreme caution. The dose of bupropion should not exceed 450 mg/day (or 150 mg/day in patients with severe hepatic cirrhosis)
PARASYMPATHOMIMETICS	**MUSCLE RELAXANTS**			
DONEPEZIL	SUXAMETHONIUM	Possible ↑ efficacy of suxamethonium	Suxamethonium is metabolized by cholinesterase; parasympathomimetics inhibit cholinesterase and so prolong the action of suxamethonium	Avoid co-administration. Ensure that the effects of suxamethonium have worn off before administering a parasympathomimetic to reverse non-depolarizing muscle relaxants. A careful risk–benefit analysis should be made before considering the use of suxamethonium for emergency anaesthesia in patients taking parasympathomimetics. The short half-life of edrophonium means that it can be used to diagnose suspected dual block with suxamethonium
PARASYMPATHOMIMETICS	NON-DEPOLARIZING	↓ efficacy of non-depolarizing muscle relaxants	The anticholinesterases oppose the action of non-depolarising muscle relaxants	Used therapeutically
PIRACETAM				
PIRACETAM	ANTICOAGULANTS – ORAL	Case report of bleeding associated with ↑ INR in a patient taking warfarin 1 month after starting piracetam	Uncertain. Piracetam inhibits platelet aggregation but it is uncertain whether it has any effect on other aspects of the clotting cascade	Warn patient to report easy bruising, etc. Monitor INR closely

Primary drug	Secondary drug	Effect	Mechanism	Precautions
RILUZOLE				
RILUZOLE	MODAFINIL	May cause ↓ riluzole levels if CYP1A2 is the predominant metabolic pathway and alternative metabolic pathways are either genetically deficient or affected	Modafinil is a moderate inducer of CYP1A2 in a concentration-dependent manner	Be aware
TETRABENAZINE				
TETRABENAZINE	ANTIDEPRESSANTS – MAOIs	Risk of confusion and agitation	Uncertain; although tetrabenazine depletes norepinephrine, if it started on a patient who is already taking MAOIs, it may stimulate the release of accumulated neurotransmitter. This will not be expected to occur if a patient starts MAOI while already taking tetrabenazine	Tetrabenazine may cause depression so should be used with caution in patients with depression. If necessary, consider using an alternative antidepressant or start an MAOI after tetrabenazine has been established
TETRABENAZINE	ANTIEMETICS – METOCLOPRAMIDE	Risk of extrapyramidal symptoms	Additive effect	Avoid co-administration
TETRABENAZINE	ANTIPARKINSON'S DRUGS – AMANTADINE	↓ antiparkinson's efficacy of amantadine	Tetrabenazine may cause extrapyramidal symptoms	Use with caution; avoid in patients <20 years
TETRABENAZINE	ANTIPSYCHOTICS	Case report of extrapyramidal symptoms when tetrabenazine was given with chlorpromazine	Uncertain	Warn patients to report any extrapyramidal symptoms

Part 3 ANTICANCER AND IMMUNOMODULATING DRUGS

Drugs used in the treatment of malignant disease include the following:

- *Cytotoxic agents*. These cause cell death either as a result of disruption of cell structure or function or by activation of apoptosis.
- *Hormone analogues and antagonists*. Malignancies dependent on or affected by hormones are treated with hormones or their antagonists as appropriate to slow cell division and rate of tumour growth.
- *Drugs that alter the immune system*. Alterations to the immune response are considered to promote the division of malignant cells. Drugs that act on the immune response (immunomodulators) are used to reduce the abnormal cell growth associated with tumours. They are used as disease-modifying therapies for inflammatory arthropathies, dermatological conditions such as psoriasis, inflammatory bowel disease and some forms of degenerative neurological disease.

Vaccines may be less effective, and live-attenuated vaccines should be avoided, during the use of immunosuppressants.

Irinotecan

SN-38, the major active metabolite of irinotecan formed from hepatic carboxylesterase, accounts for both the cytotoxic activity and the gastrointestinal side-effects. The metabolism of SN-38 is catalysed via CYP3A4 to a much less active metabolite – aminopentane carboxylic acid.

Methotrexate

As more than 80% of methotrexate is excreted unchanged in the kidneys, a minor decrease in renal function can have a profound effect on the renal clearance of methotrexate and lead to significant toxicity. When drugs that impair the renal clearance of methotrexate are used concurrently, it is mandatory to measure methotrexate levels.

Methotrexate inhibits folic acid, so leucovorin (folinic acid) is prescribed in adequate dosage to prevent excessive toxicity to the bone marrow, mucosae and liver.

Procarbazine

Procarbazine is a weak inhibitor of monoamine oxidase; adverse drug and food interactions can occur, for example with tyramine-containing foods and drinks.

Azathioprine

Potentially serious side-effects of azathioprine that are dose- and duration-dependent are haematological (leukopenia and thrombocytopenia) and gastrointestinal. Azathioprine is metabolized to 6-mercaptopurine, and both compounds are rapidly eliminated from blood and oxidized in red cells and liver. Activation of 6-mercaptopurine occurs via hypoxanthine–guanine phosphoribosyltransferase. 6-Mercaptopurine is inactivated by thiopurine *S*-methyltransferase and by xanthine oxidase.

Ciclosporin

Ciclosporin is a calcineurin immunosuppressant with a narrow therapeutic index that is widely used in organ transplantation and causes nephrotoxicity. Its bioavailability is highly variable and significantly dependent on multiple factors, for example:

- drug formulation;
- metabolism by CYP3A4;
- activity of the efflux pump P-gp, mainly in the intestine.

Therapeutic drug monitoring is essential with ciclosporin therapy with or without the concurrent administration of drugs with the potential to cause interactions.

Sirolimus

Sirolimus is a substrate and inhibitor of CYP3A4 with a narrow therapeutic index and is associated with cognitive impairment and nephrotoxicity. There is a synergistic effect when it is co-administered with ciclosporin, possibly because both are substrates of CYP3A4 (and thus compete at metabolic sites) and are P-gp substrates that may competitively inhibit each other at the efflux pump. There is considerable interindividual variability, with a 10-fold range in plasma concentration in renal transplant recipients when it is given at a dosage of 5 mg per day.

Tacrolimus

This is metabolized primarily by CYP3A4 (as well as being a moderate inhibitor of CYP3A4) and is a substrate for P-gp. It inhibits the UGT1A1 glucuronidation of substrates (by an uncertain mechanism).

It has a narrow therapeutic index and is associated with nephrotoxicity and cognitive impairment in overdose. There is less potential for interactions when it is administered topically.

Primary drug	Secondary drug	Effect	Mechanism	Precautions
CYTOTOXICS				
ALL				
ALL	ANTIPSYCHOTICS – CLOZAPINE	↑ risk of bone marrow toxicity	Additive effect	Avoid co-administration
ALL	CARDIAC GLYCOSIDES – DIGOXIN	Cytotoxics may ↓ levels of digoxin (by up to 50%) when digoxin is given in tablet form	Cytotoxic-induced damage to the mucosa of the intestine may ↓ absorption; this does not seem to be a problem with liquid or liquid-containing capsule formulations	Watch for poor response to digoxin; check levels if signs of ↓ effect and consider swapping to liquid digoxin or liquid-containing capsules
ALL	VACCINES – LIVE	Risk of contracting disease from the vaccine	↓ immunity	Avoid live vaccines for at least 6 months after completing chemotherapy

ANTICANCER AND IMMUNOMODULATING DRUGS CYTOTOXICS

Primary drug	Secondary drug	Effect	Mechanism	Precautions
ARSENIC TRIOXIDE				
ARSENIC TRIOXIDE	DRUGS THAT PROLONG THE Q–T INTERVAL			
ARSENIC TRIOXIDE	1. ANTIARRHYTHMICS – amiodarone, disopyramide, procainamide, propafenone 2. ANTIBIOTICS – macrolides (especially azithromycin, clarithromycin, parenteral erythromycin, telithromycin), quinolones (especially moxifloxacin), quinupristin/dalfopristin 3. ANTIDEPRESSANTS – TCAs, venlafaxine 4. ANTIEMETICS – dolasetron 5. ANTIFUNGALS – fluconazole, posaconazole, voriconazole 6. ANTIHISTAMINES – terfenadine, hydroxyzine, mizolastine 7. ANTIMALARIALS – artemether with lumefantrine, chloroquine, hydroxychloroquine, mefloquine, quinine 8. ANTIPROTOZOALS – pentamidine isetionate 9. ANTIPSYCHOTICS – atypicals, phenothiazines, pimozide 10. BETA-BLOCKERS – sotalol 11. BRONCHODILATORS – parenteral bronchodilators 12. CNS STIMULANTS – atomoxetine	Risk of ventricular arrhythmias, particularly torsades de pointes	Additive effect; these drugs cause prolongation of the Q–T interval	Avoid co-administration

BEXAROTENE				
BEXAROTENE	GRAPEFRUIT JUICE	Possibly ↑ efficacy and ↑ adverse effects	Possibly via inhibition of intestinal CYP3A4	Clinical significance unknown. Monitor more closely
BEXAROTENE	LIPID-LOWERING DRUGS – GEMFIBROZIL	Gemfibrozil may ↑ bexarotene levels	Uncertain at present	Avoid co-administration
BLEOMYCIN				
BLEOMYCIN	ANTICANCER AND IMMUNOMODULATING DRUGS – CISPLATIN	↑ bleomycin levels, with risk of pulmonary toxicity	Elimination of bleomycin is delayed by cisplatin due to ↓ glomerular filtration. This is most likely with accumulated doses of cisplatin in excess of 300 mg/m^2	Monitor renal function and adjust dose of bleomycin as per creatinine clearance. Monitor clinically, radiologically and with lung function tests for pulmonary toxicity
BORTEZOMIB				
BORTEZOMIB	ANTIDIABETIC DRUGS – CHLORPROPAMIDE	Likely to ↑ hypoglycaemic effect of chlorpropamide	Unknown	Watch for and warn patients about symptoms of hypoglycaemia ➢ ***For signs and symptoms of hypoglycaemia, see Clinical Features of Some Adverse Drug Interactions, Hypoglycaemia***
BUSULFAN				
BUSULFAN	ANALGESICS – PARACETAMOL	Busulfan levels may be ↑ by co-administration of paracetamol	Uncertain; paracetamol probably inhibits metabolism of busulfan	Manufacturers recommend that paracetamol should be avoided for 3 days before administering parenteral busulfan
BUSULFAN	ANTIBIOTICS			
BUSULFAN	MACROLIDES – CLARITHROMYCIN, ERYTHROMYCIN, TELITHROMYCIN	↑ plasma concentrations of busulfan and ↑ risk of toxicity of busulfan such as veno-occlusive disease and pulmonary fibrosis	Busulfan clearance may be ↓ by 25%, and the AUC of busulfan may ↑ by 1500 μmol/L	Monitor clinically for veno-occlusive disease and pulmonary toxicity in transplant patients. Monitor busulfan blood levels as AUC below 1500 μmol/L per minute tends to prevent toxicity

Primary drug	Secondary drug	Effect	Mechanism	Precautions
BUSULFAN	METRONIDAZOLE	↑ busulfan levels	Uncertain	Watch for early features of toxicity
BUSULFAN	**ANTICANCER AND IMMUNOMODULATING DRUGS**			
BUSULFAN	CYCLOPHOSPHAMIDE	↑ incidence of veno-occlusive disease and mucositis when cyclophosphamide is given <24 hours after the last dose of busulfan. Possibly also ↓ effect of cyclophosphamide	There is ↓ clearance and ↑ elimination half-life of cyclophosphamide, and ↑ concentrations of the active metabolite 4-hydroxycyclophosphamide	Administer cyclophosphamide at least 24 hours after the last dose of busulfan
BUSULFAN	TIOGUANINE	↑ risk of nodular regenerative hyperplasia of the liver, oesophageal varices and portal hypertension	Mechanism uncertain	Monitor liver function and for clinical and biochemical indices of liver toxicity (e.g. ascites, splenomegaly). Ask patients to report any symptoms suggestive of oesophageal bleeding
BUSULFAN	ANTIEPILEPTICS – FOSPHENYTOIN, PHENYTOIN	↓ plasma concentrations of busulfan (by approximately 15%)	Due to induction of glutathione *S*-transferase by fosphenytoin	Be aware. Clinical significance may be minimal
BUSULFAN	ANTIFUNGALS – ITRACONAZOLE	↑ busulfan levels, with risk of toxicity of busulfan, e.g. veno-occlusive disease and pulmonary fibrosis	Itraconazole is a potent inhibitor of CYP3A4. Busulfan clearance may be ↓ by 25%, and the AUC of busulfan may ↑ by 1500 μmol/L	Monitor clinically for veno-occlusive disease and pulmonary toxicity in transplant patients. Monitor busulfan blood levels as AUC below 1500 μmol/L per minute tends to prevent toxicity
BUSULFAN	CALCIUM CHANNEL BLOCKERS	↑ busulfan levels, with risk of toxicity of busulfan, e.g. veno-occlusive disease and pulmonary fibrosis, when co-administered with diltiazem, nifedipine or verapamil	Due to inhibition of CYP3A4-mediated metabolism of busulfan by these calcium channel blockers. Busulfan clearance may be ↓ by 25%, and the AUC of busulfan may ↑ by 1500 μmol/L	Monitor clinically for veno-occlusive disease and pulmonary toxicity in transplant patients. Monitor busulfan blood levels as AUC below 1500 μmol/L per minute tends to prevent toxicity

BUSULFAN	H2 RECEPTOR BLOCKERS – CIMETIDINE	↑ adverse effects of alkylating agent, e.g. myelosuppression	Additive toxicity	Monitor more closely; monitor FBC regularly
CAPECITABINE				
Capecitabine is metabolized to fluorouracil ➢ ***Flurorouracil/capecitabine, below***				
CARBOPLATIN ➢ ***Platinum compounds, below***				
CARMUSTINE				
CARMUSTINE	ANTICANCER AND IMMUNOMODULATING DRUGS – ETOPOSIDE (HIGH DOSE)	↑ risk of liver toxicity, which usually occurs after 1–2 months after initiating treatment without an improvement in tumour response	Possible additive hepatotoxic effects	Avoid co-administration
CARMUSTINE	ANTIEPILEPTICS - PHENOBARBITAL	↓ plasma concentrations of carmustine and ↓ anti-tumour effect in animal experiments	Attributed to induction of liver metabolizing enzymes of carmustine by phenobarbitone, particularly with long-term therapy	Avoid concurrent use. As this study did not show any interaction with phenytoin, phenytoin may be a suitable alternative antiepileptic
CARMUSTINE	H2 RECEPTOR BLOCKERS – CIMETIDINE	↑ adverse effects of alkylating agent, e.g. myelosuppression	Additive toxicity	Monitor more closely; monitor FBC regularly
CHLORAMBUCIL				
CHLORAMBUCIL	AZATHIOPRINE	↑ risk of myelosuppression and immunosuppression. Deaths have occurred following profound myelosuppression and severe sepsis	Additive myelotoxic effects Azathioprine is metabolized to 6-mercatopurine in vivo, which results in additive myelosuppression, immunosuppression and hepatotoxicity	Avoid co-administration
CHLORAMBUCIL	H2 RECEPTOR BLOCKERS – CIMETIDINE	↑ adverse effects of alkylating agent, e.g. myelosuppression	Additive toxicity	Monitor more closely; monitor FBC regularly

Primary drug	Secondary drug	Effect	Mechanism	Precautions
CISPLATIN ➢ *Platinum compounds, below*				
CRISANTASPASE (ASPARAGINASE)				
CRISANTASPASE	ANTICANCER AND IMMUNOMODULATING DRUGS			
CRISANTASPASE	METHOTREXATE	Administration prior to or concurrently may ↓ efficacy of methotrexate	Crisantaspase inhibits protein synthesis and prevents cell entry to S phase, which leads to ↓ efficacy of methotrexate	Administer crisantaspase shortly after methotrexate or 9–10 days before methotrexate
CRISANTASPASE	VINCRISTINE	↑ risk of neurotoxicity if concurrently administered or if crisantaspase is administered prior to vincristine	Uncertain but has been attributed by some to effects of crisantaspase on the metabolism of vincristine	Administer vincristine prior to crisantaspase
CYCLOPHOSPHAMIDE				
CYCLOPHOSPHAMIDE	ANTICANCER AND IMMUNOMODULATING DRUGS			
CYCLOPHOSPHAMIDE	AZATHIOPRINE	↑ risk of myelosuppression and immunosuppression. Deaths have occurred following profound myelosuppression and severe sepsis	Additive myelotoxic effects. Azathioprine is metabolized to 6-mercatopurine in vivo, which results in additive myelosuppression, immunosuppression and hepatotoxicity	Avoid co-administration
CYCLOPHOSPHAMIDE	BUSULFAN	↑ incidence of veno-occlusive disease and mucositis when cyclophosphamide is given <24 hours after the last dose of busulfan. Possibly also ↓ effect of cyclophosphamide	There is ↓ clearance and ↑ elimination half-life of cyclophosphamide, and ↑ concentrations of the active metabolite 4-hydroxycyclophosphamide	Administer cyclophosphamide at least 24 hours after the last dose of busulfan

CYCLOPHOSPHAMIDE	PACLITAXEL	↑ risk of neutropenia, thrombocytopenia and mucositis when paclitaxel is infused over 24 or 72 hours prior to cyclophosphamide	Mechanism is uncertain	Administer cyclophosphamide first and then follow with paclitaxel
CYCLOPHOSPHAMIDE	PENTOSTATIN	↑ risk of potentially fatal cardiac toxicity	Attributed to interference of adenosine metabolism by cyclophosphamide	Avoid co-administration
CYCLOPHOSPHAMIDE	TRASTUZUMAB	↑ risk of cardiac toxicity	Possibly additive cardiac toxic effect	Closely monitor cardiac function – clinically and electrocardiographically
CYCLOPHOSPHAMIDE	ANTICOAGULANTS – ORAL	Episodes of ↑ anticoagulant effect	Not understood but likely to be multifactorial	Monitor INR at least weekly until stable during administration of chemotherapy
CYCLOPHOSPHAMIDE	ANTIDIABETIC DRUGS – GLIPIZIDE	Blood sugar levels may be ↑ or ↓	Uncertain	Need to monitor blood glucose in patients with concomitant treatment at the beginning of treatment and after 1–2 weeks
CYCLOPHOSPHAMIDE	ANTIGOUT DRUGS – ALLOPURINOL	↑ risk of bone marrow suppression	Uncertain but allopurinol seems to ↑ cyclophosphamide levels	Monitor FBC closely
CYCLOPHOSPHAMIDE	CNS STIMULANTS – MODAFINIL	May cause moderate ↑ in plasma concentrations of cyclophosphamide	Modafinil is a reversible inhibitor of CYP2C19 when used in therapeutic doses	Be aware
CYCLOPHOSPHAMIDE	H2 RECEPTOR BLOCKERS – CIMETIDINE	↑ adverse effects of alkylating agent, e.g. myelosuppression	1. Additive toxicity 2. Possible minor inhibition of cyclophosphamide metabolism via CYP2C9	Avoid co-administration of cimetidine with cyclophosphamide

Primary drug	Secondary drug	Effect	Mechanism	Precautions
CYTARABINE				
CYTARABINE	ANTICANCER AND IMMUNOMODULATING DRUGS			
CYTARABINE	AZATHIOPRINE	↑ risk of myelosuppression and immunosuppression. Deaths have occurred following profound myelosuppression and severe sepsis	Additive myelotoxic effects. Azathioprine is metabolized to 6-mercatopurine in vivo, which results in additive myelosuppression, immunosuppression and hepatotoxicity	Avoid co-administration
CYTARABINE	FLUDARABINE	↑ efficacy of cytarabine	Uncertain	Watch for early features of toxicity of cytarabine
CYTARABINE	ANTIFUNGALS – FLUCYTOSINE	↓ flucytosine levels	Uncertain	Watch for poor response to flucytosine
DACARBAZINE				
DACARBAZINE	IL-2	↓ efficacy of dacarbazine	↓ AUC of dacarbazine due to ↓ volume of distribution	The clinical significance is uncertain as both drugs are used in the treatment of melanoma. It may be necessary to monitor clinically and by other appropriate measures of clinical response
DACTINOMYCIN (ACTINOMYCIN D)				
DACTINOMYCIN	AZATHIOPRINE	↑ risk of myelosuppression and immunosuppression. Deaths have occurred following profound myelosuppression and severe sepsis	Additive myelotoxic effects. Azathioprine is metabolized to 6-mercatopurine in vivo, which results in additive myelosuppression, immunosuppression and hepatotoxicity	Avoid co-administration

DASATINIB				
DASATINIB	ANTIBIOTICS – RIFAMPICIN	↓ dasatinib levels	Rifampicin ↑ metabolism of dasatinib	Avoid co-administration
DASATINIB	H2 RECEPTOR BLOCKERS – FAMOTIDINE	Possible ↓ dasatinib levels	Famotidine ↑ metabolism of dasatinib	Consider using alternative acid-suppression therapy
DASATINIB	LIPID-LOWERING DRUGS – SIMVASTATIN	Possible ↓ simvastatin levels	↑ metabolism of simvastatin	Monitor lipid profile closely and adjust simvastatin dose accordingly when starting and stopping co-administration
DAUNORUBICIN				
DAUNORUBICIN	ANTICANCER AND IMMUNOMODULATING DRUGS			
DAUNORUBICIN	AZATHIOPRINE	↑ risk of myelosuppression and immunosuppression. Deaths have occurred following profound myelosuppression and severe sepsis	Additive myelotoxic effects. Azathioprine is metabolized to 6-mercatopurine in vivo, which results in additive myelosuppression, immunosuppression and hepatotoxicity	Avoid co-administration
DAUNORUBICIN	TRASTUZUMAB	↑ risk of cardiac toxicity	Possibly additive cardiac toxic effect	Closely monitor cardiac function – clinically and electrocardiographically.
DOCETAXEL				
DOCETAXEL	ANTIBIOTICS – ERYTHROMYCIN	↑ docetaxel levels	Inhibition of CYP3A4-mediated metabolism of docetaxel is metabolized by enzymes that are moderately inhibited by erythromycin, leading to ↑ levels and possible toxicity	Cautious use, or consider use of azithromycin, which has little effect on CYP3A4 and is therefore not expected to interact with docetaxel

Primary drug	Secondary drug	Effect	Mechanism	Precautions
DOCETAXEL	ANTICANCER AND IMMUNOMODULATING DRUGS			
DOCETAXEL	AZATHIOPRINE	↑ risk of myelosuppression, immunosuppression. Deaths have occurred following profound myelosuppression and severe sepsis	Additive myelotoxic effects. Azathioprine is metabolized to 6-mercatopurine in vivo, which results in additive myelosuppression, immunosuppression and hepatotoxicity	Avoid co-administration
DOCETAXEL	CICLOSPORIN	↑ plasma concentrations of these drugs, with risk of toxic effects	Competitive inhibition of CYP3A4-mediated metabolism and P-gp transport of these drugs	Watch for toxic effects of these drugs
DOCETAXEL	CISPLATIN	↑ docetaxel levels with ↑ risk of profound myelosuppression. Concurrent use also leads to ↑ risk of neurotoxicity	↓ clearance of docetaxel when docetaxel is administered after cisplatin	Administer docetaxel first and follow it with cisplatin
DOCETAXEL	DOXORUBICIN	↑ plasma concentrations of docetaxel (↑ AUC by 50–70%) with ↑ efficacy and also ↑ risk of toxicity, particularly when docetaxel is administered after doxorubicin, compared with administration of docetaxel alone	Uncertain; possibly due to interference with hepatic microsomal enzymes	Monitor closely for ↑ incidence of bone marrow suppression, neurotoxicity, myalgia and fatigue
DOCETAXEL	TOPOTECAN	↑ risk of neutropenia when topotecan is administered on days 1–4 and docetaxel on day 4	Attributed to ↓ clearance of docetaxel (by 50%) due to inhibition of hepatic metabolism of docetaxel by CYP3A4 by topotecan	Administer docetaxel on day 1 and topotecan on days 1–4

DOCETAXEL	VINORELBINE	Administration of docetaxel after vinorelbine ↑ plasma concentrations of vinorelbine, along with ↑ risk of neutropenia compared with giving docetaxel first	Docetaxel likely causes ↓ clearance of vinorelbine	Administer docetaxel first and follow it with vinorelbine
DOCETAXEL	ANTIVIRALS – PROTEASE INHIBITORS	↑ risk of adverse effects of docetaxel	Inhibition of CYP3A4-mediated metabolism. Also inhibition of P-gp efflux of vinblastine	Use with caution. Additional monitoring required. Monitor FBC weekly
DOXORUBICIN				
DOXORUBICIN	**CYP3A4 INHIBITORS**			
DOXORUBICIN	1. ANTIBIOTICS – clarithromycin, erythromycin 2. ANTICANCER AND IMMUNOMODULATING DRUGS – imatinib mesylate 3. ANTIFUNGALS – fluconazole, itraconazole, ketoconazole, voriconazole 4. ANTIVIRALS – efavirenz, ritonavir 5. H2 RECEPTOR BLOCKERS – cimetidine 6. GRAPEFRUIT JUICE	↑ risk of myelosuppression due to ↑ plasma concentrations	Due to ↓ metabolism of doxorubicin by CYP3A4 isoenzymes owing to an inhibition of those enzymes	Monitor for ↑ myelosuppression, peripheral neuropathy, myalgias and fatigue
DOXORUBICIN	**ANTICANCER AND IMMUNOMODULATING DRUGS**			
DOXORUBICIN	AZATHIOPRINE	↑ risk of myelosuppression and immunosuppression. Deaths have occurred following profound myelosuppression and severe sepsis.	Additive myelotoxic effects. Azathioprine is metabolized to 6-mercatopurine in vivo, which results in additive myelosuppression, immunosuppression and hepatotoxicity	Avoid co-administration

Primary drug	Secondary drug	Effect	Mechanism	Precautions
DOXORUBICIN	CICLOSPORIN	High doses of ciclosporin ↑ AUC of doxorubicin by 48% and of a metabolite by 443%. Risk of severe myelosuppression and neurotoxicity	Ciclosporin inhibits P-gp and selectively inhibits cytochrome P450 isoenzymes, which results in ↓ clearance of doxorubicin	Advise patients to report symptoms such as sore throat, fever, bleeding and bruising (i.e. of myelosuppression) and confusion, headache, coma and seizures (i.e. of neurotoxicity). ↓ dosage of doxorubicin is often necessary
DOXORUBICIN	DOCETAXEL	↑ plasma concentrations of docetaxel (↑ AUC by 50–70%) with ↑ efficacy and also ↑ risk of toxicity, particularly when docetaxel is administered after doxorubicin, compared with administration of docetaxel alone	Uncertain, possibly due to interference with hepatic microsomal enzymes	Monitor closely for ↑ incidence of bone marrow suppression, neurotoxicity, myalgia and fatigue
DOXORUBICIN	MERCAPTOPURINE	↑ risk of hepatotoxicity due to mercaptopurine	Uncertain, possibly due to previous treatment with mercaptopurine	Avoid co-administration – except in clinical trials
DOXORUBICIN	PACLITAXEL	↑ risk of neutropenia, stomatitis and cardiomyopathy due to ↑ plasma concentrations of doxorubicin	↑ risk of neutropenia, stomatitis and cardiomyopathy due to ↑ plasma concentrations of doxorubicin when paclitaxel is given before doxorubicin	Doxorubicin should be administered prior to paclitaxel. The cumulative dose of doxorubicin should be limited to 360 mg/m^2 when concurrently administered with paclitaxel
DOXORUBICIN	SORAFENIB	Possible ↓ doxorubicin levels	Uncertain	Watch for poor response to doxorubicin
DOXORUBICIN	THALIDOMIDE	↑ risk (up to sixfold) of deep venous thrombosis in patients with multiple myeloma compared with those treated without doxorubicin	Uncertain. Attributed to doxorubicin contributing to the thrombogenic activity	Avoid co-administration – except in clinical trials

DOXORUBICIN	TRASTUZUMAB	When used in combination, the risk of cardiotoxicity due to trastuzumab is ↑ over fourfold	Due to additive cardiotoxic effects	Avoid co-administration – except in clinical trials
DOXORUBICIN	ANTICOAGULANTS – ORAL	Episodes of ↑ anticoagulant effect	Not understood but likely to be multifactorial	Monitor INR at least weekly until stable during administration of chemotherapy.
DOXORUBICIN	ANTIEPILEPTICS – BARBITURATES	↓ doxorubicin levels	Induction of hepatic metabolism	Monitor for ↓ efficacy of doxorubicin
DOXORUBICIN	ANTIVIRALS – ZIDOVUDINE	↑ adverse effects when doxorubicin is co-administered with zidovudine	Additive toxicity	Monitor FBC and renal function closely. ↓ doses as necessary
DOXORUBICIN	CALCIUM CHANNEL BLOCKERS	↑ serum concentrations and efficacy of doxorubicin when co-administered with verapamil, nicardipine and possibly diltiazem and nifedipine; however, no cases of doxorubicin toxicity have been reported	Uncertain; however, verapamil is known to inhibit intestinal P-gp, which may ↑ bioavailability of doxorubicin	Watch for symptoms/signs of toxicity (tachycardia, heart failure and hand–foot syndrome)
DOXORUBICIN	DRUG DEPENDENCE THERAPIES – BUPROPION	↑ plasma concentrations doxorubicin, with risk of toxic effects	Bupropion and its metabolite hydroxybupropion inhibit CYP2D6	Initiate therapy with doxorubicin at the lowest effective dose
EPIRUBICIN				
EPIRUBICIN	ANTICANCER AND IMMUNOMODULATING DRUGS – PACLITAXEL	↑ plasma concentrations of epirubicin (↑ AUC by 37% and ↓ clearance by 25%), particularly following sequential administration of paclitaxel followed by epirubicin	Attributed to altered distribution of epirubicin in the plasma and inhibition of P-gp by Cremophor, the vehicle of paclitaxel formulation, resulting in ↓ clearance	Epirubicin should always be given prior to paclitaxel

Primary drug	Secondary drug	Effect	Mechanism	Precautions
EPIRUBICIN	CALCIUM CHANNEL BLOCKERS	Cases of ↑ bone marrow suppression when verapamil added to epirubicin	Uncertain at present	Monitor FBC closely
EPIRUBICIN	H2 RECEPTOR BLOCKERS – CIMETIDINE	↑ epirubicin levels, with risk of toxicity	Attributed to inhibition of hepatic metabolism of epirubicin by cimetidine	Avoid concurrent treatment and consider using an alternative H2 receptor blocker, e.g. ranitidine, famotidine
ERLOTINIB				
ERLOTINIB	ANALGESICS – NSAIDs	Risk of gastrointestinal bleeding	Additive effect	Avoid co-administration
ERLOTINIB	ANTIBIOTICS – RIFAMPICIN	↓ erlotinib levels	Rifampicin ↑ metabolism of erlotinib	Avoid co-administration
ERLOTINIB	ANTICOAGULANTS – ORAL	Episodes of ↑ anticoagulant effect	Not understood but likely to be multifactorial	Monitor INR at least weekly until stable during administration of chemotherapy
ERLOTINIB	ANTIFUNGALS – FLUCONAZOLE, ITRACONAZOLE, KETOCONAZOLE VORICONAZOLE	↑ erlotinib levels	↓ metabolism of erlotinib	Avoid co-administration
ESTRAMUSTINE				
ESTRAMUSTINE	CALCIUM AND DAIRY PRODUCTS	↓ plasma concentrations of estramustine and risk of poor therapeutic response	Due to ↓ absorption of estramustine owing to the formation of a calcium–phosphate complex	Administer estramustine 1 hour before or 2 hours after dairy products or calcium supplements
ESTRAMUSTINE	H2 RECEPTOR BLOCKERS – CIMETIDINE	↑ adverse effects of alkylating agent, e.g. myelosuppression	Additive toxicity	Monitor more closely; monitor FBC regularly

ETOPOSIDE				
ETOPOSIDE	ANTICANCER AND IMMUNOMODULATING DRUGS			
ETOPOSIDE	AZATHIOPRINE	↑ risk of myelosuppression and immunosuppression. Deaths have occurred following profound myelosuppression and severe sepsis	Additive myelotoxic effects. Azathioprine is metabolized to 6-mercatopurine in vivo, which results in additive myelosuppression, immunosuppression and hepatotoxicity	Avoid co-administration
ETOPOSIDE (HIGH DOSE)	CARMUSTINE	↑ risk of liver toxicity, which usually occurs after 1–2 months after initiating treatment without an improvement in tumour response	Possible additive hepatotoxic effects	Avoid co-administration
ETOPOSIDE	CICLOSPORIN	↑ plasma concentrations of these drugs, with risk of toxic effects	Competitive inhibition of CYP3A4-mediated metabolism and P-gp transport of these drugs	Watch for toxic effects of these drugs
ETOPOSIDE	ANTICOAGULANTS – ORAL	Episodes of ↑ anticoagulant effect	Not understood but likely to be multifactorial	Monitor INR at least weekly until stable during administration of chemotherapy
ETOPOSIDE	ANTIEPILEPTICS – PHENYTOIN, PHENOBARBITAL	Significantly ↓ plasma concentrations of etoposide (clearance may be >170%) and considerable risk of loss of therapeutic efficacy	Due to potent induction of the hepatic microsomal enzymes that metabolize etoposide	Do not co-administer. Consider use of alternative antiepileptics that do not induce hepatic microsomal enzymes, e.g. valproic acid
ETOPOSIDE	CALCIUM CHANNEL BLOCKERS	↑ serum concentrations and risk of toxicity when verapamil is given to patients on etoposide	Verapamil inhibits CYP3A4-mediated metabolism of etoposide	Watch for symptoms/signs of toxicity (nausea, vomiting, bone marrow suppression) in patients taking calcium channel blockers

Primary drug	Secondary drug	Effect	Mechanism	Precautions
ETOPOSIDE	GRAPEFRUIT JUICE	Possibly ↓ efficacy	↓ bioavailability; unclear	Interindividual variability is considerable. Monitor more closely
FLUDARABINE				
FLUDARABINE	**ANTICANCER AND IMMUNOMODULATING DRUGS**			
FLUDARABINE	CYTARABINE	↑ efficacy of cytarabine	Uncertain	Watch for early features of toxicity of cytarabine
FLUDARABINE	PENTOSTATIN	Risk of severe and potentially fatal pulmonary toxicity	Uncertain	Avoid co-administration
FLUDARABINE	ANTIPLATELET AGENTS – DIPYRIDAMOLE	Possible ↓ efficacy of fludarabine	Uncertain	Consider using an alternative antiplatelet drug
FLUOROURACIL/CAPECITABINE/TEGAFUR				
FLUOROURACIL	ANTIBIOTICS – METRONIDAZOLE	↑ risk of toxic effects of fluorouracil (>27%), e.g. bone marrow suppression, oral ulceration, nausea and vomiting due to ↑ plasma concentrations of fluorouracil	Metronidazole ↓ clearance of fluorouracil	Avoid co-administration
FLUOROURACIL	**ANTICANCER AND IMMUNOMODULATING DRUGS**			
FLUOROURACIL	**CYTOTOXICS**			
FLUOROURACIL	HYDROXYCARBAMIDE (HYDROXYUREA)	↑ incidence of neurotoxicity (>20%)	Attributed to failure of conversion of fluorouracil to the active metabolite and an accumulation of neurotoxins	Avoid co-administration
FLUOROURACIL	FOLINATE – CALCIUM FOLINATE, CALCIUM LEVOFOLINATE	Likely ↑ toxicity of leucovorin despite ↑ cytotoxic effects	↑ cytotoxicity is attributed to maximized binding in the thymidylate synthase–fluorouracil complex (fluorouracil is thought to exert its cytotoxic effect by inhibiting thymidylate synthase, which in turn inhibits DNA synthesis)	Commonly used together for cytotoxic effects, but advise patients to report symptoms of hypersensitivity reactions (itching, wheezing) and fever

FLUOROURACIL	METHOTREXATE	↓ cytotoxic effect of methotrexate when fluorouracil is administered prior to methotrexate	Fluorouracil prevents the conversion of ↓ folates to dihydrofolate	Always administer methotrexate prior to fluorouracil
FLUOROURACIL (TOPICAL AND ORAL)	PORFIMER	↑ risk of photosensitivity reactions	Attributed to additive effects	Avoid exposure of skin and eyes to direct sunlight for 30 days after porfimer therapy
FLUOROURACIL	TEMOPORFIN	↑ risk of photosensitivity with topical fluorouracil	Uncertain; possibly additive effect (topical fluorouracil can cause local irritation, while temoporfin is a photosensitizer)	Patients on temoporfin are advised to avoid direct sunlight for at least 15 days
FLUOROURACIL	**IMMUNOMODULATING DRUGS**			
FLUOROURACIL	AZATHIOPRINE	↑ risk of myelosuppression and immunosuppression. Deaths have occurred following profound myelosuppression and severe sepsis	Additive myelotoxic effects. Azathioprine is metabolized to 6-mercatopurine in vivo, which results in additive myelosuppression, immunosuppression and hepatotoxicity	Avoid co-administration
FLUOROURACIL	THALIDOMIDE	↑ risk of thromboembolism	Mechanism is uncertain; the endothelial damaging effect of fluorouracil may possibly initiate thalidomide-mediated thrombosis	Avoid co-administration
FLUOROURACIL (continuous infusion but not bolus doses)	ANTICOAGULANTS – ORAL	Episodes of ↑ anticoagulant effect	Not understood but likely to be multifactorial	Monitor INR at least weekly until stable during administration of chemotherapy

Primary drug	Secondary drug	Effect	Mechanism	Precautions
FLUOROURACIL	ANTIDEPRESSANTS – TCAs	Possible ↑ fluorouracil levels	Inhibition of CYP2C9-mediated metabolism. The clinical significance of this depends upon whether alternative pathways of metabolism are also inhibited by co-administered drugs	Warn patients to report ↑ side-effects and monitor blood count carefully
CAPECITABINE	ANTIGOUT DRUGS – ALLOPURINOL	Possible ↓ efficacy of capecitabine	Capecitabine is a prodrug for fluorouracil; it is uncertain at which point allopurinol acts on the metabolic pathway	Manufacturers recommend avoiding co-administration
FLUOROURACIL	ANTIPROTOZOALS – LEVAMISOLE	↑ risk of hepatotoxicity and neurotoxicity despite ↑ cytotoxic effects	Antiphosphatase activity of levamisole may ↑ fluorouracil cytotoxicity	This combination has been used successfully in the treatment of colon cancer. Monitor FBC and LFTs regularly. Advise patients to report symptoms such as diarrhoea, numbness and tingling, and peeling of the skin of the hands and feet (hand–foot syndrome)
FLUOROURACIL	COLONY-STIMULATING FACTORS – FILGRASTIM	Possible ↑ risk of neutropenia	Uncertain	Monitor FBC regularly
FLUOROURACIL	FOLIC ACID	Risk of fluorouracil toxicity	Folic acid exacerbates the inhibitory effect of fluorouracil on DNA	Avoid co-administration
FLUOROURACIL	H2 RECEPTOR BLOCKERS – CIMETIDINE	Altered efficacy of fluorouracil	Inhibition of metabolism and altered action	Monitor more closely. May be of clinical benefit. No additional toxicity was noted in one study

FOLINATE				
FOLINATE – CALCIUM FOLINATE, CALCIUM LEVOFOLINATE	FLUOROURACIL	Likely ↑ toxicity of leucovorin despite ↑ cytotoxic effects	↑ cytotoxicity is attributed to maximized binding in the thymidylate synthase–fluorouracil complex (fluorouracil is thought to exert its cytotoxic effect by inhibiting thymidylate synthase, which in turn inhibits DNA synthesis)	Commonly used together for cytotoxic effects, but advise patients to report symptoms of hypersensitivity reactions (itching, wheezing) and fever
FOLINATE	RALTITREXED	Theoretical risk of ↓ efficacy of raltitrexed	Folinate antagonizes the anti-DNA effect of raltitrexed	Be aware; watch for poor response to raltitrexed
GEMCITABINE				
GEMCITABINE	ANTICANCER AND IMMUNOMODULATING DRUGS – PACLITAXEL	Possibly ↓ anti-tumour effect in breast cancer	Based on experiments on breast cell lines	Avoid co-administration except in clinical trials
GEMCITABINE	ANTICOAGULANTS – ORAL	Episodes of ↑ anticoagulant effect	Not understood but likely to be multifactorial	Monitor INR at least weekly until stable during administration of chemotherapy
HYDROXYCARBAMIDE (HYDROXYUREA)				
HYDROXYCARBAMIDE	ANTICANCER AND IMMUNOMODULATING DRUGS – FLUOROURACIL	↑ incidence of neurotoxicity (>20%)	Attributed to failure of conversion of fluorouracil to the active metabolite and an accumulation of neurotoxins	Avoid co-administration
HYDROXYCARBAMIDE	ANTIVIRALS – DIDANOSINE, ZIDOVUDINE	↑ adverse effects with didanosine and possibly zidovudine	Additive effects, enhanced antiretroviral activity via ↓ intracellular deoxynucleotides	Avoid co-administration

Primary drug	Secondary drug	Effect	Mechanism	Precautions
IDARUBICIN				
IDARUBICIN	ANTICANCER AND IMMUNOMODULATING DRUGS – TRASTUZUMAB	↑ risk of cardiotoxicity	Additive cardiotoxic effects	Avoid co-administration except in clinical trials
IFOSFAMIDE				
IFOSFAMIDE	CYP3A4 INHIBITORS			
IFOSFAMIDE	1. ANTIBIOTICS – clarithromycin, erythromycin 2. ANTIFUNGALS – fluconazole, itraconazole, ketoconazole voriconazole 3. ANTIVIRALS – efavirenz, ritonavir 4. GRAPEFRUIT JUICE 5. H2 RECEPTOR BLOCKERS – cimetidine	↓ plasma concentrations of 4-hydroxyifosfamide, the active metabolite of ifosfamide, and risk of inadequate therapeutic response	Due to inhibition of the isoenzymatic conversion to active metabolites	Monitor the efficacy of ifosfamide clinically and ↑ dose accordingly
IFOSFAMIDE	CYP3A4 INDUCERS			
IFOSFAMIDE	1. ANTIBIOTICS – rifampicin 2. ANTICANCER AND IMMUNOMODULATING DRUGS – dexamethasone 3. ANTIDEPRESSANTS – St John's wort 4. ANTIEPILEPTICS – carbamazepine, phenytoin, phenobarbital	↑ rate of biotransformation to 4-hydroxyifosfamide, the active metabolite, but there is no change in AUC of 4-hydroxyifosfamide	Due to ↑ rate of metabolism and of clearance owing to induction of CYP3A4 and CYP2D6	Be aware – clinical significance may be minimal or none

IFOSFAMIDE	ANTICANCER AND IMMUNOMODULATING DRUGS			
IFOSFAMIDE	CISPLATIN	↑ risk of neurotoxicity, haematotoxicity and tubular nephrotoxicity of ifosfamide due to ↑ plasma concentrations of ifosfamide	Cisplatin tends to cause renal damage, which results in impaired clearance of ifosfamide	Do renal function tests before initiating therapy and during concurrent therapy, and adjust dosage based on creatinine clearance values. Advise patients to drink plenty of water – vigorous hydration – and consider mesna therapy for renal protection
IFOSFAMIDE	IMATINIB MESYLATE	↓ plasma concentrations of 4-hydroxyifosfamide, the active metabolite of ifosfamide, and risk of inadequate therapeutic response	Due to inhibition of the isoenzymatic conversion to active metabolites by imatinib mesylate	Monitor the efficacy of ifosfamide clinically and ↑ dose accordingly
IFOSFAMIDE	ANTICOAGULANTS – ORAL	Episodes of ↑ anticoagulant effect	Not understood but likely to be multifactorial	Monitor INR at least weekly until stable during administration of chemotherapy
IFOSFAMIDE	CALCIUM CHANNEL BLOCKERS	↓ plasma concentrations of 4-hydroxyifosfamide, the active metabolite of ifosfamide, and risk of inadequate therapeutic response when co-administered with diltiazem, nifedipine and verapamil	Due to inhibition of the isoenzymatic conversion to active metabolites by diltiazem	Monitor the efficacy of ifosfamide clinically and ↑ dose accordingly
IFOSFAMIDE	H2 RECEPTOR BLOCKERS – CIMETIDINE	↑ adverse effects of alkylating agent, e.g. myelosuppression	Additive toxicity	Monitor more closely; monitor FBC regularly

Primary drug	Secondary drug	Effect	Mechanism	Precautions
IMATINIB				
IMATINIB	**CYP3A4 INHIBITORS**			
IMATINIB	1. ANTIBIOTICS – clarithromycin, erythromycin 2. ANTIFUNGALS – fluconazole, itraconazole, ketoconazole voriconazole 3. ANTIVIRALS – efavirenz, ritonavir 4. GRAPEFRUIT JUICE 5. H2 RECEPTOR BLOCKERS – cimetidine	↑ imatinib levels with ↑ risk of toxicity (e.g. abdominal pain, constipation, dyspnoea) and of neurotoxicity (e.g. taste disturbances, dizziness, headache, paraesthesia, peripheral neuropathy)	Due to inhibition of CYP3A4-mediated metabolism of imatinib	Monitor for clinical efficacy and for the signs of toxicity listed, along with convulsions, confusion and signs of oedema (including pulmonary oedema). Monitor electrolytes and liver function, and for cardiotoxicity
IMATINIB	**CYP3A4 INDUCERS**			
IMATINIB	1. ANTIBIOTICS – rifampicin 2. ANTICANCER AND IMMUNOMODULATING DRUGS – dexamethasone 3. ANTIDEPRESSANTS – St John's wort 4. ANTIEPILEPTICS – carbamazepine, phenobarbital, phenytoin	↓ imatinib levels	Due to induction of CYP3A4-mediated metabolism of imatinib	Monitor for clinical efficacy and adjust dose as required. Avoid co-administration of imatinib and rifampicin
IMATINIB	**CYP2C9 SUBSTRATES**			
IMATINIB	1. ANGIOTENSIN II RECEPTORS ANTAGONISTS – irbesartan, losartan, valsartan 2. ANTIDEPRESSANTS – sertraline 3. ANTIDIABETIC DRUGS – glimepride, glipizide, tolbutamide 4. ANTIEPILEPTICS – fosphenytoin, phenytoin, topiramate 5. NSAIDs – celecoxib, diclofenac, piroxicam 6. PROTON PUMP INHIBITORS – omeprazole	↑ plasma concentrations, with risk of toxic effects of these drugs	Imatinib is a potent inhibitor of CYP2C9 isoenzymes, which metabolize these drugs	Watch for the early toxic effects of these drugs. If necessary, consider using alternative drugs while the patient is being given imatinib

IMATINIB	CYP2D6 SUBSTRATES			
IMATINIB	ANALGESICS – OPIOIDS	May cause ↑ plasma concentrations, with a risk of toxic effects of codeine, dextromethorphan, hydroxycodone, methadone, morphine, oxycodone, pethidine and tramadol	Inhibition of CYP2D6-mediated metabolism of these opioids	Monitor for clinical efficacy and toxicity. Warn patients to report ↑ drowsiness, malaise or anorexia. Measure amylase and lipase levels if toxicity is suspected. Tramadol causes less respiratory depression than other opiates, but need to monitor BP and blood counts, and advise patients to report wheezing, loss of appetite and fainting attacks. Need to consider ↓ dose. Methadone may cause Q–T prolongation; the CHM has recommended that patients with heart and liver disease who are on methadone should be carefully monitored for heart conduction abnormalities such as Q–T prolongation on ECG as they may lead to sudden death. Also need to monitor patients on more than 100 mg methadone daily and thus an ↑ in plasma concentrations necessitates close monitoring of cardiac and respiratory function

Primary drug	Secondary drug	Effect	Mechanism	Precautions
IMATINIB	1. ANTIARRHYTHMICS – flecainide, mexiletine, propafenone 2. ANTI-DEPRESSANTS – fluoxetine, paroxetine, TCAs, trazodone, venlafaxine 3. ANTIPSYCHOTICS – clozapine, haloperidol, perphenazine, risperidone, thioridazine 4. BETA-BLOCKERS – metoprolol, propanolol, timolol 5. DONEPEZIL 6. METHAMPHETAMINE	Imatinib may cause ↑ plasma concentrations of these drugs, with a risk of toxic effects	Inhibition of CYP2D6-mediated metabolism of these drugs	Watch for early features of toxicity of these drugs
IMATINIB	ANTICANCER AND IMMUNOMODULATING DRUGS			
IMATINIB	CICLOSPORIN	↑ plasma concentrations of ciclosporin, with risk of nephrotoxicity, myelosuppression, neurotoxicity and excessive immunosuppression, with risk of infection and post-transplant lymphoproliferative disease	Inhibition of metabolism of ciclosporin	Monitor plasma ciclosporin levels to prevent toxicity
IMATINIB	CORTICOSTEROIDS	↑ adrenal suppressive effects of corticosteroids, which may ↑ risk of infections and produce an inadequate response to stress scenarios	Due to inhibition of metabolism of corticosteroids	Monitor cortisol levels and warn patients to report symptoms such as fever and sore throat

IMATINIB	DOXORUBICIN	↑ risk of myelosuppression due to ↑ plasma concentrations	Due to ↓ metabolism of doxorubicin by CYP3A4 isoenzymes owing to inhibition of those enzymes	Monitor for ↑ myelosuppression, peripheral neuropathy, myalgias and fatigue
IMATINIB	IFOSFAMIDE	↓ plasma concentrations of 4-hydroxyifosfamide, the active metabolite of ifosfamide, and risk of inadequate therapeutic response	Due to inhibition of the isoenzymatic conversion to active metabolites by imatinib mesylate	Monitor the efficacy of ifosfamide clinically and ↑ dose accordingly
IMATINIB	IRINOTECAN	↑ plasma concentrations of SN-38 (the active metabolite of irinotecan) and ↑ toxicity of irinotecan, e.g. diarrhoea, acute cholinergic syndrome, interstitial pulmonary disease	Inhibition of CYP3A4-mediated metabolism of SN-38	Peripheral blood counts should be checked before each course of treatment. Monitor lung function. The recommendation is to ↓ dose of irinotecan by 25%
IMATINIB	VINCA ALKALOIDS	↑ adverse effects of vinblastine and vincristine	Inhibition of CYP3A4-mediated metabolism. Also inhibition of P-gp efflux of vinblastine	Monitor FBCs and watch for early features of toxicity (pain, numbness, tingling in the fingers and toes, jaw pain, abdominal pain, constipation, ileus). Consider selecting an alternative drug
IMATINIB	ANTICOAGULANTS – ORAL	Episodes of ↑ anticoagulant effect	Not understood but likely to be multifactorial	Monitor INR at least weekly until stable during administration of chemotherapy
IMATINIB	ANTIDEPRESSANTS – TCAs	Possible ↑ imatinib levels	Inhibition of CYP2C9-mediated metabolism. The clinical significance of this depends upon whether alternative pathways of metabolism are also inhibited by co-administered drugs	Warn patients to report ↑ side-effects and monitor blood count carefully

Primary drug	Secondary drug	Effect	Mechanism	Precautions
IMATINIB	ANTIDIABETIC DRUGS – REPAGLINIDE	Likely to ↑ plasma concentrations of repaglinide and ↑ risk of hypoglycaemic episodes	Due to inhibition of CYP3A4 isoenzymes, which metabolize repaglinide	Watch for and warn patients about hypoglycaemia ➢ ***For signs and symptoms of hypoglycaemia, see Clinical Features of Some Adverse Drug Interactions, Hypoglycaemia***
IMATINIB	ANTIMIGRAINE DRUGS – ALMOTRIPTAN, ELETRIPTAN	↑ plasma concentrations of almotriptan and risk of toxic effects of almotriptan, e.g. flushing, sensations of tingling, heat, heaviness, pressure or tightness of any part of body including the throat and chest, dizziness	Almotriptan is metabolized mainly by CYP3A4 isoenzymes. Most CYP isoenzymes are inhibited by imatinib mesylate to varying degrees, and since there is an alternative pathway of metabolism by MAO-A, the toxicity responses will vary between individuals	The CSM has advised, particularly for sumatriptan, that if chest tightness or pressure is intense, the triptan should be discontinued immediately and the patient investigated for ischaemic heart disease by measuring cardiac enzymes and doing an ECG. Avoid concomitant use in patients with coronary artery disease and in those with severe or uncontrolled hypertension
IMATINIB	BETA-BLOCKERS	Imatinib may cause ↑ plasma concentrations of metoprolol, propanolol and timolol, with a risk of toxic effects	Imatinib is a potent inhibitor of CYP2D6 isoenzymes, which metabolize beta-blockers	Monitor for clinical efficacy and toxicity of beta-adrenergic blockers
IMATINIB	CALCIUM CHANNEL BLOCKERS	↑ plasma concentrations of imatinib when co-administered with diltiazem, nifedipine and verapamil. ↑ risk of toxicity (e.g. abdominal pain, constipation, dyspnoea) and of neurotoxicity (e.g. taste disturbances, dizziness, headache, paraesthesia, peripheral neuropathy)	Due to inhibition of hepatic metabolism of imatinib by the CYP3A4 isoenzymes by diltiazem	Monitor for clinical efficacy and for the signs of toxicity listed, along with convulsions, confusion and signs of oedema (including pulmonary oedema). Monitor electrolytes and liver function, and for cardiotoxicity

IMATINIB	LIPID-LOWERING DRUGS – STATINS	Imatinib may ↑ atorvastatin and simvastatin levels	Imatinib inhibits CYP3A4-mediated metabolism of simvastatin	Monitor LFTs, U&Es and CK closely
IRINOTECAN				
IRINOTECAN	**CYP3A4 INHIBITORS**			
IRINOTECAN	1. ANTIBIOTICS – clarithromycin, erythromycin 2. ANTICANCER AND IMMUNOMODULATING DRUGS – imatinib 3. ANTIFUNGALS – fluconazole, itraconazole, ketoconazole, voriconazole 4. ANTIVIRALS – efavirenz, ritonavir 5. GRAPEFRUIT JUICE 6. H2 RECEPTOR BLOCKERS – cimetidine	↑ plasma concentrations of SN-38 (↑ AUC by 100%) and ↑ toxicity of irinotecan, e.g. diarrhoea, acute cholinergic syndrome, interstitial pulmonary disease	Due to inhibition of the metabolism of irinotecan by CYP3A4 isoenzymes by ketoconazole	Peripheral blood counts should be checked before each course of treatment. Monitor lung function. Recommendation is to ↓ dose of irinotecan by 25%
IRINOTECAN	**CYP3A4 INDUCERS**			
IRINOTECAN	1. ANTIBIOTICS – rifampicin 2. ANTICANCER AND IMMUNOMODULATING DRUGS – dexamethasone 3. ANTIDEPRESSANTS – St John's wort 4. ANTIEPILEPTICS – carbamazepine, phenobarbital, phenytoin	↓ plasma concentrations of irinotecan and risk of ↓ therapeutic efficacy. The effects may last for 3 weeks after discontinuation of CYP-inducer therapy	Due to induction of CYP3A4-mediated metabolism of irinotecan	Avoid concomitant use when ever possible; if not, ↑ dose of irinotecan by 50%

Primary drug	Secondary drug	Effect	Mechanism	Precautions
IRINOTECAN	CALCIUM CHANNEL BLOCKERS	Risk of ↑ serum concentrations of irinotecan with nifedipine. No cases of toxicity reported	Inhibition of hepatic microsomal enzymes, but exact mechanism is unknown	Watch for symptoms/signs of toxicity (especially diarrhoea, an early manifestation of acute cholinergic syndrome)
LOMUSTINE				
LOMUSTINE	ANTIEPILEPTICS – PHENOBARBITAL	↓ plasma concentrations of lomustine and risk of inadequate therapeutic response	Phenobarbital induces the metabolism of lomustine by the CYP450 isoenzymes	Avoid concurrent use. If necessary, ↑ dose of lomustine and monitor therapeutic effects
LOMUSTINE	H2 RECEPTOR BLOCKERS – CIMETIDINE	↑ adverse effects of alkylating agent, e.g. myelosuppression	Additive toxicity	Monitor more closely; monitor FBC regularly
MELPHALAN				
MELPHALAN	ANTIBIOTICS – NALIDIXIC ACID	Risk of melphalan toxicity	Uncertain	Avoid co-administration
MELPHALAN	**ANTICANCER AND IMMUNOMODULATING DRUGS**			
FLUOROURACIL	AZATHIOPRINE	↑ risk of myelosuppression and immunosuppression. Deaths have occurred following profound myelosuppression and severe sepsis	Additive myelotoxic effects. Azathioprine is metabolized to 6-mercatopurine in vivo, which results in additive myelosuppression, immunosuppression and hepatotoxicity	Avoid co-administration
MELPHALAN	CICLOSPORIN	Risk of renal toxicity	Additive effect	Monitor U&Es closely
MELPHALAN	H2 RECEPTOR BLOCKERS – CIMETIDINE	↓ plasma concentrations and bioavailability of melphalan by 30% and risk of poor therapeutic response to melphalan	Cimetidine causes a change in gastric pH, which ↓ absorption of melphalan	Avoid concurrent use

MERCAPTOPURINE				
MERCAPTOPURINE	ANTIBIOTICS – CO-TRIMOXAZOLE	↑ risk of bone marrow toxicity	Additive effect	Avoid co-administration
MERCAPTOPURINE	**ANTICANCER AND IMMUNOMODULATING DRUGS**			
MERCAPTOPURINE	AMINOSALICYLATES	↑ risk of bone marrow suppression	Additive effect	Monitor FBC closely
MERCAPTOPURINE	AZATHIOPRINE	↑ risk of myelosuppression and immunosuppression. Deaths have occurred following profound myelosuppression and severe sepsis	Additive myelotoxic effects. Azathioprine is metabolized to 6-mercatopurine in vivo, which results in additive myelosuppression, immunosuppression and hepatotoxicity	Avoid co-administration
MERCAPTOPURINE	DOXORUBICIN	↑ risk of hepatotoxicity due to mercaptopurine	Uncertain, possibly due to previous treatment with mercaptopurine	Avoid co-administration – except in clinical trials
MERCAPTOPURINE	METHOTREXATE – ORAL	↑ plasma concentrations of mercaptopurine (↑ AUC by 30%) and ↑ risk of myelotoxicity	Methotrexate ↑ oral bioavailability of mercaptopurine	↓ dose of oral 6-mercaptopurine when used with doses of methotrexate >20 mg/m^2 or higher doses of methotrexate given intravenously
MERCAPTOPURINE	ANTICOAGULANTS – WARFARIN	Possible ↓ anticoagulant effect	Induction of metabolism of warfarin	Monitor INR closely
MERCAPTOPURINE	ANTIGOUT DRUGS – ALLOPURINOL	↑ mercaptopurine levels with risk of toxicity (e.g. myelosuppression, pancreatitis)	Azathioprine is metabolized to mercaptopurine. Allopurinol inhibits hepatic metabolism of mercaptopurine	↓ doses of azathioprine and mercaptopurine by up to three-quarters and monitor FBC, LFTs and amylase carefully
MESNA				
MESNA	CISPLATIN	Inactivation of cisplatin	Pharmaceutical interaction	Do not mix mesna with cisplatin infusions

Primary drug	Secondary drug	Effect	Mechanism	Precautions
METHOTREXATE				
METHOTREXATE	ANAESTHETICS – NITROUS OXIDE	↑ antifolate effect of methotrexate	↑ toxicity of methotrexate	Nitrous oxide is usually used for relatively brief durations when patients are anaesthetized, and hence this risk during anaesthesia is minimal. However, nitrous oxide may be used for analgesia for longer durations, and this should be avoided
METHOTREXATE	ANALGESICS – NSAIDs	↑ methotrexate levels, with reports of toxicity, with ibuprofen, indometacin and possibly diclofenac, flurbiprofen, ketoprofen and naproxen	Uncertain; postulated that an NSAID-induced ↓ in renal perfusion may have an effect	Consider using an alternative NSAID
METHOTREXATE	**ANTIBIOTICS**			
METHOTREXATE	CIPROFLOXACIN	↑ plasma concentrations of methotrexate, with risk of toxic effects of methotrexate, e.g. liver cirrhosis, blood dyscrasias that may be fatal, pulmonary toxicity and stomatitis. Haematopoietic suppression can occur abruptly. Other adverse effects include anorexia, dyspepsia, gastrointestinal ulceration and bleeding, and pulmonary oedema	Ciprofloxacin ↓ renal elimination of methotrexate. Ciprofloxacin is known to cause renal failure and interstitial nephritis	Although the toxic effects of methotrexate are more frequent with high doses of methotrexate, it is necessary to do a FBC and liver and renal function tests before starting treatment even with low doses, and to repeat these tests weekly until therapy is stabilized and thereafter every 2–3 months. Patients should be advised to report symptoms such as sore throat and fever immediately, and also any gastrointestinal discomfort. A profound drop in white cell count or platelet count warrants immediate stoppage of methotrexate therapy and initiation of supportive therapy. Consider a non-reacting antibiotic

METHOTREXATE	DOXYCYCLINE	↑ plasma concentrations of methotrexate, with risk of toxic effects of methotrexate, e.g. liver cirrhosis, blood dyscrasias which may be fatal, pulmonary toxicity, stomatitis. Haematopoietic suppression can occur abruptly. Other adverse effects include anorexia, dyspepsia, gastrointestinal ulceration and bleeding, and pulmonary oedema	Tetracyclines destroy the bacterial flora necessary for the breakdown of methotrexate. This results in ↑ free methotrexate concentrations. Tetracyclines are also considered to inhibit the elimination of methotrexate and allow a build-up of methotrexate in the bladder. The effects of the interaction is often delayed	Although the toxic effects of methotrexate are more frequent with high doses of methotrexate, it is necessary to do an FBC, liver and renal function tests before starting treatment even with low doses, repeating these tests weekly until therapy is stabilized, and thereafter every 2–3 months. Patients should be advised to report symptoms such as sore throat and fever immediately, and also any gastrointestinal discomfort. A profound drop in white cell count or platelet count warrants immediate stoppage of methotrexate therapy and initiation of supportive therapy
METHOTREXATE – ORAL	NEOMYCIN	↓ plasma concentrations following oral methotrexate	Oral aminoglycosides ↓ absorption of oral methotrexate by 30–50%	Separate doses of each drug by at least 2–4 hours
METHOTREXATE	PENICILLINS	↑ plasma concentrations of methotrexate and risk of toxic effects of methotrexate, e.g. myelosuppression, liver cirrhosis, pulmonary toxicity	Penicillins ↓ renal elimination of methotrexate by renal tubular secretion, which is the main route of elimination of methotrexate. Penicillins compete with methotrexate for renal elimination. Displacement from protein-binding sites may occur and is only a minor contribution to the interaction	Avoid concurrent use. If concurrent use is necessary, monitor clinically and biochemically for blood dyscrasia, liver toxicity and pulmonary toxicity. Do FBCs and LFTs prior to concurrent treatment

Primary drug	Secondary drug	Effect	Mechanism	Precautions
METHOTREXATE	SULFAMETHOXAZOLE/ TRIMETHOPRIM	↑ plasma concentrations of methotrexate and risk of toxic effects of methotrexate, e.g. myelosuppression, liver cirrhosis, pulmonary toxicity	Sulfamethoxazole displaces methotrexate from plasma protein-binding sites and also ↓ renal elimination of methotrexate. Trimethoprim inhibits dihydrofolate reductase, which leads to additive toxic effects of methotrexate	Avoid concurrent use. If concurrent use is necessary, monitor clinically and biochemically for blood dyscrasias and liver, renal and pulmonary toxicity
METHOTREXATE	SULPHONAMIDES	↑ plasma concentrations of methotrexate, with risk of toxic effects of methotrexate, e.g. liver cirrhosis, blood dyscrasias which may be fatal, pulmonary toxicity, stomatitis. Haematopoietic suppression can occur abruptly. Other adverse effects include anorexia, dyspepsia, gastrointestinal ulceration and bleeding, and pulmonary oedema	The mechanism differs from that underlying the sulfamethoxazole/trimethoprim interaction. Sulphonamides such as co-trimoxazole and sulfadiazine are known to cause renal dysfunction – interstitial nephritis and renal failure, which may ↓ excretion of methotrexate. Sulphonamides are also known to compete with methotrexate for renal elimination. Displacement from protein-binding sites of methotrexate is a minor contribution to the interaction	Although the toxic effects of methotrexate are more frequent with high doses of methotrexate, it is necessary to do an FBC, liver and renal function tests before starting treatment even with low doses, repeating these tests at 2–3 months. Patients should be advised to report symptoms such as sore throat and fever immediately, and also any gastrointestinal discomfort. A profound drop in white cell count or platelet count warrants immediate stoppage of methotrexate therapy and initiation of supportive therapy

ANTICANCER AND IMMUNOMODULATING DRUGS CYTOTOXICS

METHOTREXATE	TETRACYCLINE	↑ plasma concentrations of methotrexate, with risk of toxic effects of methotrexate, e.g. liver cirrhosis, blood dyscrasias which may be fatal, pulmonary toxicity, stomatitis. Haematopoietic suppression can occur abruptly. Other adverse effects include anorexia, dyspepsia, gastrointestinal ulceration and bleeding, and pulmonary oedema	Tetracyclines destroy the bacterial flora necessary for the breakdown of methotrexate. This results in ↑ free methotrexate concentrations. Tetracyclines are also considered to inhibit the elimination of methotrexate and allow a build-up of methotrexate in the bladder. The effect of the interaction is often delayed	Although the toxic effects of methotrexate are more frequent with high doses of methotrexate, it is necessary to do an FBC, liver and renal function tests before starting treatment even with low doses, repeating these tests at 2–3 months. Patients should be advised to report symptoms such as sore throat and fever immediately, and also any gastrointestinal discomfort. A profound drop in white cell count or platelet count warrants immediate stoppage of methotrexate therapy and initiation of supportive therapy
METHOTREXATE	**ANTICANCER AND IMMUNOMODULATING DRUGS**			
METHOTREXATE	**CYTOTOXICS**			
METHOTREXATE	CISPLATIN	↑ methotrexate levels, with ↑ risk of pulmonary toxicity	Cisplatin is the most common anticancer drug associated with renal proximal and distal tubular damage. Cisplatin could significantly ↓ renal elimination of methotrexate	It would be best to start with lower doses of methotrexate. It is necessary to assess renal function prior to and during concurrent treatment until stability is achieved. Monitor clinically and with pulmonary function tests
METHOTREXATE	CRISANTASPASE	Administration prior to or concurrently may ↓ efficacy of methotrexate	Crisantaspase inhibits protein synthesis and prevents cell entry to S phase, which leads to ↓ efficacy of methotrexate	Administer crisantaspase shortly after methotrexate or 9–10 days before methotrexate

Primary drug	Secondary drug	Effect	Mechanism	Precautions
METHOTREXATE	FLUOROURACIL	↓ cytotoxic effect of methotrexate when fluorouracil is administered prior to methotrexate	Fluorouracil prevents the conversion of reduced folates to dihydrofolate	Always administer methotrexate prior to fluorouracil
METHOTREXATE – ORAL	MERCAPTOPURINE	↑ plasma concentrations of mercaptopurine (↑ AUC by 30%) and ↑ risk of myelotoxicity	Methotrexate ↑ oral bioavailability of mercaptopurine	↓ dose of oral 6-mercaptopurine when used with doses of methotrexate $>$20 mg/m^2 or higher doses of methotrexate given intravenously
METHOTREXATE	PROCARBAZINE	↑ risk of renal impairment if methotrexate infusion is given within 48 hours of procarbazine administration. Also ↑ risk of methotrexate toxicity, particularly to the kidneys	Procarbazine has a transient effect on the kidneys, and this will delay the renal elimination of methotrexate	Do not start methotrexate infusion less than 72 hours after the last dose of procarbazine. Hydrate patients aggressively (plenty of oral fluids or intravenous fluids), alkalinize the urine to pH$>$7 and closely monitor renal function, e.g. blood urea and creatinine, before and after methotrexate infusion until methotrexate blood levels are $<$0.05 μmol/L
METHOTREXATE	RETINOIDS – ACITRETIN	↑ methotrexate levels	Uncertain	Avoid co-administration
METHOTREXATE	**IMMUNOMODULATING DRUGS**			
METHOTREXATE	AMINOSALICYLATES – SULFASALAZINE	↑ risk of hepatotoxicity with sulfasalazine	Additive hepatotoxic effects. Sulfasalazine also competes with methotrexate for renal elimination	Monitor closely for symptoms of liver failure. Check LFTs at the beginning of treatment then weekly until stable, and repeat if there is clinical suspicion of liver disease

METHOTREXATE	AZATHIOPRINE	↑ risk of hepatotoxicity	Additive hepatotoxic effects	Monitor closely for symptoms of liver failure e.g. flu-like symptoms, abdominal pain, dark urine, pruritus, jaundice, ascites and weight gain. Do LFTs at the beginning of treatment and weekly until stable, and repeat if there is clinical suspicion of liver disease
METHOTREXATE	CICLOSPORIN	↑ risk of renal toxicity and renal failure	Additive renal toxicity	Monitor renal function prior to and during therapy, and ensure an intake of at least 2 L of fluid daily. Monitor serum potassium and magnesium and correct any deficiencies
METHOTREXATE	CORTICOSTEROIDS	↑ risk of bone marrow toxicity	Additive effect	Monitor FBC regularly
METHOTREXATE	RETINOIDS – ACITRETIN	↑ risk of hepatotoxicity	Additive hepatotoxic effects	Avoid co-administration
METHOTREXATE	ANTICOAGULANTS – ORAL	Episodes of ↑ anticoagulant effect	Not understood but likely to be multifactorial	Monitor INR at least weekly until stable during administration of chemotherapy
METHOTREXATE	ANTIEPILEPTICS – PHENYTOIN	↑ plasma concentrations of phenytoin may occur and ↑ risk of toxic effects of phenytoin	High doses of methotrexate ↓ elimination of phenytoin	Monitor phenytoin levels and clinically watch for signs and symptoms of phenytoin toxicity, e.g. nausea, vomiting, insomnia, tremor, acne, hirsutism
METHOTREXATE	ANTIGOUT DRUGS – PROBENECID	↑ methotrexate levels	Probenecid ↓ elimination of methotrexate renally by interfering with tubular secretion in the proximal tubule and also ↓ protein binding of methotrexate (a relatively minor effect). Probenecid competes with methotrexate for renal elimination	Avoid co-administration if possible; if not possible, ↓ dose of methotrexate and monitor FBC closely

Primary drug	Secondary drug	Effect	Mechanism	Precautions
METHOTREXATE	ANTIMALARIALS – PYRIMETHAMINE	↑ antifolate effect of methotrexate	Pyrimethamine should not be used alone and is combined with sulfadoxine. Pyrimethamine and methotrexate synergistically induce folate deficiency	Although the toxic effects of methotrexate are more frequent with high doses of methotrexate, it is necessary to do an FBC, liver and renal function tests before starting treatment even with low doses, repeating these tests weekly until therapy is stabilized and thereafter every 2–3 months. Patients should be advised to report symptoms such as sore throat and fever immediately, and also any gastrointestinal discomfort. A profound drop in white cell count or platelet count warrants immediate stoppage of methotrexate therapy and initiation of supportive therapy
METHOTREXATE	ANTIPLATELET AGENTS – ASPIRIN	Risk of methotrexate toxicity when co-administered with high-dose aspirin. There is a risk of toxic effects of methotrexate, e.g. liver cirrhosis, blood dyscrasias which may be fatal, pulmonary toxicity, stomatitis. Haematopoietic suppression can occur abruptly. Other adverse effects include anorexia, dyspepsia, gastrointestinal ulceration and bleeding, and pulmonary oedema	Aspirin ↓ plasma protein binding of methotrexate (a relatively minor contribution to the interaction) and the renal excretion of high doses of methotrexate. Salicylates compete with methotrexate for renal elimination	Check FBC, U&Es and LFTs before starting treatment, repeating weekly until stabilized and then every 2–3 months. Patients should be advised to report symptoms such as sore throat, fever or gastrointestinal discomfort immediately. Stop methotrexate and initiate supportive therapy if the white cell or platelet count drops. Do not administer aspirin within 10 days of high-dose methotrexate treatment

ANTICANCER AND IMMUNOMODULATING DRUGS CYTOTOXICS

METHOTREXATE	ANTIVIRALS – OSELTAMIVIR	Possible ↑ efficacy/toxicity	Competition for renal excretion	Monitor more closely for signs of immunosuppression. Predicted interaction
METHOTREXATE	BRONCHODILATORS – THEOPHYLLINE	Possible ↑ in theophylline levels	Possibly inhibition of CYP2D6-mediated metabolism of theophylline	Monitor clinically for toxic effects and advise patients to seek medical attention if they have symptoms suggestive of theophylline toxicity. Measure theophylline levels before, during and after co-administration
METHOTREXATE	LIPID-LOWERING DRUGS – COLESTYRAMINE	Parenteral methotrexate levels may be ↓ by colestyramine	Colestyramine interrupts the enterohepatic circulation of methotrexate	Avoid co-administration
METHOTREXATE	PROTON PUMP INHIBITORS – OMEPRAZOLE	Likely ↑ plasma concentration of methotrexate and ↑ risk of toxic effects, e.g. blood dyscrasias, liver cirrhosis, pulmonary toxicity, renal toxicity	Attributed to omeprazole decreasing the renal elimination of methotrexate	Monitor clinically and biochemically for blood dyscrasias and liver, renal and pulmonary toxicity
MITOMYCIN				
MITOMYCIN	**ANTICANCER AND IMMUNOMODULATING DRUGS**			
MITOMYCIN	CYTOTOXICS – VINCA ALKALOIDS	↑ risk of abrupt onset of pulmonary toxicity in 3–6% of patients, when two courses of these drugs are administered concurrently	Mechanism is uncertain; possible additive pulmonary toxic effects	Monitor clinically and with lung function tests for pulmonary toxicity. Advise patients to report immediately symptoms such as shortness of breath and wheezing
MITOMYCIN	HORMONES AND HORMONE ANTAGONISTS – TAMOXIFEN	↑ incidence of anaemia and thrombocytopenia and risk of haemolytic–uraemic syndrome	Mitomycin causes subclinical endothelial damage in addition to the thrombotic effect on platelets caused by tamoxifen, which leads to haemolytic–uraemic syndrome	Monitor renal function at least twice weekly during concurrent therapy and watch clinically for bleeding episodes, e.g. nose bleeds, bleeding from the gums, skin bruising

Primary drug	Secondary drug	Effect	Mechanism	Precautions
MITOTANE				
MITOTANE	ANTICOAGULANTS – WARFARIN	Possible ↓ anticoagulant effect	Induction of metabolism of warfarin	Monitor INR closely
MITOXANTRONE				
MITOXANTRONE	AZATHIOPRINE	↑ risk of myelosuppression and immunosuppression. Deaths have occurred following profound myelosuppression and severe sepsis	Additive myelotoxic effects Azathioprine is metabolized to 6-mercatopurine in vivo, which results in additive myelosuppression, immunosuppression and hepatotoxicity	Avoid co-administration
MITOXANTRONE	CICLOSPORIN – high doses (leading to levels of ciclosporin from 3000 to 5000 ng/mL)	↑ mitoxantrone levels; no ↑ toxicity has been reported	↓ clearance (>40%) and ↑ terminal half-life (>50%) due to inhibition of P-gp in normal tissues	↓ dose of mitoxantrone of 40% has been recommended in paediatric patients. Advisable to monitor mitoxantrone levels
OXALIPLATIN ➢ ***Platinum compounds, below***				
PACLITAXEL				
PACLITAXEL	CYP3A4 INDUCERS			
PACLITAXEL	1. ANTIBIOTICS – rifampicin 2. ANTIDEPRESSANTS – St John's wort 3. ANTIEPILEPTICS – carbamazepine, phenobarbital, phenytoin	↓ plasma concentration of paclitaxel and ↓ efficacy of paclitaxel	Due to induction of hepatic metabolism of paclitaxel by the CYP isoenzymes	Monitor for clinical efficacy and need to ↑ dose if inadequate response is due to interaction

PACLITAXEL	ANTICANCER AND IMMUNOMODULATING DRUGS			
PACLITAXEL	CYTOTOXICS			
PACLITAXEL	CISPLATIN	↑ risk of profound neutropenia	Prior administration of cisplatin tends to impair renal function and ↓ clearance of paclitaxel by approximately 25%	Advise administration of paclitaxel prior to cisplatin
PACLITAXEL	CYCLOPHOSPHAMIDE	↑ risk of neutropenia, thrombocytopenia and mucositis when paclitaxel is infused over 24 or 72 hours prior to cyclophosphamide	Mechanism is uncertain	Administer cyclophosphamide first and then follow with paclitaxel
PACLITAXEL	DOXORUBICIN	↑ risk of neutropenia, stomatitis and cardiomyopathy due to ↑ plasma concentrations of doxorubicin when paclitaxel is given before doxorubicin	This is possibly due to competitive inhibition of biliary excretion of doxorubicin by paclitaxel	Doxorubicin should be administered prior to paclitaxel. The cumulative dose of doxorubicin should be limited to 360 mg/m^2 when concurrently administered with paclitaxel
PACLITAXEL	EPIRUBICIN	↑ plasma concentrations of epirubicin (↑ AUC by 37% and ↓ clearance by 25%), particularly following sequential administration of paclitaxel followed by epirubicin	Attributed to altered distribution of epirubicin in plasma and inhibition of P-gp by Cremophor, the vehicle of paclitaxel formulation, resulting in ↓ clearance	Epirubicin should always be given prior to paclitaxel
PACLITAXEL	GEMCITABINE	Possibly ↓ anti-tumour effect in breast cancer	Based on experiments on breast cell lines	Avoid co-administration except in clinical trials
PACLITAXEL	TRASTUZUMAB	↑ risk of cardiotoxicity	Possibly additive cardiac toxic effect	Closely monitor clinically and by ECGs for cardiotoxicity
PACLITAXEL	VINBLASTINE, VINCRISTINE	↓ therapeutic efficacy of paclitaxel	Antagonistic effects	Avoid co-administration

Primary drug	Secondary drug	Effect	Mechanism	Precautions
PACLITAXEL	IMMUNOMODULATING DRUGS			
PACLITAXEL	DEXAMETHASONE	↓ plasma concentrations of paclitaxel and ↓ efficacy of paclitaxel	Due to induction of hepatic metabolism of paclitaxel by the CYP isoenzymes	Monitor for clinical efficacy; need to ↑ dose if inadequate response is due to interaction
PACLITAXEL	**IMMUNOMODULATING DRUGS**			
PACLITAXEL	CICLOSPORIN	↑ plasma concentrations of these drugs, with risk of toxic effects	Competitive inhibition of CYP3A4-mediated metabolism and P-gp transport of these drugs	Watch for toxic effects of these drugs
PACLITAXEL	ANTIVIRALS – PROTEASE INHIBITORS	↑ risk of adverse effects of docetaxel and paclitaxel	Inhibition of CYP3A4-mediated metabolism. Also inhibition of P-gp efflux of vinblastine	Use with caution. Additional monitoring required. Monitor FBC weekly
PEMETREXED				
PEMETREXED	ANTIGOUT DRUGS – PROBENECID	↑ pemetrexed levels	Probable ↓ renal excretion of pemetrexed	Avoid co-administration where possible. If both need to be given, monitor FBC and renal function closely and watch for gastrointestinal disturbance and features of myopathy
PENTOSTATIN				
PENTOSTATIN	**ANTICANCER AND IMMUNOMODULATING DRUGS**			
PENTOSTATIN	CYCLOPHOSPHAMIDE	↑ risk of potentially fatal cardiac toxicity	Attributed to interference of adenosine metabolism by cyclophosphamide	Avoid co-administration
PENTOSTATIN	FLUDARABINE	Risk of severe and potentially fatal pulmonary toxicity	Uncertain	Avoid co-administration

PLATINUM COMPOUNDS – CARBOPLATIN, CISPLATIN, OXALIPLATIN				
PLATINUM COMPOUNDS	**ANTIBIOTICS**			
PLATINUM COMPOUNDS	AMINOGLYCOSIDES, CAPREOMYCIN, COLISTIN, STREPTOMYCIN, VANCOMYCIN	↑ risk of renal toxicity and renal failure and of ototoxicity. The ototoxicity tends to occur when cisplatin is administered early during the course of aminoglycoside therapy	Additive renal toxicity	Monitor renal function prior to and during therapy, and ensure an intake of at least 2 L of fluid daily. Monitor serum potassium and magnesium and correct any deficiencies. Most side-effects of aminoglycosides are dose-related, and it is necessary to ↑ interval between doses and ↓ dose of aminoglycoside if there is impaired renal function
PLATINUM COMPOUNDS	**ANTICANCER AND IMMUNOMODULATING DRUGS**			
PLATINUM COMPOUNDS	**CYTOTOXICS**			
CISPLATIN	BLEOMYCIN	↑ bleomycin levels, with risk of pulmonary toxicity	Elimination of bleomycin is delayed by cisplatin due to ↓ glomerular filtration. This is most likely with accumulated doses of cisplatin in excess of 300 mgm^2	Monitor renal function and adjust the dose of bleomycin by creatinine clearance. Monitor clinically, radiologically and with lung function tests for pulmonary toxicity
CISPLATIN	DOCETAXEL	↑ docetaxel levels, with ↑ risk of profound myelosuppression. Concurrent use also ↑ risk of neurotoxicity	↓ clearance of docetaxel when docetaxel is administered after cisplatin	Administer docetaxel first and follow with cisplatin

Primary drug	Secondary drug	Effect	Mechanism	Precautions
CISPLATIN	IFOSFAMIDE	↑ risk of neurotoxicity, haematotoxicity and tubular nephrotoxicity of ifosfamide due to ↑ plasma concentrations of ifosfamide	Cisplatin tends to cause renal damage, which results in impaired clearance of ifosfamide	Do renal function tests before initiating therapy and during concurrent therapy, and adjust the dosage based on creatinine clearance values. Advise patients to drink plenty of water – vigorous hydration – and consider mesna therapy for renal protection
CISPLATIN	MESNA	Inactivation of cisplatin	Pharmaceutical interaction	Do not mix mesna with cisplatin infusions
CISPLATIN	METHOTREXATE	↑ methotrexate levels with ↑ risk of pulmonary toxicity	Cisplatin is the most common anticancer drug associated with renal proximal and distal tubular damage. Cisplatin could significantly ↓ renal elimination of methotrexate	It would be best to start with lower doses of methotrexate. It is necessary to assess renal function prior to and during concurrent treatment until stability is achieved. Monitor clinically and with pulmonary function tests
CISPLATIN	PACLITAXEL	↑ risk of profound neutropenia	Prior administration of cisplatin tends to impair renal function and ↓ clearance of paclitaxel by approximately 25%	Advise administration of paclitaxel prior to cisplatin
CISPLATIN	TOPOTECAN	↑ risk of bone marrow suppression, especially when topotecan is administered in doses >0.75 mg/m^2 on days 1–5 and cisplatin in doses >50 mg/m^2 on day 1 before topotecan	Attributed to cisplatin inducing subclinical renal toxicity, possibly causing ↓ clearance of topotecan	Administer cisplatin on day 5 after topotecan if dose of topotecan is >0.75 mg/m^2 and cisplatin dose is >50 mg/m^2 with the use of granulocyte colony-stimulating factors
PLATINUM COMPOUNDS	VINORELBINE	↑ incidence of grade III and grade IV granulocytopenia	Additive myelosuppressive effects	Monitor blood counts at least weekly and advise patients to report symptoms such as sore throat and fever

ANTICANCER AND IMMUNOMODULATING DRUGS CYTOTOXICS

PLATINUM COMPOUNDS	IMMUNOMODULATING DRUGS			
PLATINUM COMPOUNDS	AZATHIOPRINE	↑ risk of myelosuppression and immunosuppression. Deaths have occurred following profound myelosuppression and severe sepsis	Additive myelotoxic effects. Azathioprine is metabolized to 6-mercatopurine in vivo, which results in additive myelosuppression, immunosuppression and hepatotoxicity	Avoid co-administration
PLATINUM COMPOUNDS	CICLOSPORIN	↑ risk of renal toxicity and renal failure	Additive renal toxicity	Monitor renal function prior to and during therapy, and ensure an intake of at least 2 L of fluid daily. Monitor serum potassium and magnesium and correct any deficiencies
PLATINUM COMPOUNDS	RITUXIMAB	↑ risk of severe renal failure	Uncertain; possibly due to effects of tumour lysis syndrome (which is a result of a massive breakdown of cancer cells sensitive to chemotherapy). Features include hyperkalaemia, hyperuricaemia, hyperphosphataemia and hypocalcaemia	Monitor renal function closely. Hydrate with at least 2 L of fluid before, during and after therapy. Monitor potassium and magnesium levels in particular and correct deficits. Do an ECG as arrhythmias may accompany tumour lysis syndrome
PLATINUM COMPOUNDS	TACROLIMUS	↑ risk of renal toxicity and renal failure	Additive renal toxicity	Monitor renal function prior to and during therapy, and ensure an intake of at least 2 L of fluid daily. Monitor serum potassium and magnesium and correct any deficiencies
CARBOPLATIN	ANTICOAGULANTS – ORAL	Episodes of ↑ anticoagulant effect	Not understood but likely to be multifactorial	Monitor INR at least weekly until stable during administration of chemotherapy

Primary drug	Secondary drug	Effect	Mechanism	Precautions
PLATINUM COMPOUNDS	ANTIDIABETIC DRUGS – METFORMIN	↑ risk of lactic acidosis	↓ renal excretion of metformin	Watch for lactic acidosis. The onset of lactic acidosis is often subtle with symptoms, e.g. malaise, myalgia, respiratory distress and ↑ non-specific abdominal distress. There may be hypothermia and resistant bradyarrhythmias
PLATINUM COMPOUNDS	ANTIEPILEPTICS – CARBAMAZEPINE, PHENYTOIN, VALPROIC ACID	↓ plasma concentrations of antiepileptic, which ↑ risk of seizures	Due to impaired absorption of antiepileptic	Monitor closely for seizure activity and warn patients and carers. Need to adjust dosage using parameters such as blood levels to ensure therapeutic levels
PLATINUM COMPOUNDS	ANTIFUNGALS – AMPHOTERICIN	↑ risk of renal toxicity and renal failure	Additive renal toxicity	Monitor renal function prior to and during therapy, and ensure an intake of at least 2 L of fluid daily. Monitor serum potassium and magnesium and correct any deficiencies
PLATINUM COMPOUNDS	DIURETICS – LOOP	↑ risk of auditory toxic effects with cisplatin	Loop diuretics cause tinnitus and deafness as side-effects. Additive toxic effects on auditory system likely	Monitor hearing (auditory function) regularly, particularly if patients report symptoms such as tinnitus or impaired hearing

PORFIMER				
PORFIMER	1. ACE INHIBITORS – enalapril 2. ANALGESICS – celecoxib, ibuprofen, ketoprofen, naproxen 3. ANTIARRHYTHMICS – amiodarone 4. ANTIBIOTICS – ciprofloxacin, dapsone, sulphonamides, tetracyclines 5. ANTICANCER AND IMMUNOMODULATING DRUGS – fluorouracil (topical and oral) 6. ANTIDIABETIC DRUGS – glipizide 7. ANTIMALARIALS – hydroxychloroquine, quinine 8. ANTIPSYCHOTICS – chlorpromazine, fluphenazine 9. CALCIUM CHANNEL BLOCKERS – diltiazem 10. DIURETICS – bumetanide, furosemide, hydrochlorothiazide 11. PARA-AMINOBENZOIC ACID (TOPICAL) 12. RETINOIDS – acitretin, isotretinoin 13. SALICYLATES (TOPICAL)	↑ risk of photosensitivity reactions	Attributed to additive effects	Avoid exposure of skin and eyes to direct sunlight for 30 days after porfimer therapy

Primary drug	Secondary drug	Effect	Mechanism	Precautions
PROCARBAZINE				
PROCARBAZINE	ALCOHOL	May cause a disulfiram-like reaction, additive depression of the CNS and postural hypotension	Some alcoholic beverages (beer, wine, ale) contain tyramine, which may induce hypertensive reactions	Avoid co-administration
PROCARBAZINE	ANAESTHETICS – LOCAL			
PROCARBAZINE	COCAINE	Risk of severe hypertensive episodes	The metabolism of sympathomimetics is impaired due to inhibition of MAO	Cocaine should not be administered during or within 14 days following administration of an MAOI
PROCARBAZINE	LOCAL ANAESTHETICS WITH EPINEPHRINE	Risk of severe hypertension	Due to inhibition of MAO, which metabolizes epinephrine	No sympathomimetic should be administered to patients receiving drugs that inhibit one of the metabolizing enzymes, e.g. MAO
PROCARBAZINE	SPINAL ANAESTHETICS	Risk of hypotensive episodes	Uncertain	Recommendation is to discontinue procarbazine for at least 10 days before elective spinal anaesthesia
PROCARBAZINE	ANALGESICS – OPIOIDS	Unpredictable reactions may occur associated with hypotension and respiratory depression when procarbazine is co-administered with alfentanil, fentanyl, sufentanil or morphine	Opioids cause hypotension due to arterial and venous vasodilatation, negative inotropic effects and a vagally induced bradycardia. Procarbazine can cause postural hypotension. Also attributed to an accumulation of serotonin due to inhibition of MAO	Recommended that a small test dose (one-quarter of the usual dose) be administered in initially to assess the response

ANTICANCER AND IMMUNOMODULATING DRUGS CYTOTOXICS

PROCARBAZINE	ANTICANCER AND IMMUNOMODULATING DRUGS – METHOTREXATE	↑ risk of renal impairment if methotrexate infusion is given within 48 hours of procarbazine administration. Also ↑ risk of methotrexate toxicity, particularly to the kidneys	Procarbazine has a transient effect on the kidneys, and this will delay the renal elimination of methotrexate	Do not start methotrexate infusion less than 72 hours after the last dose of procarbazine. Hydrate patients aggressively (plenty of oral fluids or intravenous fluids), alkalinize the urine to pH>7 and closely monitor renal function, e.g. blood urea and creatinine, before and after methotrexate infusion until methotrexate blood levels are <0.05 μmol/L
PROCARBAZINE	ANTICOAGULANTS – ORAL	Episodes of ↑ anticoagulant effect	Not understood but likely to be multifactorial	Monitor INR at least weekly until stable during administration of chemotherapy
PROCARBAZINE	**ANTIDEPRESSANTS**			
PROCARBAZINE	MAOIs	Concurrent therapy ↑ risk of hypertensive crisis and severe seizures	Additive effect on inhibiting MAO	Concurrent treatment should not be started on an outpatient basis. 14 days should elapse before starting these medications after procarbazine treatment

ANTICANCER AND IMMUNOMODULATING DRUGS CYTOTOXICS

Primary drug	Secondary drug	Effect	Mechanism	Precautions
PROCARBAZINE	SSRIs	↑ risk of serotonin syndrome and CNS toxicity	Additive toxicity	Monitor BP closely and also CNS side-effects. Because of the long half-life of fluoxetine and its active metabolites, at least 5 weeks should elapse between discontinuation of fluoxetine and initiation of therapy with an MAOI
PROCARBAZINE	TRYPTOPHAN	Risk of hyperreflexia, shivering, hyperventilation, hyperthermia, mania or hypomania, disorientation/confusion	Tryptophan is a precursor of a number of neurotransmitters, including serotonin. Procarbazine has MAOI activity, which inhibits the breakdown of neurotransmitters	Tryptophan should be started under specialist supervision. Recommended to start with low doses and titrate upwards with close monitoring of mental status and BP
PROCARBAZINE	ANTIDIABETIC DRUGS – INSULIN, SULPHONYLUREAS	↑ risk of hypoglycaemic episodes	Procarbazine has mild MAOI properties. MAOIs have an intrinsic hypoglycaemic effect and are considered to enhance the effect of hypoglycaemic drugs	Watch for and warn patients about symptoms of hypoglycaemia ➢ ***For signs and symptoms of hypoglycaemia, see Clinical Features of Some Adverse Drug Interactions, Hypoglycaemia***
PROCARBAZINE	ANTIEPILEPTICS – CARBAMAZEPINE, PHENOBARBITAL, PHENYTOIN, VALPROIC ACID	↑ risk of hypersensitivity reactions in patients with brain tumours	Strong correlation between the therapeutic antiepileptic level and the hypersensitivity reactions	Consider using non-enzyme-inducing agents

PROCARBAZINE	ANTIHISTAMINES – ALIMEMAZINE (TRIMEPRAZINE), CHLORPHENIRAMINE, PROMETHAZINE	1. The antimuscarinic effects (dry mouth, urinary retention, blurred vision, gastrointestinal disturbances) are ↑, as are the sedating effects of these older antihistamines 2. Excessive sedation may occur	1. MAOIs cause anticholinergic effects (including antimuscarinic effects), hence additive effects of both antimuscarinic activity and CNS depression 2. Additive effects on CNS, although on occasions chlorpheniramine may cause CNS stimulation	1. Concurrent use is not recommended. If used together, patients should be warned to report any gastrointestinal problems as paralytic ileus has been reported. Also, caution is required when performing activities needing alertness (e.g. driving, using sharp objects). Do not use OTC medications such as nasal decongestants or asthma and allergy remedies without consulting the pharmacist/doctor as these preparations may contain antihistamines
PROCARBAZINE	ANTIPARKINSON'S DRUGS – BROMOCRIPTINE	May cause ↑ serum prolactin levels and interfere with the effects of bromocriptine	Uncertain	Watch for ↓ effect of bromocriptine
PROCARBAZINE	**ANTIPSYCHOTICS**			
PROCARBAZINE	CLOZAPINE	↑ risk of bone marrow toxicity	Additive effect	Avoid co-administration
PROCARBAZINE	FLUPENTIXOL, PIMOZIDE, ZUCLOPENTHIXOL	Prolongation or greater intensity of sedative, hypotensive and anticholinergic effects	Additive effect	Avoid co-administration
PROCARBAZINE	ANXIOLYTICS AND HYPNOTICS – BUSPIRONE	Risk of elevation of BP	Additive effect; buspirone acts at serotonin receptors; procarbazine inhibits breakdown of sympathomimetics	Avoid concurrent use

Primary drug	Secondary drug	Effect	Mechanism	Precautions
PROCARBAZINE	FOODS – TYRAMINE-CONTAINING – aged cheeses, aged pickle, smoked meats (e.g. salami), yeast extracts, beer (dark more than light and tap more than bottled), red wine more than white wine, avocado, sauerkraut, marmite, banana peel, soy bean products, broad bean pods, foods containing MSG	Risk of severe tyramine reactions – hypertension, occipital headaches, vomiting, palpitations, nausea, apprehension, chills, sweating. This reaction develops 20–60 minutes after ingestion of these foods	Tyramine has both direct and indirect sympathomimetic effects, and tyramine effects of foods may be potentiated by MAOIs 10–20-fold	Prompt treatment with phentolamine (0.5 mg intravenously) or nifedipine is effective, and death is rare (0.01–0.02%). There is a recommendation that a 25 mg tablet of chlorpromazine be given to patients on MAOIs to be taken if a tyramine reaction occurs
PROCARBAZINE	SYMPATHOMIMETICS	Co-administration of ephedrine, metaraminol, methylphenidate, phenylephrine or pseudoephedrine (including nasal and ophthalmic solutions) with procarbazine may cause prolongation and ↑ intensity of cardiac stimulant effects and effects on BP, which may cause headache, arrhythmias and hypertensive or hyperpyretic crises	The metabolism of sympathomimetics is impaired due to inhibition of MAO	It is recommended that sympathomimetics not be administered during and within 14 days of stopping procarbazine. Do not use any OTC nasal decongestants (sprays or oral preparations) or asthma relief agents without consulting the pharmacist/doctor
RALTITREXED				
RALTITREXED	FOLINATE	Theoretical risk of ↓ efficacy of raltitrexed	Folinate antagonizes the anti-DNA effect of raltitrexed	Be aware; watch for poor response to raltitrexed

SORAFENIB				
SORAFENIB	ANTICOAGULANTS – ORAL	Episodes of ↑ anticoagulant effect	Not understood but likely to be multifactorial	Monitor INR at least weekly until stable during administration of chemotherapy
SORAFENIB	ANTICANCER AND IMMUNOMODULATING DRUGS – DOXORUBICIN	Possible ↓ doxorubicin levels	Uncertain	Watch for poor response to doxorubicin
SUNITINIB				
SUNITINIB	ANTIBIOTICS – RIFAMPICIN	↓ sunitinib levels	Rifampicin ↑ metabolism of sunitinib	Avoid co-administration
TEGAFUR				
Tegafur is metabolized to fluorouracil ➢ ***Fluorouracil, above***				
TEMOPORFIN				
TEMOPORFIN	FLUOROURACIL	↑ risk of photosensitivity with topical fluorouracil	Uncertain; possibly additive effect (topical fluorouracil can cause local irritation, while temoporfin is a photosensitizer)	Patients on temoporfin are advised to avoid direct sunlight for at least 15 days
THIOTEPA				
THIOTEPA	DRUG DEPENDENCE THERAPIES – BUPROPION	↑ plasma concentrations of bupropion and risk of adverse effects	Inhibition of CYP2B6	Warn patients about adverse effects and use alternatives when possible
THIOTEPA	H2 RECEPTOR BLOCKERS – CIMETIDINE	↑ adverse effects of alkylating agent, e.g. myelosuppression	Additive toxicity	Monitor more closely; monitor FBC regularly
THIOTEPA	MUSCLE RELAXANTS – DEPOLARIZING	↑ efficacy of suxamethonium	Uncertain	Be aware of this effect

Primary drug	Secondary drug	Effect	Mechanism	Precautions
TIOGUANINE (THIOGUANINE)				
TIOGUANINE	ANTICANCER AND IMMUNOMODULATING DRUGS – BUSULFAN	↑ risk of hepatic nodular regenerative hyperplasia of the liver, oesophageal varices and portal hypertension	Mechanism is uncertain	Monitor liver function and for clinical and biochemical indices of liver toxicity, e.g. ascites, splenomegaly. Ask patients to report any symptoms suggestive of oesophageal bleeding
TOPOTECAN				
TOPOTECAN	ANTICANCER AND IMMUNOMODULATING DRUGS			
TOPOTECAN	CISPLATIN	↑ risk of bone marrow suppression, especially when topotecan is administered in doses >0.75 mg/m^2 on days 1–5 and cisplatin in doses >50 mg/m^2 on day 1 before topotecan	Attributed to cisplatin-induced subclinical renal toxicity possibly causing ↓ clearance of topotecan	Administer cisplatin on day 5 after topotecan if dose of topotecan is >0.75 mg/m^2 and cisplatin dose is >50 mg/m^2 with the use of granulocyte colony-stimulating factor
TOPOTECAN	DOCETAXEL	↑ risk of neutropenia when topotecan is administered on days 1–4 and docetaxel on day 4	Attributed to ↓ clearance of docetaxel (by 50%) due to inhibition of hepatic metabolism of docetaxel by CYP3A4 by topotecan	Administer docetaxel on day 1 and topotecan on day 1–4
TOPOTECAN	ANTIEPILEPTICS – PHENYTOIN	↓ efficacy of topotecan due to ↑ plasma concentrations of topotecan lactone and its metabolites by 1.5	Due to induction of further metabolism by hepatic CYP3A4 by phenytoin	↑ dose of topotecan to obtain desired therapeutic results

TRASTUZUMAB				
TRASTUZUMAB	**ANTICANCER AND IMMUNOMODULATING DRUGS**			
TRASTUZUMAB	CICLOSPORIN, SIROLIMUS	↑ neutropenic effect of immunosuppressants	Additive effects	Warn patients to report symptoms such as sore throat and fever ➢ ***For signs and symptoms of neutropenia, see Clinical Features of Some Adverse Drug Interactions, Immunosuppression and blood dyscrasias***
TRASTUZUMAB	CYCLOPHOSPHAMIDE, DAUNORUBICIN, IDARUBICIN, PACLITAXEL	↑ risk of cardiac toxicity	Possibly additive cardiac toxic effect	Monitor cardiac function closely – clinically and electrocardiographically. Avoid co-administration of trastuzumab with idarubicin except in clinical trials
TRASTUZUMAB	DOXORUBICIN	When used in combination, the risk of cardiotoxicity due to trastuzumab is ↑ over fourfold	Due to additive cardiotoxic effects	Avoid co-administration except in clinical trials
TREOSULFAN				
TREOSULFAN	H2 RECEPTOR BLOCKERS – CIMETIDINE	↑ adverse effects of alkylating agent, e.g. myelosuppression	Additive toxicity	Monitor more closely; monitor FBC regularly
TRETINOIN ➢ ***Other immunomodulating drugs, Retinoids below***				

Primary drug	Secondary drug	Effect	Mechanism	Precautions
VINCA ALKALOIDS				
VINCA ALKALOIDS	CYP3A4 INHIBITORS			
VINCA ALKALOIDS – VINBLASTINE, VINCRISTINE, VINORELBINE	1. ANTIBIOTICS – clarithromycin, erythromycin 2. ANTICANCER AND IMMUNOMODULATING DRUGS – imatinib 3. ANTIFUNGALS – fluconazole, itraconazole, ketoconazole, voriconazole (possibly posaconazole) 4. ANTIVIRALS – efavirenz, protease inhibitors 5. GRAPEFRUIT JUICE 6. H2 RECEPTOR BLOCKERS – cimetidine	↑ adverse effects of vinblastine and vincristine	Inhibition of CYP3A4-mediated metabolism. Also inhibition of P-gp efflux of vinblastine	Monitor FBC. Watch for early features of toxicity (pain, numbness, tingling in the fingers and toes, jaw pain, abdominal pain, constipation, ileus). Consider selecting an alternative drug
VINCA ALKALOIDS	CYP3A4 INDUCERS			
VINCA ALKALOIDS – VINBLASTINE, VINCRISTINE	1. ANTIBIOTICS – rifampicin 2. ANTICANCER AND IMMUNOMODULATING DRUGS – dexamethasone 3. ANTIDEPRESSANTS – St John's wort 4. ANTIEPILEPTICS – carbamazepine, phenobarbital, phenytoin	↓ of plasma concentrations of vinblastine and vincristine, with risk of inadequate therapeutic response. Reports of ↓ AUC by 40% and elimination half life by 35%, and ↑ clearance by 63%, in patients with brain tumours taking vincristine, which could lead to dangerously inadequate therapeutic responses	Due to induction of CYP3A4-mediated metabolism	Monitor for clinical efficacy, and ↑ dose of vinblastine and vincristine as clinically indicated; in the latter case, monitor clinically and radiologically for clinical efficacy in patients with brain tumours and ↑ dose to obtain desired response

VINCA ALKALOIDS	ANTICANCER AND IMMUNOMODULATING DRUGS			
VINCA ALKALOIDS	AZATHIOPRINE	↑ risk of myelosuppression and immunosuppression. Deaths have occurred following profound myelosuppression and severe sepsis	Additive myelotoxic effects Azathioprine is metabolized to 6-mercatopurine in vivo, which results in additive myelosuppression, immunosuppression and hepatotoxicity	Avoid co-administration
VINCRISTINE	CICLOSPORIN	High doses of ciclosporin (7.5–10 mg/kg per day intravenously) tend to ↑ plasma concentrations of vincristine and ↑ risk of neurotoxicity and musculoskeletal pain	Due to a combination, to varying degrees, of inhibition of CYP3A4 metabolism and P-gp inhibition. Vinblastine and vincristine are known substrates of P-gp	Monitor for neurotoxicity and myelosuppression. The dose-limiting effect of all is myelosuppression. Monitor blood counts and clinically watch for and ask patients to report infections
VINORELBINE	CISPLATIN	↑ incidence of grade III and grade IV granulocytopenia	Additive myelosuppressive effects	Monitor blood counts at least weekly and advise patients to report symptoms such as sore throat and fever
VINCRISTINE	CRISANTASPASE	↑ risk of neurotoxicity if concurrently administered or if crisantaspase is administered prior to vincristine	Uncertain but attributed by some to effects of asparaginase on the metabolism of vincristine	Administer vincristine prior to asparaginase

Primary drug	Secondary drug	Effect	Mechanism	Precautions
VINORELBINE	DOCETAXEL	Administration of docetaxel after vinorelbine ↑ plasma concentrations of vinorelbine, along with ↑ risk of neutropenia compared with giving docetaxel first	Docetaxel likely causes ↓ clearance of vinorelbine	Administer docetaxel first and follow with vinorelbine
VINBLASTINE	MITOMYCIN-C	↑ risk of abrupt onset of pulmonary toxicity in 3–6% of patients, when two courses of these drugs are administered concurrently	Mechanism is uncertain; possible additive pulmonary toxic effects	Monitor clinically and with lung function tests for pulmonary toxicity. Advise patients to report immediately symptoms such as shortness of breath and wheezing
VINBLASTINE, VINCRISTINE	PACLITAXEL	↓ therapeutic efficacy of paclitaxel	Antagonistic effects	Avoid co-administration
VINBLASTINE	ANTIDEPRESSANTS – TCAs	Possible ↑ plasma concentrations of vinblastine	Inhibition of CYP2D6-mediated metabolism of vinblastine. The clinical significance of this depends upon whether vinblastine's alternative pathways of metabolism are also inhibited by co-administered drugs	Warn patients to report ↑ side-effects of vinblastine, and monitor blood count carefully
VINCA ALKALOIDS	**ANTIVIRALS**			
VINCA ALKALOIDS	EFAVIRENZ	↑ efficacy and ↑ adverse effects of vinca alkaloids with efavirenz	Likely ↓ CYP3A4-mediated metabolism of vinca alkaloids	Use with caution. Monitor U&Es and FBC closely

VINCA ALKALOIDS	ZIDOVUDINE	↑ adverse effects when vincristine and possibly vinblastine are co-administered with zidovudine	Additive toxicity	Use with caution. Monitor FBC and renal function closely. ↓ doses as necessary
VINCA ALKALOIDS	CALCIUM CHANNEL BLOCKERS	1. ↑ risk of bone marrow depression, neurotoxicity and ileus due to ↑ plasma concentrations of vinblastine when co-administered with diltiazem, nifedipine or verapamil 2. Verapamil ↑ vincristine levels; no cases of toxicity have been reported 3. ↑ plasma concentrations of vinorelbine and ↑ risk of bone marrow and neurotoxicity when co-administered with diltiazem, nifedipine, or verapamil	1. Inhibition of CYP3A4-mediated metabolism of vinblastine and ↓ efflux of vinblastine due to inhibition of renal P-gp 2. ↓ clearance, but exact mechanism is not known 3. Due to inhibition of CYP3A4-mediated metabolism of vinorelbine by these calcium channel blockers	1. Avoid concurrent use of CYP3A4 inhibitors and P-gp efflux inhibitors with vinblastine. Select an alternative drug of the same group with ↓ effects on enzyme inhibition and P-gp inhibition 2. Watch for symptoms/signs of toxicity 3. Monitor for clinical efficacy and monitor FBCs and for neurotoxicity (pain, numbness, tingling in the fingers and toes, jaw pain, abdominal pain, constipation, ileus)
VINCRISTINE	COLONY-STIMULATING FACTORS – FILGRASTIM, SARGRAMOSTIM	A high incidence of severe atypical neuropathy (excruciating foot pain associated with marked motor weakness)	Synergistic neurotoxicity, which was related to the cumulative dose of vincristine and the number of doses given in cycle 1	A modification in administration of two doses given on day 1, and eight instead of three doses given on days 1, 8 and 15, in the cycle has been suggested to minimize neurotoxicity
VINBLASTINE, VINCRISTINE	GRAPEFRUIT JUICE	Possibly ↑ efficacy and ↑ adverse effects	Unclear. Vinblastine and vincristine appear to be metabolized via CYP3A4. P-gp interactions may also be involved	Monitor closely for signs of toxicity

Primary drug	Secondary drug	Effect	Mechanism	Precautions
HORMONES AND HORMONE ANTAGONISTS				
ANASTRAZOLE				
ANASTRAZOLE	ANTICOAGULANTS – WARFARIN	↑ anticoagulant effect	Uncertain; possibly inhibition of hepatic enzymes. Anastrazole is a known inhibitor of CYP1A2, CYP2C9 and CYP3A4	Monitor INR at least weekly until stable at initiation and discontinuation of concurrent therapy
ANASTRAZOLE	ANTIDIABETIC DRUGS – REPAGLINIDE	Risk of hypoglycaemia	Mechanism unknown	Watch for hypoglycaemia. Warn patients about hypoglycaemia ➢ ***For signs and symptoms of hypoglycaemia, see Clinical Features of Some Adverse Drug Interactions, Hypoglycaemia***
BICALUTAMIDE				
BICALUTAMIDE	ANTICOAGULANTS – WARFARIN	↑ plasma concentrations of warfarin	Bicalutamide displaces warfarin from protein-binding sites	Monitor INR at least weekly until stable at initiation and discontinuation of concurrent therapy
FLUTAMIDE				
FLUTAMIDE	ANTICOAGULANTS – WARFARIN	↑ anticoagulant effect	Uncertain; possibly inhibition of hepatic enzymes	Monitor INR at least weekly until stable at initiation and discontinuation of concurrent therapy
LANREOTIDE				
LANREOTIDE	ANTICANCER AND IMMUNOMODULATING DRUGS – CICLOSPORIN	↓ plasma concentrations of ciclosporin and risk of transplant rejection	Lanreotide possibly induces CYP3A4-mediated metabolism of ciclosporin	Avoid co-administration if possible; if not, monitor ciclosporin levels closely

LANREOTIDE	ANTIDIABETIC DRUGS	Likely to alter hypoglycaemic agent requirements	Octreotide and lanreotide suppress pancreatic insulin and counter-regulatory hormones (glucagon, growth hormone), and delay or ↓ absorption of glucose from the intestine	Essential to monitor blood sugar at least twice a week after initiating concurrent treatment until blood sugar levels are stable. Advise self-monitoring, and warn patients about hypoglycaemia ➣ ***For signs and symptoms of hypoglycaemia, see Clinical Features of Some Adverse Drug Interactions, Hypoglycaemia***
LETROZOLE				
LETROZOLE	TAMOXIFEN	↓ plasma concentrations of letrozole (by approximately 40%) and ↓ efficacy of letrozole	Attributed to induction of enzymes metabolizing letrozole by tamoxifen	Avoid concurrent use outside clinical trials
OCTREOTIDE				
OCTREOTIDE	ANTICANCER AND IMMUNOMODULATING DRUGS – CICLOSPORIN	↓ plasma concentrations of ciclosporin and risk of transplant rejection	Octreotide is a strong inducer of CYP3A4-mediated metabolism of ciclosporin	Avoid co-administration if possible; if not, monitor ciclosporin levels closely
OCTREOTIDE	ANTIDIABETIC DRUGS	Likely to alter hypoglycaemic agent requirements	Octreotide and lanreotide suppress pancreatic insulin and counter-regulatory hormones (glucagon, growth hormone), and delay or ↓ absorption of glucose from the intestine	Essential to monitor blood sugar at least twice a week after initiating concurrent treatment until blood sugar levels are stable. Advice self monitoring. Warn patients re hypoglycaemia ➣ ***For signs and symptoms of hypoglycaemia, see Clinical Features of Some Adverse Drug Interactions, Hypoglycaemia***
OCTREOTIDE	ANTIPARKINSON'S DRUGS – BROMOCRIPTINE	↑ bromocriptine levels	Uncertain	Be aware

Primary drug	Secondary drug	Effect	Mechanism	Precautions
TAMOXIFEN				
TAMOXIFEN	ANTIBIOTICS – RIFAMPICIN	↓ plasma concentrations of tamoxifen and risk of inadequate therapeutic response	Due to induction of metabolism of tamoxifen by the CYP3A isoenzymes by rifampicin	Avoid concurrent use if possible. Otherwise monitor for clinical efficacy of tamoxifen by ↑ dose of tamoxifen
TAMOXIFEN	**ANTICANCER AND IMMUNOMODULATING DRUGS**			
TAMOXIFEN	CYTOTOXICS – MITOMYCIN	↑ incidence of anaemia and thrombocytopenia and risk of haemolytic–uraemic syndrome	Mitomycin causes subclinical endothelial damage in addition to the thrombotic effect on platelets caused by tamoxifen, which leads to the haemolytic–uraemic syndrome	Monitor renal function at least twice weekly during concurrent therapy and clinically watch for bleeding episodes, e.g. nose bleeds, bleeding from gums, skin bruising
TAMOXIFEN	HORMONES AND HORMONE ANTAGONISTS – LETROZOLE	↓ plasma concentrations of letrozole (by approximately 40%) and ↓ efficacy of letrozole	Attributed to induction of enzymes metabolizing letrozole by tamoxifen	Avoid concurrent use outside clinical trials
TAMOXIFEN	**IMMUNOMODULATING DRUGS**			
TAMOXIFEN	AZATHIOPRINE	↑ risk of myelosuppression and immunosuppression. Deaths have occurred following profound myelosuppression and severe sepsis	Additive myelotoxic effects Azathioprine is metabolized to 6-mercatopurine in vivo, which results in additive myelosuppression, immunosuppression and hepatotoxicity	Avoid co-administration
TAMOXIFEN	CICLOSPORIN	↑ plasma concentrations of ciclosporin, with risk of toxic effects	Competitive inhibition of CYP3A4-mediated metabolism and P-gp transport of these drugs	Watch for toxic effects of ciclosporin
TAMOXIFEN	CORTICOSTEROIDS	↓ plasma concentrations of tamoxifen and risk of inadequate therapeutic response	Due to induction of metabolism of tamoxifen by the CYP3A isoenzymes by dexamethasone	Avoid concurrent use if possible. Otherwise monitor for clinical efficacy of tamoxifen by ↑ dose of tamoxifen

TAMOXIFEN	ANTICOAGULANTS – WARFARIN	↑ anticoagulant effect	Uncertain; possibly inhibition of hepatic enzymes. Tamoxifen inhibits CYP3A4	Monitor INR at least weekly until stable at initiation and discontinuation of concurrent therapy
TAMOXIFEN	ANTIDEPRESSANTS – ST JOHN'S WORT	↓ plasma concentrations of tamoxifen and risk of inadequate therapeutic response	Due to induction of metabolism of tamoxifen by the CYP3A isoenzymes by St John's wort	Avoid concurrent use
TAMOXIFEN	ANTIEPILEPTICS – CARBAMAZEPINE, PHENYTOIN, PHENOBARBITAL	↓ plasma concentrations of tamoxifen and risk of inadequate therapeutic response	Due to induction of metabolism of tamoxifen by the CYP3A isoenzymes by phenytoin	Avoid concurrent use if possible. Otherwise monitor for clinical efficacy of tamoxifen by ↑ dose of tamoxifen
TAMOXIFEN	CNS STIMULANTS – MODAFINIL	May cause ↑ plasma concentrations of these substrates if CYP2C9 is the predominant metabolic pathway and the alternative pathways are either genetically deficient or affected	Modafinil is a moderate inhibitor of CYP2C9	Be aware
TOREMIFENE				
TOREMIFENE	ANTIBIOTICS – MACROLIDES	↑ plasma concentrations of toremifene with clarithromycin and erythromycin	Due to inhibition of metabolism of toremifene by the CYP3A4 isoenzymes by clarithromycin	Clinical relevance is uncertain. Necessary to monitor for clinical toxicities
TOREMIFENE	ANTICOAGULANTS – WARFARIN	↑ anticoagulant effect	Uncertain; possibly inhibition of hepatic enzymes	Monitor INR at least weekly until stable at initiation and discontinuation of concurrent therapy
TOREMIFENE	ANTIEPILEPTICS – BARBITURATES, CARBAMAZEPINE, PHENYTOIN	↓ plasma concentrations of toremifene	Due to induction of metabolism of toremifene	Watch for poor response to toremifene

Primary drug	Secondary drug	Effect	Mechanism	Precautions
TOREMIFENE	ANTIFUNGALS – AZOLES	↑ plasma concentrations of toremifene	Due to inhibition of metabolism of toremifene by the CYP3A4 isoenzymes by ketoconazole	Clinical relevance is uncertain. Necessary to monitor for clinical toxicities
TOREMIFENE	**ANTIVIRALS**			
TOREMIFENE	NNRTIs – EFAVIRENZ	↑ plasma concentrations of toremifene	Due to inhibition of metabolism of toremifene by the CYP3A4 isoenzymes by efavirenz	Clinical relevance is uncertain. Necessary to monitor for clinical toxicities
TOREMIFENE	PROTEASE INHIBITORS – RITONAVIR	↑ plasma concentrations of toremifene	Due to inhibition of metabolism of toremifene by the CYP3A4 isoenzymes by ritonavir	Clinical relevance is uncertain. Necessary to monitor for clinical toxicities
TOREMIFENE	CALCIUM CHANNEL BLOCKERS	↑ plasma concentrations of toremifene when co-administered with diltiazem, nifedipine or verapamil	Due to inhibition of CYP3A4-mediated metabolism of toremifene	Clinical relevance is uncertain. Necessary to monitor for clinical toxicities
TOREMIFENE	DIURETICS – THIAZIDES	Risk of hypercalcaemia	Additive effect	Monitor calcium levels closely. Warn patients about the symptoms of hypercalcaemia
TOREMIFENE	GRAPEFRUIT JUICE	↑ plasma concentrations of toremifene	Due to inhibition of metabolism of toremifene by the CYP3A4 isoenzymes by grapefruit juice	Clinical relevance is uncertain. Necessary to monitor for clinical toxicities
TOREMIFENE	H2 RECEPTOR BLOCKERS – CIMETIDINE	↑ plasma concentrations of toremifene	Due to inhibition of metabolism of toremifene by the CYP3A4 isoenzymes by cimetidine	Clinical relevance is uncertain. Necessary to monitor for clinical toxicities
OTHER IMMUNOMODULATING DRUGS				
ALL	VACCINES – LIVE	Risk of contracting disease from the vaccine	↓ immunity	Avoid live vaccines for at least 3 months after completing immunomodulating therapy
ACITRETIN ➢ *Other immunomodulating drugs, Retinoids below*				

ADALIMUMAB				
ADALIMUMAB	ANAKINRA	↑ risk of bone marrow suppression	Additive effect	Avoid co-administration
ALDESLEUKIN ➢ *Other immunomodulating drugs, Interleukin-2, below*				
AMINOSALICYLATES				
AMINOSALICYLATES	ANTICANCER AND IMMUNOMODULATING DRUGS			
AMINOSALICYLATES	CYTOTOXICS			
AMINOSALICYLATES	MERCAPTOPURINE	↑ risk of bone marrow suppression	Additive effect	Monitor FBC closely
AMINOSALICYLATES	METHOTREXATE	↑ risk of hepatotoxicity with sulfasalazine	Additive hepatotoxic effects. Sulfasalazine competes with methotrexate for renal elimination	Monitor closely for symptoms of liver failure. Check LFTs at beginning of treatment and then weekly until stable, and repeat if there is clinical suspicion of liver disease
SALICYLATES – TOPICAL	PORFIMER	↑ risk of photosensitivity reactions when porfimer is co-administered with hydrochlorothiazide	Attributed to additive effects	Avoid exposure of skin and eyes to direct sunlight for 30 days after porfimer therapy
AMINOSALICYLATES	IMMUNOMODULATING DRUGS			
AMINOSALICYLATES	AZATHIOPRINE	↑ blood levels of azathioprine and ↑ risk of side-effects	Due to inhibition of metabolism of purines by these aminosalicylates.	Monitor FBC closely
AMINOSALICYLATES	ANTIGOUT DRUGS – PROBENECID	Aminosalicylate levels ↑ by probenecid	Probenecid competes with aminosalicylate for active renal excretion	Watch for early features of toxicity of aminosalicylate. Consider ↓ dose of aminosalicylate
AMINOSALICYLATES	CARDIAC GLYCOSIDES – DIGOXIN	Sulfasalazine may ↓ digoxin levels. The manufacturers of balsalazide also warn against the possibility of this interaction despite of a lack of case reports	Uncertain at present	Watch for poor response to digoxin; check levels if signs of ↓ effect
AMINOSALICYLATES	FOLIC ACID	Possibly ↓ folic acid levels	Uncertain	Monitor FBC closely

Primary drug	Secondary drug	Effect	Mechanism	Precautions
ANAKINRA				
ANAKINRA				
ANAKINRA	ANTICANCER AND IMMUNOMODULATING DRUGS – ADALIMUMAB, ETANERCEPT, INFLIXIMAB	↑ risk of bone marrow suppression	Additive effect	Avoid co-administration
AZATHIOPRINE/MERCAPTOPURINE				
AZATHIOPRINE	ACE INHIBITORS	Risk of anaemia with captopril and enalapril, and leukopenia with captopril	Exact mechanism is uncertain. Azathioprine-induced impairment of haematopoiesis and ACE inhibitor induced ↓ in erythropoietin may cause additive effects. Enalapril has been used to treat post-renal transplant erythrocytosis	Monitor blood counts regularly
AZATHIOPRINE	ANTIBIOTICS – CO-TRIMOXAZOLE	↑ risk of leukopenia	Additive effects, as co-trimoxazole inhibits white cell production	Caution ➢ ***For signs and symptoms of leukopenia, see Clinical Features of Some Adverse Drug Interactions, Immunosuppression and blood dyscrasias***

ANTICANCER AND IMMUNOMODULATING DRUGS

AZATHIOPRINE	ANTICANCER AND IMMUNOMODULATING DRUGS			
AZATHIOPRINE	**CYTOTOXICS**			
AZATHIOPRINE	CHLORAMBUCIL, CISPLATIN, CYCLOPHOSPHAMIDE, CYTARABINE, DACTINOMYCIN (ACTINOMYCIN D), DAUNORUBICIN, DOCETAXEL, DOXORUBICIN, ETOPOSIDE, FLUOROURACIL, MELPHALAN, MERCAPTOPURINE, MITOXANTRONE, VINCA ALKALOIDS	↑ risk of myelosuppression and immunosuppression. Deaths have occurred following profound myelosuppression and severe sepsis	Additive myelotoxic effects. Azathioprine is metabolized to 6-mercatopurine in vivo, which results in additive myelosuppression, immunosuppression and hepatotoxicity	Avoid co-administration
AZATHIOPRINE	METHOTREXATE	↑ risk of hepatotoxicity	Additive hepatotoxic effects	Monitor closely for symptoms of liver failure, e.g. flu-like symptoms, abdominal pain, dark urine, pruritus, jaundice, ascites and weight gain. Do LFTs at the beginning of treatment and weekly until stable, and repeat if there is clinical suspicion of liver disease
AZATHIOPRINE	**HORMONES AND HORMONE ANTAGONISTS**			
AZATHIOPRINE	TAMOXIFEN	↑ risk of myelosuppression and immunosuppression. Deaths have occurred following profound myelosuppression and severe sepsis	Additive myelotoxic effects Azathioprine is metabolized to 6-mercatopurine in vivo, which results in additive myelosuppression, immunosuppression and hepatotoxicity	Avoid co-administration

Primary drug	Secondary drug	Effect	Mechanism	Precautions
AZATHIOPRINE	**IMMUNOMODULATING DRUGS**			
AZATHIOPRINE	AMINOSALICYLATES	↑ blood levels of azathioprine and ↑ risk of side-effects	Due to inhibition of metabolism of purines by these aminosalicylates	Monitor FBC closely
AZATHIOPRINE	LEFLUNOMIDE	↑ risk of serious infections (sepsis) and of opportunistic infections (*Pneumocystis jiroveci* pneumonia, tuberculosis, aspergillosis)	Additive immunosuppression	Monitor platelets, white bloods cell, haemoglobin and haematocrit at baseline and regularly – weekly, during concomitant therapy. With evidence of bone marrow suppression, discontinue leflunomide and administer colestyramine or charcoal to ↑ elimination of leflunomide ➢ ***For signs and symptoms of immunosuppression, see Clinical Features of Some Adverse Drug Interactions, Immunosuppression and blood dyscrasias***
AZATHIOPRINE	NATALIZUMAB	↑ risk of myelosuppression and immunosuppression. Deaths have occurred following profound myelosuppression and severe sepsis	Additive myelotoxic effects Azathioprine is metabolized to 6-mercatopurine in vivo, which results in additive myelosuppression, immunosuppression and hepatotoxicity	Avoid co-administration
AZATHIOPRINE	ANTICOAGULANTS – WARFARIN	Possible ↓ anticoagulant effect	Induction of metabolism of warfarin	Monitor INR closely
AZATHIOPRINE	ANTIGOUT DRUGS – ALLOPURINOL	↑ mercaptopurine levels, with risk of toxicity (e.g. myelosuppression, pancreatitis)	Azathioprine is metabolized to mercaptopurine. Allopurinol inhibits hepatic metabolism of mercaptopurine	↓ doses of azathioprine and mercaptopurine by up to three-quarters and monitor FBC, LFTs and amylase carefully

AZATHIOPRINE	ANTIVIRALS – LAMIVUDINE	↑ adverse effects with lamivudine	Unclear	Monitor closely
AZATHIOPRINE	VACCINES	↓ effectiveness of vaccines. ↑ risk of adverse/toxic effects of live vaccines (e.g. measles, mumps, rubella, oral polio, BCG, yellow fever, varicella, TY21a typhoid), e.g. vaccinal infections	Disseminated infection due to enhanced replication of vaccine virus in the presence of diminished immunocompetence	Do not vaccinate when patients are on immunosuppressants. Vaccination should be deferred for at least 3 months after discontinuing immunosuppressants/myelosuppressants. If an individual has been recently vaccinated, do not initiate therapy for at least 2 weeks after vaccination
BALSALAZIDE ➢ *Other immunomodulating drugs, Aminosalicylates, above*				
CICLOSPORIN				
CICLOSPORIN	ALISKIREN	Likely to ↑ plasma concentrations of aliskiren	Uncertain	Avoid co-administration
CICLOSPORIN	ANALGESICS – NSAIDs	1. ↑ risk of renal failure with NSAIDs 2. Diclofenac levels ↑ by ciclosporin 3. Rofecoxib ↓ plasma concentrations of ciclosporin, with risk of transplant rejection	1. Additive effect; both can cause renal insufficiency 2. Uncertain 3. Rofecoxib is a mild inducer of CYP3A4 and not a substrate of CYP3A4	1. Monitor renal function closely 2. Halve dose of diclofenac 3. Be aware. May not be clinically significant
CICLOSPORIN	**ANTIARRHYTHMICS**			
CICLOSPORIN	AMIODARONE	Ciclosporin levels may be ↑ by amiodarone; risk of nephrotoxicity	Uncertain; ciclosporin is metabolized by CYP3A4, which is markedly inhibited by amiodarone. Amiodarone also interferes with the renal elimination of ciclosporin and inhibits intestinal P-gp, which may ↑ bioavailability of ciclosporin	Monitor renal function closely; consider ↓ dose of ciclosporin when co-administering amiodarone
CICLOSPORIN	PROPAFENONE	Possible ↑ ciclosporin levels	Uncertain	Watch for signs of ciclosporin toxicity

Primary drug	Secondary drug	Effect	Mechanism	Precautions
CICLOSPORIN	**ANTIBIOTICS**			
CICLOSPORIN	AMINOGLYCOSIDES, COLISTIN	↑ risk of nephrotoxicity	Additive nephrotoxic effects	Monitor renal function
CICLOSPORIN	CO-TRIMOXAZOLE	Exacerbates hyperkalaemia induced by ciclosporin	Additive effect	Monitor serum potassium levels during co-administration ➢ ***For signs and symptoms of hyperkalaemia, see Clinical Features of Some Adverse Drug Interactions, Hyperkalaemia***
CICLOSPORIN	DAPTOMYCIN	Risk of myopathy	Additive effect	Avoid co-administration
CICLOSPORIN	MACROLIDES – CLARITHROMYCIN, ERYTHROMYCIN, TELITHROMYCIN	↑ plasma concentrations of ciclosporin, with risk of nephrotoxicity, myelosuppression, neurotoxicity, excessive immunosuppression, with risk of infection and post-transplant lymphoproliferative disease	Inhibition of CYP3A4-mediated metabolism of ciclosporin; these inhibitors vary in potency. Clarithromycin and telithromycin are classified as potent inhibitors	Avoid co-administration with clarithromycin and telithromycin. Consider alternative antibiotics but need to monitor plasma ciclosporin levels to prevent toxicity
CICLOSPORIN	**QUINOLONES**			
CICLOSPORIN	CIPROFLOXACIN	Ciprofloxacin may ↓ immunosuppressive effect (pharmacodynamic interaction)	Ciprofloxacin ↓ inhibitory effect of ciclosporin on IL-2 production to ↓ immunosuppressive effect	Avoid co-administration
CICLOSPORIN	NORFLOXACIN	↑ plasma concentrations of ciclosporin, with risk of nephrotoxicity, myelosuppression, neurotoxicity, excessive immunosuppression, with risk of infection and post-transplant lymphoproliferative disease	Inhibition of CYP3A4-mediated metabolism of ciclosporin; these inhibitors vary in potency	Monitor plasma ciclosporin levels to prevent toxicity. Monitor renal function

CICLOSPORIN	QUINUPRISTIN/ DALFOPRISTIN	↑ plasma concentrations of immunosuppressants. ↑ risk of infections and toxic effects of ciclosporin	Due to inhibition of CYP3A4-mediated metabolism of ciclosporin	Monitor renal function prior to concurrent therapy, and blood count and ciclosporin levels during therapy. Warn patients to report symptoms (fever, sore throat) immediately
CICLOSPORIN	RAPAMYCIN	↓ plasma concentrations of ciclosporin, with risk of transplant rejection	Due to induction of CYP3A4-mediated metabolism of ciclosporin by these drugs. The potency of induction varies	Monitor for signs of rejection of transplants. Monitor ciclosporin levels to ensure adequate therapeutic concentrations and ↑ dose when necessary
CICLOSPORIN	TETRACYCLINES – DOXYCYCLINE	↑ levels of ciclosporin leading to risk of nephrotoxicity, hepatotoxicity and possible neurotoxicity such as hallucinations, convulsions and coma	The mechanism is not known, but doxycycline is thought to ↑ ciclosporin levels	Concomitant use in transplant patients should be well monitored, with frequent ciclosporin levels. In non-transplant patients, renal function should be monitored closely and patients warned about potential side-effects such as back pain, flushing and gastrointestinal upset. The dose of ciclosporin should be ↓ appropriately
CICLOSPORIN	VANCOMYCIN	Risk of renal toxicity	Additive effect	Monitor renal function closely
CICLOSPORIN	**ANTICANCER AND IMMUNOMODULATING DRUGS**			
CICLOSPORIN	**CYTOTOXICS**			
CICLOSPORIN	CISPLATIN	↑ risk of renal toxicity and renal failure	Additive renal toxicity	Monitor renal function prior to and during therapy, and ensure an intake of at least 2 L of fluid daily. Monitor serum potassium and magnesium and correct any deficiencies
CICLOSPORIN	DOCETAXEL	↑ plasma concentrations of these drugs, with risk of toxic effects	Competitive inhibition of CYP3A4-mediated metabolism and P-gp transport of these drugs	Watch for toxic effects of these drugs

Primary drug	Secondary drug	Effect	Mechanism	Precautions
CICLOSPORIN	DOXORUBICIN	High doses of ciclosporin ↑ AUC of doxorubicin by 48% and of a metabolite by 443%. Risk of severe myelosuppression and neurotoxicity	Ciclosporin inhibits P-gp and cytochrome P450, which results in ↓ clearance of doxorubicin	Advise patients to report symptoms such as sore throat, fever, bleeding and bruising ➢ ***For signs and symptoms of immunosuppression, see Clinical Features of Some Adverse Drug Interactions, Immunosuppression and blood dyscrasias***
CICLOSPORIN	ETOPOSIDE	↑ plasma concentrations of these drugs, with risk of toxic effects	Competitive inhibition of CYP3A4-mediated metabolism and P-gp transport of these drugs	Watch for toxic effects of these drugs
CICLOSPORIN	IMATINIB	↑ plasma concentrations of ciclosporin, with risk of nephrotoxicity, myelosuppression, neurotoxicity, excessive immunosuppression, with risk of infection and post-transplant lymphoproliferative disease	Inhibition of metabolism of ciclosporin	Monitor plasma ciclosporin levels to prevent toxicity
CICLOSPORIN	MELPHALAN	Risk of renal toxicity	Additive effect	Monitor U&Es closely
CICLOSPORIN	METHOTREXATE	↑ risk of renal toxicity and renal failure	Additive renal toxicity	Monitor renal function prior to and during therapy, and ensure and intake of at least 2 L of fluid daily. Monitor serum potassium and magnesium and correct any deficiencies
CICLOSPORIN	MITOXANTRONE	High-dose ciclosporin (leading to levels of ciclosporin from 3000 to 5000 ng/mL) ↑ plasma concentrations of mitoxantrone	Due to inhibition by ciclosporin of P-gp leading to ↓ clearance (by >40%) and ↑ terminal half-life (>50%)	↓ dose of mitoxantrone of 40% has been recommended in paediatric patients. Advisable to monitor mitoxantrone levels

CICLOSPORIN	PACLITAXEL	↑ plasma concentrations of these drugs, with risk of toxic effects	Competitive inhibition of CYP3A4-mediated metabolism and P-gp transport of these drugs	Watch for toxic effects of these drugs
CICLOSPORIN	TRASTUZUMAB	↑ neutropenic effect of immunosuppressants	Additive effects	Warn patients to report symptoms such as sore throat and fever ➢ ***For signs and symptoms of neutropenia, see Clinical Features of Some Adverse Drug Interactions, Immunosuppression and blood dyscrasias***
CICLOSPORIN	VINCA ALKALOIDS	High doses of ciclosporin (7.5–10 mg/kg per day intravenously) ↑ plasma concentrations of vincristine. The predominant toxic effect of vincristine is peripheral neuropathy, and of the others, myelosuppression	Due to a combination, to varying degrees, of inhibition of CYP3A4 metabolism and P-gp inhibition. Vinblastine and vincristine are known substrates of P-gp	Monitor for neurotoxicity and myelosuppression. The dose-limiting effect of all vinca alkaloids is myelosuppression. Monitor blood counts and clinically watch for and ask patients to report infections
CICLOSPORIN	**HORMONES AND HORMONE ANTAGONISTS**			
CICLOSPORIN	LANREOTIDE, OCTREOTIDE	↓ plasma concentrations of ciclosporin and risk of transplant rejection	Octreotide is a strong inducer of CYP3A4-mediated metabolism of ciclosporin	Avoid co-administration if possible; if not, monitor ciclosporin levels closely
CICLOSPORIN	TAMOXIFEN	↑ plasma concentrations of ciclosporin, with risk of toxic effects	Competitive inhibition of CYP3A4-mediated metabolism and P-gp transport of these drugs	Watch for toxic effects of ciclosporin
CICLOSPORIN	**IMMUNOMODULATING DRUGS**			
CICLOSPORIN	CORTICOSTEROIDS	↓ plasma concentrations of ciclosporin, with risk of transplant rejection	Due to induction of metabolism of ciclosporin by these drugs. The potency of induction varies	Monitor for signs of rejection of transplants. Monitor ciclosporin levels to ensure adequate therapeutic concentrations and ↑ dose when necessary

Primary drug	Secondary drug	Effect	Mechanism	Precautions
CICLOSPORIN	LEFLUNOMIDE	↑ risk of serious infections (sepsis) and of opportunistic infections (*Pneumocystis jiroveci* pneumonia, tuberculosis, aspergillosis)	Additive immunosuppression	Monitor platelets, white blood cells, haemoglobin and haematocrit at baseline and regularly – weekly – during concomitant therapy. With evidence of bone marrow suppression, discontinue leflunomide and administer colestyramine and charcoal to ↑ elimination of leflunomide ➢ ***For signs and symptoms of immunosuppression, see Clinical Features of Some Adverse Drug Interactions, Immunosuppression and blood dyscrasias***
CICLOSPORIN	MYCOPHENOLATE	↓ plasma concentrations of mycophenolate and of the active metabolite mycophenolic acid	Ciclosporin is thought to interrupt the enterohepatic circulation of mycophenolate by inhibiting MRP-2 in the biliary tract, which prevents the excretion of its glucuronide	Watch for poor response to mycophenolate if ciclosporin is added; conversely, watch for early features of toxicity if ciclosporin is stopped
CICLOSPORIN	NATALIZUMAB	↑ risk of adverse effects of natalizumab and ↑ risk of concurrent infections	Additive effect	Monitor FBC closely. Warn patient to report early features suggestive of infection
CICLOSPORIN	SIROLIMUS	↑ bioavailability of sirolimus (30–40% when drug administrations are separated by 4 hours and 100% when administered together)	Due to inhibition of P-gp by ciclosporin and competition for metabolism by CYP3A4	Be aware of toxic effects of sirolimus and monitor blood levels
CICLOSPORIN	TACROLIMUS	↑ plasma concentrations of ciclosporin	Tacrolimus is probably a more powerful inhibitor of CYP3A4 than ciclosporin	Avoid co-administration

ANTICANCER AND IMMUNOMODULATING DRUGS

CICLOSPORIN	ANTICOAGULANTS – ORAL	1. ↓ ciclosporin levels when co-administered with warfarin or acenocoumarol 2. ↓ anticoagulant effect with warfarin and variable effect with acenocoumarol	Competitive metabolism by CYP3A4	1. Watch for ↓ efficacy of ciclosporin 2. Monitor INR at least weekly until stable
CICLOSPORIN	**ANTIDEPRESSANTS**			
CICLOSPORIN	ST JOHN'S WORT	↓ plasma concentrations of ciclosporin, with risk of transplant rejection	Due to induction of metabolism of ciclosporin by these drugs. The potency of induction varies. St John's wort may produce its effects due to an effect on P-gp	Avoid co-administration
CICLOSPORIN	SSRIs – FLUOXETINE	↑ plasma concentrations of ciclosporin, with risk of nephro-toxicity, myelosuppression, and neurotoxicity	Inhibition of CYP3A4-mediated metabolism of ciclosporin; these inhibitors vary in potency	Monitor plasma ciclosporin levels to prevent toxicity
CICLOSPORIN	**ANTIDIABETIC DRUGS**			
CICLOSPORIN	REPAGLINIDE	↑ plasma concentrations of repaglinide	Hepatic metabolism inhibited	Watch for hypoglycaemia ➢ ***For signs and symptoms of hypoglycaemia, see Clinical Features of Some Adverse Drug Interactions, Hypoglycaemia***
CICLOSPORIN	SULPHONYLUREAS – GLIPIZIDE	May ↑ plasma concentrations of ciclosporin	Glipizide inhibits CYP3A4-mediated metabolism of ciclosporin	Monitor plasma ciclosporin levels to prevent toxicity
CICLOSPORIN	ANTIEPILEPTICS – BARBITURATES, CARBAMAZEPINE, PHENYTOIN	↓ plasma concentrations of ciclosporin, with risk of transplant rejection	Due to induction of metabolism of ciclosporin by these drugs. The potency of induction varies	Monitor for signs of rejection of transplants. Monitor ciclosporin levels to ensure adequate therapeutic concentrations and ↑ dose when necessary

Primary drug	Secondary drug	Effect	Mechanism	Precautions
CICLOSPORIN	**ANTIFUNGALS**			
CICLOSPORIN	AMPHOTERICIN	↑ risk of nephrotoxicity	Additive nephrotoxic effects	Monitor renal function
CICLOSPORIN	AZOLES – ITRACONAZOLE, KETOCONAZOLE, VORICONAZOLE	↑ plasma concentrations of ciclosporin, with risk of nephrotoxicity, myelosuppression, neurotoxicity, excessive immunosuppression, with risk of infection and post-transplant lymphoproliferative disease	Inhibition of CYP3A4-mediated metabolism of ciclosporin; these inhibitors vary in potency. Ketoconazole and itraconazole are classified as potent inhibitors. Effect not clinically relevant with fluconazole	Avoid co-administration with itraconazole or ketoconazole. Consider alternative azole but need to monitor plasma ciclosporin levels to prevent toxicity
CICLOSPORIN	CASPOFUNGIN	1. ↓ plasma concentrations of ciclosporin, with risk of transplant rejection 2. Enhanced toxic effects of caspofungin and ↑ alanine transaminase levels	1. Due to induction of metabolism of ciclosporin by these drugs. The potency of induction varies 2. Uncertain	1. Monitor for signs of rejection of transplants. Monitor ciclosporin levels to ensure adequate therapeutic concentrations and ↑ dose when necessary 2. Monitor LFTs
CICLOSPORIN	GRISEOFULVIN	↓ plasma concentrations of ciclosporin (may be as much as 40%) and risk of rejection in patients who have received transplants	Induction of ciclosporin metabolism	Monitor ciclosporin levels closely
CICLOSPORIN	**ANTIGOUT DRUGS**			
CICLOSPORIN	ALLOPURINOL	Ciclosporin levels may be ↑	Uncertain	Monitor renal function closely
CICLOSPORIN	COLCHICINE	↑ colchicine plasma concentrations and ↑ toxic effects (hepatotoxicity, myopathy). ↑ penetration of ciclosporin through blood–brain barrier and ↑ risk of neurotoxicity	Competitive inhibition of P-gp with ↑ penetrations of ciclosporin to the tissues. Ciclosporin inhibits the transport of colchicine	Avoid co-administration
CICLOSPORIN	SULFINPYRAZONE	Cases of ↓ ciclosporin levels with transplant rejection	Uncertain	Watch for ↓ efficacy of ciclosporin

CICLOSPORIN	ANTIHYPERTENSIVE AND HEART FAILURE DRUGS			
CICLOSPORIN	ACE INHIBITORS, ANGIOTENSIN – II RECEPTOR ANTAGONISTS	↑ risk of hyperkalaemia and renal failure	Ciclosporin causes a dose-dependent ↑ in serum creatinine, urea and potassium, especially in renal dysfunction	Monitor renal function and serum potassium weekly until stable and then at least every 3–6 months
CICLOSPORIN	VASODILATOR ANTIHYPERTENSIVES	1. Co-administration of bosentan and ciclosporin leads to ↑ bosentan and ↓ ciclosporin levels 2. Risk of hypertrichosis when minoxidil is given with ciclosporin 3. ↑ sitaxentan levels	1. Additive effect; both drugs inhibit the bile sodium export pump, which is associated with hepatotoxicity 2. Additive effect 3. Uncertain	1. Avoid co-administration of bosentan and ciclosporin 2. Warn patients of the potential interaction 3. Avoid co-administration
CICLOSPORIN	ANTIMALARIALS – (HYDROXY)CHLOROQUINE	↑ plasma concentrations of ciclosporin	Likely inhibition of ciclosporin	Monitor renal function weekly
CICLOSPORIN	ANTIMUSCARINICS – DARIFENACIN	↑ levels of darifenacin	Ciclosporin inhibits P-gp and CYP3A4, which results in ↓ clearance of darifenacin	Avoid co-administration
CICLOSPORIN	ANTIOBESITY DRUGS – ORLISTAT	↓ plasma concentrations of ciclosporin and risk of transplant rejection	↓ absorption of ciclosporin	Avoid co-administration
CICLOSPORIN	**ANTIVIRALS**			
CICLOSPORIN	NNRTIs	↓ efficacy of ciclosporin	Possibly ↑ CYP3A4-mediated metabolism of ciclosporin	Monitor more closely and check levels
CICLOSPORIN	PROTEASE INHIBITORS	↑ levels with protease inhibitors	Inhibition of CYP3A4-mediated metabolism of these immunomodulating drugs	Monitor clinical effects closely and check levels
CICLOSPORIN	**OTHER ANTIVIRALS**			
CICLOSPORIN	ACICLOVIR	↑ risk of nephrotoxicity and ↑ risk of neurotoxicity with ciclosporin	Additive effect	Monitor renal function prior to concomitant therapy and monitor ciclosporin levels

Primary drug	Secondary drug	Effect	Mechanism	Precautions
CICLOSPORIN	ADEFOVIR DIPIVOXIL	Possible ↑ efficacy and side-effects	Competition for renal excretion	Monitor renal function weekly
CICLOSPORIN	FOSCARNET, GANCICLOVIR	↑ risk of nephrotoxicity	Additive nephrotoxic effects	Monitor renal function
CICLOSPORIN	**ANXIOLYTICS AND HYPNOTICS**			
CICLOSPORIN	BZDs – ALPRAZOLAM, MIDAZOLAM, DIAZEPAM	Likely ↑ plasma concentrations and risk of ↑ sedation	These BZDs are metabolized primarily by CYP3A4, which is moderately inhibited by ciclosporin	Warn patients about ↑ sedation. Consider using alternative drugs, e.g. flurazepam, quazepam. Warn about activities requiring attention ➢ ***For signs and symptoms of CNS depression, see Clinical Features of Some Adverse Drug Interactions, Central nervous system depression***
CICLOSPORIN	**BETA-BLOCKERS**			
CICLOSPORIN	ACEBUTOLOL, ATENOLOL, BETAXOLOL, BISOPROLOL, METOPROLOL, PROPANOLOL	↑ risk of hyperkalaemia	Beta-blockers cause an efflux of potassium from cells, which has been observed during ciclosporin therapy	Monitor serum potassium levels during co-administration ➢ ***For signs and symptoms of hyperkalaemia, see Clinical Features of Some Adverse Drug Interactions, Hyperkalaemia***
CICLOSPORIN	CARVEDILOL	Possible ↑ in plasma concentrations of ciclosporin	Carvedilol is metabolized primarily by CYP2D6 and CYP2D9, with a minor contribution from CYP3A4	Usually ↓ dose of ciclosporin (20%) is required
CICLOSPORIN	CALCIUM CHANNEL BLOCKERS	1. Plasma concentrations of ciclosporin are ↑ when co-administered with diltiazem, nicardipine, verapamil and possibly amlodipine and nisoldipine. However, calcium channel blockers seem to protect renal function 2. Ciclosporin ↑ nifedipine levels	1. Uncertain; presumed to be due to impaired hepatic metabolism. Also diltiazem and verapamil inhibit intestinal P-gp, which may ↑ bioavailability of ciclosporin. Uncertain mechanism of renal protection 2. Uncertain effect of ciclosporin on nifedipine	1. Monitor ciclosporin levels and ↓ dose accordingly (possibly by up to 25–50% with nicardipine) 2. Monitor BP closely and warn patients to watch for signs of nifedipine toxicity

CICLOSPORIN	CARDIAC GLYCOSIDES – DIGOXIN	↑ plasma digoxin levels, with risk of toxicity. Digoxin may ↑ ciclosporin bioavailability (15–20%)	Attributed to inhibition of intestinal and renal P-gp, which ↑ bioavailability and renal elimination. Digoxin ↑ bioavailability of ciclosporin due to substrate competition for P-gp	Watch for digoxin toxicity. Monitor plasma digoxin and ciclosporin levels
CICLOSPORIN	CNS STIMULANTS – MODAFINIL	↓ ciclosporin levels up to 50%, with risk of lack of therapeutic effect	↑ metabolism of ciclosporin. Modafinil is a moderate inducer of CYP3A4	Monitor ciclosporin levels
CICLOSPORIN	DANAZOL	↑ plasma concentrations of ciclosporin, with risk of toxic effects	Inhibition of ciclosporin metabolism	Watch for toxic effects of ciclosporin
CICLOSPORIN	**DIURETICS**			
CICLOSPORIN	LOOP DIURETICS, THIAZIDES	Risk of nephrotoxicity	Additive effect	Monitor renal function weekly
CICLOSPORIN	POTASSIUM-SPARING DIURETICS	↑ risk of hyperkalaemia	Additive effect	Monitor electrolytes closely ➢ ***For signs and symptoms of hyperkalaemia, see Clinical Features of Some Adverse Drug Interactions, Hyperkalaemia***
CICLOSPORIN	GRAPEFRUIT JUICE	↑ plasma concentrations of ciclosporin, with risk of nephrotoxicity, myelosuppression, neurotoxicity, excessive immunosuppression and post-transplant lymphoproliferative disease	Inhibition of CYP3A4-mediated metabolism of ciclosporin; these inhibitors vary in potency. Grapefruit juice is classified as a potent inhibitor	Avoid grapefruit juice while taking ciclosporin
CICLOSPORIN	H2 RECEPTOR BLOCKERS – CIMETIDINE	↑ plasma concentrations of ciclosporin, with risk of nephrotoxicity, myelosuppression, neurotoxicity, excessive immunosuppression, with risk of infection and post-transplant lymphoproliferative disease	Inhibition of CYP3A4-mediated metabolism of ciclosporin; these inhibitors vary in potency. Cimetidine is classified as a potent inhibitor	Avoid co-administration with cimetidine. Consider an alternative H2-blocker, but need to monitor plasma ciclosporin levels to prevent toxicity

Primary drug	Secondary drug	Effect	Mechanism	Precautions
CICLOSPORIN	LIPID-LOWERING DRUGS			
CICLOSPORIN	EZETIMIBE	↑ levels of both drugs when ezetimibe is co-administered with ciclosporin	Uncertain	Watch for signs of ciclosporin toxicity
CICLOSPORIN	FIBRATES	↑ risk with renal failure	Uncertain at present	Monitor renal function closely
CICLOSPORIN	STATINS – ATORVASTATIN, LOVASTATIN, ROSUVASTATIN, SIMVASTATIN	↑ plasma concentrations of these statins, with risk of myopathy and rhabdomyolysis	Ciclosporin is a moderate inhibitor of CYP3A4, which metabolizes these statins	↓ statins to lowest possible dose (do not give simvastatin in doses >10 mg). Monitor LFTs and CK closely; warn patients to report any features of rhabdomyolysis. This interaction does not occur with pravastatin
CICLOSPORIN	NANDROLONE	Cases of hepatotoxicity	Uncertain	Monitor LFTs closely
CICLOSPORIN	OESTROGENS	Possibly ↑ plasma concentrations of ciclosporin	Estradiol and immunosuppressants are substrates of CYP3A4 and P-gp. Estradiol is an inhibitor of P-gp	Monitor blood ciclosporin concentrations. Monitor renal function prior to concurrent therapy. Be aware that infections in immunocompromised patients carry a serious threat to life
CICLOSPORIN	PHOSPHODIESTERASE TYPE 5 INHIBITORS – SILDENAFIL	↑ plasma concentrations of ciclosporin, with risk of adverse effects	Competitive inhibition of CYP3A4-mediated metabolism of ciclosporin	Be aware. Sildenafil is taken intermittently and is unlikely to be of clinical significance unless concomitant therapy is long term
CICLOSPORIN	POTASSIUM	↑ risk of hyperkalaemia	Additive effect	Monitor electrolytes closely ➢ ***For signs and symptoms of hyperkalaemia, see Clinical Features of Some Adverse Drug Interactions, Hyperkalaemia***

CICLOSPORIN	PROGESTOGENS	↑ plasma concentrations of ciclosporin	Inhibition of metabolism of ciclosporin	Monitor blood ciclosporin concentrations. Monitor renal function prior to concurrent therapy. Be aware that infections in immunocompromised patients carry a serious threat to life
CICLOSPORIN	PROTON PUMP INHIBITORS – OMEPRAZOLE	Conflicting information. Possible altered efficacy of ciclosporin	Unclear	Monitor closely. Studies have reported combination use with no significant changes in ciclosporin levels
CICLOSPORIN	SYMPATHOMIMETICS	Methylphenidate may ↑ ciclosporin levels	Uncertain at present	Watch for ciclosporin toxicity; ↓ levels as necessary and monitor levels if available
CICLOSPORIN	URSODEOXYCHOLIC ACID	↑ ciclosporin levels	↑ absorption	Watch for early features of ciclosporin toxicity; monitor FBC closely
CICLOSPORIN	VACCINES	Immunosuppressants diminish effectiveness of vaccines. There is ↑ risk of adverse/toxic effects of live vaccines, and vaccinal infections may develop	Disseminated infection due to enhanced replication of vaccine virus in the presence of diminished immunocompetence	Do not vaccinate when patients are on immunosuppressants. Vaccination should be deferred for at least 3 months after discontinuing suppressants/myelosuppressants. If an individual has been recently vaccinated, do not initiate therapy for at least 2 weeks after vaccination
CORTICOSTEROIDS				
CORTICOSTEROIDS	ANALGESICS – NSAIDs	1. ↑ risk of gastrointestinal ulceration and bleeding 2. Parecoxib levels may be ↓ by dexamethasone	1. Additive effect 2. Dexamethasone induces CYP3A4-mediated metabolism of parecoxib	1. Watch for early signs of gastrointestinal upset; remember that corticosteroids may mask these features 2. Watch for poor response to parecoxib

Primary drug	Secondary drug	Effect	Mechanism	Precautions
CORTICOSTEROIDS	ANTIBIOTICS			
CORTICOSTEROIDS	MACROLIDES – CLARITHROMYCIN, ERYTHROMYCIN, TELITHROMYCIN	↑ adrenal suppressive effects of corticosteroids, which may ↑ risk of infections and produce an inadequate response to stress scenarios	Due to inhibition of metabolism of corticosteroids	Monitor cortisol levels and warn patients to report symptoms such as fever and sore throat
CORTICOSTEROIDS	RIFAMPICIN	↓ plasma concentrations of corticosteroids and risk of poor or inadequate therapeutic response, which would be undesirable if used for e.g. cerebral oedema	Due to induction of hepatic metabolism by the CYP3A4 isoenzymes	Closely monitor therapeutic response – clinically, by ophthalmoscopy and radiologically – and ↑ dose of corticosteroids for desired therapeutic effect
CORTICOSTEROIDS	ANTICANCER AND IMMUNOMODULATING DRUGS			
CORTICOSTEROIDS	CYTOTOXICS			
DEXAMETHASONE	IFOSFAMIDE	↑ rate of biotransformation to 4-hydroxyifosfamide, the active metabolite, but no change in AUC of 4-hydroxyifosfamide	Due to ↑ rate of metabolism and clearance due to induction of CYP3A4 and CYP2D6	Be aware – the clinical significance may be minimal or none
CORTICOSTEROIDS	IMATINIB	↑ adrenal suppressive effects of corticosteroids, which may ↑ risk of infections and the produce an inadequate response to stress scenarios	Due to inhibition of metabolism of corticosteroids	Monitor cortisol levels and warn patients to report symptoms such as fever and sore throat
DEXAMETHASONE	IRINOTECAN	↓ plasma concentrations of irinotecan and risk of ↓ therapeutic efficacy. The effects may last for 3 weeks after discontinuation of CYP-inducer therapy	Due to induction of CYP3A4-mediated metabolism of irinotecan	Avoid concomitant use when ever possible; if not, ↑ dose of irinotecan by 50%
CORTICOSTEROIDS	METHOTREXATE	↑ risk of bone marrow toxicity	Additive effect	Monitor FBC regularly

DEXAMETHASONE	PACLITAXEL	↓ plasma concentration s of paclitaxel and ↓ efficacy of paclitaxel	Due to induction of hepatic metabolism of paclitaxel by the CYP isoenzymes	Monitor for clinical efficacy and need to ↑ dose if inadequate response is due to interaction
DEXAMETHASONE	VINCA ALKALOIDS	↓ of plasma concentrations of vinblastine and vincristine, with risk of inadequate therapeutic response. Reports of ↓ AUC by 40% and elimination half-life by 35%, and ↑ clearance by 63%, in patients with brain tumours taking vincristine, which could lead to dangerously inadequate therapeutic responses	Due to induction of CYP3A4-mediated metabolism	Monitor for clinical efficacy, and ↑ dose of vinblastine and vincristine as clinically indicated; in the latter case, monitor clinically and radiologically for clinical efficacy in patients with brain tumours, and ↑ dose to obtain desired response
CORTICOSTEROIDS	**HORMONES AND HORMONE ANTAGONISTS**			
CORTICOSTEROIDS	TAMOXIFEN	↓ plasma concentrations of tamoxifen and risk of inadequate therapeutic response	Due to induction of metabolism of tamoxifen by the CYP3A isoenzymes by dexamethasone	Avoid concurrent use if possible. Otherwise monitor for clinical efficacy of tamoxifen by ↑ dose of tamoxifen
CORTICOSTEROIDS	**IMMUNOMODULATING DRUGS**			
CORTICOSTEROIDS	CICLOSPORIN	↓ plasma concentrations of ciclosporin, with risk of transplant rejection	Due to induction of metabolism of ciclosporin by these drugs. The potency of induction varies	Monitor for signs of rejection of transplants. Monitor ciclosporin levels to ensure adequate therapeutic concentrations, and ↑ dose when necessary
CORTICOSTEROIDS	IL-2	↓ anti-tumour effect of IL-2	Corticosteroids inhibit the release of IL-2-induced tumour necrosis factor, thus opposing the pharmacological effect of IL-2	Avoid concurrent use if possible

Primary drug	Secondary drug	Effect	Mechanism	Precautions
CORTICOSTEROIDS	MYCOPHENOLATE	↓ plasma concentrations of mycophenolate and risk of transplant rejection	Corticosteroids induce UGT enzymes and multidrug resistance-associated protein 2, involved in disposition of mycophenolate	Intervention to prevent rejection is mandatory. ↑ mycophenolate dosage to maintain therapeutic blood levels. As important is to monitor levels following steroid withdrawal to prevent adverse outcomes
CORTICOSTEROIDS	ANTICOAGULANTS – ORAL	↑ anticoagulant effect	Uncertain at present	Monitor INR at least weekly until stable
CORTICOSTEROIDS	ANTIDEPRESSANTS – ST JOHN'S WORT	↓ plasma concentrations of corticosteroids and risk of poor or inadequate therapeutic response, which would be undesirable if used for e.g. cerebral oedema	Due to induction of the hepatic metabolism by the CYP3A4 isoenzymes	Closely monitor therapeutic response – clinically, by ophthalmoscopy and radiologically – and ↑ dose of corticosteroids for desired therapeutic effect
CORTICOSTEROIDS	ANTIDIABETIC DRUGS	Often ↑ hypoglycaemic agent requirements, particularly of those with high glucocorticoid activity	Corticosteroids, particularly the glucocorticoids (betamethasone, dexamethasone, deflazacort, prednisolone > cortisone, hydrocortisone), have intrinsic hyperglycaemic activity in both diabetic and non-diabetic subjects	Monitor blood sugar during concomitant treatment, weekly if possible, or advise self-monitoring, until blood sugar levels are stable. Larger doses of insulin are often needed
CORTICOSTEROIDS	ANTIEMETICS – APREPITANT	↑ dexamethasone and methylprednisolone levels	Inhibition of CYP3A4-mediated metabolism of these corticosteroids	Be aware
CORTICOSTEROIDS	ANTIEPILEPTICS – CARBAMAZEPINE, PHENYTOIN, PHENOBARBITAL	↓ plasma concentrations of corticosteroids and risk of poor or inadequate therapeutic response, which would be undesirable if used for e.g. cerebral oedema	Due to induction of the hepatic metabolism by the CYP3A4 isoenzymes	Closely monitor therapeutic response – clinically, by ophthalmoscopy and radiologically – and ↑ dose of corticosteroids for desired therapeutic effect

ANTICANCER AND IMMUNOMODULATING DRUGS

CORTICOSTEROIDS	ANTIFUNGALS			
CORTICOSTEROIDS	AZOLES – FLUCONAZOLE, ITRACONAZOLE, KETOCONAZOLE, POSACONAZOLE, VORICONAZOLE	↑ adrenal suppressive effects of corticosteroids, which may ↑ risk of infections and produce inadequate response to stress scenarios	Due to inhibition of metabolism of corticosteroids	Monitor cortisol levels and warn patients to report symptoms such as fever and sore throat
CORTICOSTEROIDS	**OTHER ANTIFUNGALS**			
CORTICOSTEROIDS	AMPHOTERICIN	Risk of hyperkalaemia	Additive effect	Avoid co-administration
DEXAMETHASONE	CASPOFUNGIN	↓ caspofungin levels, with risk of therapeutic failure	Induction of caspofungin metabolism	↑ dose of caspofungin to 70 mg daily
CORTICOSTEROIDS	**ANTIHYPERTENSIVES AND HEART FAILURE DRUGS**			
CORTICOSTEROIDS	ANTIHYPERTENSIVES AND HEART FAILURE DRUGS	↓ hypotensive effect	Corticosteroids cause sodium and water retention leading to ↑ BP	Monitor BP at least weekly until stable
CORTICOSTEROIDS	VASODILATOR ANTIHYPERTENSIVES	Risk of hyperglycaemia when diazoxide co-administered is with corticosteroids	Additive effect; both drugs have a hyperglycaemic effect	Monitor blood glucose closely, particularly with diabetics
DEXAMETHASONE	ANTIMIGRAINE DRUGS – ALMOTRIPTAN, ELETRIPTAN	Possible ↓ plasma concentrations of almotriptan and risk of inadequate therapeutic efficacy	One of the major metabolizing enzymes of almotriptan; CYP3A4 isoenzymes are induced by rifampicin. As there are alternative metabolic pathways, the effect may not be significant and could vary from individual to individual	Be aware of possibility of ↓ response to triptan and consider ↑ dose if considered due to interaction
CORTICOSTEROIDS	ANTIPLATELET AGENTS – ASPIRIN	Corticosteroids ↓ aspirin levels, and therefore there is a risk of salicylate toxicity when withdrawing corticosteroids. Risk of gastric ulceration when aspirin is co-administered with corticosteroids	Uncertain	Watch for features of salicylate toxicity when withdrawing corticosteroids. Use aspirin in the lowest dose. Remember that corticosteroids may mask the features of peptic ulceration

Primary drug	Secondary drug	Effect	Mechanism	Precautions
CORTICOSTEROIDS	ANTIVIRALS			
CORTICOSTEROIDS	NNRTIs INHIBITORS – EFAVIRENZ	↑ adrenal suppressive effects of corticosteroids, which may ↑ risk of infections and the produce an inadequate response to stress scenarios	Due to inhibition of metabolism of corticosteroids	Monitor cortisol levels and warn patients to report symptoms such as fever and sore throat
CORTICOSTEROIDS	PROTEASE INHIBITORS – RITONAVIR	↑ plasma levels of betamethasone, dexamethasone, hydrocortisone, prednisolone and both inhaled and intranasal budesonide and fluticasone with ritonavir (with or without lopinavir)	Inhibition of CYP3A4-mediated metabolism	Monitor closely for signs of corticosteroid toxicity and immunosupression, and ↓ dose as necessary. Consider using inhaled beclometasone
CORTICOSTEROIDS	BETA-BLOCKERS	↓ efficacy of beta-blockers	Mineralocorticoids cause ↑ BP as a result of sodium and water retention	Watch for poor response to beta-blockers
CORTICOSTEROIDS	BRONCHODILATORS – BETA AGONISTS (HIGH-DOSE), THEOPHYLLINE	Risk of hypokalaemia	Additive effect. The CSM notes that this effect occurs with beta-2 agonists, theophyllines and corticosteroids, all of which may be given during severe asthma; hypoxia exacerbates this effect	Monitor blood potassium levels prior to concomitant administration and during therapy (monitor 1–2-hourly during parenteral administration). Administer potassium supplements to prevent hypokalaemia, which may also be worsened by hypoxia during severe attacks of asthma
CORTICOSTEROIDS	CALCIUM	↓ calcium levels	↓ intestinal absorption and ↑ excretion	Separate doses as much as possible

CORTICOSTEROIDS	CALCIUM CHANNEL BLOCKERS	1. Antihypertensive effect of calcium channel blockers are antagonized by corticosteroids 2. ↑ adrenal suppressive effects of corticosteroids, methylprednisolone and prednisolone when co-administered with diltiazem, nifedipine and verapamil. This may ↑ risk of infections and produce an inadequate response to stress scenarios	1. Mineralocorticoids cause sodium and water retention, which antagonizes the hypotensive effects of calcium channel blockers 2. Due to inhibition of metabolism of these corticosteroids	1. Monitor BP at least weekly until stable 2. Monitor cortisol levels and warn patients to report symptoms such as fever and sore throat
CORTICOSTEROIDS	CARDIAC GLYCOSIDES – DIGOXIN	Risk of digoxin toxicity due to hypokalaemia	Corticosteroids may cause hypokalaemia	Monitor potassium levels closely. Monitor digoxin levels; watch for digoxin toxicity
CORTICOSTEROIDS	CNS STIMULANTS – MODAFINIL	May ↓ modafinil levels	Induction of CYP3A4, which has a partial role in the metabolism of modafinil	Be aware
CORTICOSTEROIDS	DRUG DEPENDENCE THERAPIES – BUPROPION	↑ risk of seizures. This risk is marked in elderly people, in patients with a history of seizures, with addiction to opiates/cocaine/stimulants, and in diabetics treated with oral hypoglycaemics or insulin	Bupropion is associated with a dose-related risk of seizures. These drugs, which lower seizure threshold, are individually epileptogenic. Additive effects occur when combined	Extreme caution. The dose of bupropion should not exceed 450 mg/day (or 150 mg/day in patients with severe hepatic cirrhosis)
CORTICOSTEROIDS	GRAPEFRUIT JUICE	↑ adrenal suppressive effects of corticosteroids, which may ↑ risk of infections and produce an inadequate response to stress scenarios	Due to inhibition of metabolism of corticosteroids	Monitor cortisol levels and warn patients to report symptoms such as fever and sore throat

Primary drug	Secondary drug	Effect	Mechanism	Precautions
CORTICOSTEROIDS	H2 RECEPTOR BLOCKERS – CIMETIDINE	↑ adrenal suppressive effects of corticosteroids, which may ↑ risk of infections and produce an inadequate response to stress scenarios	Due to inhibition of metabolism of corticosteroids	Monitor cortisol levels and warn patients to report symptoms such as fever and sore throat
CORTICOSTEROIDS	NITRATES	Antihypertensive effect of calcium channel blockers are antagonized by corticosteroids	Mineralocorticoids cause sodium and water retention, which antagonizes the hypotensive effects of calcium channel blockers	Monitor BP at least weekly until stable
CORTICOSTEROIDS	OESTROGENS	Possibly ↑ corticosteroid levels	Uncertain	Warn patients to report symptoms such as fever and sore throat
CORTICOSTEROIDS	SODIUM PHENYLBUTYRATE	Possibly ↓ efficacy of sodium phenylbutyrate	These drugs are associated with ↑ ammonia levels	Avoid co-administration
CORTICOSTEROIDS	SOMATROPIN	Possible ↓ efficacy of somatropin	Uncertain	Watch for poor response to somatropin
CORTICOSTEROIDS	SYMPATHOMIMETICS – EPHEDRINE	Ephedrine may ↓ dexamethasone levels	Uncertain at present	Watch for poor response to dexamethasone. Uncertain at present if other corticosteroids are similarly affected
ETANERCEPT				
ETANERCEPT	ANAKINRA	↑ risk of bone marrow suppression	Additive effect	Avoid co-administration
GOLD (SODIUM AUROTHIOMALATE)				
GOLD	ACE INHIBITORS	Cases of ↓ BP	Additive vasodilating effects	Monitor BP at least weekly until stable. Warn patients to report symptoms of hypotension (light-headedness, dizziness on standing, etc.). If a reaction occurs, consider changing to an alternative gold formulation or stopping ACE inhibitor
HYDROXYCHLOROQUINE ➢ *Drugs to Treat Infections, Antimalarials*				

INFLIXIMAB				
INFLIXIMAB	ANAKINRA	↑ risk of bone marrow suppression	Additive effect	Avoid co-administration
INTERFERONS – (peg)interferon alfa, interferon beta, interferon gamma				
INTERFERON ALFA	ACE INHIBITORS	Risk of severe granulocytopenia	Possibly due to synergistic haematological toxicity	Monitor blood counts frequently; warn patients to report promptly any symptoms of infection
INTERFERON ALPHA	ANTICOAGULANTS – ORAL	↑ anticoagulant effect	Uncertain at present	Monitor INR at least weekly until stable
INTERFERON	ANTIVIRALS			
INTERFERON	TELBIVUDINE	Peripheral neuropathy	Unclear	Use with caution
INTERFERON	ZIDOVUDINE	↑ adverse effects with zidovudine	Additive toxicity	Monitor FBC and renal function closely. ↓ doses as necessary. Use of pyrimethamine as prophylaxis seems to be tolerated
INTERFERON ALFA	BRONCHODILATORS – THEOPHYLLINE	↑ theophylline levels	Inhibition of theophylline metabolism	Monitor theophylline levels before, during and after co-administration
INTERFERON GAMMA	CARDIAC GLYCOSIDES – DIGOXIN	↑ plasma concentrations of digoxin may occur with interferon gamma	Interferon gamma ↓ P-gp-mediated renal and biliary excretion of digoxin	Monitor digoxin levels; watch for digoxin toxicity
INTERFERON	DRUG DEPENDENCE THERAPIES – BUPROPION	↑ risk of seizures. This risk is marked in elderly people, in patients with history of seizures, with addiction to opiates/cocaine/stimulants, and in diabetics treated with oral hypoglycaemics or insulin	Bupropion is associated with dose-related risk of seizures. These drugs, which lower seizure threshold, are individually epileptogenic. Additive effects occur when combined	Extreme caution. The dose of bupropion should not exceed 450 mg/day (or 150 mg/day in patients with severe hepatic cirrhosis)
INTERFERON GAMMA	VACCINES	Immunosuppressants diminish the effectiveness of vaccines. There is ↑ risk of adverse/toxic effects of live vaccines, and vaccinal infections may develop	Disseminated infection due to enhanced replication of vaccine virus in the presence of diminished immunocompetence	Do not vaccinate when patients are on immunosuppressants. Vaccination should be deferred for at least 3 months after discontinuing suppressants/myelosuppressants. If an individual has been recently vaccinated, do not initiate therapy for at least 2 weeks after vaccination

Primary drug	Secondary drug	Effect	Mechanism	Precautions
INTERLEUKIN-2 (ALDESLEUKIN)				
IL-2	ANTICANCER AND IMMUNOMODULATING DRUGS			
IL-2	CYTOTOXICS – DACARBAZINE	↓ efficacy of dacarbazine	↓ AUC of dacarbazine due to ↓ volume of distribution	The clinical significance is uncertain as both drugs are used in the treatment of melanoma. It may be necessary to monitor clinically and by other appropriate measures of clinical response
IL-2	IMMUNOMODULATING DRUGS – CORTICOSTEROIDS	↓ efficacy of inteleukin-2	Corticosteroids inhibits release of aldesleukin-induced tumour necrosis factor, thus opposing the action of aldesleukin	Avoid concurrent use if possible
IL-2	ANTIHYPERTENSIVE AND HEART FAILURE DRUGS	↑ hypotensive effect	Additive hypotensive effect; may be used therapeutically. Aldesleukin causes ↓ vascular resistance and ↑ capillary permeability	Monitor BP at least weekly until stable. Warn patients to report symptoms of hypotension (light-headedness, dizziness on standing, etc.)
IL-2	ANTIVIRALS			
IL-2	NUCLEOSIDE REVERSE TRANSCRIPTASE INHIBITORS – TENOFOVIR	↑ adverse effects with tenofovir	Uncertain	Avoid if possible; otherwise monitor renal function weekly
IL-2	PROTEASE INHIBITORS	↑ protease inhibitor levels, with risk of toxicity	Aldesleukin induces formation of IL-6, which inhibits the metabolism of protease inhibitors by the CYP3A4 isoenzymes	Warn patients to report symptoms such as nausea, vomiting, flatulence, dizziness and rashes. Monitor blood sugar at initiation of and on discontinuing treatment
IL-2	BETA-BLOCKERS, CALCIUM CHANNEL BLOCKERS, DIURETICS, NITRATES, POTASSIUM CHANNEL ACTIVATORS	↑ hypotensive effect	Additive hypotensive effect; may be used therapeutically. Aldesleukin causes ↓ vascular resistance and ↑ capillary permeability	Monitor BP at least weekly until stable. Warn patients to report symptoms of hypotension (light-headedness, dizziness on standing, etc.)

LEFLUNOMIDE				
LEFLUNOMIDE	**ANTICANCER AND IMMUNOMODULATING DRUGS**			
LEFLUNOMIDE	AZATHIOPRINE	↑ risk of serious infections (sepsis) and of opportunistic infections (*Pneumocystis jiroveci* pneumonia, tuberculosis, aspergillosis)	Additive immunosuppression	Monitor platelets, white blood cells, haemoglobin and haematocrit at baseline and regularly – weekly – during concomitant therapy. With evidence of bone marrow suppression, discontinue leflunomide and administer colestyramine and charcoal to ↑ elimination of leflunomide ➢ ***For signs and symptoms of immunosuppression, see Clinical Features of Some Adverse Drug Interactions, Immunosuppression and blood dyscrasias***
LEFLUNOMIDE	CICLOSPORIN	↑ risk of serious infections (sepsis) and of opportunistic infections (*Pneumocystis jiroveci* pneumonia, tuberculosis, aspergillosis)	Additive immunosuppression	Monitor platelets, white blood cells, haemoglobin and haematocrit at baseline and regularly – weekly – during concomitant therapy. With evidence of bone marrow suppression, discontinue leflunomide and administer colestyramine and charcoal to ↑ elimination of leflunomide ➢ ***For signs and symptoms of immunosuppression, see Clinical Features of Some Adverse Drug Interactions, Immunosuppression and blood dyscrasias***

Primary drug	Secondary drug	Effect	Mechanism	Precautions
LEFLUNOMIDE	MYCOPHENOLATE	↑ risk of serious infections (sepsis) and of opportunistic infections (*Pneumocystis jiroveci* pneumonia, tuberculosis, aspergillosis)	Additive immunosuppression	Monitor platelets, white blood cells, haemoglobin and haematocrit at baseline and regularly – weekly – during concomitant therapy. With evidence of bone marrow suppression, discontinue leflunomide and administer colestyramine and charcoal to ↑ elimination of leflunomide ➢ ***For signs and symptoms of immunosuppression, see Clinical Features of Some Adverse Drug Interactions, Immunosuppression and blood dyscrasias***
LEFLUNOMIDE	ANTICOAGULANTS – ORAL	↑ anticoagulant effect	Uncertain at present	Monitor INR at least weekly until stable
LEFLUNOMIDE	ANTIDEPRESSANTS – TCAs	Possible ↑ leflunomide levels	Inhibition of CYP2C9-mediated metabolism. The clinical significance of this depends upon whether alternative pathways of metabolism are also inhibited by co-administered drugs	Warn patients to report ↑ side-effects and monitor blood count carefully
LEFLUNOMIDE	ANTIDIABETIC DRUGS – TOLBUTAMIDE	Possible ↑ effect of tolbutamide	Uncertain	Monitor blood sugar closely. Watch for and warn patients about symptoms of hypoglycaemia ➢ ***For signs and symptoms of hypoglycaemia, see Clinical Features of Some Adverse Drug Interactions, Hypoglycaemia***
LEFLUNOMIDE	LIPID-LOWERING DRUGS – CHOLESTYRAMINE	↓ levels of leflunomide	↓ absorption	Avoid co-administration

MESALAZINE ➢ *Other immunomodulating drugs, Aminosalicylates, above*				
MYCOPHENOLATE				
MYCOPHENOLATE	ANALGESICS – NSAIDs	↑ risk of nephrotoxicity	Additive effect	Monitor renal function closely
MYCOPHENOLATE	ANTACIDS	↓ plasma concentrations of mycophenolate (may be 30%)	↓ absorption	Do not co-administer simultaneously – separate by at least 4 hours
MYCOPHENOLATE	**ANTIBIOTICS**			
MYCOPHENOLATE	CO-TRIMOXAZOLE	Exacerbates neutropenia caused by mycophenolate	Additive effect	➢ ***For signs and symptoms of neutropenia, see Clinical Features of Some Adverse Drug Interactions, Immunosuppression and blood dyscrasias***
MYCOPHENOLATE	METRONIDAZOLE, NORFLOXACIN, RIFAMPICIN	Significant ↓ plasma mycophenolate concentrations (>60% with rifampicin)	Inhibition of metabolism of mycophenolate	Avoid co-administration
MYCOPHENOLATE	ANTIVIRALS – ACICLOVIR, GANCICLOVIR	↑ plasma concentrations of both drugs. Toxic effects of both drugs likely	Attributed to competition for renal tubular excretion	Monitor blood counts ➢ ***For signs and symptoms of immunosuppression, see Clinical Features of Some Adverse Drug Interactions, Immunosuppression and blood dyscrasias***
MYCOPHENOLATE	**ANTICANCER AND IMMUNOMODULATING DRUGS**			
MYCOPHENOLATE	**IMMUNOMODULATING DRUGS**			
MYCOPHENOLATE	CICLOSPORIN	↓ plasma concentrations of mycophenolate and of its active metabolite mycophenolic acid	Ciclosporin is thought to interrupt the enterohepatic circulation of mycophenolate by inhibiting MRP-2 in the biliary tract, which prevents the excretion of its glucuronide	Watch for poor response to mycophenolate if ciclosporin is added; conversely, watch for early features of toxicity if ciclosporin is stopped

Primary drug	Secondary drug	Effect	Mechanism	Precautions
MYCOPHENOLATE	CORTICOSTEROIDS	↓ plasma concentrations of mycophenolate and risk of transplant rejection	Corticosteroids induce UGT enzymes and multidrug resistance associated protein 2, involved in disposition of mycophenolate	Intervention to prevent rejection is mandatory. ↑ tacrolimus dosage to maintain therapeutic blood levels (see below). As important is to monitor levels following steroid withdrawal to prevent adverse outcomes
MYCOPHENOLATE	LEFLUNOMIDE	↑ risk of serious infections (sepsis) and of opportunistic infections (*Pneumocystis jiroveci* pneumonia, tuberculosis, aspergillosis)	Additive immunosuppression	Monitor platelets, white blood cells, haemoglobin and haematocrit at baseline and regularly – weekly – during concomitant therapy. With evidence of bone marrow suppression, discontinue leflunomide and administer cholestyramine and charcoal to ↑ elimination of leflunomide ➢ ***For signs and symptoms of immunosuppression, see Clinical Features of Some Adverse Drug Interactions, Immunosuppression and blood dyscrasias***
MYCOPHENOLATE	NATALIZUMAB	↑ risk of infections including progressive multifocal leukoencephalopathy, a potentially fatal virus infection of the brain	Due to additive immunosuppressant effects. Natalizumab inhibits migration of leukocytes into the CNS	Avoid co-administration
MYCOPHENOLATE	ANTIVIRALS – ACICLOVIR, GANCICLOVIR	Possible ↑ efficacy	Competition for renal excretion	Monitor renal function, particularly if on >4 g valaciclovir. ↓ dose of aciclovir if there is a background of renal failure
MYCOPHENOLATE	IRON – ORAL	↓ plasma concentrations of mycophenolate and risk of transplant rejection	↓ absorption	Avoid co-administration

MYCOPHENOLATE	LIPID-LOWERING DRUGS – COLESTYRAMINE	↓ plasma concentrations of mycophenolate by approximately 40%. Risk of therapeutic failure	Due to interruption of enterohepatic circulation due to binding of recirculating mycophenolate with cholestyramine in intestine	Avoid co-administration
MYCOPHENOLATE	OESTROGENS	Possible altered efficacy of contraceptive	Unclear	Clinical significance uncertain. It would seem wise to advise patients to use an alternative form of contraception during and for 1 month after stopping co-administration of these drugs
MYCOPHENOLATE	SEVELAMER	↓ plasma concentrations of mycophenolate	Attributed to binding of mycophenolate to calcium free phosphate binders	Separate administration by at least 2 hours
MYCOPHENOLATE	VACCINES	Immunosuppressants diminish effectiveness of vaccines. ↑ risk of adverse/toxic effects of live vaccines, and vaccinal infections may develop	Disseminated infection due to enhanced replication of vaccine virus in the presence of diminished immunocompetence	Do not vaccinate when patients are on immunosuppressants. Vaccination should be deferred for at least 3 months after discontinuing immunosuppressants/myelosuppressants. If an individual has recently been vaccinated, do not initiate therapy for at least 2 weeks after vaccination
NATALIZUMAB				
NATALIZUMAB	AZATHIOPRINE	↑ risk of myelosuppression, immunosuppression. Deaths have occurred following profound myelosuppression and severe sepsis	Additive myelotoxic effects Azathioprine is metabolized to 6-mercatopurine in vivo, which results in additive myelosuppression, immunosuppression and hepatotoxicity	Avoid co-administration

Primary drug	Secondary drug	Effect	Mechanism	Precautions
NATALIZUMAB	CICLOSPORIN	↑ risk of adverse effects of natalizumab and ↑ risk of concurrent infections	Additive effect	Monitor FBC closely. Warn patients to report early features suggestive of infection
NATALIZUMAB	MYCOPHENOLATE	↑ risk of infections, including progressive multifocal leuko-encephalopathy, a potentially fatal virus infection of the brain	Due to additive immunosuppres-sant effects. Natalizumab inhibits migration of leukocytes in to the CNS	Avoid co-administration
OLSALAZINE ➢ ***Other immunomodulating drugs, Aminosalicylates, above***				
PENICILLAMINE				
PENICILLAMINE	ANALGESICS – NSAIDs	↑ risk of nephrotoxicity	Additive effect	Monitor renal function closely
PENICILLAMINE	ANTACIDS	↓ penicillamine levels	↓ absorption of penicillamine	Avoid co-administration
PENICILLAMINE	ANTIPSYCHOTICS – CLOZAPINE	Risk of bone marrow suppression	Additive effect	Avoid co-administration
PENICILLAMINE	CARDIAC GLYCOSIDES – DIGOXIN	Plasma concentrations of digoxin may be ↓ by penicillamine	Uncertain at present	Watch for poor response to digoxin
PENICILLAMINE	IRON – ORAL	↓ penicillamine levels	↓ absorption of penicillamine	Avoid co-administration
PENICILLAMINE	ZINC	↓ penicillamine and zinc levels	Mutual ↓ absorption	Avoid co-administration
RETINOIDS – acitretin, (iso)tretinoin				
RETINOIDS	ANTIBIOTICS	Risk of benign intracranial hypertension with tetracycline	Unknown	Avoid co-administration
RETINOIDS	ANTICANCER AND IMMUNOMODULATING DRUGS			
ACITRETIN	METHOTREXATE	↑ risk of hepatotoxicity	Additive hepatotoxic effects	Avoid co-administration
RETINOIDS	PORFIMER	↑ risk of photosensitivity reactions when porfimer is co-administered with hydrochlorothiazide	Attributed to additive effects	Avoid exposure of skin and eyes to direct sunlight for 30 days after porfimer therapy

RETINOIDS – TRETINOIN	CALCIUM CHANNEL BLOCKERS	↓ plasma tretinoin levels and risk of ↓ anti-tumour activity when co-administered with diltiazem, nifedipine or verapamil	Due to induction of CYP3A4-mediated metabolism of tretinoin	Avoid co-administration if possible
RETINOIDS	VITAMIN A	Risk of vitamin A toxicity	Additive effect; tretinoin is a form of vitamin A	Avoid co-administration
RITUXIMAB				
RITUXIMAB	CISPLATIN	↑ risk of severe renal failure	Uncertain, possibly due to effects of tumour lysis syndrome (which is a result of massive breakdown of cancer cells sensitive to chemotherapy). Features include hyperkalaemia, hyperuricaemia, hyperphosphataemia and hypocalcaemia	Monitor renal function closely. Hydrate with at least 2 L of fluid before, during and after therapy. Monitor potassium and magnesium levels in particular and correct deficits. Do an ECG as arrhythmias may accompany tumour lysis syndrome
SIROLIMUS				
SIROLIMUS	ANALGESICS – NSAIDs	↑ risk of nephrotoxicity	Additive effect	Monitor renal function closely
SIROLIMUS	ANTIBIOTICS			
SIROLIMUS	CO-TRIMOXAZOLE	Exacerbates neutropenia caused by sirolimus	Additive effect	Monitor blood count closely ➢ ***For signs and symptoms of neutropenia, see Clinical Features of Some Adverse Drug Interactions, Immunosuppression and blood dyscrasias***
SIROLIMUS	MACROLIDES – CLARITHROMYCIN, ERYTHROMYCIN, TELITHROMYCIN	↑ sirolimus levels	Inhibition of metabolism of sirolimus	Avoid co-administration

Primary drug	Secondary drug	Effect	Mechanism	Precautions
SIROLIMUS	**ANTICANCER AND IMMUNOMODULATING DRUGS**			
SIROLIMUS	CYTOTOXICS – TRASTUZUMAB	↑ neutropenic effect of immunosuppressants	Additive effect	Warn patients to report symptoms such as sore throat and fever ➢ ***For signs and symptoms of neutropenia, see Clinical Features of Some Adverse Drug Interactions, Immunosuppression and blood dyscrasias***
SIROLIMUS	IMMUNOMODULATING DRUGS – CICLOSPORIN	↑ bioavailability of sirolimus (30–40% when drug administrations are separated by 4 hours and 100% when administered together)	Due to inhibition of P-gp by ciclosporin and competition for metabolism by CYP3A4	Be aware of toxic effects of sirolimus and monitor blood levels
SIROLIMUS	ANTIFUNGALS – AZOLES	↑ sirolimus levels	Inhibition of metabolism of sirolimus	Avoid co-administration
SIROLIMUS	ANTIVIRALS – PROTEASE INHIBITORS	↑ levels with protease inhibitors	Inhibition of CYP3A4-mediated metabolism of these immunomodulating drugs	Monitor clinical effects closely; check levels
SIROLIMUS	CALCIUM CHANNEL BLOCKERS	Plasma concentrations of sirolimus are ↑ when given with diltiazem Plasma concentrations of both drugs are ↑ when verapamil and sirolimus are co-administered	Diltiazem and verapamil inhibit intestinal CYP3A, which is the main site of sirolimus metabolism	Watch for side-effects of sirolimus when it is co-administered with diltiazem or verapamil; monitor renal and hepatic function. Monitor PR and BP closely when sirolimus is given with verapamil
SIROLIMUS	GRAPEFRUIT JUICE	Possibly ↑ efficacy and ↑ adverse effects	Possibly ↑ bioavailability via inhibition of intestinal CYP3A4 and effects of P-gp	Avoid co-administration

SIROLIMUS	H2 RECEPTOR BLOCKERS	↑ adverse effects of sirolimus, e.g. thrombocytopenia, hepatotoxicity	Sirolimus is metabolized primarily by CYP3A4 isoenzymes, which are inhibited by cimetidine. Cimetidine is also an inhibitor of CYP2D6, CYP2C19 and CYP1A2	Consider alternative acid suppression, e.g. alginate suspension or rabeprazole. Not thought to be clinically significant, although ensure close monitoring of immunosuppressant levels and renal function
SULFASALAZINE ➢ ***Other immunomodulating drugs, Aminosalicylates, above***				
TACROLIMUS				
TACROLIMUS	ANALGESICS – NSAIDs	↑ risk of nephrotoxicity	Additive effect	Monitor renal function closely
TACROLIMUS	**ANTIBIOTICS**			
TACROLIMUS	AMINOGLYCOSIDES	Risk of renal toxicity	Additive effect	Monitor renal function closely
TACROLIMUS	CHLORAMPHENICOL	Toxic blood levels of tacrolimus, usually on the second day of starting chloramphenicol	Attributed to impaired clearance of tacrolimus by chloramphenicol.	Dose ↓ of nearly 80% of tacrolimus may be required to prevent toxicity. Watch for adverse effects. Monitor tacrolimus plasma concentrations
TACROLIMUS	CO-TRIMOXAZOLE	Exacerbates hyperkalaemia induced by tacrolimus	Additive hyperkalaemic effects	Monitor electrolytes closely ➢ ***For signs and symptoms of hyperkalaemia, see Clinical Features of Some Adverse Drug Interactions, Hyperkalaemia***
TACROLIMUS	MACROLIDES	↑ plasma concentrations of tacrolimus, with risk of toxic effect	Clarithromycin, erythromycin and telithromycin inhibit the CYP3A4-mediated metabolism of tacrolimus. Azithromycin, mildly if at all, inhibits CYP3A4; marked ↑ in tacrolimus levels is attributed to inhibition of P-gp	Be aware, and monitor tacrolimus plasma concentrations

Primary drug	Secondary drug	Effect	Mechanism	Precautions
TACROLIMUS	RIFAMPICIN	↓ tacrolimus levels	Induction of CYP3A4-mediated metabolism of tacrolimus	Avoid co-administration
TACROLIMUS	VANCOMYCIN	Risk of renal toxicity	Additive effect	Monitor renal function closely
TACROLIMUS	**ANTICANCER AND IMMUNOMODULATING DRUGS**			
TACROLIMUS	CYTOTOXICS – CISPLATIN	↑ risk of renal toxicity and renal failure	Additive renal toxicity	Monitor renal function prior to and during therapy, and ensure an intake of at least 2 L of fluid daily. Monitor serum potassium and magnesium and correct any deficiencies
TACROLIMUS	IMMUNOMODULATING DRUGS – CICLOSPORIN	↑ plasma concentrations of ciclosporin	Tacrolimus is probably a more powerful inhibitor of CYP3A4 than ciclosporin	Avoid co-administration
TACROLIMUS	ANTIDEPRESSANTS – ST JOHN'S WORT	↓ tacrolimus levels	Induction of CYP3A4-mediated metabolism of tacrolimus	Avoid co-administration
TACROLIMUS	ANTIDIABETIC DRUGS – METFORMIN	↑ level of metformin	↓ renal excretion of metformin	Watch for andf warn patients about hypoglycaemia ➢ ***For signs and symptoms of hypoglycaemia, see Clinical Features of Some Adverse Drug Interactions, Hypoglycaemia***
TACROLIMUS	ANTIEPILEPTICS – PHENOBARBITAL, PHENYTOIN	↓ tacrolimus levels	Induction of CYP3A4-mediated metabolism of tacrolimus	Avoid co-administration
TACROLIMUS	**ANTIFUNGALS**			
TACROLIMUS	AMPHOTERICIN	Risk of renal toxicity	Additive effect	Monitor renal function closely
TACROLIMUS	AZOLES	↑ levels with azoles	Inhibition of CYP3A4-mediated metabolism of tacrolimus	Monitor clinical effects closely, check levels
TACROLIMUS	CASPOFUNGIN	↓ tacrolimus levels	Induction of CYP3A4-mediated metabolism of tacrolimus	Avoid co-administration

TACROLIMUS	ANTIHYPERTENSIVES AND HEART FAILURE DRUGS – ANGIOTENSIN II RECEPTOR ANTAGONISTS	↑ risk of hyperkalaemia	Uncertain	Monitor serum potassium weekly until stable and then every 6 months
TACROLIMUS	**ANTIVIRALS**			
TACROLIMUS	ADEFOVIR DIPIVOXIL	Possible ↑ efficacy and side-effects	Competition for renal excretion	Monitor renal function weekly
TACROLIMUS	GANCICLOVIR/ VALGANCICLOVIR	Possible ↑ nephrotoxicity/ neurotoxicity	Additive side-effects	Monitor more closely; check tacrolimus levels
TACROLIMUS	PROTEASE INHIBITORS	↑ levels with protease inhibitors	Inhibition of CYP3A4-mediated metabolism of tacrolimus	Monitor clinical effects closely; check levels
TACROLIMUS	CALCIUM CHANNEL BLOCKERS	Plasma concentrations of tacrolimus are ↑ when given with diltiazem, felodipine and nifedipine; however, they appear to protect renal function	Uncertain, but presumed to be due to inhibition of CYP3A4-mediated tacrolimus metabolism	Watch for side-effects of tacrolimus; monitor ECG, blood count and renal and hepatic function
TACROLIMUS	CARDIAC GLYCOSIDES – DIGOXIN	Digoxin toxicity (pharmacodynamic)	Possibly due to tacrolimus-induced hyperkalaemia and hypomagnesaemia	Watch for digoxin toxicity. Monitor potassium and magnesium levels
TACROLIMUS	DANAZOL	Cases of ↑ tacrolimus levels	Uncertain	Watch for early features of tacrolimus toxicity
TACROLIMUS	DIURETICS – POTASSIUM-SPARING DIURETICS AND ALDOSTERONE ANTAGONISTS	Risk of hyperkalaemia	Additive effect	Monitor potassium levels closely
TACROLIMUS	ECHINACEA	May ↓ immunosuppressant effect	Considered to improve immunity and is usually taken in the long term	Be aware
TACROLIMUS	GRAPEFRUIT JUICE	↑ efficacy and ↑ adverse effects of tacrolimus	Unclear but probably due to inhibition of metabolism	Avoid concomitant use. Measure levels if toxicity is suspected, ↓ dose as necessary and monitor levels closely

Primary drug	Secondary drug	Effect	Mechanism	Precautions
TACROLIMUS	H2 RECEPTOR BLOCKERS	↑ adverse effects of tacrolimus, e.g. thrombocytopenia, hepatotoxicity	Tacrolimus is metabolized primarily by CYP3A4 isoenzymes, which are inhibited by cimetidine. Cimetidine is also an inhibitor of CYP2D6, CYP2C19 and CYP1A2. Sirolimus has multiple pathways of metabolism that would be inhibited by cimetidine	Consider alternative acid suppression, e.g. alginate suspension or rabeprazole. Not thought to be clinically significant, although ensure close monitoring of immunosuppressant levels and renal function
TACROLIMUS	LIPID-LOWERING DRUGS – STATINS	Single case report of rhabdomyolysis when simvastatin was added to tacrolimus	Uncertain at present	Monitor LFTs and CK closely; warn patients to report any features of rhabdomyolysis
TACROLIMUS	OESTROGENS	May ↑ plasma tacrolimus concentrations	Due to inhibition of CYP3A4	Be aware. Monitor plasma tacrolimus concentrations and watch for adverse effects
TACROLIMUS	POTASSIUM	Risk of hyperkalaemia	Additive effect	Monitor potassium levels closely
TACROLIMUS	PROTON PUMP INHIBITORS	Possible ↑ efficacy and adverse effects of immunosuppression	Altered metabolism from CYP2C19 to CYP3A4 in patients with low CYP2C19 levels	Monitor levels more closely
THALIDOMIDE				
THALIDOMIDE	**ANTICANCER AND IMMUNOMODULATING DRUGS**			
THALIDOMIDE	**CYTOTOXICS**			
THALIDOMIDE	DOXORUBICIN	↑ risk (up to sixfold) of deep venous thrombosis in patients with multiple myeloma compared with those treated without doxorubicin	Uncertain. Attributed to doxorubicin contributing to the thrombogenic activity	Avoid co-administration except in clinical trials
THALIDOMIDE	FLUOROURACIL	↑ risk of thromboembolism	Mechanism is uncertain; possibly the endothelium-damaging effect of fluorouracil may initiate thalidomide-mediated thrombosis	Avoid co-administration

Part 4 ANTICOAGULANTS

Warfarin

Warfarin is a racemic mixture of *S*- and *R*-warfarin enantiomers, with the *S*-enantiomer possessing significantly (5–6 times) more anticoagulant properties. *S*-warfarin is metabolized primarily by CYP2C9 and *R*-warfarin by CYP1A2, CYP2C19 and CYP3A4.

Major mechanisms of interaction

- *Additional anticlotting effects*. Drugs that affect any aspect of clotting, including antiplatelet agents, will increase the risk of bleeding.
- *Gastrointestinal injury*. Any drug that damages the mucosa of the gastrointestinal tract will increase the risk of bleeding from these lesions if anticoagulants are given.
- *Altered gut vitamin K synthesis*. Vitamin K antagonizes the effects of warfarin. External sources of vitamin K include the diet and intestinal flora, the latter only becoming significant in those with a low dietary intake of the vitamin. Broad-spectrum antibiotics that may reduce intestinal bacteria may alter the effect of warfarin.
- Altered warfarin metabolism. CYP2C9-mediated metabolism of the more potent isomer, *S*-warfarin, may be induced or inhibited. The less potent *R*-warfarin has several alternative metabolic pathways; therefore, inhibition of a particular metabolizing isoenzyme often has minimal clinical effect.

Parenteral anticoagulants

Heparin binds to antithrombin (a protease inhibitor that inactivates factors IIa, IXa, Xa and XIa) and markedly accelerates its inhibitory effect on coagulation. In addition, heparin inhibits platelet function. The newer low-molecular-weight heparins augment antithrombin activity preferentially against factor Xa and do not prolong the APTT like standard (unfractionated) heparin does.

ANTICOAGULANTS ANTICOAGULANTS – ORAL

Primary drug	Secondary drug	Effect	Mechanism	Precautions
ANTICOAGULANTS – ORAL				
ANTICOAGULANTS – ORAL	ALCOHOL	Fluctuations in anticoagulant effect in heavy drinkers or patients with liver disease who drink alcohol	Alcohol may reduce the half-life of oral anticoagulants by inducing hepatic enzymes. They may also alter hepatic synthesis of clotting factors	Caution should be taken when prescribing oral anticoagulants to alcoholics, particularly those who binge drink or have liver damage
ANTICOAGULANTS – ORAL	**ANALGESICS**			
ANTICOAGULANTS – ORAL	NSAIDs	1. Risk of gastrointestinal bleeding with all NSAIDs 2. Possible ↑ anti-coagulant effect with celecoxib, etoricoxib, flurbiprofen, piroxicam and sulindac	1. NSAIDs irritate the gastric mucosa and can cause bleeding, which is exacerbated by anticoagulants 2. Uncertain but possibly a combination of impaired hepatic metabolism and displacement of anticoagulants from their plasma proteins.	1. Extreme caution when co-administering; monitor patients closely 2. Monitor INR closely
ANTICOAGULANTS – ORAL	OPIOIDS	Cases of ↑ anticoagulant effect with tramadol	Uncertain at present	Monitor INR at least weekly until stable
ANTICOAGULANTS – ORAL	PARACETAMOL	Possible ↑ anticoagulant effect when paracetamol is taken regularly (but not occasionally)	Uncertain; possibly due to competitive inhibition of CYP-mediated metabolism of warfarin	Monitor INR closely for the first 1–2 weeks of starting or stopping regular paracetamol
ANTICOAGULANTS – ORAL	**ANTIARRHYTHMICS**			
ANTICOAGULANTS – ORAL	AMIODARONE	Cases of bleeding within 4 weeks of starting amiodarone in patients previously stabilized on warfarin. The effect was seen to last up to 16 weeks after stopping amiodarone	Amiodarone inhibits CYP2C9- and CYP3A4-mediated metabolism of warfarin	Reduce the dose of anticoagulant by 30–50% and monitor INR closely for at least the first month of starting amiodarone and for 4 months after stopping amiodarone. If the INR suddenly ↑ after being initially stabilized, check TSH

ANTICOAGULANTS – ORAL	PROPAFENONE	Warfarin levels may be ↑ by propafenone	Propafenone seems to inhibit warfarin metabolism	Monitor INR at least weekly until stable
ANTICOAGULANTS – ORAL	**ANTIBIOTICS**			
ANTICOAGULANTS – ORAL	AMINOGLYCOSIDES – NEOMYCIN	Elevated prothrombin times and ↑ risk of bleeding	The mechanism is not fully understood, but it is thought that neomycin may reduce the number of vitamin K-producing bacteria in the gastrointestinal tract and/or that absorption of vitamin K may be ↓ by neomycin	The INR should be monitored in all patients starting or stopping neomycin therapy. Patients more at risk are those with an inadequate diet
ANTICOAGULANTS – ORAL	CEPHALOSPORINS	Certain cephalosporins (cefaclor, cefixime, ceftriaxone) may ↑ efficacy of oral anticoagulants	These cephalosporins have vitamin K antagonistic activity, which adds to the action of oral anticoagulants.	Monitor INR closely; any significant ↑ INR may require vitamin K therapy. If possible, use an alternative cephalosporin
ANTICOAGULANTS – ORAL	METRONIDAZOLE, SULPHONAMIDES, TRIMETHOPRIM	↑ anticoagulant effect	Inhibition of CYP2C9-mediated metabolism of oral anticoagulants	Monitor INR every 2–3 days
ANTICOAGULANTS – ORAL	CHLORAMPHENICOL, MACROLIDES, PENICILLINS, QUINOLONES	Occasional episodes of ↑ anti-coagulant effect	Uncertain at present	Monitor INR every 2–3 days
ANTICOAGULANTS – ORAL	RIFAMPICIN	↓ anticoagulant effect	Rifampicin induces CYP2C9-mediated metabolism of warfarin	Monitor INR closely for at least 1 week after starting rifampicin and up to 5 weeks after stopping it. During co-administration, the warfarin dose may need to be markedly ↑

Primary drug	Secondary drug	Effect	Mechanism	Precautions
ANTICOAGULANTS – ORAL	TETRACYCLINES	Additive effects of warfarin and oxytetracycline leading to prolongation of the prothrombin time or INR and bleeding	Tetracyclines have been associated with ↓ prothrombin activity, causing hypoprothrombinaemia and bleeding. Tetracyclines may also decrease the intestinal flora of the gut, depleting the body of vitamin K2; this may only be significant if the patient's diet is low in vitamin K1	Monitor INR closely and adjust the dose of warfarin accordingly. Patients should be alert for signs of overanti-coagulation, bleeding from the gums when brushing their teeth, nose bleeds, unusual bruising and weakness
ANTICOAGULANTS – ORAL	**ANTICANCER AND IMMUNOMODULATING DRUGS**			
ANTICOAGULANTS – ORAL	**CYTOTOXICS**			
ANTICOAGULANTS – ORAL	CYTOTOXICS – CAPECITABINE, CARBOPLATIN, CYCLOPHOSPHAMIDE, DOXORUBICIN, ERLOTINIB, ETOPOSIDE, FLUORO-URACIL (continuous infusion but not bolus doses), GEMCITABINE, IFOSFAMIDE, IMATINIB, METHOTREXATE, PROCAR-BAZINE, SORAFENIB, TEGAFUR WITH URACIL	Episodes of ↑ anticoagulant effect	Not understood but likely to be multifactorial, including CYP interactions (e.g. capecitabine/imatinib inhibit CYP2C9, ifosfamide inhibits CYP3A4), ↓ protein binding of warfarin (e.g. etoposide, flutamide) and ↓ absorption of anticoagulant or vitamin K	Monitor INR at least weekly until stable during administration of chemotherapy
ANTICOAGULANTS – ORAL	AZATHIOPRINE, MERCAPTOPURINE, MITOTANE	Possible ↓ anticoagulant effect	Induction of metabolism of warfarin	Monitor INR closely

ANTICOAGULANTS – ORAL	HORMONES AND HORMONE ANTAGONISTS			
ANTICOAGULANTS – ORAL	BICALUTAMIDE	↑ plasma concentrations of warfarin	Bicalutamide displaces warfarin from protein-binding sites	Monitor INR at least weekly until stable at initiation and discontinuation of concurrent therapy
ANTICOAGULANTS – ORAL	FLUTAMIDE, TAMOXIFEN, POSSIBLY ANASTRAZOLE AND TOREMIFENE	↑ anticoagulant effect	Uncertain; possibly inhibition of hepatic enzymes. Anastrazole is a known inhibitor of CYP1A2, CYP2C9 and CYP3A4. Tamoxifen inhibits CYP3A4	Monitor INR at least weekly until stable at initiation and discontinuation of concurrent therapy
ANTICOAGULANTS – ORAL	**IMMUNOMODULATING DRUGS**			
ANTICOAGULANTS – ORAL	CICLOSPORIN	1. ↓ ciclosporin levels when co-administered with warfarin or acenocoumarol 2. ↓ anticoagulant effect with warfarin and variable effect with acenocoumarol	Competitive metabolism by CYP3A4	1. Watch for ↓ efficacy of ciclosporin 2. Monitor INR at least weekly until stable
ANTICOAGULANTS – ORAL	ACITRETIN, CORTICOSTEROIDS, INTERFERON ALFA, LEFLUNOMIDE	↑ anticoagulant effect	Uncertain at present	Monitor INR at least weekly until stable
ANTICOAGULANTS – ORAL	ANTIDEMENTIA DRUGS – MEMANTINE	Possible ↑ anticoagulant effect	Uncertain at present	Monitor INR at least weekly until stable
ANTICOAGULANTS – ORAL	**ANTIDEPRESSANTS**			
ANTICOAGULANTS – ORAL	MIRTAZAPINE	↑ anticoagulant effect of warfarin	Inhibition of metabolism of warfarin	Monitor INR at least weekly until stable
ANTICOAGULANTS – ORAL	ST JOHN'S WORT	↓ warfarin levels	Induction of metabolism	Avoid co-administration
ANTICOAGULANTS – ORAL	SSRIs	Possible increase in anticoagulant effect with citalopram, fluoxetine, fluvoxamine and paroxetine	Uncertain at present	Monitor INR at least weekly until stable

Primary drug	Secondary drug	Effect	Mechanism	Precautions
ANTICOAGULANTS – ORAL	TCAs	Cases of both ↑ and ↓ effect of warfarin	Uncertain at present	Monitor INR at least weekly until stable
ANTICOAGULANTS – ORAL	ANTIDIABETIC DRUGS – SULPHONYLUREAS	Cases reported of hypoglycaemia when coumarins are started in patients on tolbutamide. Conversely, there are several case reports of bleeding when patients taking tolbutamide are started on oral anticoagulants	Oral anticoagulants inhibit hepatic metabolism of tolbutamide and ↑ its half-life threefold. Tolbutamide possibly alters the plasma protein binding of anticoagulants	Use alternative sulphonylurea or another class of hypoglycaemic
ANTICOAGULANTS – ORAL	**ANTIEPILEPTICS**			
ANTICOAGULANTS – ORAL	BARBITURATES	↓ anticoagulant effect. This reaches a maximum after 3 weeks and can last up to 6 weeks after stopping the barbiturates	Barbiturates induce CYP2B6- and CYP2C9-mediated metabolism of warfarin	Monitor INR carefully. Dose of anticoagulant may need to be ↑ by up to 60%
ANTICOAGULANTS – ORAL	CARBAMAZEPINE	Carbamazepine ↓ effect of warfarin	Uncertain; carbamazepine probably ↑ hepatic metabolism of warfarin	Monitor INR at least weekly until stable
ANTICOAGULANTS – ORAL	PHENYTOIN	Possible ↑ anticoagulant effect	Possibly due to inhibition of CYP2C9-mediated metabolism of warfarin and induction of CYP1A2, which plays a role in activation of coumarins	Monitor INR at least weekly until stable
ANTICOAGULANTS – ORAL	**ANTIFUNGALS**			
ANTICOAGULANTS – ORAL	AZOLES – FLUCONAZOLE, ITRACONAZOLE, KETOCONAZOLE, MICONAZOLE, VORICONAZOLE	↑ anticoagulant effect with azole antifungals. There have been cases of bleeding when topical miconazole (oral gel or pessaries) have been used by patients on warfarin. Posaconazole may be a safer alternative	Itraconazole potently inhibits CYP3A4, which metabolizes both *R*-warfarin (also metabolized by CYP1A2) and the more active *S*-warfarin (also metabolized by CYP2C9)	Necessary to monitor the effects of warfarin closely (weekly INR) and to warn patients to report any symptoms of bleeding ➢ ***For signs and symptoms of hypoglycaemia, see Clinical Features of Some Adverse Drug Interactions, Bleeding disorders***

ANTICOAGULANTS – ORAL	GRISEOFULVIN	Possible ↓ anticoagulant effect coumarins and phenindione	Uncertain at present	Necessary to monitor the effects of warfarin closely (weekly INR) and to warn patients to report any symptoms of bleeding ➢ ***For signs and symptoms of hypoglycaemia, see Clinical Features of Some Adverse Drug Interactions, Bleeding disorders***
ANTICOAGULANTS – ORAL	**ANTIGOUT DRUGS**			
ANTICOAGULANTS – ORAL	ALLOPURINOL	Uncommon instances of ↑ anti-coagulant effect in patients on warfarin who have started allopurinol	Allopurinol possibly ↓ hepatic metabolism of warfarin but is considerable individual variation	Monitor INR at least weekly until stable
ANTICOAGULANTS – ORAL	SULFINPYRAZONE	↑ anticoagulant effect	Uncertain; possibly displacement of anticoagulant from plasma proteins, possibly inhibition of CYP2C9-mediated metabolism of warfarin	Monitor INR at least weekly until stable
ANTICOAGULANTS – ORAL	ANTIHYPERTENSIVES AND HEART FAILURE DRUGS – VASODILATOR ANTIHYPERTENSIVES	1. Bosentan may ↓ warfarin levels 2. Iloprost and sitaxentan may ↑ warfarin levels	1. Uncertain; postulated that bosentan induces CYP3A4 and CYP2C9 2. Uncertain	Monitor INR closely
ANTICOAGULANTS – ORAL	ANTIOBESITY DRUGS – ORLISTAT	↓ anticoagulant effect	Probably ↓ absorption of coumarins	Monitor INR closely until stable
ANTICOAGULANTS – ORAL	ANTIPARKINSON'S DRUGS – ENTACAPONE	↑ anticoagulant effect	Uncertain at present	Monitor INR at least weekly until stable

Primary drug	Secondary drug	Effect	Mechanism	Precautions
ANTICOAGULANTS – ORAL	**ANTIPLATELET AGENTS**			
ANTICOAGULANTS – ORAL	ASPIRIN	Risk of bleeding when high-dose aspirin is co-administered with anticoagulants; less risk with low-dose aspirin	Antiplatelet effects of aspirin add to the anticoagulant effects. Aspirin also irritates the gastric mucosa	Avoid co-administration of anticoagulants and high-dose aspirin. Patients on warfarin should be warned that many OTC and some herbal remedies contain aspirin
ANTICOAGULANTS – ORAL	CLOPIDOGREL	Risk of bleeding when clopidogrel co-administered with anticoagulants	Additive effect on different parts of the clotting mechanism	Closely monitor effects; watch for signs of excess bleeding
ANTICOAGULANTS – ORAL	DIPYRIDAMOLE	Cases of mild bleeding when dipyridamole added to warfarin	Antiplatelet effects of dipyridamole add to the anticoagulant effects	Warn patients to report early signs of bleeding
ANTICOAGULANTS – ORAL	ANTIPROTOZOALS – LEVAMISOLE	Possible ↑ anticoagulant effect	Uncertain	Monitor INR closely
ANTICOAGULANTS – ORAL	**ANTIVIRALS**			
ANTICOAGULANTS – ORAL	NNRTIs	↓ efficacy of warfarin with nevirapine	Altered metabolism. *S*-warfarin is metabolized by CYP2D6, *R*-warfarin by CYP3A4	Monitor INR every 3–7 days when starting or altering treatment and adjust dose by 10% as necessary. May need an approximately twofold increase in dose
ANTICOAGULANTS – ORAL	PROTEASE INHIBITORS	1. Anticoagulant effect altered (cases of both ↑ and ↓) when ritonavir and possibly saquinavir are given with warfarin 2. Possibly ↓ anticoagulant effect when ritonavir and nelfinavir are given with acenocoumarol	Uncertain. Ritonavir inhibits CYP3A4 and CYP2C9 while inducing CYP1A2	Monitor INR at least weekly until stable

ANTICOAGULANTS – ORAL	APREPITANT	Possible ↓ in INR when aprepitant is added to warfarin	Aprepitant ↑ CYP2C9-mediated metabolism of warfarin	Monitor INR carefully for 2 weeks after completing each course of aprepitant
ANTICOAGULANTS – ORAL	CNS STIMULANTS – MODAFINIL	May cause moderate ↑ plasma concentrations of warfarin	Modafinil is a reversible inhibitor of CYP2C9 and CYP2C19 when used in therapeutic doses	Be aware
ANTICOAGULANTS – ORAL	CRANBERRY JUICE	Cases of markedly ↑ anticoagulant effect (including fatal haemorrhage) with regular cranberry juice ingestion	Uncertain; possibly due to inhibition of CYP-mediated metabolism of warfarin	Patients taking warfarin should avoid cranberry juice
ANTICOAGULANTS – ORAL	DANAZOL	Possible ↓ anticoagulant effect	Uncertain	Monitor INR at least weekly until stable
ANTICOAGULANTS – ORAL	DISULFIRAM	↑ anticoagulant effect	Uncertain at present	Monitor INR at least weekly until stable
ANTICOAGULANTS – ORAL	GLUCAGON	↑ anticoagulant effect	Uncertain at present	Monitor INR after administration of glucagon
ANTICOAGULANTS – ORAL	GLUCOSAMINE	↑ anticoagulant effect	Uncertain at present	Avoid co-administration
ANTICOAGULANTS – ORAL	GRAPEFRUIT JUICE	↑ efficacy and ↑ adverse effects of warfarin e.g. ↑ INR, haemorrhage	Unclear. Possibly via inhibition of intestinal CYP3A4	Monitor INR more closely. Avoid concomitant use if unstable INR
ANTICOAGULANTS – ORAL	H2 RECEPTOR BLOCKERS	↑ anticoagulant effect with cimetidine and possibly famotidine	Inhibition of metabolism via CYP1A2, CYP2C9 and CYP2C19	Use alternative acid suppression, e.g. other H2 antagonist or protein pump inhibitor (not esomeprazole, lansoprazole or omeprazole) or monitor INR more closely; ↓ dose may be required. Take acid suppression regularly not PRN if affects INR control
ANTICOAGULANTS – ORAL	LEUKOTRIENE ANTAGONISTS	Zafirlukast ↑ anticoagulant effect	Zafirlukast inhibits CYP2C9-mediated metabolism of warfarin	Monitor INR at least weekly until stable

Primary drug	Secondary drug	Effect	Mechanism	Precautions
ANTICOAGULANTS – ORAL	**LIPID-LOWERING DRUGS**			
ANTICOAGULANTS – ORAL	ANION EXCHANGE RESINS	↓ anticoagulant effect with colestyramine	↓ absorption of warfarin	Give warfarin 1 hour before or 4–6 hours after colestyramine
ANTICOAGULANTS – ORAL	FIBRATES	↑ efficacy of warfarin and phenindione	Uncertain; postulated that fibrates displace anticoagulants from their binding sites	Monitor INR closely
ANTICOAGULANTS – ORAL	STATINS	Possible ↑ anticoagulant effect with fluvastatin and simvastatin	Uncertain; possibly due to inhibition of CYP2C9-mediated metabolism of warfarin	Monitor INR at least weekly until stable
ANTICOAGULANTS – ORAL	NANDROLONE	Episodes of bleeding when patients on oral anticoagulants are started on anabolic steroids	Not understood	Reduce the dose of anticoagulant by 50% and monitor INR closely until stabilized
ANTICOAGULANTS – ORAL	OESTROGENS	↑ anticoagulant effect	Uncertain at present	Oestrogens are usually not recommended in those with a history of thromboembolism; if they are used, monitor INR closely
ANTICOAGULANTS – ORAL	PERIPHERAL VASODILATORS	Cases of major haemorrhage when pentoxifylline is given with acenocoumarol	Uncertain; possibly additive effect (pentoxifylline has an antiplatelet action)	Monitor INR closely
ANTICOAGULANTS – ORAL	PIRACETAM	Case of bleeding associated with ↑ INR in a patient taking warfarin 1 month after starting piracetam	Uncertain. Piracetam inhibits platelet aggregation but uncertain whether it has any effect on other aspects of the clotting cascade	Warn patient to report easy bruising, etc. Monitor INR closely
ANTICOAGULANTS – ORAL	PROGESTOGENS	↓ anticoagulant effect	Uncertain at present	Monitor INR closely

ANTICOAGULANTS – ORAL	PROTON PUMP INHIBITORS	Possibly ↑ anticoagulant effect when esomeprazole, lansoprazole or omeprazole is added to warfarin	Uncertain at present. Omeprazole and lansoprazole are known to induce CYP1A2, which plays a role in activation of coumarins	Monitor INR more closely. ↓ dose may be required. If 10%, 20% or 30% over range, omit dose for 1, 2 or 3 days respectively; consider ↓ maintenance dose by 10%. Regular dosing of a proton pump inhibitor is preferable if affects INR significantly. Not reported with pantoprazole or rabeprazole
ANTICOAGULANTS – ORAL	RALOXIFENE	Possible ↓ anticoagulant effect, which may take several weeks to develop	Uncertain at present	Monitor INR closely for several weeks
ANTICOAGULANTS – ORAL	SUCRALFATE	Possible ↓ anticoagulant effect	↓ absorption of warfarin	Monitor INR at least weekly until stable
ANTICOAGULANTS – ORAL	SYMPATHOMIMETICS – INDIRECT	Methylphenidate may increase the efficacy of warfarin	Uncertain at present	Monitor INR at least weekly until stable
ANTICOAGULANTS – ORAL	TESTOSTERONE	Possible ↑ anticoagulant effect	Uncertain	Monitor INR at least weekly until stable
ANTICOAGULANTS – ORAL	THYROID HORMONES	Possible ↑ anticoagulant effect	Uncertain	Monitor INR at least weekly until stable
ANTICOAGULANTS – ORAL	VITAMIN E	Case of ↑ anticoagulant effect	Uncertain	Monitor INR closely for 1–2 weeks after starting and stopping vitamin E
ANTICOAGULANTS – PARENTERAL				
FONDAPARINUX				
FONDAPARINUX	ANTICOAGULANTS – PARENTERAL	↑ risk of bleeding when heparins are given with fondaparinux	Combined anticoagulant effect	Manufacturers recommend avoiding co-administration

Primary drug	Secondary drug	Effect	Mechanism	Precautions
HEPARINS				
HEPARINS	ALISKIREN	Risk of hyperkalaemia with heparin	Additive effect	Monitor serum potassium closely
HEPARINS	ANALESICS – NSAIDs	1. Risk of prolonged bleeding when ketorolac is co-administered with dalteparin (but not enoxaparin), and intravenous diclofenac is given with heparins 2. ↑ risk of hyperkalaemia when ketorolac is given with heparin	1. Uncertain 2. Heparin inhibits aldosterone secretion, causing hyperkalaemia	1. Avoid co-administration 2. Monitor potassium levels closely
HEPARINS	ANTICOAGULANTS – PARENTERAL	↑ risk of bleeding when heparins are given with fondaparinux	Combined anticoagulant effect	Manufacturers recommend avoiding co-administration
HEPARINS	**ANTIHYPERTENSIVES AND HEART FAILURE DRUGS**			
HEPARINS	ACE INHIBITORS, ANGIOTENSIN II RECEPTOR ANTAGONISTS	↑ risk of hyperkalaemia	Heparin inhibits aldosterone secretion, causing hyperkalaemia	Monitor potassium levels closely
HEPARINS	VASODILATOR ANTIHYPERTENSIVES	Possible ↑ risk of bleeding with iloprost	Anticoagulant effects of heparins ↑ by an mechanism that is uncertain at present	Monitor APTT closely
HEPARINS	ANTIOBESITY DRUGS – SIBUTRAMINE	Possible ↑ risk of bleeding	Uncertain	Monitor APTT closely.
HEPARINS	ANTIPLATELET AGENTS	↑ risk of bleeding when heparins are co-administered with glycoprotein IIb/IIIa inhibitors, dipyridamole, clopidogrel or high-dose aspirin	Additive effect on different parts of the clotting mechanism. Aspirin also irritates the gastric mucosa	Closely monitor effects; watch for signs of excess bleeding. Avoid co-administration of heparins with high-dose aspirin

HEPARINS	DROTRECOGIN ALFA (recombinant activated protein C)	↑ risk of bleeding	Drotrecogin alfa ↓ prothrombin production and has fibrinolytic/antithrombotic effects	Avoid co-administration of drotrecogin alfa with high-dose heparin (>15 IU/kg per hour). Carefully consider the risk–benefit ratio when giving lower doses of heparin
HEPARINS	NITRATES	Possible ↓ efficacy of heparin with GTN infusion	Uncertain	Monitor APTT closely
HEPARINS	THROMBOLYTICS	Heparin requirements are ↑ when administered after streptokinase	Uncertain at present.	Monitor APTT closely when starting heparin after streptokinase
HIRUDINS				
HIRUDINS	THROMBOLYTICS	↑ risk of bleeding complications when alteplase or streptokinase is co-administered with lepirudin	Additive effect on clotting cascade	Watch for bleeding complications. Risk–benefit analysis is needed before co-administering; this will involve availability of alternative therapies such as primary angioplasty
THROMBOLYTICS				
THROMBOLYTICS	**ANTICOAGULANTS – PARENTERAL**			
THROMBOLYTICS	HEPARINS	Heparin requirements are ↑ when administered after streptokinase	Uncertain at present	Monitor APTT closely when starting heparin after streptokinase.
THROMBOLYTICS	HIRUDINS	↑ risk of bleeding complications when alteplase or streptokinase co-administered with lepirudin.	Additive effect on clotting cascade	Watch for bleeding complications. Risk–benefit analysis is needed before co-administering; this will involve the availability of alternative therapies such as primary angioplasty

ANTICOAGULANTS THROMBOLYTICS

Primary drug	Secondary drug	Effect	Mechanism	Precautions
THROMBOLYTICS	ANTIPLATELET AGENTS			
THROMBOLYTICS	ASPIRIN	↑ risk of intracerebral bleeding when streptokinase is co-administered with higher-dose (300 mg) aspirin	Additive effect	Avoid co-ingestion when streptokinase is given for cerebral infarction; use low-dose aspirin when co-administered for myocardial infarction
THROMBOLYTICS	GLYCOPROTEIN IIb/IIIa INHIBITORS	1. ↑ risk of major haemorrhage when co-administered with alteplase 2. Possible ↑ risk of bleeding complications when streptokinase is co-administered with eptifibatide	1. Uncertain; other thrombolytics do not seem to interact 2. Additive effect	1. Avoid co-administration 2. Watch for bleeding complications. Risk–benefit analysis is needed before co-administering; this will involve the availability of alternative therapies such as primary angioplasty
THROMBOLYTICS	THROMBOLYTICS	Repeated doses of streptokinase are ineffective and is ↑ risk of allergic reactions	Anti-streptococcal antibodies are formed within a few days of administering a dose; these neutralize subsequent doses	Do not give more than one dose of streptokinase

ANTICOAGULANTS THROMBOLYTICS

Part 5 ANTIDIABETIC DRUGS

Insulin

Insulin cannot be taken as a pill as it is broken down during digestion, similar to protein in food. Therefore it is injected under the skin (subcutaneously). There are more than 20 different preparations of insulin available, but essentially there are four classes determined by the speed of onset, the time of reaching the peak plasma concentration and the duration of activity in the body:

- *Rapid-acting insulin* reaches the blood within 15 minutes of injection, peak levels occur between 30 and 90 minutes, and the duration of action is usually 5 hours.
- *Short-acting (regular) insulin* reaches the blood within 30 minutes of injection, peaks in 2–4 hours and acts for 4–8 hours
- *Intermediate-acting (NPH and lente) insulin* reaches the blood 2–6 hours after injection, peaks in 4–14 hours and acts for 14–20 hours.
- Long-acting (ultralente) insulin reaches the blood in 6–14 hours, usually does not peak or has a short peak at 10–16 hours and acts for 20–24 hours.

Some insulins come mixed together, for example regular and NPH. All insulins contain additives to keep them fresh or to make them act better or last longer. The main issue is that, with long-acting insulins, the risk of adverse interactions tends to last for a long time and management is necessary until the drug's action wears off.

Metformin

Metformin increases the sensitivity of the peripheral insulin receptors. It is well absorbed orally and does not undergo hepatic metabolism (therefore being unaffected by CYP inducers and inhibitors). It is completely excreted in the urine and not significantly bound to plasma proteins.

Sulphonylureas

Sulphonylureas stimulate the release of insulin and undergo extensive first-pass hepatic metabolism by the cytochrome P450 system (and therefore adverse drug interactions with inducers and inhibitors of cytochrome P450). They are highly protein-bound. Chlorpropramide is the only sulphonylurea with significant renal excretion.

Acarbose

The gastrointestinal tract is the main site of action of acarbose, which is metabolized exclusively within the gastrointestinal tract, principally by intestinal bacteria; this process may be adversely affected by antibiotics that alter the intestinal bacterial flora. Acarbose affects the absorption of some drugs (e.g. digoxin).

Meglitinide derivatives

Repaglinide and nateglinide are rapidly and completely absorbed from the gastrointestinal tract and are highly bound to plasma proteins. Repaglinide undergoes extensive first-pass hepatic metabolism (by cytochrome P450) and is excreted mainly from the gastrointestinal tract. Nateglinide is predominantly metabolized by the cytochrome P450 system in the liver and predominantly excreted in the urine. Nateglinide is a potent inhibitor of CYP2C9.

Thiazolidinediones

Pioglitazone and rosiglitazone are well absorbed orally and highly protein-bound. Multiple CYP isoforms are involved in their hepatic and, to a lesser degree, extrahepatic metabolism. Pioglitazone may be a weak inducer of CYP enzymes.

Sitagliplitin

Approximately 80% of the drug is excreted unchanged in the urine, the primary enzyme responsible for the limited metabolism being CYP3A4, with a limited contribution from CYP2C8. Sitagliptin does not inhibit or induce cytochrome enzymes. It is a substrate of P-glycoprotein but not an inhibitor.

Primary drug	Secondary drug	Effect	Mechanism	Precautions
INSULIN				
INSULIN	ALCOHOL	Tends to mask signs of hypoglycaemia and ↑ risk of hypoglycaemic episodes	Inhibits glucose production and release from many sources, including the liver	Watch for and warn patients about symptoms of hypoglycaemia ➢ ***For signs and symptoms of hypoglycaemia, see Clinical Features of Some Adverse Drug Interactions, Hypoglycaemia***
INSULIN	ANTIARRHYTHMICS – DISOPYRAMIDE	↑ risk of hypoglycaemic episodes – particularly in patients with impaired renal function. Hypoglycaemic attacks may occur even when plasma levels of disopyramide are within the normal range (attacks occurring with plasma disopyramide levels of 1–4 ng/mL)	Disopyramide and its metabolite mono-isopropyl disopyramide ↑ secretion of insulin (considered to be due to inhibition of potassium-ATP channels). Suggestion that disopyramide causes an impairment of the counterregulatory (homeostatic) mechanisms that follow hypoglycaemia	In patients receiving antidiabetic drugs, start with the lowest dose of disopyramide if there is no alternative. Measure creatinine clearance. If creatinine clearance is 40 mL/min or less, the dose of disopyramide should not exceed 100 mg and should be administered once daily if creatinine clearance is <15 ml/min. Watch for and warn patients about symptoms of hypoglycaemia ➢ ***For signs and symptoms of hypoglycaemia, see Clinical Features of Some Adverse Drug Interactions, Hypoglycaemia***
INSULIN	**ANTIBIOTICS**			
INSULIN	ISONIAZID	↓ efficacy of antidiabetic drugs	Isoniazid causes hyperglycaemia, the mechanism being uncertain at present	Monitor capillary blood glucose closely; ↑ doses of antidiabetic drugs may be needed

ANTIDIABETIC DRUGS INSULIN

Primary drug	Secondary drug	Effect	Mechanism	Precautions
INSULIN	**QUINOLONES**			
INSULIN	LEVOFLOXACIN	Altered insulin requirements	Both hyperglycaemia and hypoglycaemia	Altered glycaemic control requires frequent monitoring
INSULIN	OFLOXACIN	↑ risk of hypoglycaemic episodes	Mechanism underlying hypoglycaemia is not known	Watch for and warn patients about symptoms of hypoglycaemia ➢ ***For signs and symptoms of hypoglycaemia, see Clinical Features of Some Adverse Drug Interactions, Hypoglycaemia***
INSULIN	**ANTICANCER AND IMMUNOMODULATING DRUGS**			
INSULIN	CYTOTOXICS – PROCARBAZINE	↑ risk of hypoglycaemic episodes	Procarbazine has mild MAO properties. MAOIs have an intrinsic hypoglycaemic effect and are considered to enhance the effect of hypoglycaemic drugs	Watch for and warn patients about symptoms of hypoglycaemia ➢ ***For signs and symptoms of hypoglycaemia, see Clinical Features of Some Adverse Drug Interactions, Hypoglycaemia***
INSULIN	HORMONE ANTAGONISTS – OCTREOTIDE, LANREOTIDE	Likely to alter insulin requirements	Octreotide and lanreotide suppress pancreatic insulin and counter-regulatory hormones (glucagon, growth hormone) and delay or ↓ absorption of glucose from the intestine	Essential to monitor blood sugar at least twice a week after initiating concurrent treatment until blood sugar levels are stable. Advise self-monitoring. Warn patients re hypoglycaemia ➢ ***For signs and symptoms of hypoglycaemia, see Clinical Features of Some Adverse Drug Interactions, Hypoglycaemia***

INSULIN	IMMUNOMODULATING DRUGS – CORTICOSTEROIDS	Often ↑ insulin requirements, particularly with those with high glucocorticoid activity	Corticosteroids, particularly the glucocorticoids (betamethasone, dexamethasone, deflazacort, prednisolone > cortisone, hydrocortisone), have intrinsic hyperglycaemic activity in both diabetic and non-diabetic subjects	Monitor blood sugar during concomitant treatment, weekly if possible, or advise self-monitoring, until blood sugar levels are stable. Larger doses of insulin are often needed
INSULIN	**ANTIDEPRESSANTS**			
INSULIN	MAOIs	↑ risk of hypoglycaemic episodes	MAOIs have an intrinsic hypoglycaemic effect and are considered to enhance the effect of hypoglycaemic drugs	Watch for and warn patients about symptoms of hypoglycaemia ➢ ***For signs and symptoms of hypoglycaemia, see Clinical Features of Some Adverse Drug Interactions, Hypoglycaemia***
INSULIN	SSRIs	Fluctuations in blood sugar are very likely, with both hypoglycaemic and hyperglycaemic events being reported in diabetics receiving hypoglycaemic treatment. ↑ plasma concentrations of sulphonylureas (e.g. tolbutamide) may occur	Brain serotonin and corticotropin-releasing hormone systems participate in the control of blood sugar levels. An ↑ (usually acute) in brain serotonergic activity induces a hyperglycaemic response. Fluvoxamine is a potent inhibitor and fluoxetine a less potent inhibitor of CYP2C9, which metabolizes sulphonylureas	Both hyper- and hypoglycaemic responses have been reported with SSRIs, and there is a need to monitor blood glucose closely prior to, during and after discontinuing SSRI treatment ➢ ***For signs and symptoms of hypoglycaemia and hyperglycaemia, see Clinical Features of Some Adverse Drug Interactions, Hypoglycaemia, Hyperglycaemia***

ANTIDIABETIC DRUGS INSULIN

ANTIDIABETIC DRUGS INSULIN

Primary drug	Secondary drug	Effect	Mechanism	Precautions
INSULIN	TCAs	Likely to impair control of diabetes	TCAs may ↑ serum glucose levels by up to 150%, and ↑ appetite (particularly carbohydrate craving) and ↓ metabolic rate	Be aware and monitor blood sugar weekly until stable. They are generally considered safe unless diabetes is poorly controlled or is associated with significant cardiac or renal disease. Amitriptyline, imipramine and citalopram are also used to treat painful diabetic neuropathy
INSULIN	ANTIDIABETIC DRUGS	↑ risk of hypoglycaemic episodes	Due to additive effects by similar or differing mechanisms to lower blood sugar	Combinations may be used therapeutically. Warn patients about hypoglycaemia ➢ ***For signs and symptoms of hypoglycaemia, see Clinical Features of Some Adverse Drug Interactions, Hypoglycaemia***
INSULIN	**ANTIHYPERTENSIVES AND HEART FAILURE DRUGS**			
INSULIN	ACE INHIBITORS	↑ risk of hypoglycaemic episodes	Mechanism uncertain. ACE inhibitors possibly ↑ insulin sensitivity and glucose utilization. Altered renal function may also be factor. ACE inhibitors may ↑ bradykinin levels, which ↓ production of glucose by the liver. Hypoglycaemia is reported as a (rare) side-effect of ACE inhibitors. Suggested that occurrence of hypoglycaemia is greater with captopril than enalapril. Captopril and enalapril are used in the treatment of diabetic nephropathy	Concurrent treatment need not be avoided and is often beneficial in type II diabetes. Watch for and warn patients about symptoms of hypoglycaemia. Be aware that the risk of hypoglycaemia is greater in elderly people and in patients with poor glycaemic control ➢ ***For signs and symptoms of hypoglycaemia, see Clinical Features of Some Adverse Drug Interactions, Hypoglycaemia***

INSULIN	ADRENERGIC NEURONE BLOCKERS	↑ hypoglycaemic effect	Catecholamines are diabetogenic; guanethidine blocks the release of catecholamines from nerve endings	Monitor blood glucose closely
INSULIN	VASODILATOR ANTIHYPERTENSIVES – DIAZOXIDE	May ↑ insulin requirement	Diazoxide causes hyperglycaemia by inhibiting insulin release and probably by a catecholamine-induced extrahepatic effect. Used in the treatment of hypoglycaemia due to insulinomas	Larger doses of insulin are often required, and there is a need to monitor blood sugar until adequate control of blood sugar is achieved
INSULIN	ANTIOBESITY DRUGS – ORLISTAT, RIMONABANT, SIBUTRAMINE	Tendency for blood glucose levels to fluctuate	These agents change dietary intake of carbohydrates and other foods, and the risk of such fluctuations in blood glucose is greater if there is a concurrent dietary regimen. A side-effect of orlistat is hypoglycaemia	These agents are used often in patients with type II diabetes who are on hypoglycaemic therapy. Need to monitor blood sugars twice weekly until stable. Advise self-monitoring and watch for and warn about symptoms of hypoglycaemia ➢ ***For signs and symptoms of hypoglycaemia, see Clinical Features of Some Adverse Drug Interactions, Hypoglycaemia***
INSULIN	ANTIPARKINSON'S DRUGS – RASAGILINE, SELEGILINE	↑ risk of hypoglycaemic episodes	These drugs are MAO-B inhibitors. MAOIs have an intrinsic hypoglycaemic effect and are considered to enhance the effect of hypoglycaemic drugs	Watch for and warn patients about symptoms of hypoglycaemia ➢ ***For signs and symptoms of hypoglycaemia, see Clinical Features of Some Adverse Drug Interactions, Hypoglycaemia***
INSULIN	ANTIPLATELET AGENTS – ASPIRIN	Risk of hypoglycaemia when high-dose aspirin (3.5–7.5 g/day) is given with antidiabetic drugs	Additive effect; aspirin has a hypoglycaemic effect	Avoid high-dose aspirin

Primary drug	Secondary drug	Effect	Mechanism	Precautions
INSULIN	ANTIPROTOZOALS – PENTAMIDINE	Altered insulin requirement	Attributed to pancreatic beta cell toxicity	Altered glycaemic control; need to monitor blood sugar until stable and following withdrawal of pentamidine
INSULIN	ANTIPSYCHOTICS – CLOZAPINE	May cause ↑ blood sugar and loss of control of blood sugar	Clozapine can cause resistance to the action of insulin	Watch for diabetes mellitus in patients on long-term clozapine treatment
INSULIN	ANTIVIRALS – PROTEASE INHIBITORS	↓ efficacy of insulin	Several mechanisms considered include insulin resistance, impaired insulin-stimulated glucose uptake by skeletal muscle cells, ↓ insulin binding to receptors, and inhibition of intrinsic transport activity of glucose transporters in the body	Necessary to establish baseline values for blood sugar before initiating therapy with a protease inhibitor. Atazanavir, darunavir, fosamprenavir or tipranavir may be safer ➢ ***For signs and symptoms of hyperglycaemia, see Clinical Features of Some Adverse Drug Interactions, Hyperglycaemia***
INSULIN	APROTININ	↑ availability of insulin and risk of hypoglycaemic episodes	Aprotinin ↑ availability of insulin injected subcutaneously. The mechanism is uncertain	Watch for and warn patients about symptoms of hypoglycaemia ➢ ***For signs and symptoms of hypoglycaemia, see Clinical Features of Some Adverse Drug Interactions, Hypoglycaemia***

INSULIN	BETA-BLOCKERS			
INSULIN	BETA-BLOCKERS	Beta-blockers may mask the symptoms and signs of hypoglycaemia. They also ↓ insulin sensitivity; however, beta-blockers that also have vasodilating properties (carvedilol, celiprolol, labetalol, nebivolol) seem to ↑ sensitivity to insulin	Beta-blockers ↓ glucose tolerance and interfere with the metabolic and autonomic responses to hypoglycaemia	Warn patients about the masking of signs of hypoglycaemia. Vasodilating beta-blockers are preferred in patients with diabetes, and all beta-blockers should be avoided in those having frequent hypoglycaemic attacks. Monitor capillary blood glucose closely, especially during initiation of therapy ➢ ***For signs and symptoms of hypoglycaemia, see Clinical Features of Some Adverse Drug Interactions, Hypoglycaemia***
INSULIN	BETA-BLOCKERS – PINDOLOL, PROPRANOLOL, TIMOLOL EYE DROPS	Hypoglycaemia has occurred in patients on insulin also taking oral propanolol and pindolol, propanolol, and timolol eye drops	These beta-blockers inhibit the rebound in blood glucose that occurs as a response to a fall in blood glucose levels	Cardioselective beta-blockers are preferred, and all beta-blockers should be avoided in those having frequent hypoglycaemic attacks. Monitor capillary blood glucose closely, especially during initiation of therapy ➢ ***For signs and symptoms of hypoglycaemia, see Clinical Features of Some Adverse Drug Interactions, Hypoglycaemia***
INSULIN	BRONCHODILATORS – BETA-AGONISTS	↑ risk of hyperglycaemia. ↑ risk of hypoglycaemia in the fetus when administered during pregnancy even with normal maternal blood sugar levels. ↑ risk of ketoacidosis when administered intravenously	By inducing glycogenolysis, beta-adrenergic agonists cause an elevation of blood sugar in adults. In the fetus, these agents cause a depletion of fetal glycogen stores	Monitor blood sugar closely during concomitant administration until blood sugar levels are stable. Be cautious during use in pregnancy. Formoterol and salmeterol are long-acting beta-agonists

ANTIDIABETIC DRUGS INSULIN

ANTIDIABETIC DRUGS INSULIN

Primary drug	Secondary drug	Effect	Mechanism	Precautions
INSULIN	CALCIUM CHANNEL BLOCKERS – DILTIAZEM, NIFEDIPINE	Single case reports of impaired glucose intolerance requiring ↑ insulin requirements with diltiazem and nifedipine	Uncertain at present	Evidence suggests that calcium channel blockers are safe in diabetics; monitor blood glucose levels when starting calcium channel blockers
INSULIN	MUSCLE RELAXANTS – BACLOFEN	↓ hypoglycaemic effect of insulin	Due to these drugs causing hyperglycaemia, the mechanism being uncertain at present	↑ doses of insulin are often required for adequate glycaemic control
INSULIN	NANDROLONE	↑ effect of antidiabetic drugs	Uncertain	Monitor blood sugar closely
INSULIN	NIACIN	↓ hypoglycaemic effect of insulin	Due to these drugs causing hyperglycaemia, the mechanism being uncertain at present	↑ doses of insulin are often required for adequate glycaemic control
INSULIN	NICOTINE	↓ hypoglycaemic effect of insulin	Due to these drugs causing hyperglycaemia, the mechanism being uncertain at present	↑ doses of insulin are often required for adequate glycaemic control
INSULIN	OESTROGENS	Altered glycaemic control	Uncertain at present	Monitor blood glucose closely
INSULIN	PROGESTOGENS	Altered glycaemic control	Uncertain at present	Monitor blood glucose closely
INSULIN	SOMATROPIN	↓ hypoglycaemic effect of insulin	Due to these drugs causing hyperglycaemia, the mechanism being uncertain at present	↑ doses of insulin are often required for adequate glycaemic control
INSULIN	SYMPATHOMIMETICS – EPINEPHRINE	May ↑ insulin requirement	Epinephrine causes the release of glucose from the liver and is an important defence/homeostatic mechanism. Hyperglycaemia due to an antagonistic effect	Larger doses of insulin may be needed during the period of epinephrine use, which is usually in the short term or in emergency situations
INSULIN	TESTOSTERONE	↑ hypoglycaemic effect and ↑ risk of hypoglycaemic episodes	Exact mechanism is uncertain. Low testosterone levels are associated with type II diabetes. Experimental work has suggested that testosterone may play a role in glucose efflux from cells	Warn patients about symptoms of hypoglycaemia ➢ ***For signs and symptoms of hypoglycaemia, see Clinical Features of Some Adverse Drug Interactions, Hypoglycaemia***

INSULIN	THYROID HORMONES	↓ hypoglycaemic effect of insulin	Due to these drugs causing hyperglycaemia, the mechanism being uncertain at present	↑ doses of insulin are often required for adequate glycaemic control
METFORMIN				
METFORMIN	ALCOHOL	Enhanced effect of metformin and ↑ risk of lactic acidosis. May mask signs and symptoms of hypoglycaemia	Alcohol is known to potentiate the effect of metformin on lactate metabolism. Inhibits glucose production and release, from many sources including the liver and release	Watch for and warn patients about symptoms of hypoglycaemia. The onset of lactic acidosis is often subtle with symptoms of malaise, myalgia, respiratory distress and ↑ non-specific abdominal distress. There may be hypothermia and resistant bradyarrhythmias ➢ ***For signs and symptoms of hypoglycaemia, see Clinical Features of Some Adverse Drug Interactions, Hypoglycaemia***
METFORMIN	**ANALGESICS**			
METFORMIN	NSAIDs	Possibility of ↑ plasma levels of metformin if there is renal impairment due to NSAIDs. Phenylbutazone is likely to ↓ renal elimination of metformin and ↑ plasma levels.	These drugs are often used in the long term. NSAIDs can cause renal dysfunction. As metformin is not protein-bound, as the sulphonylureas are, displacement from such binding sites is unlikely	Do not use metformin if serum creatinine is >1.5 mg/dL in males and >1.4 mg/dL in females, or creatinine clearance is <30 mL per minute. Use with caution in patients who have a creatinine clearance of 30–60 mL/min. Warn patients about hypoglycaemia ➢ ***For signs and symptoms of hypoglycaemia, see Clinical Features of Some Adverse Drug Interactions, Hypoglycaemia***

ANTIDIABETIC DRUGS METFORMIN

Primary drug	Secondary drug	Effect	Mechanism	Precautions
METFORMIN	MORPHINE	↑ level of metformin and risk of lactic acidosis. The onset of lactic acidosis is often subtle with symptoms of malaise, myalgia, respiratory distress and ↑ non-specific abdominal distress. There may be hypothermia and resistant bradyarrhythmias	Metformin is not metabolized in humans and is not protein-bound. Competition for renal tubular excretion is the basis for ↑ activity or retention of metformin	A theoretical possibility. Need to consider ↓ of metformin dose or avoidance of co-administration. Warn patients about hypoglycaemia ➢ ***For signs and symptoms of hypoglycaemia, see Clinical Features of Some Adverse Drug Interactions, Hypoglycaemia***
METFORMIN	ANTIARRHYTHMICS – DISOPYRAMIDE	↑ risk of hypoglycaemic episodes	Disopyramide and its metabolite mono-isopropyl disopyramide ↑ secretion of insulin (considered to be due to inhibition of potassium-ATP channels). Suggestion that disopyramide causes an impairment of the counterregulatory (homeostatic) mechanisms that follow hypoglycaemia	The risk of this interaction is high. Recommended that if disopyramide is absolutely necessary, doses in the lower range (1–4 ng/mL) be used. Watch for and warn patients about symptoms of hypoglycaemia ➢ ***For signs and symptoms of hypoglycaemia, see Clinical Features of Some Adverse Drug Interactions, Hypoglycaemia***
METFORMIN	**ANTIBIOTICS**			
METFORMIN	AMINOGLYCOSIDES	Risk of hypoglycaemia due to ↑ plasma concentrations of metformin	Mechanism uncertain. Metformin does not undergo hepatic metabolism. Renal tubular secretion is the major route of metformin elimination. Aminoglycosides are also principally excreted via the kidney, and nephrotoxicity is an important side-effect	Watch and monitor for hypoglycaemia, and warn patients about it ➢ ***For signs and symptoms of hypoglycaemia, see Clinical Features of Some Adverse Drug Interactions, Hypoglycaemia***

METFORMIN	ISONIAZID	↓ efficacy of antidiabetic drugs	Isoniazid causes hyperglycaemia, the mechanism being uncertain at present	Monitor capillary blood glucose closely; ↑ doses of antidiabetic drugs may be needed
METFORMIN	QUINOLONES	↑ risk of hypoglycaemic episodes	Mechanism uncertain. Ciprofloxacin is a potent inhibitor of CYP1A2. Norfloxacin is a weak inhibitor of CYP1A2, but these may inhibit other CYP isoenzymes to varying degrees	Watch for and warn patients about symptoms of hypoglycaemia ➢ ***For signs and symptoms of hypoglycaemia, see Clinical Features of Some Adverse Drug Interactions, Hypoglycaemia***
METFORMIN	**ANTICANCER AND IMMUNOMODULATING DRUGS**			
METFORMIN	CYTOTOXICS – PLATINUM COMPOUNDS	↑ risk of lactic acidosis	Renal excretion of metformin is ↓	Watch for lactic acidosis. The onset of lactic acidosis is often subtle with symptoms of malaise, myalgia, respiratory distress and ↑ non-specific abdominal distress. There may be hypothermia and resistant bradyarrhythmias
METFORMIN	HORMONES AND HORMONE ANTAGONISTS – LANREOTIDE, OCTREOTIDE	Likely to alter metformin requirements	Octreotide and lanreotide suppress pancreatic insulin and counter-regulatory hormones (glucagon, growth hormone) and delay or ↓ absorption of glucose from the intestine	Essential to monitor blood sugar at least twice a week after initiating concurrent treatment until blood sugar levels are stable. Advise self-monitoring. Warn patients about hypoglycaemia ➢ ***For signs and symptoms of hypoglycaemia, see Clinical Features of Some Adverse Drug Interactions, Hypoglycaemia***

ANTIDIABETIC DRUGS METFORMIN

Primary drug	Secondary drug	Effect	Mechanism	Precautions
METFORMIN	IMMUNOMODULATING DRUGS			
METFORMIN	CORTICOSTEROIDS	Often ↑ requirements of hypoglycaemic agent, particularly with high glucocorticoid activity steroids	Corticosteroids, particularly the glucocorticoids (betamethasone, dexamethasone, deflazacort, prednisolone > cortisone, hydrocortisone), have intrinsic hyperglycaemic activity in both diabetic and non-diabetic subjects	Monitor blood sugar during concomitant treatment, weekly if possible, or advise self-monitoring, until blood sugar levels are stable. Larger doses of glimepiride are often needed
METFORMIN	TACROLIMUS	↑ level of metformin	↓ renal excretion of metformin	Watch for and warn patients about hypoglycaemia ➢ ***For signs and symptoms of hypoglycaemia, see Clinical Features of Some Adverse Drug Interactions, Hypoglycaemia***
METFORMIN	**ANTIDEPRESSANTS**			
METFORMIN	SSRIs	Fluctuations in blood sugar are very likely, with both hypoglycaemic and hyperglycaemic events being reported in diabetics receiving hypoglycaemic treatment. ↑ plasma concentrations of sulphonylureas (e.g. tolbutamide) may occur	Brain serotonin and corticotropin-releasing hormone systems participate in the control of blood sugar levels. ↑ (usually acute) in brain serotonergic activity induces a hyperglycaemic response. Fluvoxamine is a potent inhibitor and fluoxetine a less potent inhibitor of CYP2C9, which metabolizes sulphonylureas	Both hyper- and hypoglycaemic responses have been reported with SSRIs, and there is a need to monitor blood glucose closely prior to, during and after discontinuing SSRI treatment ➢ ***For signs and symptoms of hypoglycaemia, see Clinical Features of Some Adverse Drug Interactions, Hypoglycaemia***

ANTIDIABETIC DRUGS METFORMIN

METFORMIN	TCAs	Likely to impair control of diabetes	TCAs may ↑ serum glucose levels by up to 150%, ↑ appetite (particularly carbohydrate craving) and ↓ metabolic rate	Be aware and monitor blood sugar weekly until stable. They are generally considered safe unless diabetes is poorly controlled or is associated with significant cardiac or renal disease. Amitriptyline, imipramine and citalopram are also used to treat painful diabetic neuropathy
METFORMIN	**ANTIEPILEPTICS**			
METFORMIN	HYDANTOINS	↓ hypoglycaemic efficacy	Hydantoins are considered to ↓ release of insulin	Monitor capillary blood glucose closely; higher doses of antidiabetic drugs will be needed
METFORMIN	TOPIRAMATE	↑ level of metformin	Unknown mechanism	Watch for and warn patients about hypoglycaemia ➢ ***For signs and symptoms of hypoglycaemia, see Clinical Features of Some Adverse Drug Interactions, Hypoglycaemia***
METFORMIN	ANTIGOUT DRUGS – PROBENECID	↑ level of metformin and risk of lactic acidosis. The onset of lactic acidosis is often subtle with symptoms of malaise, myalgia, respiratory distress and ↑ non-specific abdominal distress. There may be hypothermia and resistant bradyarrhythmias	↓ renal excretion of metformin	Watch for hypoglycaemia and lactic acidosis. Warn patients about hypoglycaemia ➢ ***For signs and symptoms of hypoglycaemia, see Clinical Features of Some Adverse Drug Interactions, Hypoglycaemia***
METFORMIN	ANTIHISTAMINES – KETOTIFEN	↓ platelet count	Unknown	Avoid co-administration (manufacturers' recommendation)

Primary drug	Secondary drug	Effect	Mechanism	Precautions
METFORMIN	**ANTIHYPERTENSIVES AND HEART FAILURE DRUGS**			
METFORMIN	ACE INHIBITORS	↑ risk of hypoglycaemic episodes	Mechanism uncertain. ACE inhibitors possibly ↑ insulin sensitivity and glucose utilization. Altered renal function may also be factor. ACE inhibitors may ↑ bradykinin levels, which ↓ production of glucose by the liver. Hypoglycaemia is reported as a (rare) side-effect of ACE inhibitors. Suggested that occurrence of hypoglycaemia is greater with captopril than enalapril. Captopril and enalapril are used in the treatment of diabetic nephropathy	Concurrent treatment need not be avoided and is often beneficial in type II diabetes. Watch for and warn patients about symptoms of hypoglycaemia. Be aware that the risk of hypoglycaemia is greater in the elderly and in those with poor glycaemic control ➢ ***For signs and symptoms of hypoglycaemia, see Clinical Features of Some Adverse Drug Interactions, Hypoglycaemia***
METFORMIN	ADRENERGIC NEURONE BLOCKERS	↑ hypoglycaemic effect	Catecholamines are diabetogenic; guanethidine blocks the release of catecholamines from nerve endings	Monitor blood glucose closely
METFORMIN	VASODILATOR ANTIHYPERTENSIVES – DIAZOXIDE	May ↑ metformin requirements	Diazoxide causes hyperglycaemia by inhibiting insulin release and probably by a catecholamine-induced extrahepatic effect. Used in the treatment of hypoglycaemia due to insulinomas	Larger doses of metformin are often required; need to monitor blood sugar until adequate control of blood sugar is achieved
METFORMIN	ANTIPLATELET AGENTS – ASPIRIN	Risk of hypoglycaemia when high-dose aspirin (3.5–7.5 g/day) is given with antidiabetic drugs	Additive effect; aspirin has a hypoglycaemic effect	Avoid high-dose aspirin

METFORMIN	**ANTIPSYCHOTICS**			
METFORMIN	CLOZAPINE	May cause ↑ blood sugar and loss of control of blood sugar	Clozapine can cause resistance to the action of insulin	Watch and monitor for diabetes mellitus in patients on long-term clozapine treatment
METFORMIN	PHENOTHIAZINES	May ↑ blood sugar-lowering effect and risk of hypoglycaemic episodes. Likely to occur with doses exceeding 100 mg/day	Phenothiazines such as chlorpromazine inhibit the release of epinephrine and ↑ risk of hypoglycaemia. May inhibit the release of insulin	Chlorpromazine is nearly always used in the long term. Watch for and warn patients about symptoms of hypoglycaemia ➢ ***For signs and symptoms of hypoglycaemia, see Clinical Features of Some Adverse Drug Interactions, Hypoglycaemia***
METFORMIN	ANTIVIRALS – CIDOFOVIR	↑ risk of lactic acidosis	↓ renal excretion of metformin	Watch for lactic acidosis. The onset of lactic acidosis is often subtle with symptoms of malaise, myalgia, respiratory distress and ↑ non-specific abdominal distress. There may be hypothermia and resistant bradyarrhythmias
METFORMIN	BETA-BLOCKERS	Beta-blockers may mask the symptoms and signs of hypoglycaemia, such as tachycardia and tremor; there have even been cases of bradycardia and ↑ BP during hypoglycaemic episodes in patients on beta-blockers	Beta-blockers prevent or inhibit the normal physiological response to hypoglycaemia by interfering with catecholamine-induced mobilization – glycogenolysis and mobilization of glucose – thereby prolonging the time taken by the body to achieve normal (euglycaemic) blood sugar levels	Warn patients about the masking of signs of hypoglycaemia. Cardioselective beta-blockers are preferred, and all beta-blockers should be avoided in those having frequent hypoglycaemic attacks; otherwise monitor glycaemic control, especially during initiation of therapy ➢ ***For signs and symptoms of hypoglycaemia, see Clinical Features of Some Adverse Drug Interactions, Hypoglycaemia***

ANTIDIABETIC DRUGS METFORMIN

ANTIDIABETIC DRUGS METFORMIN

Primary drug	Secondary drug	Effect	Mechanism	Precautions
METFORMIN	BRONCHODILATORS – BETA AGONISTS	↑ risk of hyperglycaemia. If administered during pregnancy, there is a risk of hypoglycaemia in the fetus, independent of maternal blood glucose levels. ↑ risk of ketoacidosis when administered intravenously	By inducing glycogenolysis, beta-adrenergic agonists cause elevation of blood sugar in adults. In the fetus, these agents cause a depletion of fetal glycogen stores	Monitor blood sugar closely during concomitant administration until blood sugar levels are stable. Be cautious during use in pregnancy. Formoterol and salmeterol are long-acting beta-agonists
METFORMIN	DIURETICS – AMILORIDE	↑ metformin levels and risk of lactic acidosis	Metformin is not metabolized in humans and is not protein-bound. Competition for renal tubular excretion is the basis for ↑ activity or retention of metformin	A theoretical possibility. Need to consider ↓ dose of metformin or avoidance of co-administration
METFORMIN	H2 RECEPTOR BLOCKERS – CIMETIDINE, RANITIDINE	↑ level of metformin and risk of lactic acidosis. The onset of lactic acidosis is often subtle with symptoms of malaise, myalgia, respiratory distress and ↑ non-specific abdominal distress. There may be hypothermia and resistant bradyarrhythmias	Metformin is not metabolized in humans and is not protein-bound. Competition for renal tubular excretion is the basis for ↑ activity or retention of metformin. Cimetidine competes for the excretory pathway	A theoretical possibility. Need to consider ↓ dose of metformin or avoidance of co-administration. Warn patients about hypoglycaemia ➢ ***For signs and symptoms of hypoglycaemia, see Clinical Features of Some Adverse Drug Interactions, Hypoglycaemia***
METFORMIN	MUSCLE RELAXANTS – BACLOFEN	↓ hypoglycaemic effect of metformin	Due to these drugs causing hyperglycaemia, the mechanism being uncertain at present	↑ doses of metformin are often required for adequate glycaemic control
METFORMIN	NANDROLONE	↑ effect of antidiabetic drugs	Uncertain	Monitor blood sugar closely
METFORMIN	NIACIN	↓ hypoglycaemic effect of metformin	Due to these drugs causing hyperglycaemia, the mechanism being uncertain at present	↑ doses of metformin are often required for adequate glycaemic control

METFORMIN	NICOTINIC ACID	↓ hypoglycaemic effect of metformin	Due to these drugs causing hyperglycaemia, the mechanism being uncertain at present	↑ doses of metformin are often required for adequate glycaemic control
METFORMIN	SOMATROPIN	↓ hypoglycaemic effect of metformin	Due to these drugs causing hyperglycaemia, the mechanism being uncertain at present	↑ doses of metformin are often required for adequate glycaemic control
METFORMIN	SYMPATHOMIMETICS – EPINEPHRINE	May ↑ antidiabetic requirements	Epinephrine causes the release of glucose from the liver and is an important defence/homeostatic mechanism. Hyperglycaemia due to an antagonistic effect	Larger doses of antidiabetic therapy may be needed during the period of epinephrine use, which is usually in the short term or in emergency situations
METFORMIN	TESTOSTERONE	↑ hypoglycaemic effect and ↑ risk of hypoglycaemic episodes	Exact mechanism is uncertain. Low testosterone levels are associated with type II diabetes. Experimental work has suggested that testosterone may play a role in glucose efflux from cells	Warn patients about symptoms of hypoglycaemia ➢ ***For signs and symptoms of hypoglycaemia, see Clinical Features of Some Adverse Drug Interactions, Hypoglycaemia***
METFORMIN	THYROID HORMONES	↓ hypoglycaemic effect of metformin	Due to these drugs causing hyperglycaemia, the mechanism being uncertain at present	↑ doses of metformin are often required for adequate glycaemic control
SULPHONYLUREAS				
SULPHONYLUREAS	ALCOHOL	Tends to mask signs of hypoglycaemia and ↑ risk of hypoglycaemic episodes	Inhibits glucose production and release, from many sources including the liver and release	Watch for and warn patients about symptoms of hypoglycaemia ➢ ***For signs and symptoms of hypoglycaemia, see Clinical Features of Some Adverse Drug Interactions, Hypoglycaemia***

ANTIDIABETIC DRUGS SULPHONYLUREAS

Primary drug	Secondary drug	Effect	Mechanism	Precautions
SULPHONYLUREAS	ANALGESICS – NSAIDs	Enhanced hypoglycaemic effect of sulphonylureas with most NSAIDs, which are highly protein bound. There have been reports of hyperglycaemia and hypoglycaemia (e.g. with diclofenac)	Attributed to displacement of sulphonylureas from protein binding sites, thus ↑ plasma concentration. Some NSAIDs may impair the renal elimination of sulphonylureas, particularly chlorpropamide	Be aware. There are conflicting reports. Suggestions that sulindac and diclofenac with misoprostol may interact minimally
SULPHONYLUREAS	ANTIARRHYTHMICS – DISOPYRAMIDE	↑ risk of hypoglycaemic episodes – particularly in patients with impaired renal function. Hypoglycaemic attacks may occur even when plasma levels of disopyramide are within the normal range (attacks occurring with plasma disopyramide levels of 1–4 ng/mL)	Disopyramide and its metabolite mono-isopropyl disopyramide ↑ secretion of insulin (considered to be due to inhibition of potassium-ATP channels). Suggestion that disopyramide causes an impairment of the counterregulatory (homeostatic) mechanisms that follow hypoglycaemia	In patients receiving antidiabetic drugs, start with the lowest dose of disopyramide if there is no alternative. Measure creatinine clearance. If creatinine clearance is 40 mL/min or less, the dose of disopyramide should not exceed 100 mg and should be administered once daily if creatinine clearance is <15 ml/min. Watch for and warn patients about symptoms of hypoglycaemia ➢ ***For signs and symptoms of hypoglycaemia, see Clinical Features of Some Adverse Drug Interactions, Hypoglycaemia***
SULPHONYLUREAS	**ANTIBIOTICS**			
SULPHONYLUREAS	CHLORAMPHENICOL	Possibly ↓ hypoglycaemic effect of sulphonylureas	Mechanism uncertain. Chloramphenicol is an inhibitor of CYP3A4	Be aware
SULPHONYLUREAS	ISONIAZID	↓ efficacy of antidiabetic drugs	Isoniazid causes hyperglycaemia, the mechanism being uncertain at present	Monitor capillary blood glucose closely; ↑ doses of antidiabetic drugs may be needed

SULPHONYLUREAS	QUINOLONES	↑ risk of hypoglycaemic episodes	Mechanism uncertain. Ciprofloxacin is a potent inhibitor of CYP1A2. Norfloxacin is a weak inhibitor of CYP1A2, but the quinolones may inhibit other CYP isoenzymes to varying degrees	Watch for and warn patients about symptoms of hypoglycaemia ➢ ***For signs and symptoms of hypoglycaemia, see Clinical Features of Some Adverse Drug Interactions, Hypoglycaemia***
SULPHONYLUREAS	RIFAMPICIN	↓ hypoglycaemic efficacy	Plasma levels of sulphonylureas are ↓ by induction of CYP-mediated metabolism	Watch for and warn patients about symptoms of hyperglycaemia ➢ ***For signs and symptoms of hypoglycaemia, see Clinical Features of Some Adverse Drug Interactions, Hypoglycaemia***
SULPHONYLUREAS	**ANTICANCER AND IMMUNOMODULATING DRUGS**			
SULPHONYLUREAS	**CYTOTOXICS**			
CHLORPROPAMIDE	BORTEZOMIB	Likely to ↑ hypoglycaemic effect of chlorpropamide	Unknown	Watch for and warn patients about symptoms of hypoglycaemia ➢ ***For signs and symptoms of hypoglycaemia, see Clinical Features of Some Adverse Drug Interactions, Hypoglycaemia***
GLIPIZIDE	CYCLOPHOSPHAMIDE	Blood sugar levels may be ↑ or ↓	Uncertain	Need to monitor blood glucose in patients with concomitant treatment at the beginning of treatment and after 1–2 weeks
SULPHONAMIDES – GLIMEPIRIDE, GLIPIZIDE, TOLBUTAMIDE	IMATINIB	↑ plasma concentrations, with risk of toxic effects of these drugs	Imatinib is a potent inhibitor of CYP2C9 isoenzymes, which metabolize these drugs	Watch for the early toxic effects of these drugs. If necessary, consider using alternative drugs while the patient is being given imatinib

Primary drug	Secondary drug	Effect	Mechanism	Precautions
GLIPIZIDE	PORFIMER	↑ risk of photosensitivity reactions	Attributed to additive effects	Avoid exposure of skin and eyes to direct sunlight for 30 days after porfimer therapy
SULPHONYLUREAS	PROCARBAZINE	↑ risk of hypoglycaemic episodes	MAOIs have an intrinsic hypoglycaemic effect. MAOIs are considered to enhance the effect of hypoglycaemic drugs	Watch for and warn patients about symptoms of hypoglycaemia ➢ ***For signs and symptoms of hypoglycaemia, see Clinical Features of Some Adverse Drug Interactions, Hypoglycaemia***
SULPHONYLUREAS	**HORMONES AND HORMONE ANTAGONISTS**			
SULPHONYLUREAS	LANREOTIDE, OCTREOTIDE	Likely to alter insulin requirements	Octreotide and lanreotide suppress pancreatic insulin and counterregulatory hormones (glucagon, growth hormone) and delay or ↓ absorption of glucose from the intestine	Essential to monitor blood sugar at least twice a week after initiating concurrent treatment until blood sugar levels are stable. Advise self-monitoring
SULPHONYLUREAS	**IMMUNOMODULATING DRUGS**			
GLIPIZIDE	CICLOSPORIN	May ↑ plasma concentrations of ciclosporin	Glipizide inhibits CYP3A4-mediated metabolism of ciclosporin	Monitor plasma ciclosporin levels to prevent toxicity
SULPHONYLUREAS	CORTICOSTEROIDS	Often ↑ requirements of hypoglycaemic agent, particularly with high glucocorticoid activity steroids	Corticosteroids, particularly the glucocorticoids (betamethasone, dexamethasone, deflazacort, prednisolone > cortisone, hydrocortisone), have intrinsic hyperglycaemic activity in both diabetic and non-diabetic subjects	Monitor blood sugar during concomitant treatment, weekly if possible, or advise self-monitoring, until blood sugar levels are stable. Larger doses of glimepiride are often needed

ANTIDIABETIC DRUGS SULPHONYLUREAS

TOLBUTAMIDE	LEFLUNOMIDE	Possible ↑ effect of tolbutamide	Uncertain	Monitor blood sugar closely. Watch for and warn patients about symptoms of hypoglycaemia ➢ ***For signs and symptoms of hypoglycaemia, see Clinical Features of Some Adverse Drug Interactions, Hypoglycaemia***
SULPHONYLUREAS	ANTICOAGULANTS – ORAL	Cases reported of hypoglycaemia when coumarins started in patients on tolbutamide. Conversely, there are several case reports of bleeding when tolbutamide was started in patients on oral anticoagulants	Oral anticoagulants inhibit hepatic metabolism of tolbutamide and ↑ its half-life threefold. Tolbutamide possibly alters the plasma protein binding of anticoagulants	Use an alternative sulphonylurea or another class of hypoglycaemic
SULPHONYLUREAS	**ANTIDEPRESSANTS**			
SULPHONYLUREAS	MAOIs	↑ risk of hypoglycaemic episodes	MAOIs have an intrinsic hypoglycaemic effect and are considered to enhance the effect of hypoglycaemic drugs	Watch for and warn patients about symptoms of hypoglycaemia ➢ ***For signs and symptoms of hypoglycaemia, see Clinical Features of Some Adverse Drug Interactions, Hypoglycaemia***
SULPHONYLUREAS	SSRIs	Fluctuations in blood sugar are very likely, with both hypoglycaemic and hyperglycaemic events being reported in diabetics receiving hypoglycaemic treatment. ↑ plasma concentrations of sulphonylureas (e.g. tolbutamide) may occur	Brain serotonin and corticotropin-releasing hormone systems participate in the control of blood sugar levels. ↑ (usually acute) in brain serotonergic activity induces a hyperglycaemic response. Fluvoxamine is a potent inhibitor and fluoxetine a less potent inhibitor of CYP2C9, which metabolizes sulphonylureas	Both hyper- and hypoglycaemic responses have been reported with SSRIs; there is a need to monitor blood glucose closely prior to, during and after discontinuing SSRI treatment ➢ ***For signs and symptoms of hypoglycaemia and hyperglycaemia, see Clinical Features of Some Adverse Drug Interactions, Hypoglycaemia, Hyperglycaemia***

ANTIDIABETIC DRUGS SULPHONYLUREAS

Primary drug	Secondary drug	Effect	Mechanism	Precautions
SULPHONYLUREAS	ST JOHN'S WORT	↓ hypoglycaemic efficacy	Plasma levels of sulphonylureas are ↓ by induction of CYP-mediated metabolism	Watch for and warn patients about symptoms of hyperglycaemia ➢ ***For signs and symptoms of hyperglycaemia, see Clinical Features of Some Adverse Drug Interactions, Hyperglycaemia***
SULPHONYLUREAS	TCAs	Likely to impair control of diabetes	TCAs may ↑ serum glucose levels by up to 150%, ↑ appetite (particularly carbohydrate craving) and ↓ metabolic rate	Be aware and monitor blood sugar weekly until stable. They are generally considered safe unless diabetes is poorly controlled or is associated with significant cardiac or renal disease. Amitriptyline, imipramine and citalopram are also used to treat painful diabetic neuropathy
SULPHONYLUREAS	ANTIDIABETIC DRUGS	↑ risk of hypoglycaemic episodes	Due to additive effects by similar or differing mechanisms to lower blood sugar	Combinations may be used therapeutically. Warn patients about hypoglycaemia ➢ ***For signs and symptoms of hypoglycaemia, see Clinical Features of Some Adverse Drug Interactions, Hypoglycaemia***
TOLBUTAMIDE	ANTIEMETICS – APREPITANT	↓ tolbutamide levels	Aprepitant ↑ CYP2C9-mediated metabolism of tolbutamide	Monitor blood glucose closely
SULPHONYLUREAS	**ANTIEPILEPTICS**			
SULPHONYLUREAS	BARBITURATES	↓ hypoglycaemic efficacy	Plasma levels of sulphonylureas are ↓ by induction of CYP-mediated metabolism	Watch for and warn patients about symptoms of hyperglycaemia ➢ ***For signs and symptoms of hyperglycaemia, see Clinical Features of Some Adverse Drug Interactions, Hyperglycaemia***

ANTIDIABETIC DRUGS SULPHONYLUREAS

GLIPIZIDE	CARBAMAZEPINE	↓ blood sugar-lowering effect of glipizide due to ↓ blood levels	↑ metabolism of glipizide due to ↑ activity of the enzymes that metabolize glipizide by carbamazepine	A higher dose of glipizide may be needed for adequate control of high blood sugar
SULPHONYLUREAS	HYDANTOINS	↓ hypoglycaemic efficacy	Hydantoins are considered to ↓ release of insulin	Monitor capillary blood glucose closely; higher doses of antidiabetic drugs are needed
SULPHONYLUREAS	ANTIFUNGALS – ITRACONAZOLE, FLUCONAZOLE, MICONAZOLE, VORICONAZOLE	↑ risk of hypoglycaemic episodes	Inhibition of CYP2C9-mediated metabolism of sulphonylureas	Watch for and warn patients about symptoms of hypoglycaemia ➢ ***For signs and symptoms of hypoglycaemia, see Clinical Features of Some Adverse Drug Interactions, Hypoglycaemia***
SULPHONYLUREAS	**ANTIGOUT DRUGS**			
SULPHONYLUREAS	PROBENECID	↑ risk of hypoglycaemic episodes due to ↑ plasma levels of glimepiride	Attributed to ↓ renal excretion of sulphonylureas by probenecid. Probenecid is also an inhibitor of CYP2C9 isoenzymes	Watch for and warn patients about symptoms of hypoglycaemia ➢ ***For signs and symptoms of hypoglycaemia, see Clinical Features of Some Adverse Drug Interactions, Hypoglycaemia***
SULPHONYLUREAS	SULFINPYRAZONE	↑ hypoglycaemic effect of sulphonylureas	Uncertain	Monitor blood glucose regularly

Primary drug	Secondary drug	Effect	Mechanism	Precautions
SULPHONYLUREAS	ANTIHYPERTENSIVES AND HEART FAILURE DRUGS			
SULPHONYLUREAS	ACE INHIBITORS	↑ risk of hypoglycaemic episodes	Mechanism uncertain. ACE inhibitors possibly ↑ insulin sensitivity and glucose utilization. Altered renal function may also be factor. ACE inhibitors may ↑ bradykinin levels, which ↓ production of glucose by the liver. Hypoglycaemia is reported as a (rare) side-effect of ACE inhibitors. Suggested that the occurrence of hypoglycaemia is greater with captopril than enalapril. Captopril and enalapril are used in the treatment of diabetic nephropathy	Concurrent treatment need not be avoided and is often beneficial in type II diabetes. Watch for and warn patients about symptoms of hypoglycaemia. Be aware that the risk of hypoglycaemia is greater in elderly people and in patients with poor glycaemic control ➢ ***For signs and symptoms of hypoglycaemia, see Clinical Features of Some Adverse Drug Interactions, Hypoglycaemia***
SULPHONYLUREAS	ADRENERGIC NEURONE BLOCKERS	↑ hypoglycaemic effect	Catecholamines are diabetogenic; guanethidine blocks the release of catecholamines from nerve endings	Monitor blood glucose closely
SULPHONYLUREAS – TOLBUTAMIDE	ANGIOTENSIN II RECEPTOR ANTAGONISTS – IRBESARTAN	Possible ↑ hypotensive effect of irbesartan	Tolbutamide competitively inhibits CYP2C9-mediated metabolism of irbesartan	Monitor BP at least weekly until stable. Warn patients to report symptoms of hypotension (light-headedness, dizziness on standing, etc.)
SULPHONYLUREAS	VASODILATOR ANTIHYPERTENSIVES – BOSENTAN	1. Risk of hepatotoxicity when bosentan is given with glibenclamide 2. ↑ risk of hypoglycaemic episodes when bosentan is given with glimepiride or tolbutamide	1. Additive effect: both drugs inhibit the bile sodium export pump 2. Bosentan may inhibit CYP2C9-mediated metabolism of sulphonylureas	1. Avoid co-administration 2. Monitor blood glucose levels closely. Warn patients about the signs and symptoms of hypoglycaemia ➢ ***For signs and symptoms of hypoglycaemia, see Clinical Features of Some Adverse Drug Interactions, Hypoglycaemia***

ANTIDIABETIC DRUGS SULPHONYLUREAS

SULPHONYLUREAS	DIAZOXIDE	May ↑ sulphonylurea requirements	Diazoxide causes hyperglycaemia by inhibiting insulin release and probably by a catecholamine-induced extrahepatic effect. Sulphonylureas act by ↑ insulin release. Used in the treatment of hypoglycaemia due to insulinomas	Larger doses of sulphonylureas are often required; need to monitor blood sugar until adequate control of blood sugar is achieved
SULPHONYLUREAS	ANTIOBESITY DRUGS – ORLISTAT, RIMONABANT, SIBUTRAMINE	Tendency for blood glucose levels to fluctuate. There may be a tendency to enhance the hypoglycaemic effect	These agents change dietary intake of carbohydrates and other foods, and the risk of fluctuations of blood glucose is greater if there is a concurrent dietary regimen. A side-effect of orlistat is hypoglycaemia	These agents are used often in type II diabetics on hypoglycaemic therapy. Need to monitor blood sugars twice weekly until stable. Advise self-monitoring. Warn patients about hypoglycaemia ➢ ***For signs and symptoms of hypoglycaemia, see Clinical Features of Some Adverse Drug Interactions, Hypoglycaemia***
SULPHONYLUREAS	ANTIPARKINSON'S DRUGS – RASAGILINE, SELEGILINE	↑ risk of hypoglycaemic episodes	These drugs are MAO-B inhibitors. MAOIs have an intrinsic hypoglycaemic effect and are considered to enhance the effect of hypoglycaemic drugs	Watch for and warn patients about symptoms of hypoglycaemia ➢ ***For signs and symptoms of hypoglycaemia, see Clinical Features of Some Adverse Drug Interactions, Hypoglycaemia***
SULPHONYLUREAS	ANTIPLATELET AGENTS – ASPIRIN	Risk of hypoglycaemia when high-dose aspirin (3.5–7.5 g/day) is given with antidiabetic drugs	Additive effect; aspirin has a hypoglycaemic effect	Avoid high-dose aspirin
SULPHONYLUREAS	ANTIPROTOZOALS – PENTAMIDINE	May alter sulphonylurea requirements due to altered glycaemic control	Attributed to pancreatic beta cell toxicity	Need to monitor blood sugar until stable and following withdrawal of pentamidine

Primary drug	Secondary drug	Effect	Mechanism	Precautions
SULPHONYLUREAS	**ANTIPSYCHOTICS**			
SULPHONYLUREAS	CLOZAPINE	May cause ↑ blood sugar and loss of control of blood sugar	Clozapine can cause resistance to the action of insulin	Watch/monitor for diabetes mellitus in subjects on long-term clozapine treatment
SULPHONYLUREAS	PHENOTHIAZINES	May ↑ blood sugar-lowering effect and risk of hypoglycaemic episodes. Likely to occur with doses exceeding 100 mg/day per day	Phenothiazines such as chlorpromazine inhibit the release of epinephrine and ↑ risk of hypoglycaemia. May inhibit release of insulin, which is the mechanism by which sulphonylureas act	Chlorpromazine is nearly always used in the long term. Watch for and warn patients about symptoms of hypoglycaemia ➢ ***For signs and symptoms of hypoglycaemia, see Clinical Features of Some Adverse Drug Interactions, Hypoglycaemia***
SULPHONYLUREAS	ANTIVIRALS – PROTEASE INHIBITORS	↑ adverse effects of tolbutamide with ritonavir (e.g. myelosuppression, peripheral neuropathy, mucositis)	Uncertain	Monitor blood sugar closely
SULPHONYLUREAS	APROTININ	↑ availability of insulin and risk of hypoglycaemic episodes	Aprotinin ↑ availability of insulin injected subcutaneously. The mechanism is uncertain. Sulphonylureas augment insulin release	Watch for and warn patients about symptoms of hypoglycaemia ➢ ***For signs and symptoms of hypoglycaemia, see Clinical Features of Some Adverse Drug Interactions, Hypoglycaemia***
SULPHONYLUREAS	BETA-BLOCKERS	Beta-blockers may mask the symptoms and signs of hypoglycaemia, such as tachycardia and tremor; there have even been cases of bradycardia and ↑ BP during hypoglycaemic episodes in patients on beta-blockers	Beta-blockers prevent or inhibit the normal physiological response to hypoglycaemia by interfering with catecholamine-induced mobilization – glycogenolysis and mobilization of glucose –thereby prolonging the time taken by the body to achieve normal (euglycaemic) blood sugar levels	Warn patients about the masking of signs of hypoglycaemia. Cardioselective beta-blockers are preferred, and all beta-blockers should be avoided in patients having frequent hypoglycaemic attacks; otherwise monitor glycaemic control, especially during initiation of therapy ➢ ***For signs and symptoms of hypoglycaemia, see Clinical Features of Some Adverse Drug Interactions, Hypoglycaemia***

SULPHONYLUREAS	BRONCHODILATORS – BETA-AGONISTS	↑ risk of hyperglycaemia. If administered during pregnancy, there is a risk of hypoglycaemia in the fetus, independent of maternal blood glucose levels. ↑ risk of ketoacidosis when administered intravenously	By inducing glycogenolysis, beta-adrenergic agonists cause elevation of blood sugar in adults. In the fetus, these agents cause a depletion of fetal glycogen stores	Monitor blood sugar closely during concomitant administration until blood sugar levels are stable. Be cautious during use in pregnancy. Formoterol and salmeterol are long-acting beta-agonists
SULPHONYLUREAS	CNS STIMULANTS – MODAFINIL	May cause ↑ plasma concentrations of sulphonylureas if CYP2C9 is the predominant metabolic pathway and the alternative pathways are either genetically deficient or affected	Modafinil is a moderate inhibitor of CYP2C9	Be aware
SULPHONYLUREAS	**DIURETICS**			
CHLORPROPAMIDE	POTASSIUM-SPARING DIURETICS AND ALDOSTERONE ANTAGONISTS	Risk of hyponatraemia when chlorpropamide is given to a patient taking both potassium-sparing diuretics/aldosterone antagonists and thiazides	Additive effect; chlorpropamide enhances ADH secretion	Monitor serum sodium regularly
SULPHONYLUREAS	**THIAZIDES**			
SULPHONYLUREAS	THIAZIDES	↓ hypoglycaemic efficacy	Hyperglycaemia due to antagonistic effect	Monitor blood glucose regularly until stable. A higher dose of oral antidiabetic is often needed
CHLORPROPAMIDE	THIAZIDES	Risk of hyponatraemia when chlorpropamide is given to a patient taking both potassium-sparing diuretics/aldosterone antagonists and thiazides	Additive effect; chlorpropamide enhances ADH secretion	Monitor serum sodium regularly

ANTIDIABETIC DRUGS SULPHONYLUREAS

Primary drug	Secondary drug	Effect	Mechanism	Precautions
GLIMEPIRIDE	H2 RECEPTOR BLOCKERS – CIMETIDINE, RANITIDINE	↑ plasma concentrations of glimepiride and ↑ risk of hypoglycaemic episodes	Cimetidine and ranitidine ↓ renal elimination of glimepiride and ↑ intestinal absorption of glimepiride. Cimetidine is also an inhibitor of CYP2D6 and CYP3A4	Consider alternative acid suppression, e.g. proton pump inhibitor (not omeprazole), and monitor more closely
SULPHONYLUREAS	**LIPID-LOWERING DRUGS**			
GLIPIZIDE	ANION EXCHANGE RESINS	Glipizide absorption may be ↓ by colestyramine	Colestyramine interrupts the entero-hepatic circulation of glipizide	Avoid co-administration
TOLBUTAMIDE	FIBRATES	Fibrates may ↑ efficacy of sulphonylureas	Uncertain; postulated that fibrates displace sulphonylureas from plasma proteins and ↓ their hepatic metabolism. In addition, fenofibrate may inhibit CYP2C9-mediated metabolism of tolbutamide	Monitor blood glucose levels closely. Warn patients about hypoglycaemia ➢ ***For signs and symptoms of hypoglycaemia, see Clinical Features of Some Adverse Drug Interactions, Hypoglycaemia***
SULPHONYLUREAS	MUSCLE RELAXANTS – BACLOFEN	↓ hypoglycaemic effect of sulphonylureas	Due to these drugs causing hyperglycaemia, the mechanism being uncertain at present	↑ doses of sulphonylureas are often required for adequate glycaemic control
SULPHONYLUREAS	NANDROLONE	↑ effect of antidiabetic drugs	Uncertain	Monitor blood sugar closely
SULPHONYLUREAS	NIACIN	↓ hypoglycaemic effect of sulphonylureas	Due to these drugs causing hyperglycaemia, the mechanism being uncertain at present	↑ doses of sulphonylureas are often required for adequate glycaemic control
SULPHONYLUREAS	NICOTINE	↓ hypoglycaemic effect of sulphonylureas	Due to these drugs causing hyperglycaemia, the mechanism being uncertain at present	↑ doses of sulphonylureas are often required for adequate glycaemic control
SULPHONYLUREAS	OESTROGENS	Altered glycaemic control	Uncertain at present	Monitor blood glucose closely
SULPHONYLUREAS	PROGESTOGENS	Altered glycaemic control	Uncertain at present	Monitor blood glucose closely

SULPHONYLUREAS	PROTON PUMP INHIBITORS	Possible ↑ efficacy and adverse effects of sulphonylurea, e.g. hypoglycaemia	Possible ↑ absorption	Monitor capillary blood glucose more closely; ↓ dose may be required
SULPHONYLUREAS	SOMATROPIN	↓ hypoglycaemic effect of sulphonylureas	Due to these drugs causing hyperglycaemia, the mechanism being uncertain at present	↑ doses of sulphonylureas are often required for adequate glycaemic control
SULPHONYLUREAS	SYMPATHOMIMETICS – EPINEPHRINE	May ↑ antidiabetic therapy requirement	Epinephrine causes the release of glucose from the liver and is an important defence/homeostatic mechanism. Hyperglycaemia due to antagonistic effect	Larger doses of antidiabetic therapy may be needed during the period of epinephrine use, which is usually in the short term or in emergency situations
SULPHONYLUREAS	TESTOSTERONE	↑ hypoglycaemic effect and ↑ of hypoglycaemic episodes	Exact mechanism is uncertain. Low testosterone levels are associated with type II diabetes. Experimental work has suggested that testosterone may play a role in glucose efflux from cells	Warn patients about symptoms of hypoglycaemia ➢ ***For signs and symptoms of hypoglycaemia, see Clinical Features of Some Adverse Drug Interactions, Hypoglycaemia***
SULPHONYLUREAS	THYROID HORMONES	↓ hypoglycaemic effect of sulphonylureas	Due to these drugs causing hyperglycaemia, the mechanism being uncertain at present	↑ doses of sulphonylureas are often required for adequate glycaemic control
OTHER ANTIDIABETIC DRUGS				
ACARBOSE				
ACARBOSE	ALCOHOL	Tends to mask signs of hypoglycaemia and ↑ risk of hypoglycaemic episodes	Inhibits glucose production and release from many sources, including the liver	Watch for and warn patients about symptoms of hypoglycaemia ➢ ***For signs and symptoms of hypoglycaemia, see Clinical Features of Some Adverse Drug Interactions, Hypoglycaemia***

Primary drug	Secondary drug	Effect	Mechanism	Precautions
ACARBOSE	**ANTIBIOTICS**			
ACARBOSE	AMINOGLYCOSIDES – NEOMYCIN	↑ postprandial hypoglycaemia and ↑ gastrointestinal effects as a result of concurrent use of acarbose and neomycin	Neomycin is known to cause a drop in blood glucose levels after meals; when used concomitantly with acarbose this ↓ may be ↑. Neomycin also exacerbates the adverse gastrointestinal effects caused by acarbose	Blood glucose levels should be closely monitored; if gastrointestinal signs are severe, the dose of acarbose should be ↓
ACARBOSE	QUINOLONES – CIPROFLOXACIN, NORFLOXACIN, OFLOXACIN	↑ risk of hypoglycaemic episodes	Mechanism uncertain. Ciprofloxacin is a potent inhibitor of CYP1A2. Norfloxacin is a weak inhibitor of CYP1A2, but these drugs may inhibit other CYP isoenzymes to varying degrees	Watch for and warn patients about symptoms of hypoglycaemia ➢ ***For signs and symptoms of hypoglycaemia, see Clinical Features of Some Adverse Drug Interactions, Hypoglycaemia***
ACARBOSE	**ANTIDEPRESSANTS**			
ACARBOSE	SSRIs	Fluctuations in blood sugar are very likely, with both hypoglycaemic and hyperglycaemic events being reported in diabetics receiving hypoglycaemic treatment. ↑ plasma concentrations of sulphonylureas (e.g. tolbutamide) may occur	Brain serotonin and corticotropin-releasing hormone systems participate in the control of blood sugar levels. ↑ (usually acute) in brain serotonergic activity induces a hyperglycaemic response. Fluvoxamine is a potent inhibitor and fluoxetine a less potent inhibitor of CYP2C9, which metabolizes sulphonylureas	Both hyper- and hypoglycaemic responses have been reported with SSRIs; there is a need to monitor blood glucose closely prior to, during and after discontinuing SSRI treatment ➢ ***For signs and symptoms of hypoglycaemia and hpyerglycaemia, see Clinical Features of Some Adverse Drug Interactions, Hypoglycaemia, Hpyerglycaemia***

ACARBOSE	TCAs	Likely to impair control of diabetes	TCAs may ↑ serum glucose levels by up to 150%, ↑ appetite (particularly carbohydrate craving) and ↓ metabolic rate	Be aware and monitor blood sugar weekly until stable. They are generally considered safe unless diabetes is poorly controlled or is associated with significant cardiac or renal disease. Amitriptyline, imipramine and citalopram are also used to treat painful diabetic neuropathy
ACARBOSE	ANTIDIABETIC DRUGS	↑ risk of hypoglycaemic episodes	Due to additive effects by similar or differing mechanisms to lower blood sugar	Combinations are often used and useful. Warn patients about hypoglycaemia ➢ ***For signs and symptoms of hypoglycaemia, see Clinical Features of Some Adverse Drug Interactions, Hypoglycaemia***
ACARBOSE	ANTIEPILEPTICS – VALPROATE	Case of ↓ valproate levels	Uncertain	Monitor valproate levels
ACARBOSE	ANTIHYPERTENSIVES AND HEART FAILURE DRUGS – ADRENERGIC NEURONE BLOCKERS	↑ hypoglycaemic effect	Catecholamines are diabetogenic; guanethidine blocks the release of catecholamines from nerve endings	Monitor blood glucose closely
ACARBOSE	ANTIOBESITY DRUGS – ORLISTAT, RIMONABANT, SIBUTRAMINE	Tendency for blood glucose levels to fluctuate	These agents change dietary intake of carbohydrates and other foods, and the risk of fluctuations in blood glucose is greater if there is a concurrent dietary regimen. A side-effect of orlistat is hypoglycaemia	These agents are used often in patients with type II diabetes who are on hypoglycaemic therapy. Need to monitor blood sugars twice weekly until stable. Advise self-monitoring. Watch for and warn patients about symptoms of hypoglycaemia. Avoid co-administration of acarbose and orlistat ➢ ***For signs and symptoms of hypoglycaemia, see Clinical Features of Some Adverse Drug Interactions, Hypoglycaemia***

Primary drug	Secondary drug	Effect	Mechanism	Precautions
ACARBOSE	ANTIPLATELET AGENTS - ASPIRIN	Risk of hypoglycaemia when high-dose aspirin (3.5–7.5 g/day) given with antidiabetic drugs	Additive effect; aspirin has a hypoglycaemic effect	Avoid high-dose aspirin
ACARBOSE	ANTIPROTOZOALS – PENTAMIDINE	May alter acarbose requirements due altered glycaemic control	Attributed to pancreatic beta cell toxicity	Need to monitor blood sugar until stable and following withdrawal of pentamidine
ACARBOSE	CARDIAC GLYCOSIDES	Acarbose may ↓ plasma levels of digoxin	Uncertain; possibly ↓ absorption of digoxin	Monitor digoxin levels; watch for ↓ levels
ACARBOSE	H2 RECEPTOR BLOCKERS – RANITIDINE	↓ blood levels of ranitidine	Possibly due to ↓ absorption of ranitidine	Be aware
ACARBOSE	LIPID-LOWERING DRUGS – ANION EXCHANGE RESINS	↑ hypoglycaemic effect of acarbose	Uncertain	Monitor blood glucose during co-administration and after discontinuation of concurrent therapy
ACARBOSE	MUSCLE RELAXANTS – BACLOFEN	↓ hypoglycaemic effect	Due to these drugs causing hyperglycaemia, the mechanism being uncertain at present	↑ doses of antidiabetic drugs are often required for adequate glycaemic control
ACARBOSE	NANDROLONE	↑ effect of antidiabetic drugs	Uncertain	Monitor blood sugar closely
ACARBOSE	NIACIN	↓ hypoglycaemic effect	Due to these drugs causing hyperglycaemia, the mechanism being uncertain at present	↑ doses of antidiabetic drugs are often required for adequate glycaemic control
ACARBOSE	NICOTINE	↓ hypoglycaemic effect	Due to these drugs causing hyperglycaemia, the mechanism being uncertain at present	↑ doses of antidiabetic drugs are often required for adequate glycaemic control
ACARBOSE	OESTROGENS	Altered glycaemic control	Uncertain at present	Monitor blood glucose closely
ACARBOSE	PANCREATIN	Theoretical risk of ↓ efficacy of acarbose	↓ absorption	Watch for poor response to acarbose; monitor capillary blood glucose closely

ACARBOSE	PROGESTOGENS	Altered glycaemic control	Uncertain at present	Monitor blood glucose closely
ACARBOSE	SOMATROPIN	↓ hypoglycaemic effect	Due to these drugs causing hyperglycaemia, the mechanism being uncertain at present	↑ doses of antidiabetic drugs are often required for adequate glycaemic control
ACARBOSE	THYROID HORMONES	↓ hypoglycaemic effect	Due to these drugs causing hyperglycaemia, the mechanism being uncertain at present	↑ doses of antidiabetic drugs are often required for adequate glycaemic control
MEGLITINIDE DERIVATIVES – NATEGLINIDE, REPAGLINIDE				
NATEGLINIDE, REPAGLINIDE	ALCOHOL	Tends to mask signs of hypoglycaemia and ↑ risk of hypoglycaemic episodes	Inhibits glucose production and release from many sources, including the liver and release	Watch for and warn patients about symptoms of hypoglycaemia ➢ ***For signs and symptoms of hypoglycaemia, see Clinical Features of Some Adverse Drug Interactions, Hypoglycaemia***
NATEGLINIDE, REPAGLINIDE	ANTIARRHYTHMICS – DISOPYRAMIDE	↑ risk of hypoglycaemic episodes – particularly in patients with impaired renal function. Hypoglycaemic attacks may occur even when plasma levels of disopyramide are within the normal range (attacks occurring with plasma disopyramide levels of 1–4 ng/mL)	Disopyramide and its metabolite mono-isopropyl disopyramide ↑ secretion of insulin (considered to be due to inhibition of potassium-ATP channels). Suggestion that disopyramide causes an impairment of the counterregulatory (homeostatic) mechanisms that follow hypoglycaemia	In patients receiving antidiabetic drugs, start with the lowest dose of disopyramide if there is no alternative. Measure creatinine clearance. If creatinine clearance is 40 mL/min or less, the dose of disopyramide should not exceed 100 mg and should be administered once daily if creatinine clearance is <15 ml/min. Watch for and warn patients about symptoms of hypoglycaemia ➢ ***For signs and symptoms of hypoglycaemia, see Clinical Features of Some Adverse Drug Interactions, Hypoglycaemia***

Primary drug	Secondary drug	Effect	Mechanism	Precautions
NATEGLINIDE, REPAGLINIDE	**ANTIBIOTICS**			
NATEGLINIDE, REPAGLINIDE	ISONIAZID	↓ efficacy of antidiabetic drugs	Isoniazid causes hyperglycaemia, the mechanism being uncertain at present	Monitor capillary blood glucose closely; ↑ doses of antidiabetic drugs may be needed
REPAGLINIDE	MACROLIDES – ERYTHROMYCIN, CLARITHROMYCIN, TELITHROMYCIN	Likely to ↑ plasma concentrations of repaglinide and ↑ risk of hypoglycaemic episodes. ↑ risk of gastrointestinal side-effects with clarithromycin	Due to inhibition of CYP3A4 isoenzymes, which metabolize repaglinide. These drugs vary in potency as inhibitors (clarithromycin is a potent inhibitor), and ↑ plasma concentrations will vary. Clarithromycin ↑ plasma concentrations by 60% However, the alternative pathway – CYP2C8 – is unaffected by these inhibitors	Watch for and warn patients about hypoglycaemia ➢ ***For signs and symptoms of hypoglycaemia, see Clinical Features of Some Adverse Drug Interactions, Hypoglycaemia***
NATEGLINIDE, REPAGLINIDE	QUINOLONES – CIPROFLOXACIN, LEVOFLOXACIN, NORFLOXACIN, OFLOXACIN	↑ risk of hypoglycaemic episodes	Mechanism uncertain. Ciprofloxacin is a potent inhibitor of CYP1A2. Norfloxacin is a weak inhibitor of CYP1A2, but these drugs may inhibit other CYP isoenzymes to varying degrees	Watch for and warn patients about symptoms of hypoglycaemia ➢ ***For signs and symptoms of hypoglycaemia, see Clinical Features of Some Adverse Drug Interactions, Hypoglycaemia***
REPAGLINIDE	RIFAMPICIN	↓ plasma concentrations of repaglinide likely. Rifampicin ↓ AUC of repaglinide by 25%	Due to inducing CYP3A4 isoenzymes, which metabolize repaglinide. However, the alternative pathway – CYP2C8 – is unaffected by these inducers except by rifampicin	The interaction is likely to be most severe with rifampicin. Be aware and monitor for hyperglycaemia ➢ ***For signs and symptoms of hyperglycaemia, see Clinical Features of Some Adverse Drug Interactions, Hyperglycaemia***

REPAGLINIDE	TRIMETHOPRIM	↑ repaglinide levels (by approximately 40%); risk of hypoglycaemia	Hepatic metabolism inhibited	Manufacturers do not recommend concurrent use
NATEGLINIDE, REPAGLINIDE	**ANTICANCER AND IMMUNOMODULATING DRUGS**			
REPAGLINIDE	**CYTOTOXICS**			
REPAGLINIDE	IMATINIB	Likely to ↑ plasma concentrations of repaglinide and ↑ risk of hypoglycaemic episodes	Due to inhibition of CYP3A4 isoenzymes, which metabolize repaglinide	Watch for and warn patients about hypoglycaemia ➢ ***For signs and symptoms of hypoglycaemia, see Clinical Features of Some Adverse Drug Interactions, Hypoglycaemia***
NATEGLINIDE, REPAGLINIDE	**HORMONES AND HORMONE ANTAGONISTS**			
REPAGLINIDE	ANASTRAZOLE	Risk of hypoglycaemia	Mechanism unknown	Watch for and warn patients about hypoglycaemia ➢ ***For signs and symptoms of hypoglycaemia, see Clinical Features of Some Adverse Drug Interactions, Hypoglycaemia***
NATEGLINIDE, REPAGLINIDE	LANREOTIDE, OCTREOTIDE	Likely to alter antidiabetic requirements	Octreotide and lanreotide suppress pancreatic insulin and counter-regulatory hormones (glucagon, growth hormone) and delay or ↓ absorption of glucose from the intestine	Essential to monitor blood sugar at least twice a week after initiating concurrent treatment until blood sugar levels are stable. Advise self-monitoring. Warn patients about hypoglycaemia ➢ ***For signs and symptoms of hypoglycaemia, see Clinical Features of Some Adverse Drug Interactions, Hypoglycaemia***

Primary drug	Secondary drug	Effect	Mechanism	Precautions
REPAGLINIDE	**IMMUNOMODULATING DRUGS**			
REPAGLINIDE	CICLOSPORIN	↑ repaglinide levels, with ↑ risk of hypoglycaemia	Hepatic metabolism inhibited	Watch for and warn patients about hypoglycaemia ➢ ***For signs and symptoms of hypoglycaemia, see Clinical Features of Some Adverse Drug Interactions, Hypoglycaemia***
NATEGLINIDE, REPAGLINIDE	**ANTIDEPRESSANTS**			
NATEGLINIDE, REPAGLINIDE	SSRIs	Fluctuations in blood sugar are very likely, with both hypoglycaemic and hyperglycaemic events being reported in diabetics receiving hypoglycaemic treatment. ↑ plasma concentrations of sulphonylureas (e.g. tolbutamide) may occur	Brain serotonin and corticotropin-releasing hormone systems participate in the control of blood sugar levels. ↑ (usually acute) in brain serotonergic activity induces a hyperglycaemic response. Fluvoxamine is a potent inhibitor and fluoxetine a less potent inhibitor of CYP2C9, which metabolizes sulphonylureas	Both hyper- and hypoglycaemic responses have been reported with SSRIs; there is a need to monitor blood glucose closely prior to, during and after discontinuing SSRI treatment ➢ ***For signs and symptoms of hypoglycaemia and hpyerglycaemia, see Clinical Features of Some Adverse Drug Interactions, Hypoglycaemia, Hyperglycaemia***
REPAGLINIDE	ST JOHN'S WORT	↓ plasma concentrations of repaglinide likely	Due to inducing CYP3A4 isoenzymes, which metabolize repaglinide. However, the alternative pathway – CYP2C8 – is unaffected by these inducers	Be aware and monitor for hyperglycaemia ➢ ***For signs and symptoms of hyperglycaemia, see Clinical Features of Some Adverse Drug Interactions, Hyperglycaemia***
NATEGLINIDE, REPAGLINIDE	TCAs	Likely to impair control of diabetes	TCAs may ↑ serum glucose levels by up to 150%, ↑ appetite (particularly carbohydrate craving) and ↓ metabolic rate	Be aware and monitor blood sugar weekly until stable. They are generally considered safe unless diabetes is poorly controlled or is associated with significant cardiac or renal disease. Amitriptyline, imipramine and citalopram are also used to treat painful diabetic neuropathy

NATEGLINIDE, REPAGLINIDE	ANTIDIABETIC DRUGS	↑ risk of hypoglycaemic episodes	Due to additive effects by similar or differing mechanisms to lower blood sugar	Combinations are often used and useful. Warn patients about hypoglycaemia ➢ ***For signs and symptoms of hypoglycaemia, see Clinical Features of Some Adverse Drug Interactions, Hypoglycaemia***
REPAGLINIDE	ANTIEPILEPTICS – CARBAMAZEPINE, PHENOBARBITONE, HYDANTOINS	↓ plasma concentrations of repaglinide likely	Due to inducing CYP3A4 isoenzymes, which metabolize repaglinide. However, the alternative pathway – CYP2C8 – is unaffected by these inducers	Be aware and monitor for hyperglycaemia ➢ ***For signs and symptoms of hyperglycaemia, see Clinical Features of Some Adverse Drug Interactions, Hyperglycaemia***
NATEGLINIDE, REPAGLINIDE	**ANTIFUNGALS**			
NATEGLINIDE, REPAGLINIDE	AZOLES – KETOCONAZOLE, FLUCONAZOLE, ITRACONAZOLE, VORICONAZOLE	Likely to ↑ plasma concentrations of repaglinide and ↑ risk of hypoglycaemic episodes.	Due to inhibition of CYP3A4-mediated metabolism. These drugs vary in potency as inhibitors (ketoconazole and itraconazole are potent inhibitors) and ↑ plasma concentrations will vary	Watch for and warn patients of hypoglycaemia ➢ ***For signs and symptoms of hypoglycaemia, see Clinical Features of Some Adverse Drug Interactions, Hypoglycaemia***
REPAGLINIDE	GRISEOFULVIN	↓ repaglinide levels	Hepatic metabolism is induced	Watch for and warn patients of hypoglycaemia ➢ ***For signs and symptoms of hypoglycaemia, see Clinical Features of Some Adverse Drug Interactions, Hypoglycaemia***
NATEGLINIDE	ANTIGOUT DRUGS – SULPHINPYRAZONE	↑ blood levels of nateglinide	Sulfinpyrazone is a selective CYP2C9 inhibitor	Need to monitor blood sugar weekly in patients receiving both drugs. Watch for and warn patients of hypoglycaemia ➢ ***For signs and symptoms of hypoglycaemia, see Clinical Features of Some Adverse Drug Interactions, Hypoglycaemia***

Primary drug	Secondary drug	Effect	Mechanism	Precautions
NATEGLINIDE, REPAGLINIDE	**ANTIHYPERTENSIVES AND HEART FAILURE DRUGS**			
NATEGLINIDE, REPAGLINIDE	ACE INHIBITORS	↑ risk of hypoglycaemic episodes	Mechanism uncertain. ACE inhibitors possibly ↑ insulin sensitivity and glucose utilization. Altered renal function may also be factor. ACE inhibitors may ↑ bradykinin levels, which ↓ production of glucose by the liver. Hypoglycaemia is reported as a (rare) side-effect of ACE inhibitors. Suggested that the occurrence of hypoglycaemia is greater with captopril than enalapril. Captopril and enalapril are used in the treatment of diabetic nephropathy	Concurrent treatment need not be avoided and is often beneficial in type II diabetes. Watch for and warn patients of hypoglycaemia. Be aware that the risk of hypoglycaemia is greater in elderly people and in patients with poor glycaemic control ➢ ***For signs and symptoms of hypoglycaemia, see Clinical Features of Some Adverse Drug Interactions, Hypoglycaemia***
NATEGLINIDE, REPAGLINIDE	ADRENERGIC NEURONE BLOCKERS	↑ hypoglycaemic effect	Catecholamines are diabetogenic; guanethidine blocks release of catecholamines from nerve endings	Monitor blood glucose closely
NATEGLINIDE, REPAGLINIDE	VASODILATOR ANTIHYPERTENSIVES – DIAZOXIDE	May ↑ antidiabetic requirements	Diazoxide causes hyperglycaemia by inhibiting insulin release and probably by a catecholamine-induced extrahepatic effect. Used in the treatment of hypoglycaemia due to insulinomas	Larger doses of antidiabetic drugs are often required; need to monitor blood sugar until adequate control of blood sugar is achieved

NATEGLINIDE, REPAGLINIDE	ANTIOBESITY DRUGS – ORLISTAT, RIMONABANT, SIBUTRAMINE	Tendency for blood glucose levels to fluctuate	These agents change dietary intake of carbohydrates and other foods, and the risk of fluctuations in blood glucose is greater if there is a concurrent dietary regimen. A side-effect of orlistat is hypoglycaemia	These agents are used often in patients with type II diabetes who are on hypoglycaemic therapy. Need to monitor blood sugars twice weekly until stable. Advise self-monitoring. Watch for and warn patients about symptoms of hypoglycaemia ➢ ***For signs and symptoms of hypoglycaemia, see Clinical Features of Some Adverse Drug Interactions, Hypoglycaemia***
NATEGLINIDE, REPAGLINIDE	ANTIPLATELET AGENTS – ASPIRIN	Risk of hypoglycaemia when high-dose aspirin (3.5–7.5 g/day) is given with antidiabetic drugs	Additive effect; aspirin has a hypoglycaemic effect	Avoid high-dose aspirin
NATEGLINIDE, REPAGLINIDE	ANTIPROTOZOALS – PENTAMIDINE	May alter antidiabetic requirements due to altered glycaemic control	Attributed to pancreatic beta cell toxicity	Need to monitor blood sugar until stable and following withdrawal of pentamidine
NATEGLINIDE, REPAGLINIDE	**ANTIPSYCHOTICS**			
REPAGLINIDE	PHENOTHIAZINES, CLOZAPINE, OLANZAPINE	↓ hypoglycaemic effect	Antagonistic effect	Higher doses of repaglinide needed
NATEGLINIDE, REPAGLINIDE	RISPERIDONE	↑ risk of hypoglycaemic episodes	Attributed to a synergistic effect	Watch for and warn patients about symptoms of hypoglycaemia ➢ ***For signs and symptoms of hypoglycaemia, see Clinical Features of Some Adverse Drug Interactions, Hypoglycaemia***

Primary drug	Secondary drug	Effect	Mechanism	Precautions
NATEGLINIDE, REPAGLINIDE	ANTIVIRALS			
REPAGLINIDE	NNRTIs – EFAVIRENZ	Likely to ↑ plasma concentrations of repaglinide and ↑ risk of hypoglycaemic episodes	Due to inhibition of CYP3A4 isoenzymes, which metabolize repaglinide	Watch for and warn patients about hypoglycaemia ➢ ***For signs and symptoms of hypoglycaemia, see Clinical Features of Some Adverse Drug Interactions, Hypoglycaemia***
NATEGLINIDE, REPAGLINIDE	PROTEASE INHIBITORS	↑ levels of these antidiabetic drugs	Inhibition of CYP2C9- and CYP3A4-mediated metabolism of nateglinide, and CYP3A4-mediated metabolism of repaglinide	Monitor blood sugar closely
NATEGLINIDE, REPAGLINIDE	BETA-BLOCKERS	Beta-blockers may mask the symptoms and signs of hypoglycaemia. They also ↓ insulin sensitivity; however, beta-blockers that also have vasodilating properties (carvedilol, celiprolol, labetalol, nebivolol) seem to ↑ sensitivity to insulin	Beta-blockers ↓ glucose tolerance and interfere with metabolic and autonomic responses to hypoglycaemia	Warn patients about the masking of signs of hypoglycaemia. Vasodilating beta-blockers are preferred in patients with diabetes, and all beta-blockers should be avoided in those having frequent hypoglycaemic attacks. Monitor capillary blood glucose closely, especially during initiation of therapy ➢ ***For signs and symptoms of hypoglycaemia, see Clinical Features of Some Adverse Drug Interactions, Hypoglycaemia***

REPAGLINIDE	CALCIUM CHANNEL BLOCKERS	Likely to ↑ plasma concentrations of repaglinide and ↑ risk of hypoglycaemic episodes	Inhibition of CYP3A4-mediated metabolism of repaglinide	Watch for and warn patients about hypoglycaemia ➢ ***For signs and symptoms of hypoglycaemia, see Clinical Features of Some Adverse Drug Interactions, Hypoglycaemia***
NATEGLINIDE	CNS STIMULANTS – MODAFINIL	May cause ↑ plasma concentrations of nateglinide if CYP2C9 is the predominant metabolic pathway and the alternative pathways are either genetically deficient or affected	Modafinil is a moderate inhibitor of CYP2C9	Be aware
REPAGLINIDE	DIURETICS – POTASSIUM-SPARING	↓ hypoglycaemic effect	Antagonistic effect	Higher doses of repaglinide are needed
REPAGLINIDE	GRAPEFRUIT JUICE	Possibly ↑ repaglinide levels	Due to inhibition of CYP3A4 isoenzymes, which metabolize repaglinide	Uncertain if clinically significant. May need to monitor blood glucose more closely
NATEGLINIDE, REPAGLINIDE	H2 RECEPTOR BLOCKERS – CIMETIDINE	Likely to ↑ plasma concentrations of these antidiabetic drugs and ↑ risk of hypoglycaemic episodes	Due to inhibition of CYP3A4-mediated metabolism of nateglinide and repaglinide	Watch for and warn patients about hypoglycaemia ➢ ***For signs and symptoms of hypoglycaemia, see Clinical Features of Some Adverse Drug Interactions, Hypoglycaemia***
NATEGLINIDE, REPAGLINIDE	**LIPID-LOWERING DRUGS**			
REPAGLINIDE	FIBRATES – GEMFIBROZIL	Nearly eightfold ↑ in repaglinide levels. Risk of severe and prolonged hypoglycaemia	Hepatic metabolism inhibited	The European Agency for the Evaluation of Medicinal products contraindicated concurrent use in 2003. Bezafibrate and fenofibrate are suitable alternatives if a fibric acid derivative is required

Primary drug	Secondary drug	Effect	Mechanism	Precautions
NATEGLINIDE, REPAGLINIDE	**STATINS**			
NATEGLINIDE, REPAGLINIDE	STATINS	↑ incidence of adverse effects such as myalgia. There was ↑ maximum concentration of repaglinide by 25%, with high variability	Uncertain. Statins are also substrates for CYP3A4, and competition for metabolism by the enzyme system may be a factor	Clinical significance of the effect is uncertain but it is necessary to be aware of it. Warn patients about adverse effects of statins and repaglinide
REPAGLINIDE	EZETIMIBE/SIMVASTATIN	↑ repaglinide levels, risk of hypoglycaemia	Hepatic metabolism inhibited	Watch for and warn patients about hypoglycaemia ➢ ***For signs and symptoms of hypoglycaemia, see Clinical Features of Some Adverse Drug Interactions, Hypoglycaemia***
REPAGLINIDE	MONTELUKAST	↑ repaglinide levels; risk of hypoglycaemia	Hepatic metabolism inhibited	Watch for and warn patients about hypoglycaemia ➢ ***For signs and symptoms of hypoglycaemia, see Clinical Features of Some Adverse Drug Interactions, Hypoglycaemia***
NATEGLINIDE, REPAGLINIDE	MUSCLE RELAXANTS – BACLOFEN	↓ hypoglycaemic effect	Due to these drugs causing hyperglycaemia, the mechanism being uncertain at present	↑ doses of antidiabetic are often required for adequate glycaemic control
NATEGLINIDE, REPAGLINIDE	NANDROLONE	↑ effect of antidiabetic drugs	Uncertain	Monitor blood sugar closely
NATEGLINIDE, REPAGLINIDE	NIACIN	↓ hypoglycaemic effect	Due to these drugs causing hyperglycaemia, the mechanism being uncertain at present	↑ doses of antidiabetic are often required for adequate glycaemic control
NATEGLINIDE, REPAGLINIDE	NICOTINE	↓ hypoglycaemic effect	Due to these drugs causing hyperglycaemia, the mechanism being uncertain at present	↑ doses of antidiabetic are often required for adequate glycaemic control

NATEGLINIDE, REPAGLINIDE	OESTROGENS	Altered glycaemic control	Uncertain at present	Monitor blood glucose closely
NATEGLINIDE, REPAGLINIDE	PROGESTOGENS	Altered glycaemic control	Uncertain at present	Monitor blood glucose closely
NATEGLINIDE, REPAGLINIDE	SOMATROPIN	↓ hypoglycaemic effect	Due to these drugs causing hyperglycaemia, the mechanism being uncertain at present	↑ doses of antidiabetic are often required for adequate glycaemic control
NATEGLINIDE, REPAGLINIDE	THYROID HORMONES	↓ hypoglycaemic effect	Due to these drugs causing hyperglycaemia, the mechanism being uncertain at present	↑ doses of antidiabetic are often required for adequate glycaemic control
THIAZOLIDINEDIONES – PIOGLITAZONE, ROSIGLITAZONE				
PIOGLITAZONE, ROSIGLITAZONE	ALCOHOL	Tends to mask signs of hypoglycaemia and ↑ risk of hypoglycaemic episodes	Inhibits glucose production and release from many sources, including the liver and release.	Watch for and warn patients about hypoglycaemia ➢ ***For signs and symptoms of hypoglycaemia, see Clinical Features of Some Adverse Drug Interactions, Hypoglycaemia***
PIOGLITAZONE, ROSIGLITAZONE	ANTIARRHYTHMICS – DISOPYRAMIDE	↑ risk of hypoglycaemic episodes – particularly in patients with impaired renal function. Hypoglycaemic attacks may occur even when plasma levels of disopyramide are within the normal range (attacks occurring with plasma disopyramide levels of 1–4 ng/mL)	Disopyramide and its metabolite mono-isopropyl disopyramide ↑ secretion of insulin (considered to be due to inhibition of potassium-ATP channels). Suggestion that disopyramide causes an impairment of the counterregulatory (homeostatic) mechanisms that follow hypoglycaemia	In patients receiving antidiabetic drugs, start with the lowest dose of disopyramide if there is no alternative. Measure creatinine clearance. If creatinine clearance is 40 mL/min or less, the dose of disopyramide should not exceed 100 mg and should be administered once daily if creatinine clearance is <15 ml/min. Watch for and warn patients about symptoms of hypoglycaemia ➢ ***For signs and symptoms of hypoglycaemia, see Clinical Features of Some Adverse Drug Interactions, Hypoglycaemia***

Primary drug	Secondary drug	Effect	Mechanism	Precautions
PIOGLITAZONE, ROSIGLITAZONE	**ANTIBIOTICS**			
PIOGLITAZONE, ROSIGLITAZONE	ISONIAZID	↓ efficacy of antidiabetic drugs	Isoniazid causes hyperglycaemia, the mechanism being uncertain at present.	Monitor capillary blood glucose closely; ↑ doses of antidiabetic drugs may be needed
PIOGLITAZONE, ROSIGLITAZONE	QUINOLONES – CIPROFLOXACIN, NORFLOXACIN, OFLOXACIN	↑ risk of hypoglycaemic episodes	Mechanism uncertain. Ciprofloxacin is a potent inhibitor of CYP1A2. Norfloxacin is a weak inhibitor of CYP1A2, but these may inhibit other CYP isoenzymes to varying degrees	Watch for and warn patients about hypoglycaemia ➢ ***For signs and symptoms of hypoglycaemia, see Clinical Features of Some Adverse Drug Interactions, Hypoglycaemia***
PIOGLITAZONE, ROSIGLITAZONE	RIFAMPICIN	Significant ↓ in blood levels of rosiglitazone. Metabolism and clearance is ↑, the latter threefold	Rosiglitazone is metabolized primarily by CYP2C8, with a minor contribution from CYP2C9. Rifampicin is a potent inducer of CYP2C8 and CYP2C9 and ↑ the formation of *N*-desmethyl-rosiglitazone by about 40%	May need to use an alternative drug or ↑ dose of rosiglitazone
PIOGLITAZONE, ROSIGLITAZONE	TRIMETHOPRIM	↑ in blood levels of rosiglitazone by nearly 40%	Trimethoprim is a relatively selective inhibitor of CYP2C8	Watch for hypoglycaemic events and ↓ dose of rosiglitazone after repeated blood sugar measurements. Warn patients about hypoglycaemia ➢ ***For signs and symptoms of hypoglycaemia, see Clinical Features of Some Adverse Drug Interactions, Hypoglycaemia***

PIOGLITAZONE, ROSIGLITAZONE	**ANTIDEPRESSANTS**			
PIOGLITAZONE, ROSIGLITAZONE	SSRIs	Fluctuations in blood sugar are very likely, with both hypoglycaemic and hyperglycaemic events being reported in diabetics receiving hypoglycaemic treatment. ↑ plasma concentrations of sulphonylureas (e.g. tolbutamide) may occur	Brain serotonin and corticotropin-releasing hormone systems participate in the control of blood sugar levels. ↑ (usually acute) in brain serotonergic activity induces a hyperglycaemic response. Fluvoxamine is a potent inhibitor and fluoxetine a less potent inhibitor of CYP2C9, which metabolizes sulphonylureas	Both hyper- and hypoglycaemic responses have been reported with SSRIs, and there is a need to monitor blood glucose closely prior to, during and after discontinuing SSRI treatment ➢ ***For signs and symptoms of hypoglycaemia and hpyerglycaemia, see Clinical Features of Some Adverse Drug Interactions, Hypoglycaemia, Hyperglycaemia***
PIOGLITAZONE, ROSIGLITAZONE	TCAs	Likely to impair control of diabetes	TCAs may ↑ serum glucose levels by up to 150%, ↑ appetite (particularly carbohydrate craving) and ↓ metabolic rate	Be aware and monitor blood sugar weekly until stable. They are generally considered safe unless diabetes is poorly controlled or is associated with significant cardiac or renal disease. Amitriptyline, imipramine and citalopram are also used to treat painful diabetic neuropathy
PIOGLITAZONE, ROSIGLITAZONE	**ANTIHYPERTENSIVES AND HEART FAILURE DRUGS**			
PIOGLITAZONE, ROSIGLITAZONE	ADRENERGIC NEURONE BLOCKERS	↑ hypoglycaemic effect	Catecholamines are diabetogenic; guanethidine blocks the release of catecholamines from nerve endings	Monitor blood glucose closely

Primary drug	Secondary drug	Effect	Mechanism	Precautions
PIOGLITAZONE, ROSIGLITAZONE	VASODILATOR ANTIHYPERTENSIVES – DIAZOXIDE	May ↑ antidiabetic requirements	Diazoxide causes hyperglycaemia by inhibiting insulin release and probably by a catecholamine-induced extrahepatic effect. Sulphonylureas act by ↑ insulin release. Used in the treatment of hypoglycaemia due to insulinomas	Larger doses of insulin are often required, and need to monitor blood sugar until adequate control of blood sugar is achieved
PIOGLITAZONE, ROSIGLITAZONE	ANTIPLATELET AGENTS – ASPIRIN	Risk of hypoglycaemia when high-dose aspirin (3.5–7.5 g/day) is given with antidiabetic drugs	Additive effect; aspirin has a hypoglycaemic effect	Avoid high-dose aspirin
PIOGLITAZONE	ANTIVIRALS – PROTEASE INHIBITORS	↑ levels of these antidiabetic drugs	Inhibition of CYP3A4-mediated metabolism of pioglitazone	Monitor blood sugar closely
PIOGLITAZONE, ROSIGLITAZONE	BETA-BLOCKERS	Beta-blockers may mask the symptoms and signs of hypoglycaemia. They also ↓ insulin sensitivity; however, beta-blockers that also have vasodilating properties (carvedilol, celiprolol, labetalol, nebivolol) seem to ↑ sensitivity to insulin	Beta-blockers ↓ glucose tolerance and interfere with the metabolic and autonomic responses to hypoglycaemia	Warn patients about the masking of signs of hypoglycaemia. Vasodilating beta-blockers are preferred in patients with diabetes, and all beta-blockers should be avoided in those having frequent hypoglycaemic attacks. Monitor capillary blood glucose closely, especially during initiation of therapy ➢ ***For signs and symptoms of hypoglycaemia, see Clinical Features of Some Adverse Drug Interactions, Hypoglycaemia***

PIOGLITAZONE, ROSIGLITAZONE	CNS STIMULANTS			
PIOGLITAZONE	MODAFINIL	May ↓ modafinil levels	Induction of CYP3A4, which has a partial role in the metabolism of modafinil	Be aware
ROSIGLITAZONE	MODAFINIL	May cause ↑ plasma concentrations of rosiglitazone if CYP2C9 is the predominant metabolic pathway and the alternative pathways are either genetically deficient or affected	Modafinil is a moderate inhibitor of CYP2C9	Be aware
ROSIGLITAZONE	LIPID-LOWERING DRUGS – GEMFIBROZIL	↑ in blood levels of rosiglitazone – often doubled	Gemfibrozil is a relatively selective inhibitor of CYP2C8	Watch for hypoglycaemic events and ↓ dose of rosiglitazone after repeated blood sugar measurements. Warn patients about hypoglycaemia ➢ ***For signs and symptoms of hypoglycaemia, see Clinical Features of Some Adverse Drug Interactions, Hypoglycaemia***
PIOGLITAZONE, ROSIGLITAZONE	MUSCLE RELAXANTS – BACLOFEN	↓ hypoglycaemic effect	Due to these drugs causing hyperglycaemia, the mechanism being uncertain at present	↑ doses of antidiabetic are often required for adequate glycaemic control
PIOGLITAZONE, ROSIGLITAZONE	NANDROLONE	↑ effect of antidiabetic drugs	Uncertain	Monitor blood sugar closely
PIOGLITAZONE, ROSIGLITAZONE	NIACIN	↓ hypoglycaemic effect	Due to these drugs causing hyperglycaemia, the mechanism being uncertain at present	↑ doses of antidiabetic are often required for adequate glycaemic control

Primary drug	Secondary drug	Effect	Mechanism	Precautions
PIOGLITAZONE, ROSIGLITAZONE	NICOTINE	↓ hypoglycaemic effect	Due to these drugs causing hyperglycaemia, the mechanism being uncertain at present	↑ doses of antidiabetic are often required for adequate glycaemic control
PIOGLITAZONE, ROSIGLITAZONE	OESTROGENS	Altered glycaemic control	Uncertain at present	Monitor blood glucose closely
PIOGLITAZONE, ROSIGLITAZONE	PROGESTOGENS	Altered glycaemic control	Uncertain at present	Monitor blood glucose closely
PIOGLITAZONE, ROSIGLITAZONE	SOMATROPIN	↓ hypoglycaemic effect	Due to these drugs causing hyperglycaemia, the mechanism being uncertain at present	↑ doses of antidiabetic are often required for adequate glycaemic control
PIOGLITAZONE, ROSIGLITAZONE	THYROID HORMONES	↓ hypoglycaemic effect	Due to these drugs causing hyperglycaemia, the mechanism being uncertain at present	↑ doses of antidiabetic are often required for adequate glycaemic control

ANTIDIABETIC DRUGS OTHER ANTIDIABETIC DRUGS

Part 6 OTHER ENDOCRINE DRUGS

Primary drug	Secondary drug	Effect	Mechanism	Precautions
BISPHOSPHONATES				
ALENDRONATE	ANALGESICS – NSAIDs	Risk of oesophagitis/peptic ulceration	Additive effect	Avoid co-administration
BISPHOSPHONATES	ANTACIDS	↓ bisphosphonate levels	↓ absorption	Separate doses by at least 30 minutes
SODIUM CLODRONATE	ANTIBIOTICS – AMINOGLYCOSIDES	Risk of symptomatic hypocalcaemia	Uncertain	Monitor calcium levels closely
BISPHOSPHONATES	CALCIUM	↓ bisphosphonate levels	↓ absorption	Separate doses by at least 30 minutes
BISPHOSPHONATES	IRON	↓ bisphosphonate levels when given oral iron	↓ absorption	Separate doses by as much as possible
DANAZOL ➢ *Drugs Used in Obstetrics and Gynaecology*				
DESMOPRESSIN				
DESMOPRESSIN	ANALGESICS – NSAIDs	↑ efficacy of desmopressin with indometacin	Uncertain	Monitor U&Es and BP closely
DESMOPRESSIN	ANTIDIARRHOEA DRUGS – LOPERAMIDE	↑ desmopressin levels when given orally	Delayed intestinal transit time ↑ absorption of desmopressin	Watch for early features of desmopressin toxicity (e.g. abdominal pain, headaches)
DIAZOXIDE ➢ *Cardiovascular Drugs, Antiypertensives and heart failure drugs*				
DUTASTERIDE ➢ *Urological Drugs*				
FEMALE SEX HORMONES ➢ *Drugs Used in Obstetrics and Gynaecology*				
GESTRINONE ➢ *Drugs Used in Obstetrics and Gynaecology*				
GLUCAGON				
GLUCAGON	ANTICOAGULANTS – ORAL	↑ anticoagulant effect	Uncertain at present	Monitor INR after administration of glucagon

NANDROLONE				
NANDROLONE	ANTICOAGULANTS – ORAL	Episodes of bleeding when patients on oral anticoagulants are started on anabolic steroids	Not understood	↓ dose of anticoagulant by 50% and monitor INR closely until stabilized
NANDROLONE	ANTICANCER AND IMMUNOMODULATING DRUGS – CICLOSPORIN	Cases of hepatotoxicity	Uncertain	Monitor LFTs closely
NANDROLONE	ANTIDIABETIC DRUGS	↑ effect of antidiabetic drugs	Uncertain	Monitor blood sugar closely
SOMATROPIN (GROWTH HORMONE)				
SOMATROPIN	ANTICANCER AND IMMUNOMODULATING DRUGS – CORTICOSTEROIDS	Possible ↓ efficacy of somatropin	Uncertain	Watch for poor response to somatropin
SOMATROPIN	ANTIDIABETIC DRUGS	↓ hypoglycaemic effect of insulin	Due to these a drugs causing hyperglycaemia, the mechanism being uncertain at present	↑ doses of antidiabetic agents are often required for adequate glycaemic control
SOMATROPIN	OESTROGENS	Possible ↓ efficacy of somatropin	Uncertain	↑ dose of somatropin may be needed
STEROID REPLACEMENT THERAPY ➢ *Anticancer and Immunomodulating Drugs, Other immunomodulating drugs*				
STRONTIUM RANELATE				
STRONTIUM RANELATE	ANTIBIOTICS – QUINOLONES, TETRACYCLINES	↓ levels of these antibiotics	↓ absorption	Avoid co-administration
TESTOSTERONE				
TESTOSTERONE	ANTICOAGULANTS – ORAL	Possible ↑ anticoagulant effect	Uncertain	Monitor INR at least weekly until stable

OTHER ENDOCRINE DRUGS TESTOSTERONE

Primary drug	Secondary drug	Effect	Mechanism	Precautions
TESTOSTERONE	ANTIDIABETIC DRUGS	↑ hypoglycaemic effect and ↑ risk of hypoglycaemic episodes	Exact mechanism is uncertain. Low testosterone levels are associated with type II diabetes. Experimental work has suggested that testosterone may play a role in glucose efflux from cells	Warn patients about symptoms of hypoglycaemia ➢ ***For signs and symptoms of hypoglycaemia, see Clinical Features of Some Adverse Drug Interactions, Hypoglycaemia***
THYROID HORMONES				
THYROID HORMONES	ANAESTHETICS – GENERAL – KETAMINE	Cases of tachycardia and hypertension when ketamine was given to patients on thyroxine; this required treatment with propanolol	Uncertain	Monitor PR and BP closely
THYROID HORMONES	ANTIARRHYTHMICS – AMIODARONE	Risk of either under- or overtreatment of thyroid function	Amiodarone contains iodine and has been reported to cause both hyper- and hypothyroidism	Monitor triiodothyronine, thyroxine and TSH levels at least 6-monthly
THYROID HORMONES	ANTIBIOTICS			
THYROID HORMONES	QUINOLONES – CIPROFLOXACIN	↓ levels of levothyroxine and possible therapeutic failure	The mechanism has not been elucidated; the concurrent administration of ciprofloxacin with levothyroxine may interfere with the absorption of levothyroxine and result in lower than expected levels	The interaction may be minimized by separating dosing of the two agents; ciprofloxacin should be taken several hours before or after taking levothyroxine
THYROID HORMONES	RIFAMPICIN	↓ levothyroxine levels	Induction of metabolism	Monitor TFTs regularly and consider ↑ dose of levothyroxine
THYROID HORMONES	ANTICOAGULANTS – ORAL	Possible ↑ anticoagulant effect	Uncertain	Monitor INR at least weekly until stable

THYROID HORMONES	ANTIDEPRESSANTS – TCAs	Possible ↑ antidepressant effect	Uncertain	May be beneficial but reported cases of nausea and dizziness; warn patients to report these symptoms
THYROID HORMONES	ANTIDIABETIC DRUGS	↓ hypoglycaemic effect	Due to these a drugs causing hyperglycaemia, the mechanism being uncertain at present	↑ doses of antidiabetic drug are often required for adequate glycaemic control
THYROID HORMONES	ANTIEPILEPTICS – BARBITURATES, CARBAMAZEPINE, PHENYTOIN	↓ levothyroxine levels	Induction of metabolism	Monitor TFTs regularly and consider ↑ dose of levothyroxine
THYROID HORMONES	ANTIVIRALS – PROTEASE INHIBITORS	↓ efficacy of levothyroxine by ritonavir (with or without lopinavir) and possibly indinavir and nelfinavir	Uncertain; possibly ↑ metabolism via induction of glucuronosyl transferases	Monitor thyroid function closely
THYROID HORMONES	BRONCHODILATORS – THEOPHYLLINE	Altered theophylline levels (↑ or ↓) when thyroid status was altered therapeutically	Uncertain	Monitor theophylline levels closely during changes in treatment of abnormal thyroid function. Watch for early features of theophylline toxicity
THYROID HORMONES	CALCIUM	↓ levothyroxine levels	↓ absorption	Separate doses by at least 4 hours. Monitor TFTs regularly and consider ↑ dose of levothyroxine
THYROID HORMONES	H2 RECEPTOR BLOCKERS – CIMETIDINE	↓ efficacy of levothyroxine	↓ absorption	Clinical significance unclear. Monitor requirement for ↑ levothyroxine dose
THYROID HORMONES	IRON	↓ levothyroxine levels with oral iron	↓ absorption	Separate doses by at least 2 hours. Monitor TFTs regularly and consider ↑ dose of levothyroxine
THYROID HORMONES	LIPID-LOWERING DRUGS – ANION EXCHANGE RESINS	↓ efficacy of thyroid hormones	↓ absorption	Separate doses by at least 4–6 hours. Monitor TFTs

OTHER ENDOCRINE DRUGS TRILOSTANE

Primary drug	Secondary drug	Effect	Mechanism	Precautions
THYROID HORMONES	SODIUM POLYSTYRENE SULPHONATE	↓ levothyroxine levels	↓ absorption	Monitor TFTs regularly and consider ↑ dose of levothyroxine
THYROID HORMONES	SUCRALFATE	↓ thyroxine levels	↓ absorption	Give thyroxine 2–3 hours before sucralfate
TRILOSTANE				
TRILOSTANE	DIURETICS – POTASSIUM-SPARING	Risk of hyperkalaemia	Additive effect	Monitor potassium levels regularly during co-administration

Part 7 ANALGESICS

Opioids

Opioid drugs act at opioid receptors distributed throughout the central/peripheral nervous system, causing a wide range of physiological, behavioural and cognitive effects. The main adverse drug interactions are due to additive depressive effects on the CNS, which results in loss of consciousness, respiratory depression and hypotension.

Non-steroidal anti-inflammatory drugs

Non-steroidal anti-inflammatory drugs inhibit cyclooxygenase, the enzyme that limits the conversion of arachidonic acid to cyclic endoperoxide, an intermediate in prostaglandin production. This blocks the binding of agents released by the prostaglandin cascade to nociceptive receptors.

The main drug interactions result from additive adverse effects such as:

- increased or additive gastrointestinal bleeding or ulceration;
- precipitation of heart failure due to salt and fluid retention;
- additive renal toxicity.

The co-administration of more than one NSAID does not produce synergism of the analgesic effect but significantly increases the risk of gastrointestinal toxicity and liver and kidney damage so should be avoided.

Some NSAIDs (e.g. diclofenac, ibuprofen, naproxen, piroxicam) are actively metabolized by CYP2C9, which may be a site of possible interaction with inhibitors and inducers of this isoenzyme.

Aspirin

Aspirin produces an antipyretic and anti-inflammatory effect primarily by irreversibly inhibiting cyclooxygenase (thus having similar effects to NSAIDs). It possesses an antiplatelet effect that may have additive effect with other drugs with a similar effect (e.g. selective serotonin reuptake inhibitors) and those which affect other aspects of blood clotting. The risk of interactions and adverse effects are reduced by using a lower dose (e.g. 75 mg); fortunately, a full antiplatelet effect is seen at this dose. This is considered in Part 1, Cardiovascular Drugs.

Paracetamol (acetaminophen)

This is a non-narcotic, non-salicylate analgesic with few anti-inflammatory effects that acts by inhibiting prostaglandin synthesis in the CNS (hence being antipyretic and analgesic). It is metabolized by CYP1A2.

Nefopam

Nefopam is a centrally acting non-opioid analgesic used for mild to moderate pain; its mechanism of action is uncertain but may be due to an inhibition of serotonin, noradrenaline and dopamine reuptake. It is considered by some to act on GABA B receptors and is likely to interact with other drugs affecting these neurotransmitters.

Ketamine

Ketamine is an intravenous anaesthetic that is a potent analgesic at subanaesthetic doses. It is considered in Part 9 with general anaesthetics.

Interactions of herbal medicines with analgesics

NSAIDs, particularly aspirin, have the potential to interact with herbal supplements:

- They interact with supplements known to possess antiplatelet activity (gingko, garlic, ginger, bilberry, dong quai, feverfew, ginseng, turmeric, meadowsweet, willow).
- They also interact with supplements containing coumarin (chamomile, motherwort, horse chestnut, fenugreek, red clover).
- The hepatotoxicity of paracetamol may be increased when it is concomitantly used with hepatotoxic herbs (echinacea, kava, herbs containing salicylates such as willow and meadowsweet).
- There may be side-effects from the concomitant use of opioids with sedative herbal supplements; use with, for example, valerian, kava or chamomile may lead to additive depression of the CNS.
- The analgesic effect of opioids may be inhibited by ginseng.

Analgesics in over-the-counter medicines

The opioids (e.g. codeine, dextromethorphan), NSAIDs, aspirin and paracetamol found in many over-the-counter drugs have the potential for adverse drug interactions. For more details, see Over-the-Counter Drugs.

Primary drug	Secondary drug	Effect	Mechanism	Precautions
ACETAMINOPHEN	➢ *Paracetamol, below*			
NEFOPAM				
NEFOPAM	ADDITIVE ANTIMUSCARINIC EFFECTS			
NEFOPAM	1. ANTIARRHYTHMICS – disopyramide, propafenone 2. ANTIDEPRESSANTS – TCAs 3. ANTIEMETICS – cyclizine 4. ANTIHISTAMINES – chlorphenamine, cyproheptadine, hydroxyzine 5. ANTIMUSCARINICS – atropine, benzatropine, cyclopentolate, dicycloverine, flavoxate, homatropine, hyoscine, orphenadrine, oxybutynin, procyclidine, propantheline, tolterodine, trihexyphenidyl or tropicamide. 6. ANTIPARKINSON'S DRUGS – dopaminergics 7. ANTIPSYCHOTICS – phenothiazines, clozapine, pimozide 8. MUSCLE RELAXANTS – baclofen 9. NITRATES – isosorbide dinitrate	↑ risk of antimuscarinic side-effects. **NB ↓ efficacy of sublingual nitrate tablets**	Additive effect; both drugs cause antimuscarinic side-effects. **Antimuscarinic effects ↓ saliva production, which ↓ dissolution of the tablet**	Warn patients of this additive effect. **Consider using sublingual nitrate spray**

ANALGESICS NEFOPAM

Primary drug	Secondary drug	Effect	Mechanism	Precautions
NEFOPAM	**ANTIDEPRESSANTS**			
NEFOPAM	TCAs	Risk of seizures with TCAs	Additive effect; both drugs lower the seizure threshold	Avoid co-administration
NEFOPAM	MAOIs	Risk of arrhythmias	Additive effect; both drugs have sympathomimetic effects	Avoid co-administration
NON-STEROIDAL ANTI-INFLAMMATORY DRUGS (NSAIDs)				
NSAIDs	**ANALGESICS**			
NSAIDs	ANTACIDS	1. Magnesium hydroxide ↑ absorption of ibuprofen, flurbiprofen, mefenamic acid and tolfenamic acid 2. Aluminium-containing antacids ↓ absorption of these NSAIDs	Uncertain	These effects are ↓ by taking these drugs with food
NSAIDs	NSAIDs	↑ risk of gastrointestinal bleeding	Additive effect.	Avoid co-administration
PARECOXIB	ANTIARRHYTHMICS – FLECAINIDE, PROPAFENONE	Possible ↑ flecainide or propafenone levels	Parecoxib weakly inhibits CYP2D6	Monitor PR and BP closely. If possible, use only short courses of NSAID
NSAIDs	**ANTIBIOTICS**			
INDOMETACIN	AMINOGLYCOSIDES	↑ amikacin, gentamicin, and vancomycin levels in neonates	Uncertain; indometacin possibly ↓ renal clearance of these aminoglycosides	Halve the dose of antibiotic. Uncertain whether this applies to adults but suggest check levels. Otherwise use an alternative NSAID
INDOMETACIN	CEPHALOSPORINS	Indometacin ↑ ceftazidime levels in neonates	Indometacin ↓ clearance of ceftazidime	↓ dose of ceftazidime
NSAIDs	QUINOLONES	Reports of convulsions when NSAIDs are added to quinolones in epileptic patients	Unknown	Take care in co-administering epileptics and NSAIDs in epileptic patients

ANALGESICS NON-STEROIDAL ANTI-INFLAMMATORY DRUGS

NSAIDs	RIFAMPICIN	Rifampicin ↓ diclofenac, celecoxib, etoricoxib and parecoxib levels	Rifampicin ↑ CYP2C9-mediated metabolism of these NSAIDs	Monitor analgesic effects; consider using alternative NSAIDs
NSAIDs	**ANTICANCER AND IMMUNOMODULATING DRUGS**			
NSAIDs	CYTOTOXICS	1. ↑ risk of bleeding with erlotinib 2. ↑ plasma concentrations of celecoxib, diclofenac and piroxicam, with risk of toxic effects when co-administered with imatinib 3. ↑ risk of photosensitivity reactions when porfimer is co-administered with celecoxib, ibuprofen, ketoprofen or naproxen	1. Additive effect 2. Imatinib is a potent inhibitor of CYP2C9, which metabolizes celecoxib, diclofenac and piroxicam 3. Attributed to additive effects	1. Avoid co-administration 2. Monitor for toxic effects of celecoxib (flatulence, insomnia, pharyngitis, stomatitis, palpitations, paraesthesia), diclofenac (nausea, diarrhoea, gastrointestinal bleeding, rashes, angioedema, renal damage) and piroxicam (e.g. gastrointestinal effects). It is necessary to monitor effects 2 weeks after initiating treatment with piroxicam, and the use of a gastroprotective agent is advised by CSM 3. Avoid exposure of skin and eyes to direct sunlight for 30 days after porfimer therapy
NSAIDs	**IMMUNOMODULATING DRUGS**			
NSAIDs	CICLOPSORIN	1. ↑ risk of renal failure with NSAIDs 2. Diclofenac levels ↑ by ciclosporin 3. Rofecoxib ↓ plasma concentrations of ciclosporin, with risk of transplant rejection	1. Additive effect; both can cause renal insufficiency 2. Uncertain 3. Rofecoxib is a mild inducer of CYP3A4 and not a substrate of CYP3A4	1. Monitor renal function closely 2. Halve the dose of diclofenac 3. Be aware. May not be clinically significant
NSAIDs	CORTICOSTEROIDS	1. ↑ risk of gastrointestinal ulceration and bleeding 2. Parecoxib levels may be ↓ by dexamethasone	1. Additive effect 2. Dexamethasone induces CYP3A4-mediated metabolism of parecoxib	1. Watch for early signs of gastro-intestinal upset; remember that corticosteroids may mask these features 2. Watch for poor response to parecoxib

ANALGESICS NON-STEROIDAL ANTI-INFLAMMATORY DRUGS

Primary drug	Secondary drug	Effect	Mechanism	Precautions
NSAIDs	METHOTREXATE	↑ methotrexate levels, with reports of toxicity, with ibuprofen, indometacin and possibly diclofenac, flurbiprofen, ketoprofen, meloxicam and naproxen	Uncertain; postulated that an NSAID-induced ↓ in renal perfusion may have an effect	Consider using an alternative NSAID
NSAIDs	MYCOPHENOLATE, PENICILLAMINE, SIROLIMUS, TACROLIMUS	↑ risk of nephrotoxicity	Additive effect	Monitor renal function closely
NSAIDs	**ANTICOAGULANTS**			
NSAIDs	ANTICOAGULANTS – ORAL	1. Risk of gastrointestinal bleeding with all NSAIDs 2. Possible ↑ anticoagulant effect with celecoxib, etoricoxib, flurbiprofen, piroxicam and sulindac	1. NSAIDs irritate the gastric mucosa and can cause bleeding, which is exacerbated by anticoagulants 2. Uncertain but possibly a combination of impaired hepatic metabolism and displacement of anticoagulants from their plasma proteins	1. Extreme caution when co-administering; monitor patients closely 2. Monitor INR closely
NSAIDs	ANTICOAGULANTS – PARENTERAL	1. Risk of prolonged bleeding when ketorolac is co-administered with dalteparin (but not enoxaparin), and intravenous diclofenac is given with heparins 2. ↑ risk of hyperkalaemia when ketorolac is given with heparin	1. Uncertain 2. Heparin inhibits aldosterone secretion, causing hyperkalaemia	1. Avoid co-administration 2. Monitor potassium levels closely
NSAIDs	**ANTIDEPRESSANTS**			
NSAIDs	LITHIUM	NSAIDs may ↑ lithium levels; cases of toxicity have been reported	Uncertain; possibly NSAIDs ↓ renal clearance of lithium	Monitor lithium levels closely
NSAIDs	SSRIs, VENLAFAXINE	Slight ↑ risk of bleeding	Unknown	Warn patients to watch for early signs of bleeding

ANALGESICS NON-STEROIDAL ANTI-INFLAMMATORY DRUGS

NSAIDs	**ANTIDIABETIC DRUGS**			
NSAIDs	METFORMIN	Possibility of ↑ plasma levels of metformin if there is renal impairment due to NSAIDs. Phenylbutazone is likely to ↓ renal elimination of metformin and ↑ plasma levels	These drugs are often used in the long term. NSAIDs can cause renal dysfunction. As metformin is not protein-bound, as are the sulphonylureas, displacement from such binding sites is unlikely	Do not use metformin if serum creatinine is >1.5 mg/dL in males and >1.4 mg/dL in females, or creatinine clearance is <30 mL/min. Use with caution in patients who have a creatinine clearance of 30–60 mL/min. Warn patients about hypoglycaemia ➢ ***For signs and symptoms of hypoglycaemia, see Clinical Features of Some Adverse Drug Interactions, Hypoglycaemia***
NSAIDs	SULPHONYLUREAS	Enhanced hypoglycaemic effect of sulphonylureas with most NSAIDs, which are highly protein bound. There have been reports of hyper-glycaemia and hypoglycaemia (e.g. with diclofenac)	Attributed to displacement of sulphonylureas from protein-binding sites, thus increasing the plasma concentration. Some NSAIDs may impair the renal elimination of sulphonylureas, particularly chlorpropamide	Be aware. Conflicting reports. Suggestions that sulindac and Arthrotec may interact minimally
NSAIDs	ANTIEMETICS	1. Metoclopramide speeds up the onset of action of tolfenamic acid 2. Metoclopramide ↓ efficacy of ketoprofen	Metoclopramide promotes gastric emptying 1. Tolfenamic acid reaches its main site of absorption in the small intestine more rapidly 2. Ketoprofen has low solubility and has less time to dissolve in the stomach; therefore less ketoprofen is absorbed	1. This interaction can be used beneficially to hasten the onset of analgesia 2. Take ketoprofen at least 2 hours before metoclopramide

Primary drug	Secondary drug	Effect	Mechanism	Precautions
NSAIDs	ANTIEPILEPTICS	1. Parecoxib levels may be ↓ by carbamazepine and phenytoin 2. Report of ↑ phenytoin levels when celecoxib added	1. Carbamazepine and phenytoin induce CYP3A4-mediated metabolism of parecoxib 2. Uncertain; possibly competitive inhibition of CYP2C9-mediated metabolism of phenytoin	1. Watch for poor response to parecoxib 2. Monitor phenytoin levels
NSAIDs	ANTIFUNGALS – FLUCONAZOLE	Fluconazole ↑ celecoxib and possibly parecoxib levels	Fluconazole inhibits CYP2C9-mediated metabolism of celecoxib and parecoxib	Halve the dose of celecoxib and start parecoxib at the lowest dose
NSAIDs	ANTIGOUT DRUGS – PROBENECID	↑ levels of indometacin, ketorolac and possibly dexketoprofen, ketoprofen, naproxen, tenoxicam and tiaprofenic acid	Probenecid competitively inhibits renal metabolism of these NSAIDs	Watch for signs of toxicity of these NSAIDs. Consider using an alternative NSAID. The manufacturers of ketorolac advise avoiding co-administration of ketorolac and probenecid
NSAIDs	**ANTIHYPERTENSIVES AND HEART FAILURE DRUGS**			
NSAIDs	ANTIHYPERTENSIVES AND HEART FAILURE DRUGS	↓ hypotensive effect, especially with indometacin. The effect is variable among different ACE inhibitors and NSAIDs, but is most notable between captopril and indometacin	NSAIDs cause sodium and water retention and raise BP by inhibiting vasodilating renal prostaglandins. ACE inhibitors metabolize tissue kinins (e.g. bradykinin), and this may be the basis for indometacin attenuating the hypotensive effect of captopril	Monitor BP at least weekly until stable. Avoid co-administering indometacin with captopril
NSAIDs	ACE INHIBITORS, ANGIOTENSIN II RECEPTOR ANTAGONISTS	1. ↑ risk of renal impairment with NSAIDs and ACE inhibitors 2. ↑ risk of hyperkalaemia with ketorolac	1. Additive effect 2. Ketorolac causes hyperkalaemia, and ACE inhibitors can ↓ renal function	1. Monitor renal function and BP closely. Benefits often outweigh risks for short-term NSAID use 2. Ketorolac is licensed only for short-term control of perioperative pain. Monitor serum potassium daily

NSAIDs	VASODILATOR ANTIHYPERTENSIVES	Etoricoxib may ↑ minoxidil levels	Etoricoxib inhibits sulphotransferase activity	Monitor BP closely
NSAIDs	ANTIOBESITY DRUGS – SIBUTRAMINE	↑ risk of bleeding	Additive effect	Avoid co-administration
NSAIDs	**ANTIPLATELET AGENTS**			
NSAIDs	ASPIRIN	1. Risk of gastrointestinal bleeding when aspirin, even low dose, is co-administered with NSAIDs 2. Ibuprofen ↓ antiplatelet effect of aspirin	1. Additive effect 2. Ibuprofen competitively inhibits binding of aspirin to platelets	1. Avoid co-administration 2. Avoid co-administration
NSAIDs	CLOPIDOGREL	1. Risk of gastrointestinal bleeding when clopidogrel is co-administered with NSAIDs 2. Case report of intracerebral haemorrhage when clopidogrel is given with celecoxib	1. NSAIDs may cause gastric mucosal irritation/ulceration; clopidogrel inhibits platelet aggregation 2. Uncertain; possible that celecoxib inhibits CYP2D6-mediated metabolism of clopidogrel	1. Warn patients to report immediately any gastrointestinal symptoms; use NSAIDs for as short a course as possible 2. Avoid co-ingestion of clopidogrel and celecoxib
NSAIDs	ANTIPSYCHOTICS	1. Reports of ↑ sedation when indometacin was added to haloperidol 2. Risk of agranulocytosis when azapropazone is given with clozapine	1. Unknown 2. Unknown	1. Avoid co-administration 2. Avoid co-administration
NSAIDs	**ANTIVIRALS**			
NSAIDs	NUCLEOSIDE REVERSE TRANSCRIPTASE INHIBITORS	Risk of haematological effects of zidovudine with NSAIDs	Unknown	Avoid co-administration
NSAIDs	PROTEASE INHIBITORS	Ritonavir ↑ piroxicam levels	Uncertain; ritonavir is known to inhibit CYP2C9, for which NSAIDs are substrates	Avoid co-administration

ANALGESICS NON-STEROIDAL ANTI-INFLAMMATORY DRUGS

Primary drug	Secondary drug	Effect	Mechanism	Precautions
NSAIDs	**BETA-BLOCKERS**			
NSAIDs	BETA-BLOCKERS	↓ hypotensive efficacy of beta-blockers with indometacin, piroxicam, and possibly ibuprofen and naproxen. Other NSAIDs do not seem to show this effect	Additive toxic effects on kidney, salt and water retention by NSAIDs. NSAIDs can raise BP by inhibiting the renal synthesis of vasodilating prostaglandins. Uncertain why this effect is specific to these NSAIDs	Watch for ↓ response to beta-blockers with indometacin, piroxicam, ibuprofen and naproxen
PARECOXIB	METOPROLOL	Risk of ↑ hypotensive efficacy of metoprolol	Metoprolol is metabolized by CYP2D6, which is inhibited by valdecoxib	Monitor BP at least weekly until stable. Warn patients to report symptoms of hypotension (light-headedness, dizziness on standing, etc.)
NSAIDs	BISPHOSPHONATES – ALENDRONATE	Risk of oesophagitis/peptic ulceration	Additive effect	Avoid co-administration
NSAIDs	BRONCHODILATORS – BETA-2 AGONISTS	Etoricoxib may ↑ oral salbutamol levels	Etoricoxib inhibits sulphotransferase activity	Monitor PR and BP closely
NSAIDs	CALCIUM CHANNEL BLOCKERS	↓ antihypertensive effect of calcium channel blockers	NSAIDs cause salt retention and vasoconstriction at possibly both renal and endothelial sites	Monitor BP at least weekly until stable
NSAIDs	CARDIAC GLYCOSIDES	Diclofenac, indometacin and possibly fenbufen, ibuprofen and tiaprofenic ↑ plasma concentrations of digoxin and ↑ risk of precipitating cardiac failure and renal dysfunction	Uncertain. Postulated that NSAID-induced renal impairment plays a role; however, since all NSAIDs have this effect, it is not understood why only certain NSAIDs actually influence digoxin levels	Monitor renal function closely; watch for digoxin toxicity and check levels if necessary

NSAIDs	CNS STIMULANTS			
INDOMETACIN	MODAFINIL	May cause ↑ indometacin levels if CYP2C9 is the predominant metabolic pathway and the alternative pathways are either genetically deficient or affected	Modafinil is a moderate inhibitor of CYP2C9	Be aware
NAPROXEN	MODAFINIL	May cause ↓ naproxen levels if CYP1A2 is the predominant metabolic pathway and alternative metabolic pathways are either genetically deficient or affected	Modafinil is moderate inducer of CYP1A2 in a concentration-dependent manner	Be aware
NSAIDs	DESMOPRESSIN	↑ efficacy of desmopressin with indometacin	Uncertain	Monitor U&Es and BP closely
NSAIDs	DIURETICS – POTASSIUM-SPARING AND ALDOSTERONE ANTAGONISTS	Risk of hyperkalaemia with NSAIDs	Renal insufficiency caused by NSAIDs can exacerbate potassium retention by these diuretics	Monitor renal function and potassium closely
NSAIDs – CELECOXIB	DRUG DEPENDENCE THERAPIES – BUPROPION	↑ plasma concentrations of these substrates, with risk of toxic effects	Bupropion and its metabolite hydroxybupropion inhibit CYP2D6	Initiate therapy of these drugs at the lowest effective dose
NSAIDs	LIPID-LOWERING DRUGS	Colestyramine ↓ absorption of some NSAIDs	Colestyramine binds NSAIDs in the intestine, reducing their absorption; it also binds those NSAIDs with a significant enterohepatic recirculation (meloxicam, piroxicam, sulindac. tenoxicam)	Give NSAID 1 hour before or 4–6 hours after colestyramine; however, meloxicam, piroxicam, sulindac or tenoxicam should not be given with colestyramine

Primary drug	Secondary drug	Effect	Mechanism	Precautions
NSAIDs	MIFEPRISTONE	↓ efficacy of mifepristone	NSAIDs have an antiprostaglandin effect	Avoid co-administration
NSAIDs	MUSCLE RELAXANTS – SKELETAL	↑ baclofen levels with ibuprofen	↓ renal excretion of baclofen	Avoid co-administration
NSAIDs	NITRATES	Hypotensive effects of hydralazine, minoxidil and nitroprusside are antagonized by NSAIDs	NSAIDs cause salt and water retention in the kidney and can raise BP due to ↓ production of vasodilating renal prostaglandins	Monitor BP at least weekly until stable
NSAIDs	OESTROGENS	Etoricoxib may ↑ ethinylestradiol levels	Etoricoxib inhibits sulphotransferase activity	Consider using a formulation with a lower dose of ethinylestradiol
NSAIDs	PERIPHERAL VASODILATORS	Risk of bleeding when pentoxifylline is given with ketorolac post surgery	Possibly additive antiplatelet effect	Avoid co-administration
NSAIDs	PROGESTOGENS	↑ risk of hyperkalaemia	Drospirenone (component of the Yasmin brand of combined contraceptive pill) is a progestogen derived from spironolactone that can cause potassium retention	Monitor serum potassium weekly until stable, and then every 6 months
OPIOIDS				
OPIOIDS	ALCOHOL	↑ sedation	Additive effect	Warn patient
OPIOIDS	**ANTIARRHYTHMICS**			
METHADONE, TRAMADOL	FLECAINIDE, PROCAINAMIDE, PROPAFENONE	Possible ↑ flecainide, procainamide and propafenone levels	Methadone and tramadol inhibit CYP2D6	Monitor PR and BP closely

OPIOIDS	MEXILETINE	1. Absorption of oral mexiletine is ↓ by co-administration with morphine or diamorphine 2. Methadone may ↑ mexiletine levels	1. Uncertain but thought to be due to an opioid-induced delay in gastric emptying 2. Methadone inhibits CYP2D6-mediated metabolism of mexiletine	1. Watch for poor response to mexiletine; consider starting at a higher or using the intravenous route 2. Monitor PR, BP and ECG closely; watch for mexiletine toxicity
OPIOIDS	**ANTIBIOTICS**			
OPIOIDS	CIPROFLOXACIN	1. Effects of methadone ↑ by ciprofloxacin 2. ↓ levels of ciprofloxacin with opioids	1. Ciprofloxacin inhibits CYP1A2-, CYP2D6- and CYP3A4-mediated metabolism of methadone 2. Uncertain	1. Watch for ↑ effects of methadone 2. Avoid opioid premedication when ciprofloxacin is used as surgical prophylaxis
OPIOIDS	MACROLIDES	Effects of alfentanil ↑ by erythromycin	Erythromycin inhibits metabolism of alfentanil	Be aware that the effects of alfentanil (especially when given as an infusion) may be prolonged by erythromycin
OPIOIDS	RIFAMPICIN	↓ effect of alfentanil, codeine, methadone and morphine	Rifampicin ↑ hepatic metabolism of these opioids (alfentanil by CYP3A4, codeine by CYP2D6, morphine unknown). Rifampicin is also known to induce intestinal P-gp, which may ↓ bioavailability of oral morphine	Be aware that alfentanil, codeine, methadone and morphine doses may need to be ↑

ANALGESICS OPIOIDS

Primary drug	Secondary drug	Effect	Mechanism	Precautions
OPIOIDS	ANTICANCER AND IMMUNOMODULATING DRUGS – CYTOTOXICS	1. Imatinib may cause ↑ plasma concentrations, with a risk of toxic effects of codeine, dextromethorphan, hydroxycodone, methadone, morphine, oxycodone, pethidine and tramadol 2. Unpredictable reactions may occur associated with hypotension and respiratory depression when procarbazine is co-administered with alfentanil, fentanyl, sufentanil or morphine	1. Imatinib is a potent inhibitor of CYP2D6 isoenzymes, which metabolize these opioids 2. Opioids cause hypotension due to arterial and venous vasodilatation, negative inotropic effects and a vagally induced bradycardia. Procarbazine can cause postural hypotension. Also attributed to accumulation of serotonin due to inhibition of MAO	1. Monitor for clinical efficacy and toxicity. Warn patients to report ↑ drowsiness, malaise and anorexia. Measure amylase and lipase if toxicity is suspected. Tramadol causes less respiratory depression than other opiates, but need to monitor BP and blood counts and advise patients to report wheezing, loss of appetite and fainting attacks. Need to consider reducing dose. Methadone may cause Q–T prolongation; the CSM has recommended that patients with heart and liver disease on methadone should be carefully monitored for heart conduction abnormalities such as Q–T prolongation on ECG, which may lead to sudden death. Also need to monitor patients on more than 100 mg methadone daily, and thus ↑ plasma concentrations necessitates close monitoring of cardiac and respiratory function 2. Recommended that a small test dose (one-quarter of the usual dose) be administered initially to assess response
OPIOIDS	ANTICOAGULANTS – ORAL	Cases of ↑ anticoagulant effect with tramadol	Unknown	Monitor INR at least weekly until stable

DEXTROMETHORPHAN	ANTIDEMENTIA DRUGS – MEMANTINE	↑ CNS side-effects	Additive effects on NMDA receptors	Avoid co-administration
OPIOIDS	**ANTIDEPRESSANTS**			
OPIOIDS	MAOIs	Additive depression of CNS ranging from drowsiness to coma and respiratory depression	Synergistic depressant effects on CNS function	Necessary to warn patients, particularly regards activities that require attention, e.g. driving or using machinery and equipment that could cause self-harm
PETHIDINE, MORPHINE, PHENOPERIDINE, DEXTROMETHORPHAN	MAOIs	Two types of reactions are reported: 1. Risk of serotonin syndrome with dextromethorphan, pethidine or tramadol and MAOIs 2. Depressive – respiratory depression, hypotension, coma	Type I reactions are attributed to an inhibition of reuptake of serotonin; this more common with pethidine, phenoperidine and dextromethorphan. Type II reactions, attributed to MAOI inhibition of metabolism of opioids, are more common with morphine	Avoid co-administration; do not give dextromethorphan, pethidine or tramadol for at least 2 weeks after cessation of MAOI
OPIOIDS	SSRIs	1. Possible ↓ analgesic effect of oxycodone and tramadol 2. ↑ serotonin effects, including possible cases of serotonin syndrome, when opioids (oxycodone, pethidine, pentazocine, tramadol) are co-administered with SSRIs (fluoxetine, sertraline) 3. SSRIs may ↑ codeine, fentanyl, methadone, pethidine and tramadol levels	1. Uncertain. Paroxetine inhibits CYP2D6, which is required to produce the active form of tramadol 2. Uncertain 3. SSRIs inhibit CYP2D6-mediated metabolism of these opioids	1. Consider using an alternative opioid 2. Look for signs of ↑ serotonin activity, particularly on initiating therapy 3. Watch for excessive narcotization

Primary drug	Secondary drug	Effect	Mechanism	Precautions
OPIOIDS	TCAs	1. Risk of ↑ respiratory depression and sedation 2. ↑ levels of morphine 3. Cases of seizures when tramadol is co-administered with TCAs 4.TCAs may ↑ codeine, fentanyl, pethidine and tramadol levels	1. Additive effect 2. Uncertain; likely to ↑ bioavailability of morphine 3. Unknown 4. TCAs inhibit CYP2D6-mediated metabolism of these opioids	1. Warn patients of this effect. Titrate doses carefully 2. Warn patients of this effect. Titrate doses carefully 3. Consider an alternative opioid 4. Watch for excessive narcotization
OPIOIDS	OTHER – DULOXETINE	↑ serotonin effects, including possible cases of serotonin syndrome, when opioids (oxycodone, pethidine, pentazocine, tramadol) are given	Uncertain	Look for signs of ↑ serotonin activity, particularly on initiating therapy
MORPHINE	ANTIDIABETIC DRUGS – METFORMIN	↑ level of metformin and risk of lactic acidosis. The onset of lactic acidosis is often subtle with symptoms of malaise, myalgia, respiratory distress and increasing non-specific abdominal distress. There may be hypothermia and resistant bradyarrhythmias	Metformin is not metabolized in humans and is not protein bound. Competition for renal tubular excretion is the basis for ↑ activity or retention of metformin	Theoretical possibility. Requires ↓ of metformin dose to be considered or to avoid co-administration. Warn patients re hypoglycaemia ➢ ***For signs and symptoms of hypoglycaemia, see Clinical Features of Some Adverse Drug Interactions, Hypoglycaemia***
OPIOIDS	ANTIEMETICS	1. Ondansetron seems to ↓ analgesic effect of tramadol 2. ↓ efficacy of domperidone on gut motility by opioids 3. Metoclopramide ↑ speed of onset and effect of oral morphine	1. Uncertain; tramadol exerts its analgesic properties via serotoninergic pathways in addition to stimulation of opioid receptors. Ondansetron is a serotonin receptor antagonist 2. Antagonist effect 3. Uncertain; possibly metoclopramide promotes absorption of morphine by increasing gastric emptying	1. Avoid co-administration. Although increasing the dose of tramadol restored the analgesic effect, it also caused a poor response to an antiemetic 2. Caution with co-administration 3. Be aware that the effects of oral morphine are ↑

ANALGESICS OPIOIDS

OPIOIDS	ANTIEPILEPTICS	1. Barbiturates ↑ sedative effects of opioids 2. ↓ efficacy of fentanyl and methadone with carbamazepine, phenobarbital, phenytoin or primidone 3. Carbamazepine ↓ tramadol levels 4. Risk of pethidine toxicity	1. Additive sedative effect 2. ↑ hepatic metabolism of fentanyl and methadone, and possibly an effect at the opioid receptor 3. Carbamazepine ↑ metabolism of tramadol 4. Phenytoin induces metabolism of pethidine, which causes ↑ level of a neurotoxic metabolite	1. Monitor respiratory rate and conscious levels 2. Be aware that the dose of fentanyl and methadone may need to be ↑ 3. Watch for poor effect of tramadol. Consider using an alternative opioid 4. Co-administer with caution; the effect may be ↓ by administering pethidine intravenously
OPIOIDS	ANTIFUNGALS	1, Ketoconazole ↑ effect of buprenorphine 2. Fluconazole and itraconazole ↑ the effect of alfentanil 3. Fluconazole and possibly voriconazole ↑ effect of methadone; this is a recognized pharmacokinetic effect but of uncertain clinical significance	1. Ketoconazole ↓ the CYP3A4-mediated metabolism of buprenorphine 2. ↓ clearance of alfentanil 3. ↓ hepatic metabolism	1. The dose of buprenorphine needs to be ↓ (by up to 50%) 2. ↓ dose of alfentanil 3. Watch for ↑ effects of methadone
OPIOIDS	ANTIHISTAMINES	Promethazine ↑ analgesic and anaesthetic effects of opioids. However, it has an additive sedative effect	Unknown	Monitor vital signs closely during co-administration
OPIOIDS	ANTIMALARIALS – QUININE	↑ codeine, fentanyl, pethidine and tramadol levels	Quinine inhibits CYP2D6	Watch for excessive narcotization
PETHIDINE, TRAMADOL	ANTIPARKINSON'S DRUGS – RASAGILINE, SELEGILINE	1. Risk of neurological toxicity when pethidine is co-administered with rasagiline 2. Risk of hyper-pyrexia when pethidine and possibly tramadol is co-administered with selegiline	Unknown	1. Avoid co-administration; do not use pethidine for at least 2 weeks after stopping rasagiline 2. Avoid co-administration

Primary drug	Secondary drug	Effect	Mechanism	Precautions
OPIOIDS	ANTIPSYCHOTICS	Risk of ↑ respiratory depression, sedation and ↓ BP. This effect seems to be particularly marked with clozapine	Additive effects	Warn patients of these effects. Monitor BP closely. Titrate doses carefully
TRAMADOL	ANTIPSYCHOTICS	↑ risk of fits	Additive effects	Consider using an alternative analgesic
OPIOIDS	**ANTIVIRALS**			
METHADONE	NNRTIs	Methadone levels may be significantly ↓ by efavirenz and nevirapine	↑ CYP3A4- and 2B6-mediated metabolism of methadone	Monitor closely for opioid withdrawal; ↑ dose as necessary. Likely to need dose titration of methadone (mean 22% but up to 186% ↑)
METHADONE	NUCLEOSIDE REVERSE TRANSCRIPTASE INHIBITORS	↓ efficacy of methadone when co-administered with abacavir	Uncertain; possibly enzyme induction	Monitor for opioid withdrawal and consider increasing dose
OPIOIDS	**PROTEASE INHIBITORS**			
ALFENTANIL, BUPRENORPHINE, FENTANYL, TRAMADOL	PROTEASE INHIBITORS	Possibly ↑ adverse effects when buprenorphine is co-administered with indinavir, ritonavir (with or without lopinavir) or saquinavir	Inhibition of CYP3A4 (CYP2D6 in the case of tramadol)	Halve the starting dose and titrate to effect. For single injection of fentanyl, monitor sedation and respiratory function closely. If continued use of fentanyl, ↓ dose may be required. Concomitant use of ritonavir and transdermal fentanyl is not recommended
CODEINE, DIHYDROCODEINE	PROTEASE INHIBITORS	↓ efficacy of codeine and dihydrocodeine when given with ritonavir	Inhibition of CYP2D6-mediated metabolism of codeine to its active metabolites	Use an alternative opioid

METHADONE, PETHIDINE	PROTEASE INHIBITORS	↓ efficacy of methadone, with risk of withdrawal, when co-administered with amprenavir, nelfinavir, ritonavir (with or without lopinavir) or saquinavir	Uncertain; possibly due to induction of CYP3A4 and CYP2D6	Monitor closely for opioid withdrawal, and ↑ dose of methadone as necessary. This advice includes co-administration of methadone with low-dose ritonavir. Short-term use of pethidine is unlikely to cause a problem
OPIOIDS	**ANXIOLYTICS AND HYPNOTICS**			
OPIOIDS	ANXIOLYTICS AND HYPNOTICS	1. ↑ sedation with BZDs 2. Respiratory depressant effect of morphine antagonized by lorazepam	1. Additive effect; both drugs are sedatives 2. Uncertain	1. Closely monitor vital signs during co-administration 2. Although this effect may be considered to be beneficial, risk of additive effects should be borne in mind if the combination of an opioid and BZDs is used for sedation for painful procedures
OPIOIDS	ANXIOLYTICS AND HYPNOTICS – SODIUM OXYBATE	Risk of CNS depression – coma, respiratory depression	Additive effect	Avoid co-administration
OPIOIDS	BETA-BLOCKERS	1. Risk of ↑ plasma concentrations and effects of labetalol, metoprolol and propranolol; ↑ systemic effects of timolol eye drops 2. ↑ plasma concentrations of esmolol when morphine added 3. ↑ plasma concentrations of metoprolol and propranolol when dextro-propoxyphene added	1. Methadone inhibits CYP2D6 which metabolizes these beta-blockers 2. Unknown 3. ↓ hepatic clearance of metoprolol and propanolol	1. Monitor BP at least weekly until stable 2. Monitor BP closely 3. Monitor BP at least weekly until stable. Warn patients to report symptoms of hypotension (light-headedness, dizziness on standing, etc.)

ANALGESICS OPIOIDS

Primary drug	Secondary drug	Effect	Mechanism	Precautions
OPIOIDS	CALCIUM CHANNEL BLOCKERS	Diltiazem prolongs the action of alfentanil	Diltiazem inhibits CYP3A4-mediated metabolism of alfentanil	Watch for the prolonged action of alfentanil in patients taking calcium channel blockers; case reports of delayed extubation in patients recovering from anaesthetics involving large doses of alfentanil in patients on diltiazem
OPIOIDS	CARDIAC GLYCOSIDES	↑ concentrations of digoxin may occur with tramadol	Unknown	Watch for digoxin toxicity; check levels and ↓ dose of digoxin as necessary
OPIOIDS	CNS STIMULANTS – ATOMOXETINE	Risk of arrhythmias with methadone and possible risk of fits with tramadol	Uncertain	Avoid co-administration of atomoxetine with methadone or tramadol
OPIOIDS	DRUG DEPENDENCE THERAPIES – BUPROPION	↑ plasma concentrations of these substrates, with risk of toxic effects	Bupropion and its metabolite hydroxybupropion inhibit CYP2D6	Initiate therapy of these drugs at the lowest effective dose
OPIOIDS	**H2 RECEPTOR BLOCKERS**			
ALFENTANIL, FENTANYL, PETHIDINE, TRAMADOL	CIMETIDINE	Cimetidine may ↑ fentanyl, pethidine and tramadol levels	Cimetidine inhibits CYP2D6-mediated metabolism of these opioids. Ranitidine weakly inhibits CYP2D6	Watch for excessive narcotization
CODEINE	CIMETIDINE	Cimetidine may ↓ efficacy of codeine	Cimetidine inhibits CYP2D6-mediated conversion of codeine to its active metabolite. Ranitidine weakly inhibits CYP2D6	Watch for poor response to codeine. Consider using an alternative opioid or acid suppression therapy
OPIOIDS	OESTROGENS	Effect of morphine may be ↓ by combined oral contraceptives	Hepatic metabolism of morphine is ↑	Be aware that morphine dose may need to be ↑. Consider using an alternative opioid such as pethidine
OPIOIDS	PROGESTOGENS	Gestodene ↑ effect of buprenorphine	Gestodene ↓ the CYP3A4-mediated metabolism of buprenorphine	The dose of buprenorphine needs to be ↓ (by up to 50%)

OPIOIDS	SYMPATHOMIMETICS – INDIRECT	Dexamfetamine and methylphenidate ↑ analgesic effects and ↓ sedation of opioids, when used for chronic pain	Uncertain; complex interaction between the sympathetic nervous system and opioid receptors	Opioid requirements may be ↓ when patients also take indirect sympathomimetics
PARACETAMOL				
PARACETAMOL	ANTIARRHYTHMICS	Disopyramide and propafenone may slow the onset of action of intermittent-dose paracetamol	Anticholinergic effects delay gastric emptying and absorption	Warn patients that the action of paracetamol may be delayed. This will not be the case when paracetamol is taken regularly
PARACETAMOL	ANTIBIOTICS			
PARACETAMOL	ISONIAZID	Risk of paracetamol toxicity at regular, therapeutic doses when co-administered with isoniazid	Uncertain; it seems that formation of toxic metabolites is ↑ in fast acetylators when isoniazid levels ↓ (i.e. at the end of a dosing period)	There have been cases of hepatic pathology; regular paracetamol should be avoided in patients taking isoniazid
PARACETAMOL	RIFAMPICIN	Rifampicin ↓ paracetamol levels	Rifampicin ↑ glucuronidation of paracetamol	Warn patients that paracetamol may be less effective
PARACETAMOL	ANTICANCER AND IMMUNOMODULATING DRUGS – BUSULFAN	Busulfan levels may be ↑ by co-administration of paracetamol	Uncertain; paracetamol probably inhibits metabolism of busulfan	Manufacturers recommend that paracetamol should be avoided for 3 days before administering parenteral busulfan
PARACETAMOL	ANTICOAGULANTS – ORAL	Possible ↑ anticoagulant effect when paracetamol is taken regularly (but not occasionally)	Uncertain; possibly due to competitive inhibition of CYP-mediated metabolism of warfarin	Monitor INR closely for the first 1–2 weeks of starting or stopping regular paracetamol
PARACETAMOL	ANTIDEPRESSANTS – TCAs	TCAs may slow the onset of action of intermittent-dose paracetamol	Anticholinergic effects delay gastric emptying and absorption	Warn patients that the action of paracetamol may be delayed. This will not be the case when paracetamol is taken regularly
PARACETAMOL	ANTIEMETICS	Cyclizine may slow the onset of action of intermittent-dose paracetamol	Anticholinergic effects delay gastric emptying and absorption	Warn patients that the action of paracetamol may be delayed. This will not be the case when paracetamol is taken regularly

ANALGESICS PARACETAMOL

Primary drug	Secondary drug	Effect	Mechanism	Precautions
PARACETAMOL	ANTIHISTAMINES	Chlorphenamine, cyproheptadine and hydroxyzine may slow the onset of action of intermittent-dose paracetamol	Anticholinergic effects delay gastric emptying and absorption	Warn patients that the action of paracetamol may be delayed. This will not be the case when paracetamol is taken regularly
PARACETAMOL	ANTIMUSCARINICS	Atropine, benzatropine, orphenadrine, procyclidine and trihexyphenidyl may slow the onset of action of intermittent-dose paracetamol	Anticholinergic effects delay gastric emptying and absorption	Warn patients that the action of paracetamol may be delayed. This will not be the case when paracetamol is taken regularly
PARACETAMOL	ANTIPARKINSON'S DRUGS – DOPAMINERGICS	Amantadine, bromocriptine, levodopa, pergolide, pramipexole and selegiline may slow the onset of action of intermittent-dose paracetamol	Anticholinergic effects delay gastric emptying and absorption	Warn patients that the action of paracetamol may be delayed. This will not be the case when paracetamol is taken regularly
PARACETAMOL	ANTIVIRALS	Cases of hepatotoxicity have been reported when paracetamol was added to either didanosine or zidovudine	Uncertain; possible additive hepatotoxic effect	Monitor liver function regularly during co-administration
PARACETAMOL	CNS STIMULANTS – MODAFINIL	May cause ↓ paracetamol levels if CYP1A2 is the predominant metabolic pathway and alternative metabolic pathways are either genetically deficient or affected	Modafinil is moderate inducer of CYP1A2 in a concentration-dependent manner	Be aware
PARACETAMOL	LIPID-LOWERING DRUGS	Colestyramine ↓ paracetamol by 60% when they are given together	Colestyramine binds paracetamol in the intestine	Give colestyramine and paracetamol at least 1 hour apart
PARACETAMOL	MUSCLE RELAXANTS – SKELETAL	Baclofen may slow the onset of action of intermittent-dose paracetamol	Anticholinergic effects delay gastric emptying and absorption	Warn patients that the action of paracetamol may be delayed. This will not be the case when paracetamol is taken regularly

Part 8 MUSCULOSKELETAL DRUGS

Antigout drugs

Colchicine is a known substrate for P-gp, and inhibitors of P-gp can cause colchicine toxicity.

Skeletal muscle relaxants

Muscle relaxation is caused by various mechanisms, such as depression of ACh synthesis (e.g. hemicholinium), storage (vesamicol) and release (magnesium, botulinum toxin) and depression of muscle activity by drugs such as dantrolene and baclofen.

Carisoprodol

This is a centrally acting skeletal muscle relaxant whose active metabolite is meprobamate. It is metabolized primarily by CYP2C19.

Dantrolene

Dantrolene sodium produces its effects by affecting the contractile response of the skeletal muscle at a site beyond the neuromuscular junction, probably by interfering with the release of calcium ions from the sarcoplasmic reticulum.

Tizanidine

Tizanidine is an agonist at alpha-2 adrenergic receptor sites. It is considered to reduce spasticity by increasing the presynaptic inhibition of motor neurones, mainly influencing polysynaptic pathways, thus decreasing the facilitation of spinal motor neurones. It undergoes extensive first-pass metabolism, and the primary isoenzyme involved is CYP1A2.

Primary drug	Secondary drug	Effect	Mechanism	Precautions
ANTIGOUT DRUGS				
ALLOPURINOL				
ALLOPURINOL	ANTIBIOTICS			
ALLOPURINOL	AMOXICILLIN, AMPICILLIN	Possible ↑ risk of rash with amoxicillin and ampicillin (over 20% incidence in one study)	Uncertain	Reassure patients that the rash is unlikely to have clinical significance
ALLOPURINOL	PYRAZINAMIDE	↓ efficacy of antigout drugs	Pyrazinamide can induce hyperuricaemia	Pyrazinamide should not be used in patients with gout
ALLOPURINOL	ANTICANCER AND IMMUNOMODULATING DRUGS			
ALLOPURINOL	AZATHIOPRINE/ MERCAPTOPURINE	↑ mercaptopurine levels, with risk of toxicity (e.g. myelosuppression, pancreatitis)	Azathioprine is metabolized to mercaptopurine. Allopurinol inhibits hepatic metabolism of mercaptopurine	↓ doses of azathioprine and mercaptopurine by up to three-quarters and monitor FBC, LFTs and amylase carefully
ALLOPURINOL	CAPECITABINE/ FLUOROURACIL	Possible ↓ efficacy of capecitabine	Capecitabine is a prodrug for fluorouracil; uncertain at which point allopurinol acts on the metabolic pathway	Manufacturers recommend avoiding co-administration
ALLOPURINOL	CICLOSPORIN	Ciclosporin levels may be ↑	Uncertain	Monitor renal function closely
ALLOPURINOL	CYCLOPHOSPHAMIDE	↑ risk of bone marrow suppression	Uncertain but allopurinol seems to ↑ cyclophosphamide levels	Monitor FBC closely
ALLOPURINOL	ANTICOAGULANTS – ORAL	Uncommon instances of ↑ anti-coagulant effect in patients on warfarin who started allopurinol	Allopurinol possibly ↓ hepatic metabolism of warfarin but considerable individual variation	Monitor INR closely when allopurinol is first started

ALLOPURINOL	ANTIEPILEPTICS			
ALLOPURINOL	CARBAMAZEPINE	High-dose allopurinol (600 mg/day) may ↑ carbamazepine levels over a period of several weeks. 300 mg/day allopurinol does not seem to have this effect	Uncertain	Monitor carbamazepine levels in patients taking long-term, high-dose allopurinol
ALLOPURINOL	PHENYTOIN	Phenytoin levels may be ↑ in some patients	Uncertain	Monitor phenytoin levels
ALLOPURINOL	ANTIHYPERTENSIVES AND HEART FAILURE DRUGS – ACE INHIBITORS	Risk of serious hypersensitivity with captopril and enalapril	Uncertain. Both drugs can cause hypersensitivity reactions	Warn patient to look for clinical features of hypersensitivity and Stevens–Johnson syndrome
ALLOPURINOL	ANTIVIRALS – DIDANOSINE	Didanosine levels may be ↑	Uncertain	Watch for the early signs of toxicity
ALLOPURINOL	BRONCHODILATORS – THEOPHYLLINE	↑ theophylline levels	Allopurinol inhibits xanthine oxidase	Watch for early features of toxicity of theophylline (headache, nausea)
ALLOPURINOL	DIURETICS – THIAZIDES	Possible ↑ risk of severe allergic reactions when allopurinol is given with thiazides in the presence of renal impairment	Uncertain	Caution in co-administering allopurinol with thiazides in the presence of renal insufficiency
COLCHICINE				
COLCHICINE	**ANTIBIOTICS**			
COLCHICINE	MACROLIDES	Case reports of colchicine toxicity when macrolides were added	Uncertain; macrolides possibly inhibit hepatic metabolism of colchicine. Clarithromycin and erythromycin both inhibit intestinal P-gp, which may ↑ bioavailability of colchicine	Monitor FBC and renal function closely
COLCHICINE	PYRAZINAMIDE	↓ efficacy of antigout drugs	Pyrazinamide can induce hyperuricaemia	Pyrazinamide should not be used in patients with gout

Primary drug	Secondary drug	Effect	Mechanism	Precautions
COLCHICINE	ANTICANCER AND IMMUNOMODULATING DRUGS – CICLOSPORIN	↑ colchicine plasma concentrations and ↑ toxic effects (hepatotoxicity, myopathy). ↑ penetration of ciclosporin through blood–brain barrier and ↑ risk of neurotoxicity	Competitive inhibition of P-gp with ↑ penetrations of ciclosporin to tissues. Ciclosporin inhibits transport of colchicine	Avoid concurrent use
PROBENECID				
PROBENECID	ACE INHIBITORS	↑ plasma concentrations of captopril and enalapril; uncertain clinical significance	Renal excretion of captopril and enalapril ↓ by probenecid	Monitor BP closely
PROBENECID	ANALGESICS – NSAIDS	Probenecid ↑ levels of indometacin and ketorolac and possibly dexketoprofen, ketoprofen, naproxen, tenoxicam and tiaprofenic acid	Probenecid competitively inhibits renal metabolism of these NSAIDs	Watch for signs of toxicity of these NSAIDs. Consider using an alternative NSAID. The manufacturers of ketorolac advise avoiding co-administration of ketorolac and probenecid
PROBENECID	**ANTIBIOTICS**			
PROBENECID	CEPHALOSPORINS	↑ cephalosporin levels	Uncertain	Watch for ↑ incidence of side-effects of antibiotic
PROBENECID	DAPSONE	↑ dapsone levels, with risk of bone marrow suppression	Uncertain	Monitor FBC closely
PROBENECID	MEROPENEM	↑ meropenem levels	Uncertain	Manufacturers recommend avoiding co-administration
PROBENECID	NITROFURANTOIN	↓ efficacy of nitrofurantoin in urinary tract infections	↓ urinary excretion	Watch for poor response to nitrofurantoin
PROBENECID	PENICILLINS	↑ penicillin levels	Uncertain	Watch for ↑ incidence of side-effects of antibiotic
PROBENECID	PYRAZINAMIDE	↓ efficacy of antigout drugs	Pyrazinamide can induce hyperuricaemia	Pyrazinamide should not be used in patients with gout

PROBENECID	QUINOLONES – CIPROFLOXACIN, LEVOFLOXACIN, NALIDIXIC ACID, NORFLOXACIN	↑ ciprofloxacin, nalidixic acid and norfloxacin levels	Uncertain	Watch for ↑ incidence of side-effects. Moxifloxacin, ofloxacin and sparfloxacin do not seem to interact and could be used as alternative therapy
PROBENECID	**ANTICANCER AND IMMUNOMODULATING DRUGS**			
PROBENECID	AMINOSALICYLATES	Aminosalicylate levels are ↑ by probenecid	Probenecid competes with aminosalicylate for active renal excretion	Watch for early features of toxicity of aminosalicylate. Consider ↓ dose of aminosalicylate
PROBENECID	METHOTREXATE	↑ methotrexate levels	Probenecid ↓ elimination of methotrexate renally by interfering with tubular secretion in the proximal tubule and also ↓ protein binding of methotrexate (a relatively minor effect). Probenecid competes with methotrexate for renal elimination	Avoid co-administration if possible; if not possible, ↓ dose of methotrexate and monitor FBC closely
PROBENECID	PEMETREXED	↑ pemetrexed levels	Probable ↓ renal excretion of pemetrexed	Avoid co-administration where possible. If both need to be given, monitor FBC and renal function closely and watch for gastrointestinal disturbances and features of myopathy
PROBENECID	**ANTIDIABETIC DRUGS**			
PROBENECID	METFORMIN	↑ level of metformin and risk of lactic acidosis. The onset of lactic acidosis is often subtle with symptoms of malaise, myalgia, respiratory distress and ↑ non-specific abdominal distress. There may be hypothermia and resistant bradyarrhythmias	↓ renal excretion of metformin	Watch for hypoglycaemia and lactic acidosis. Warn patients about hypoglycaemia ➢ ***For signs and symptoms of hypoglycaemia, see Clinical Features of Some Adverse Drug Interactions, Hypoglycaemia***

Primary drug	Secondary drug	Effect	Mechanism	Precautions
PROBENECID	SULPHONYLUREAS	↑ risk of hypoglycaemic episodes due to ↑ plasma levels of glimepride	Attributed to ↓ renal excretion of sulphonylureas by probenecid. Probenecid is also an inhibitor of CYP2C9 isoenzymes	Watch for and warn patients about symptoms of hypoglycaemia ➢ ***For signs and symptoms of hypoglycaemia, see Clinical Features of Some Adverse Drug Interactions, Hypoglycaemia***
PROBENECID	ANTIPLATELET AGENTS	Aspirin possibly ↓ efficacy of probenecid	Uncertain	Watch for poor response to probenecid
PROBENECID	**ANTIVIRALS**			
PROBENECID	ANTIVIRALS	↑ levels of aciclovir, valaciclovir and ganciclovir	Competitive inhibition of renal excretion	Care with co-administering probenecid with *high-dose* antivirals
PROBENECID	ZIDOVUDINE	↑ levels of zidovudine with cases of toxicity	↓ hepatic metabolism of zidovudine	Avoid co-administration if possible; if not possible, ↓ dose of zidovudine
PROBENECID	SODIUM PHENYLBUTYRATE	Possibly ↑ sodium phenylbutyrate levels	Possibly ↓ excretion of sodium phenylbutyrate	Watch for signs of sodium phenylbutyrate toxicity. Monitor FBC, U&Es and ECG
SULFINPYRAZONE				
SULFINPYRAZONE	**ANTIBIOTICS**			
SULFINPYRAZONE	NITROFURANTOIN	↓ renal excretion of nitrofurantoin, which ↓ its efficacy in urinary tract infections	Uncertain	Watch for poor response to nitrofurantoin
SULFINPYRAZONE	PENICILLINS	↑ penicillin levels	Uncertain	Watch for ↑ incidence of side-effects
SULFINPYRAZONE	PYRAZINAMIDE	↓ efficacy of antigout drugs	Pyrazinamide can induce hyperuricaemia	Pyrazinamide should not be used in patients with gout
SULFINPYRAZONE	ANTICANCER AND IMMUNOMODULATING DRUGS – CICLOSPORIN	Cases of ↓ ciclosporin levels with transplant rejection	Uncertain	Watch for ↓ efficacy of ciclosporin

SULFINPYRAZONE	ANTICOAGULANTS – ORAL	↑ anticoagulant effect	Uncertain; possibly displacement of anticoagulant from plasma proteins, possibly inhibition of CYP2C9-mediated metabolism of warfarin	Monitor INR at least weekly until stable
SULFINPYRAZONE	**ANTIDIABETIC DRUGS**			
SULPHINPYRAZONE	NATEGLINIDE	↑ blood levels of nateglinide	Sulphinpyrazone is a selective CYP2C9 inhibitor	Need to monitor blood sugar weekly in patients receiving both drugs. Warn patients about hypoglycaemia ➢ ***For signs and symptoms of hypoglycaemia, see Clinical Features of Some Adverse Drug Interactions, Hypoglycaemia***
SULFINPYRAZONE	SULPHONYLUREAS	↑ hypoglycaemic effect of sulphonylureas	Uncertain	Monitor blood glucose regularly
SULFINPYRAZONE	ANTIEPILEPTICS	Phenytoin levels may be ↑ in some patients	Uncertain	Monitor phenytoin levels
SULFINPYRAZONE	ANTIPLATELET AGENTS	High-dose aspirin antagonizes the urate-lowering effect of sulfinpyrazone	Salicylates block the sulfinpyrazone-induced inhibition of renal tubular reabsorption of urate	Avoid long-term co-administration of high-dose aspirin with sulfinpyrazone. Low-dose aspirin does not seem to have this effect
SULFINPYRAZONE	BETA-BLOCKERS	Antihypertensive effects of oxprenolol ↓ by sulfinpyrazone	Unknown	Monitor PR and BP closely; consider starting an alternative beta-blocker
SULFINPYRAZONE	BRONCHODILATORS – THEOPHYLLINE	↓ theophylline levels	Due to ↑ demethylation and hydroxylation, and thus ↑ clearance of theophylline	May need to ↑ dose of theophylline by 25%
SULFINPYRAZONE	CALCIUM CHANNEL BLOCKERS	Serum concentrations of verapamil are significantly ↓ when it is co-administered with sulfinpyrazone	Uncertain, but presumed to be due to ↑ hepatic metabolism	Monitor PR and BP closely; watch for poor response to verapamil

MUSCULOSKELETAL DRUGS SKELETAL MUSCLE RELAXANTS

Primary drug	Secondary drug	Effect	Mechanism	Precautions
DRUGS AFFECTING BONE METABOLISM ➢ *Other Endocrine Drugs*				
DRUGS TREATING INFLAMMATORY ARTHROPATHIES				
Corticosteroids ➢ *Anticancer and Immunomodulating Drugs, Other immunomodulating drugs*				
Disease-modifying Drugs ➢ *Anticancer and Immunomodulating Drugs; Drugs to Treat Infections, Antimalarial drugs*				
Non-steroidal anti-inflammatory drugs ➢ *Analgesics, Non-steroidal anti-inflammatory drugs*				
SKELETAL MUSCLE RELAXANTS				
BACLOFEN	ADDITIVE ANTIMUSCARINIC EFFECTS			
BACLOFEN	1. ANALGESICS – nefopam 2. ANTIARRHYTHMICS – disopyramide, propafenone 3. ANTIDEPRESSANTS – TCAs 4. ANTIEMETICS – cyclizine 5. ANTIHISTAMINES – chlorphenamine, cyproheptadine, hydroxyzine 6. ANTIMUSCARINICS – atropine, benzatropine, cyclopentolate, dicycloverine, flavoxate, homatropine, hyoscine, orphenadrine, oxybutynin, procyclidine, propantheline, tolterodine, trihexyphenidyl, tropicamide 7. ANTIPARKINSON'S DRUGS – dopaminergics 8. ANTIPSYCHOTICS – phenothiazines, clozapine, pimozide 9. NITRATES	↑ risk of antimuscarinic side-effects. **NB ↓ efficacy of sublingual nitrate tablets**	Additive effect; both drugs cause antimuscarinic side-effects. **Antimuscarinic effects ↓ saliva production, which ↓ dissolution of the tablet**	Warn patient of this additive effect. **Consider using sublingual nitrate spray**

BACLOFEN, TIZANIDINE	ADDITIVE HYPOTENSIVE EFFECTS			
BACLOFEN, TIZANIDINE	1. ANAESTHETICS – general 2. ANTICANCER AND IMMUNOMODULATING DRUGS – IL-2 3. ANTIDEPRESSANTS – MAOIs 4. ANTIHYPERTENSIVES AND HEART FAILURE DRUGS 5. ANTIPSYCHOTICS 6. ANXIOLYTICS AND HYPNOTICS 7. BETA-BLOCKERS 8. CALCIUM CHANNEL BLOCKERS 9. DIURETICS 10. NITRATES 11. PERIPHERAL VASODILATORS – moxisylyte (thymoxamine) 12. POTASSIUM CHANNEL ACTIVATORS	↑ hypotensive effect	Additive hypotensive effect. Tizanidine also has a negative chronotropic effect and may cause additive bradycardia with beta-blockers and calcium channel blockers	Monitor BP at least weekly until stable. Warn patients to report symptoms of hypotension (light-headedness, dizziness on standing, etc.)
BACLOFEN, METHOCARBAMOL, TIZANIDINE	ALCOHOL	↑ sedation	Additive effect	Warn patients; advise them to drink alcohol only in moderation and not to drive if they have drunk any alcohol and are taking these muscle relaxants
BACLOFEN, TIZANIDINE	ANAESTHETICS – GENERAL	↑ hypotensive effect	Additive hypotensive effect. Tizanidine also has a negative chronotropic effect and may cause additive bradycardia with beta-blockers and calcium channel blockers	Monitor BP closely, especially during induction of anaesthesia

MUSCULOSKELETAL DRUGS SKELETAL MUSCLE RELAXANTS

MUSCULOSKELETAL DRUGS SKELETAL MUSCLE RELAXANTS

Primary drug	Secondary drug	Effect	Mechanism	Precautions
BACLOFEN	ANALGESICS			
BACLOFEN	NSAIDs	↑ baclofen levels with ibuprofen	↓ renal excretion of baclofen	Avoid co-administration
BACLOFEN	PARACETAMOL	Baclofen may slow the onset of action of intermittent-dose paracetamol	Anticholinergic effects delay gastric emptying and absorption	Warn patients that the action of paracetamol may be delayed. This will not be the case when paracetamol is taken regularly
TIZANIDINE	ANTIBIOTICS – CIPROFLOXACIN	↑ tizanidine levels	Tizanidine is a substrate for CYP1A2; ciprofloxacin is a potent inhibitor of CYP1A2 and is thought to inhibit its presystemic metabolism, resulting in ↑ absorption and ↑ levels of tizanidine	Avoid co-administration
BACLOFEN	ANTIDEPRESSANTS – LITHIUM	Enhancement of hyperkinesias associated with lithium	Uncertain	Consider alternative skeletal muscle relaxant
BACLOFEN	ANTIDIABETIC DRUGS	↓ hypoglycaemic effect	Due to these a drugs causing hyperglycaemia, the mechanism being uncertain at present	↑ doses of antidiabetic drugs are often required for adequate glycaemic control
DANTROLENE	ANTIEMETICS – METOCLOPRAMIDE	Possibly ↑ dantrolene levels	Uncertain	Be aware; monitor BP and LFTs closely
BACLOFEN	ANTIPARKINSON'S DRUGS – LEVODOPA	Reports of CNS agitation and ↓ efficacy of levodopa	Uncertain	Avoid co-administration
BACLOFEN, METHOCARBAMOL, TIZANIDINE	ANXIOLYTICS AND HYPNOTICS	↑ sedation	Additive effect	Warn patients; advise them to drink alcohol only in moderation and not to drive if they have drunk any alcohol and are taking these muscle relaxants

BACLOFEN, TIZANIDINE	BETA-BLOCKERS	↑ hypotensive effect with baclofen and tizanidine. Risk of bradycardia with tizanidine	Additive hypotensive effect. Tizanidine has a negative inotropic and chronotropic effect	Monitor BP at least weekly until stable. Warn patients to report symptoms of hypotension (light-headedness, dizziness on standing, etc.)
DANTROLENE	CALCIUM CHANNEL BLOCKERS	Risk of arrhythmias when diltiazem is given with intravenous dantrolene. Risk of ↓ BP, myocardial depression and hyperkalaemia when verapamil is given with intravenous dantrolene	Uncertain at present	Extreme caution must be exercised when administering parenteral dantrolene to patients on diltiazem or verapamil. Monitor BP and cardiac rhythm closely; watch for hyperkalaemia
TIZANIDINE	CARDIAC GLYCOSIDES – DIGOXIN	Risk of bradycardia when tizanidine is given with digoxin	Tizanidine has a negative inotropic effect	Monitor PR closely
SKELETAL MUSCLE RELAXANTS	**CNS STIMULANTS**			
TIZANIDINE	MODAFINIL	Possibly ↓ tizanidine levels	Modafinil is moderate inducer of CYP1A2 in a concentration-dependent manner	Be aware. Watch for poor response to tizanidine
CARISOPRODOL	MODAFINIL	May cause moderate ↑ in carisoprodol levels	Modafinil is a reversible inhibitor of CYP2C19 when used in therapeutic doses	Be aware

MUSCULOSKELETAL DRUGS SKELETAL MUSCLE RELAXANTS

Part 9 ANAESTHETIC DRUGS

General anaesthetics

General anaesthetics are volatile agents intended to produce loss of consciousness and can cause additive CNS depressant effects with drugs having this effect (e.g. opioid analgesics or antiemetics administered postoperatively). Patients undergoing day-case surgery should be warned about this effect (and should be warned to avoid alcohol for at least 24 hours). General anaesthetics have negative inotropic and/or vasodilating properties that may lead to hypotension, likely to be exacerbated by the co-administration of other drugs with hypotensive effects. They are also likely to increase risk of arrhythmias (due to inherent Q–T prolongation effects and sensitization of the myocardium to circulating catecholamines).

Local anaesthetics

Local anaesthetics reversibly prevent the transmission of nerve impulses by binding to sodium channels (preventing depolarization) and produce analgesia without loss of consciousness.

Additives to local anaesthetic solutions used include the following:

- *Epinephrine*. This causes local vasoconstriction, which reduces blood loss from the area and decreases rate of removal of local anaesthetic, which in turn increases the duration of action and, in the case of lidocaine, the safe dose that can be administered.
- *Bicarbonate*. This maintains the local anaesthetic in an unionized form, which promotes the movement of local anaesthetic into the neurone/axon, thereby increasing the speed of onset of action.
- *Glucose*. Glucose increases the baricity of the solution to greater than that of CSF to provide greater control of spread when it is administered intrathecally.

Toxicity relates to the effects of local anaesthetics on ion channels in excitable membranes in the CNS (producing tingling of the lips, slurred speech, decreased levels of consciousness and seizures) and cardiovascular system (causing arrhythmias and decreased myocardial contractility).

Ester local anaesthetics (procaine, tetracaine) are metabolized by pseudocholinesterase. Drugs or chemicals (e.g. organophosphate insecticides, nerve gases, various other drugs) that depress pseudocholinesterase levels can prolong duration of action.

Muscle relaxants – depolarizing and non-depolarizing

Suxamethonium is a depolarizing short-acting muscle relaxant that is rapidly hydrolysed by pseudocholinesterase, and drugs or chemicals that inhibit this enzyme may prolong its action.

Non-depolarizing muscle relaxants compete with the neurotransmitter ACh for sites at the postsynaptic nicotinic receptor on the muscle. Most non-depolarizing muscle relaxants are metabolized in the liver, with the exception of atracurium, which undergoes spontaneous breakdown (Hoffman degradation). Additive effects are associated with several medications that have effects on neuromuscular transmission (e.g. aminoglycosides). In addition, non-depolarizing muscle relaxants are subject to adverse interactions by drugs interfering with the synthesis and/or release of ACh and with drugs that have an affinity for the postsynaptic nicotinic receptors on muscle.

ANAESTHETIC DRUGS ANAESTHETICS – GENERAL

Primary drug	Secondary drug	Effect	Mechanism	Precautions
ANAESTHETICS – GENERAL				
INHALATIONAL	ANTIARRHYTHMICS – AMIODARONE	Amiodarone may ↑ myocardial depressant effects of inhalational anaesthetics	Additive effect	Monitor PR, BP and ECG closely
INTRAVENOUS – THIOPENTONE	ANTIBIOTICS – SULPHONAMIDES	↑ effect of thiopentone but ↓ duration of action	Uncertain; possibly displacement from protein-binding sites	Be aware that ↓ dose may be needed
NITROUS OXIDE	ANTICANCER AND IMMUNOMODULATING DRUGS – METHOTREXATE	↑ antifolate effect of methotrexate	↑ toxicity of methotrexate	Nitrous oxide is usually used for relatively brief durations when patients are anaesthetized, and hence this risk during anaesthesia is minimal. However, nitrous oxide may be used for analgesia for longer durations, and this should be avoided
ANAESTHETICS – GENERAL	**ANTIDEPRESSANTS**			
ANAESTHETICS – GENERAL	MAOIs	Some cases of both ↑ and ↓ BP on induction of anaesthesia. Mostly no significant changes	Uncertain	Some recommend stopping MAOIs 2 weeks before surgery. Others suggest no need for this; monitor BP closely, especially during induction of anaesthesia
ANAESTHETICS – GENERAL	TCAs	A few cases of arrhythmias	Uncertain	Monitor ECG, PR and BP closely
INTRAVENOUS – KETAMINE	ANTIDEMENTIA DRUGS – MEMANTINE	↑ CNS side-effects	Additive effects on NMDA receptors	Avoid co-administration
INTRAVENOUS	ANTIHYPERTENSIVES AND HEART FAILURE DRUGS	Risk of severe hypotensive episodes during induction of anaesthesia	Most general anaesthetics are myocardial depressants and vasodilators. Additive hypotensive effect	Monitor BP closely, especially during induction of anaesthesia

VOLATILE AGENTS	ANTIPARKINSON'S DRUGS – LEVODOPA	Possible risk of arrhythmias	Uncertain	Monitor EGC and BP closely. Consider using intravenous agents for maintenance of anaesthesia
INTRAVENOUS – THIOPENTONE	ANTIPLATELET AGENTS – ASPIRIN	↓ requirements of thiopentone when aspirin (1 g) used during premedication	Uncertain at present	Be aware of possible ↓ dose requirements for thiopentone
ANAESTHETICS – GENERAL	ANTIPSYCHOTICS	Risk of hypotension	Additive effect	Monitor BP closely, especially during induction of anaesthesia
INTRAVENOUS ANAESTHETICS (e.g. thiopentone sodium, propofol)	BETA-BLOCKERS	Risk of severe hypotensive episodes during induction of anaesthesia (including patients taking timolol eye drops)	Most intravenous anaesthetic agents are myocardial depressants and vasodilators, and additive ↓ BP may occur	Monitor BP closely, especially during induction of anaesthesia
ANAESTHETICS – GENERAL	**BRONCHODILATORS**			
INHALATIONAL – HALOTHANE	TERBUTALINE, THEOPHYLLINE	Cases of arrhythmias when these bronchodilators are co-administered with halothane	Possibly due to sensitization of the myocardium to circulating catecholamines by the volatile anaesthetics to varying degrees	Risk of cardiac events is higher with halothane. Desflurane is irritant to the upper respiratory tract, and ↑ secretions can occur and are best avoided in patients with bronchial asthma. Sevoflurane is non-irritant and unlikely to cause serious adverse effects
INTRAVENOUS – KETAMINE	THEOPHYLLINE	Risk of fits	Uncertain	A careful risk–benefit assessment should be made before using ketamine. However, there are significant benefits for the use of ketamine to anaesthetize patients for emergency management of life-threatening asthma

Primary drug	Secondary drug	Effect	Mechanism	Precautions
INHALATIONAL	CALCIUM CHANNEL BLOCKERS	↑ hypotensive effects of dihydropyridines, and hypotensive/bradycardic effects of diltiazem and verapamil	Additive hypotensive and negative inotropic effects. General anaesthetics tend to be myocardial depressants and vasodilators; they also ↓ sinus automaticity and AV conduction	Monitor BP and ECG closely
INHALATIONAL AND INTRAVENOUS ANAESTHETICS	DIURETICS	↑ hypotensive effect	Additive effect as the anaesthetics cause varying degrees of myocardial depression and/or vasodilatation, while diuretics tend to ↓ circulatory volume	Monitor BP closely, especially during induction of anaesthesia
HALOTHANE	ERGOT DERIVATIVES	↓ efficacy of ergometrine on uterus	Halothane ↓ muscle tone of the pregnant uterus; generally, its use in obstetric anaesthesia is not recommended as it ↑ risk of postpartum haemorrhage, for which ergot derivatives are commonly used	Use alternative form of anaesthesia for surgery requiring use of ergotamine
ANAESTHETICS – GENERAL	MUSCLE RELAXANTS – BACLOFEN, TIZANIDINE	↑ hypotensive effect	Additive hypotensive effect. Tizanidine also has a negative chronotropic effect and may cause additive bradycardia with beta-blockers and calcium channel blockers	Monitor BP closely, especially during induction of anaesthesia
ANAESTHETICS – GENERAL	NITRATES	↑ hypotensive effect	Additive effect (vasodilatation and/or depression of myocardial contractility)	Monitor BP closely, especially during induction of anaesthesia

ANAESTHETIC DRUGS ANAESTHETICS – GENERAL

INHALATIONAL – HALOTHANE	OXYTOCICS	Report of arrhythmias and cardiovascular collapse when halothane was given to patients taking oxytocin	Uncertain; possibly additive effect. High-dose oxytocin may cause hypotension and arrhythmias	Monitor PR, BP and ECG closely; give oxytocin in the lowest possible dose. Otherwise consider using an alternative inhalational anaesthetic
ANAESTHETICS – GENERAL	PERIPHERAL VASODILATORS – MOXISYLYTE	↑ hypotensive effect	Additive effect	Monitor BP closely, especially during induction of anaesthesia
ANAESTHETICS – GENERAL	POTASSIUM CHANNEL ACTIVATORS	↑ hypotensive effect	Additive effect	Monitor BP closely
ANAESTHETICS – GENERAL	**SYMPATHOMIMETICS**			
ANAESTHETICS – GENERAL	DIRECTLY ACTING SYMPATHOMIMETICS (e.g. epinephrine)	1. Risk of arrhythmias when inhalational anaesthetics are co-administered with epinephrine or norepinephrine 2. Case report of marked ↑ BP when phenylephrine eye drops were given during general anaesthesia	1. The arrhythmogenic threshold with injected epinephrine is lower with halothane than isoflurane or enflurane, which is attributed to sensitization to beta-adrenoceptor stimulation 2. Uncertain. Phenylephrine produces its effects by acting on alpha-adrenergic receptors; possible that these effects are enhanced	1. Use epinephrine in the smallest possible dose (when using 1:100 000 infiltration to ↓ intraoperative bleeding, no more than 10 mL/10 minutes and less than 30 mL/hour should be given) 2. Avoid use of phenylephrine eye drops during anaesthesia
ANAESTHETICS – GENERAL	INDIRECTLY ACTING SYMPATHOMIMETICS (e.g. methylphenidate)	1. Risk of arrhythmias when inhalational anaesthetics are co-administered with methylphenidate 2. Case report of ↓ sedative effect of midazolam and ketamine by methylphenidate	1. Uncertain; attributed by some to sensitization of the myocardium to sympathomimetics by inhalational anaesthetics 2. Uncertain at present; possibly due to CNS stimulation caused by methylphenidate (hence its use in narcolepsy)	Avoid giving methylphenidate on the day of elective surgery

Primary drug	Secondary drug	Effect	Mechanism	Precautions
INTRAVENOUS – KETAMINE	THYROID HORMONES	Case reports of tachycardia and hypertension when ketamine was given to patients on thyroxine; treatment with propanolol	Uncertain	Monitor PR and BP closely
ANAESTHETICS – LOCAL				
PHARMACEUTICAL INTERACTIONS				
LIDOCAINE SOLUTIONS	AMPHOTERICIN, AMPICILLIN, PHENYTOIN, SULFADIAZINE	Precipitation of drugs, which may not be immediately apparent	A pharmaceutical interaction	Do not mix in the same infusion or syringe
PROCAINE SOLUTIONS	AMINOPHYLLINE, AMPHOTERICIN, BARBITURATES, MAGNESIUM SULPHATE, PHENYTOIN, SODIUM BICARBONATE	Precipitation of drugs, which may not be immediately apparent	A pharmaceutical interaction	Do not mix in the same infusion or syringe
PROCAINE SOLUTIONS	CALCIUM, MAGNESIUM AND SODIUM SALT-CONTAINING SOLUTIONS	A temperature-dependent incompatibility that causes a physicochemical reaction	A pharmaceutical interaction	Do not mix in the same infusion or syringe
OTHER INTERACTIONS				
ANAESTHETICS – LOCAL	ANTIARRHYTHMICS			
ANAESTHETICS – LOCAL	ADENOSINE	↑ myocardial depression	Additive effect; local anaesthetics and adenosine are myocardial depressants	Monitor PR, BP and ECG closely
ANAESTHETICS – LOCAL	AMIODARONE, DISOPYRAMIDE, FLECAINIDE, MEXILETINE, PROCAINAMIDE, PROPAFENONE	Risk of ↓ BP	Additive myocardial depression	Particular care should be taken to avoid inadvertent intravenous administration during bupivacaine infiltration; monitor PR, BP and ECG during epidural administration of bupivacaine

LIDOCAINE	MEXILETINE	Mexiletine ↑ lidocaine levels (with cases of toxicity when lidocaine is given intravenously)	Mexiletine displaces lidocaine from its tissue binding sites; it also seems to ↓ its clearance but the exact mechanism is uncertain at present	Watch for the early symptoms/signs of lidocaine toxicity (perioral paraesthesia)
LIDOCAINE	PROCAINAMIDE	Case report of neurotoxicity when intravenous lidocaine administered with procainamide. No significant interaction expected when lidocaine is used for local anaesthetic infiltration	Likely to be an additive effect; both may cause neurotoxicity in overdose	Care should be taken when administering lidocaine as an infusion for patients taking procainamide
ANAESTHETICS – LOCAL	**ANTIBIOTICS**			
LIDOCAINE	QUINUPRISTIN/ DALFOPRISTIN	Risk of arrhythmias	Additive effect when lidocaine given intravenously	Avoid co-administration of quinupristin/dalfopristin with intravenous lidocaine
PRILOCAINE	SULPHONAMIDES	Risk of methaemoglobinaemia; a case report of methaemoglobinaemia with topical prilocaine in a patient taking sulphonamides	Additive effect	Avoid co-administration
ANAESTHETICS – LOCAL	**ANTICANCER AND IMMUNOMODULATING DRUGS**			
LOCAL ANAESTHETICS WITH EPINEPHRINE	PROCARBAZINE	Risk of severe hypertension	Due to inhibition of MAO, which metabolizes epinephrine	
SPINAL ANAESTHETICS	PROCARBAZINE	Risk of hypotensive episodes	Uncertain	Recommendation is to discontinue procarbazine for at least 10 days before elective spinal anaesthesia

Primary drug	Secondary drug	Effect	Mechanism	Precautions
ROPIVACAINE	ANTIDEPRESSANTS – FLUVOXAMINE	↑ plasma concentrations and prolonged effects of ropivacaine, a local anaesthetic related to bupivacaine but less potent and cardiotoxic than bupivacaine. Adverse effects include nausea, vomiting, tachycardia, headache and rigors	Fluvoxamine inhibits metabolism of ropivacaine	Be aware of the possibility of prolonged effects and of toxicity. Take note of any numbness or tingling around the lips and mouth or slurring of speech after administration as they may be warning signs of more severe toxic effects such as seizures or loss of consciousness
ANAESTHETICS – LOCAL	**ANTIHYPERTENSIVES AND HEART FAILURE DRUGS**			
ANAESTHETICS – LOCAL	ACE INHIBITORS	Risk of profound ↓ BP with epidural bupivacaine in patients on captopril	Additive hypotensive effect; epidural bupivacaine causes vasodilatation in the lower limbs	Monitor BP closely. Ensure that the patient is preloaded with fluids
LOCAL ANAESTHETICS	ADRENERGIC NEURONE BLOCKERS – GUANETHIDINE	↓ clinical efficacy of guanethidine when used in the treatment of complex regional pain syndrome type I	The local anaesthetic ↓ reuptake of guanethidine	Be aware. Consider use of a local anaesthetic that minimally inhibits reuptake, e.g. lidocaine, when possible
ANAESTHETICS – LOCAL	ANTIVIRALS – PROTEASE INHIBITORS	↑ adverse effects of lidocaine with lopinavir and ritonavir	Uncertain; ↑ bioavailability	Caution; consider using an alternative local anaesthetic
ANAESTHETICS – LOCAL	**BETA-BLOCKERS**			
↑ BP is likely when epinephrine-containing local anaesthetics are used in patients on treatment with beta-adrenergic blockers **Remember that ↑ BP can occur when epinephrine-containing local anaesthetics are used with patients on beta-blockers** ➢ ***Sympathomimetics, below***				
BUPIVACAINE	BETA-BLOCKERS	Risk of bupivacaine toxicity	Beta-blockers, particularly propranolol, inhibit the hepatic microsomal metabolism of bupivacaine	Watch for bupivacaine toxicity – monitor ECG and BP

LIDOCAINE	BETA-BLOCKERS	1. Risk of bradycardia (occasionally severe), ↓ BP and heart failure with intravenous lidocaine 2. Risk of lidocaine toxicity due to ↑ plasma concentrations of lidocaine, particularly with propranolol and nadolol 3. ↑ plasma concentrations of propranolol and possibly some other beta-blockers	1. Additive negative inotropic and chronotropic effects 2. Uncertain, but possibly a combination of beta-blocker-induced ↓ hepatic blood flow (due to ↓ cardiac output) and inhibition of metabolism of lidocaine 3. Attributed to inhibition of metabolism by lidocaine	1. Monitor PR, BP and ECG closely; watch for development of heart failure when intravenous lidocaine is administered to patients on beta-blockers 2. Watch for lidocaine toxicity 3. Be aware. Regional anaesthetics should be used cautiously in patients with bradycardia. Beta-blockers could cause dangerous hypertension due to stimulation of alpha-receptors if adrenaline is used with local anaesthetic
ANAESTHETICS – LOCAL	CALCIUM CHANNEL BLOCKERS	Case reports of severe ↓ BP when a bupivacaine epidural was administered to patients on calcium channel blockers	Additive hypotensive effect; both bupivacaine and calcium channel blockers are cardiodepressant. In addition, epidural anaesthesia causes sympathetic block in the lower limbs, which leads to vasodilatation and ↓ BP	Monitor BP closely. Preload intravenous fluids prior to the epidural
ANAESTHETICS, LOCAL – ROPIVACAINE	CNS STIMULANTS – MODAFINIL	May cause ↓ plasma concentrations of these substrates if CYP1A2 is the predominant metabolic pathway and alternative metabolic pathways are either genetically deficient or affected	Modafinil is moderate inducer of CYP1A2 in a concentration-dependent manner	Be aware
PROCAINE	ECOTHIOPATE	↑ plasma concentrations and risk of unconsciousness, and cardiovascular collapse with injections of prilocaine	Ecothiopate inhibits pseudocholinesterase, which metabolizes prilocaine	Do not co-administer. Use an alternative local anaesthetic not subject to metabolism by pseudocholinesterases

Primary drug	Secondary drug	Effect	Mechanism	Precautions
LIDOCAINE	H2 RECEPTOR BLOCKERS – CIMETIDINE, RANITIDINE	↑ efficacy and adverse effects of local anaesthetic, e.g. light-headedness, paraesthesia	Unknown for most local anaesthetics. Lidocaine ↑ bio-availability	Uncertain. Monitor more closely. No toxicity reported to date with bupivacaine. If using intravenous lidocaine, monitor closely for symptoms of toxicity; ↓ dose may be required
PROCAINE	LARONIDASE	Possibly ↓ efficacy of laronidase	Uncertain	Avoid co-administration
ANAESTHETICS – LOCAL	**MUSCLE RELAXANTS**			
PROCAINE	DEPOLARIZING	Possibly ↑ plasma concentrations of both drugs, with risk of toxic effects	Due to competition for metabolism by pseudocholinesterase	Avoid co-administration
LIDOCAINE	DEPOLARIZING	↑ efficacy of suxamethonium with intravenous lidocaine	Uncertain	Monitor neuromuscular blockade carefully

ANTICHOLINESTERASES ➢ *Drugs Acting on the Nervous System, Drugs used to treat neuromuscular dseases and movement disorders*

ANTIMUSCARINICS ➢ *Drugs Acting on the Nervous System, Antiparkinson's drugs*

BENZODIAZEPINES ➢ *Drugs Acting on the Nervous System, Anxiolytics and hypnotics*

DANTROLENE ➢ *Musculoskeletal Drugs, Skeletal muscle relaxants*

MUSCLE RELAXANTS – DEPOLARIZING AND NON-DEPOLARIZING

Primary drug	Secondary drug	Effect	Mechanism	Precautions
MUSCLE RELAXANTS	**ANAESTHETICS – LOCAL**			
DEPOLARIZING	LIDOCAINE	↑ efficacy of suxamethonium with intravenous lidocaine	Uncertain	Monitor neuromuscular blockade carefully
DEPOLARIZING	PROCAINE	Possibly ↑ plasma concentrations of both drugs, with risk of toxic effects	Due to competition for metabolism by pseudocholinesterase	Avoid co-administration
MUSCLE RELAXANTS – DEPOLARIZING	ANTIARRHYTHMICS – PROCAINAMIDE	Possibility of ↑ neuromuscular blockade	Uncertain; procainamide may ↓ plasma cholinesterase levels	Be aware of the possibility of a prolonged effect of suxamethonium when it is administered to patients taking procainamide

MUSCLE RELAXANTS	ANTIBIOTICS			
DEPOLARIZING, NON-DEPOLARIZING	AMINOGLYCOSIDES	↑ neuromuscular block	Aminoglycosides ↓ release of ACh at neuromuscular junctions by altering the influx of calcium. It is also thought to alter the sensitivity of the postsynaptic receptors/membrane, with ↓ transmission. These effects are additive to those of non-depolarizing muscle relaxants/neuromuscular blockers, which essentially prevents ACh acting on postsynaptic nicotinic receptors	Monitor neuromuscular blockade closely. Aminoglycosides vary in their potency to block neuromuscular junctions, with neomycin having the highest potency, then streptomycin, gentamicin and kanamycin
DEPOLARIZING, NON-DEPOLARIZING	CLINDAMYCIN, COLISTIN, PIPERACILLIN	↑ efficacy of muscle relaxants	Piperacillin has some neuromuscular blocking activity	Monitor neuromuscular blockade carefully
DEPOLARIZING, NON-DEPOLARIZING	VANCOMYCIN	1. ↑ efficacy of these muscle relaxants 2. Possible risk of hypersensitivity reactions	1. Vancomycin has some neuromuscular blocking activity 2. Animal studies suggest additive effect on histamine release	1. Monitor neuromuscular blockade carefully 2. Be aware
DEPOLARIZING	ANTICANCER AND IMMUNOMODULATING DRUGS – THIOTEPA	↑ efficacy of suxamethonium	Uncertain	Be aware of this effect
NON-DEPOLARIZING	ANTIDEPRESSANTS – LITHIUM	Antagonism of effects of non-depolarizing muscle relaxants	Uncertain	Monitor intraoperative muscle relaxation closely; may need ↑ doses of muscle relaxants
SUXAMETHONIUM	ANTIEMETICS – METOCLOPRAMIDE	Possible ↑ efficacy of suxamethonium	Uncertain	Be aware and monitor effects of suxamethonium closely

ANAESTHETIC DRUGS MUSCLE RELAXANTS

ANAESTHETIC DRUGS MUSCLE RELAXANTS

Primary drug	Secondary drug	Effect	Mechanism	Precautions
NON-DEPOLARIZING	BETA-BLOCKERS	1. Modest ↑ efficacy of muscle relaxants, particularly with propanolol 2. Risk of ↓ BP with atracurium and alcuronium	1 and 2. Uncertain	1. Watch for prolonged muscular paralysis after use of muscle relaxants 2. Monitor BP at least weekly until stable
MUSCLE RELAXANTS	**BRONCHODILATORS**			
SUXAMETHONIUM	BAMBUTEROL	↑ effect of suxamethonium	Bambuterol is an inhibitor of pseudocholinesterase, which hydrolyses suxamethonium	Be cautious of prolonged periods of respiratory muscle paralysis and monitor respiration closely until complete recovery
PANCURONIUM	THEOPHYLLINE	Antagonism of neuromuscular blockade	Uncertain	Larger doses of pancuronium may be needed to obtain the desired muscle relaxation during anaesthesia; other non-depolarizing muscle relaxants do not seem to be affected
MUSCLE RELAXANTS	**CALCIUM CHANNEL BLOCKERS**			
DEPOLARIZING	CALCIUM CHANNEL BLOCKERS	↑ effect of suxamethonium with parenteral, but not oral, calcium channel blockers	Uncertain; postulated that ACh release at the synapse is calcium-dependent. ↓ calcium concentrations at the nerve ending may ↓ ACh release, which in turn prolongs the nerve blockade	Monitor nerve blockade carefully particularly during short procedures
NON-DEPOLARIZING	CALCIUM CHANNEL BLOCKERS	↑ effect of non-depolarizing muscle relaxants with parenteral calcium channel blockers; the effect is less certain with oral therapy. In two cohort studies, vecuronium requirements were halved in patients on diltiazem. Nimodipine does not seem to share this effect	Uncertain; postulated that ACh release at the synapse is calcium dependent. ↓ calcium concentrations at the nerve ending may ↓ ACh release, which in turn prolongs the nerve blockade	Monitor nerve blockade carefully in patients on calcium channel blockers, particularly near to the end of surgery, when muscle relaxation may be prolonged and difficult to reverse

MUSCLE RELAXANTS	CARDIAC GLYCOSIDES			
DEPOLARIZING	DIGOXIN	Risk of ventricular arrhythmias when suxamethonium is given to patients taking digoxin	Uncertain; postulated that the mechanism involves a rapid efflux of potassium from cells	Use caution and monitor the ECG closely if suxamethonium needs to be used in patients taking digoxin
NON-DEPOLARIZING	DIGOXIN	Case reports of S–T segment/T wave changes and sinus/atrial tachycardia when pancuronium was given to patients on digoxin	Uncertain	Avoid pancuronium in patients taking digoxin
VECURONIUM	H2 RECEPTOR BLOCKERS – CIMETIDINE	↑ efficacy of vecuronium	Unclear	Potential for slightly prolonged recovery time (minutes)
DEPOLARIZING AND NON-DEPOLARIZING	MAGNESIUM (PARENTERAL)	↑ efficacy of these muscle relaxants, with risk of prolonged neuromuscular blockade	Additive effect; magnesium inhibits ACh release and ↓ postsynaptic receptor sensitivity	Monitor nerve blockade closely
MUSCLE RELAXANTS	**PARASYMPATHOMIMETICS**			
SUXAMETHONIUM	DONEPEZIL	Possible ↑ efficacy of suxamethonium	Suxamethonium is metabolized by cholinesterase; parasympathomimetics inhibit cholinesterase and so prolong the action of suxamethonium	Avoid co-administration. Ensure that the effects of suxamethonium have worn off before administering a parasympathomimetic to reverse non-depolarizing muscle relaxants. A careful risk–benefit analysis should be made before considering the use of suxamethonium
NON-DEPOLARIZING	PARASYMPATHOMIMETICS	↓ efficacy of non-depolarizing muscle relaxants	Anticholinesterases oppose the action of non-depolarizing muscle relaxants	Used therapeutically
VECURONIUM	PROTON PUMP INHIBITORS – LANSOPRAZOLE	Possible ↑ efficacy and adverse effects of vecuronium	Unclear	Altered duration of action. May need ↑ recovery time

OPIOIDS ➢ *Analgesics, Opioids*

ANAESTHETIC DRUGS OPIOIDS

Part 10 DRUGS TO TREAT INFECTIONS

Antibiotics

Penicillins

Penicillins are rapidly eliminated, particularly by glomerular filtration and renal tubular secretion. With some (e.g. cloxacillin), metabolic transformation occurs, especially in anuric patients. When renal function is impaired, 7–10% of the antibiotic will be inactivated by the liver per hour. Adverse drug reactions are:

- *immunologically mediated*: hypersensitivity/allergic reactions – type I – mediated by immunoglobulin E;
- *type II reactions*: a cytotoxic reaction such as haemolysis;
- *dose- or concentration-dependent*:
  - the augmentation of body sodium or potassium content with salt and water overload with large doses as the formulations for injection contain the salts of one of these cations;
  - seizures, penicillin G being most epileptogenic;
  - impaired platelet aggregation, which is most severe with ticarcillin but may occur with piperacillin, mezlocillin and penicillin.

Macrolides

Macrolides, particularly erythromycin and clarithromycin, inhibit CYP3A4. With erythromycin, the inhibition of CYP3A4 is non-competitive due to irreversible binding with the isoenzyme to form an inactive complex. Thus, unlike the case with inhibitors with a short half-life (e.g. cimetidine), the offset of inhibition is slow since new enzyme must be synthesized to replace the inactive complexes. Azithromycin, clarithromycin and erythromycin can prolong the Q–T interval and must not be co-administered with other Q–T-prolonging drugs.

Quinolones

A significant fraction of each drug is excreted unchanged in the urine (by glomerular filtration and tubular secretion, e.g. norfloxacin and ciprofloxacin). Sparfloxacin and trovafloxacin have significant non-renal elimination pathways. Hepatic metabolism also takes place (e.g. nalidixic acid being converted to an active metabolite).

All tetracyclines are excreted in the urine and faeces. The primary route for most is the kidney (by glomerular filtration). Doxycycline is excreted in the faeces as an inactive conjugate or perhaps as a chelate, and does not accumulate in the blood in significant amounts in patients with renal failure.

Chloramphenicol

The major route of elimination is hepatic metabolism. The variability in the metabolism and pharmacokinetics in neonates, infants and children necessitates monitoring of drug concentrations in the plasma, particularly when it is co-administered with phenytoin, phenobarbital or rifampin.

Fusidic Acid

Fusidic acid is eliminated primarily by the biliary excretion of various conjugates and CYP oxidative metabolism. It inhibits CYP3A4 isoforms.

Aminoglycosides

The same spectrum of toxicity (ototoxicity and nephrotoxicity) is shared by all members of the group. The more important and frequent interactions are pharmacodynamic. Streptomycin and gentamicin produce predominantly vestibular effects, whereas amikacin, kanamycin and neomycin primarily affect auditory function. All are rapidly excreted by the kidney.

Cephalosporins

These resemble the penicillins structurally, in mode of action and in general lack of toxicity. They are primarily excreted by the kidney by tubular secretion and some also by glomerular filtration (e.g. cephalothin) or only by glomerular filtration (e.g. cefazolin). Cefoperazone is excreted by the bile. Cefotaxime undergoes hepatic biotransformation to active metabolites. Hypersensitivity reactions are qualitatively similar to those of the penicillins, but the epileptogenic potential is less.

Carbapenems

These are structurally related to penicillins and are excreted predominantly by renal tubular secretion. The risk of seizures with imipenem is 0.2%. They are toxic to the proximal renal tubule cells.

Monobactams

Aztreonam – intramuscular or intravenous – is excreted unchanged by glomerular filtration and renal tubular secretion. It lacks the allergenic tricyclic nuclear structure of penicillins, cephalosporins and carbapenem beta-lactams.

Oxazolidones

The elimination of linezolid is by non-renal means (and does not involve CYP isoenzymes). It has weak MAOI activity. Myelosuppression, both dose- and time-dependent, occurs in 2–10% of patients with therapeutic doses. Linezolid interacts with serotonergic and adrenergic drugs.

Streptogramins

Quinupristin–dalfopristin (combined in a 3:7 ratio) inhibits CYP3A4 isoenzymes. At doses over 10 mg/kg, it prolongs the Q–T interval.

Polymyxins

Colistin is completely excreted unchanged in the urine. It is potentially nephrotoxic and ototoxic. Respiratory paralysis due to muscle weakness is rare but cannot be reversed by neostigmine (compared with aminoglycosides).

Glycopeptides

Vancomycin and teicoplanin are completely excreted unchanged in the urine by glomerular filtration. Vancomycin also partly undergoes hepatic metabolism. They are ototoxic and nephrotoxic.

Telithromycin

The ketolide telithromycin is metabolized by CYP3A4 isoenzymes and tends to cause prolongation of the Q–T interval.

Rifampin, rifabutin and rifapentine

Rifampin induces CYP2B6, CYP2C8, CYP2C9 and CYP3A4 (in both gut and liver), UDGPTs, glutathione *S*-transferases and P-gp. CYP3A4 is more efficiently induced than other CYPs. Rifampicin is the most potent inducer of CYP3A4 isoenzymes, followed by rifapentine and rifabutin.

Antifungals

Amphotericin

This is metabolized to a limited extent, being excreted unchanged in the urine or in the bile. It may have adverse effects on the kidneys and in high doses can cause arrhythmias.

Azoles

These antifungals are inhibitors of the CYP3A4 isoenzyme but the inhibiting potencies of azoles vary: itraconazole and ketoconazole are considered to be more potent than posaconazole and voriconazole, which in turn are more potent than fluconazole. Fluconazole, itraconazole and voriconazole also inhibit CYP2C9 and CYP2C19.

Fluconazole is mainly excreted unchanged in the urine and is thus not under the influence of the induction or inhibition of a metabolic pathway. Itraconazole is predominantly metabolized by CYP3A4 and is the only azole with an active metabolite. Itraconazole is also a substrate of P-gp and an inhibitor of P-gp activity.

Ketoconazole is a substrate of CYP3A4.

Posaconazole metabolism involves phase II reactions – glucuronidation.

Voriconazole is a substrate of CYP2C19 and to a lesser extent of CYP2C9 and CYP3A4 and is unique because of its saturable metabolism; thus when the dose is increased, a larger than proportional increase in drug exposure is seen.

Flucytosine

Flucytosine is eliminated unchanged in the urine.

Griseofulvin

Griseofulvin is metabolized in the liver; its half-life is approximately 24 hours (so interactions can last a long time). It is a weak inducer of CYP1A2, CYP2C9 and CYP3A4.

Terbinafine

This is a substrate of CYP1A2, CYP2C9/19 and CYP3A4 and a strong inhibitor of CYP2D6.

Antiprotozoal agents

Note that antimalarials are also antiprotozoals but have been described in a separate section.

Antibiotics with antiprotozoal activity are not included in this chapter. These include clindamycin, co-trimoxazole–trimethoprim, dapsone, doxycycline and metronidazole.

Antivirals

Anti-HIV drugs

Nucleoside reverse transcriptase inhibitors are not significantly metabolized by the CYP system.

Protease inhibitors are metabolized by CYP3A4, and ritonavir is also metabolized by CYP2D6. Ritonavir inhibits CYP3A4, CYP2D6, CYP2C9 and CYP2C19. Amprenavir, indinavir and nelfinavir are moderately potent CYP3A4 inhibitors.

Of the *NNRTIs*, nevirapine induces CYP3A4 while efavirenz can both inhibit and induce CYP3A4. Nevirapine and efavirenz are potent inducers of CYP3A4, while efavirenz may inhibit CYP2C9 and CYP2C19.

DRUGS TO TREAT INFECTIONS ANTIBIOTICS – AMINOGLYCOSIDES

Primary drug	Secondary drug	Effect	Mechanism	Precautions
ANTIBIOTICS – AMINOGLYCOSIDES				
GENTAMICIN	AGALSIDASE BETA	Possibly ↓ clinical effect of agalsidase beta	Uncertain	Avoid co-administration
AMINOGLYCOSIDES	ANALGESICS – INDOMETACIN	↑ amikacin, gentamicin and vancomycin levels in neonates	Uncertain; indometacin possibly ↓ renal clearance of these aminoglycosides	Halve the dose of antibiotic. Uncertain if this applies to adults but suggest check levels. Otherwise use an alternative NSAID
AMINOGLYCOSIDES	**ANTIBIOTICS**			
AMINOGLYCOSIDES	CEPHALOSPORINS	Possible ↑ risk of nephrotoxicity	Additive effect; cephalosporins are rarely associated with interstitial nephritis	Renal function should be carefully monitored
AMINOGLYCOSIDES	COLISTIN	↑ risk of nephrotoxicity	Additive effect	Renal function should be carefully monitored
NEOMYCIN	PENICILLIN V	↓ levels of phenoxymethylpenicillin and possible therapeutic failure	↓ absorption of phenoxymethyl-penicillin due to malabsorption syndrome caused by neomycin	Patients should be monitored for efficacy of phenoxymethylpenicillin
AMINOGLYCOSIDES	TEICOPLANIN, VANCOMYCIN	↑ risk of nephrotoxicity and ototoxicity	Additive effect	Hearing and renal function should be carefully monitored
AMINOGLYCOSIDES	**ANTICANCER AND IMMUNOMODULATING DRUGS**			
AMINOGLYCOSIDES	CICLOSPORIN	↑ risk of nephrotoxicity	Additive nephrotoxic effects	Monitor renal function
NEOMYCIN	METHOTREXATE – ORAL	↓ plasma concentrations following oral methotrexate	Oral aminoglycosides ↓ absorption of oral methotrexate by 30–50%	Separate doses of each drug by at least 2–4 hours

AMINOGLYCOSIDES, CAPREOMYCIN, STREPTOMYCIN,	PLATINUM COMPOUNDS	↑ risk of renal toxicity and renal failure, and of ototoxicity. The ototoxicity tends to occur when cisplatin is administered early during the course of aminoglycoside therapy	Additive renal toxicity	Monitor renal function prior to and during therapy, and ensure an intake of at least 2 L of fluid daily. Monitor serum potassium and magnesium and correct any deficiencies. Most side-effects of aminoglycosides are dose related, and it is necessary to ↑ interval between doses and ↓ dose of aminoglycoside if there is impaired renal function
AMINOGLYCOSIDES	TACROLIMUS	Risk of renal toxicity	Additive effect	Monitor renal function closely
NEOMYCIN	ANTICOAGULANTS – ORAL	Elevated prothrombin times and ↑ risk of bleeding	The mechanism is not fully understood; however, it is thought that neomycin may ↓ number of vitamin K-producing bacteria in the gastrointestinal tract and/or that the absorption of vitamin K may be ↓ by the neomycin	The INR should be monitored in all patients starting or stopping neomycin therapy. Patients more at risk are those with an inadequate diet
AMINOGLYCOSIDES	**ANTIDIABETIC DRUGS**			
AMINOGLYCOSIDES	ACARBOSE	↑ postprandial hypoglycaemia and ↑ gastrointestinal effects as a result of the concurrent use of acarbose and neomycin	Neomycin is known to cause ↓ blood glucose levels after meals; when used concomitantly with acarbose, this effect may be ↑. Neomycin also exacerbates the adverse gastrointestinal effects caused by acarbose	Blood glucose levels should be closely monitored; if gastrointestinal signs are severe, the dose of acarbose should be ↓

DRUGS TO TREAT INFECTIONS ANTIBIOTICS – AMINOGLYCOSIDES

Primary drug	Secondary drug	Effect	Mechanism	Precautions
AMINOGLYCOSIDES	METFORMIN	Risk of hypoglycaemia due to ↑ plasma concentrations of metformin	Mechanism uncertain. Metformin does not undergo hepatic metabolism. Renal tubular secretion is the major route of metformin elimination. Aminoglycosides are also principally excreted via the kidney, and nephrotoxicity is an important side-effect	Watch/monitor and warn patients about hypoglycaemia ➢ ***For signs and symptoms of hypoglycaemia, see Clinical Features of Some Adverse Drug Interactions, Hypoglycaemia***
AMINOGLYCOSIDES	ANTIFUNGALS – AMPHOTERICIN	Risk of renal failure	Additive effect	Monitor renal function closely
AMINOGLYCOSIDES	**ANTIVIRALS**			
AMINOGLYCOSIDES	ADEFOVIR DIPIVOXIL	Possible ↑ efficacy and side-effects	Competition for renal excretion	Monitor renal function weekly
AMINOGLYCOSIDES	FOSCARNET SODIUM	Possible ↑ nephrotoxicity	Additive side-effect	Monitor renal function closely
AMINOGLYCOSIDES	NUCLEOSIDE REVERSE TRANSCRIPTASE INHIBITORS	Possibly ↑ risk of nephrotoxicity	Additive effect	Avoid co-administration if possible; otherwise monitor renal function weekly
AMINOGLYCOSIDES	BISPHOSPHONATES – SODIUM CLODRONATE	Risk of symptomatic hypocalcaemia	Uncertain	Monitor calcium levels closely
AMINOGLYCOSIDES	CARDIAC GLYCOSIDES – DIGOXIN	1. Gentamicin may ↑ plasma concentrations of digoxin 2. Neomycin may ↓ plasma concentrations of digoxin	1. Uncertain; postulated to be due to impaired renal clearance of digoxin 2. Neomycin ↓ absorption of digoxin; this may be offset in some patients by ↓ breakdown of digoxin by intestinal bacterial	1. Monitor digoxin levels; watch for ↑ levels, particularly in diabetics and in the presence of renal insufficiency 2. Monitor digoxin levels; watch for poor response to digoxin
AMINOGLYCOSIDES	DIURETICS – LOOP	↑ risk of ototoxicity and possible deafness as a result of concomitant use of furosemide and gentamicin	Both furosemide and gentamicin are associated with ototoxicity; this risk is ↑ if they are used together	If used concurrently, patients should be monitored for any hearing impairment

DRUGS TO TREAT INFECTIONS ANTIBIOTICS – AMINOGLYCOSIDES

AMINOGLYCOSIDES	MUSCLE RELAXANTS – DEPOLARIZING AND NON-DEPOLARIZING	↑ neuromuscular block	Aminoglycosides ↓ release of ACh at neuromuscular junctions by altering the influx of calcium. It is also thought that it alters the sensitivity of the postsynaptic membrane, with ↓ transmission. These effects are additive to those of the neuromuscular blockers	Monitor neuromuscular blockade closely. Aminoglycosides vary in their potency to block neuromuscular junctions, with neomycin having the highest potency, then streptomycin, gentamicin and kanamycin
AMINOGLYCOSIDES	PARASYMPATHOMIMETICS – NEOSTIGMINE, PYRIDOSTIGMINE	↓ efficacy of neostigmine and pyridostigmine	Uncertain	Watch for poor response to these parasympathomimetics and ↑ dose accordingly
ANTIBIOTICS – BETA-LACTAMS				
CEPHALOSPORINS				
CEFPODOXIME, CEFUROXIME	ANTACIDS	↓ levels of these antibiotics	↓ absorption	Take azithromycin at least 1 hour before or 2 hours after an antacid. Take these cephalosporins at least 2 hours after an antacid. Separate quinolones and antacids by 2–6 hours. Separate tetracyclines and antacids by 2–3 hours
CEPHALOSPORINS	ANALGESICS – INDOMETACIN	Indometacin ↑ ceftazidime levels in neonates	Indometacin ↓ clearance of ceftazidime	The dose of ceftazidime needs to be ↓
CEPHALOSPORINS	ANTIBIOTICS – AMINOGLYCOSIDES	Possible ↑ risk of nephrotoxicity	Additive effect; cephalosporins are rarely associated with interstitial nephritis	Renal function should be carefully monitored
CEPHALOSPORINS	ANTICOAGULANTS – ORAL	Certain cephalosporins (cefaclor, cefixime, ceftriaxone) may ↑ efficacy of oral anticoagulants	These cephalosporins have vitamin K antagonistic activity, which adds to the action of oral anticoagulants	Monitor INR closely; significant ↑ in INR may require vitamin K therapy. If possible, use an alternative cephalosporin

Primary drug	Secondary drug	Effect	Mechanism	Precautions
CEPHALOSPORINS	ANTIGOUT DRUGS – PROBENECID	↑ cephalosporin levels	Uncertain	Watch for ↑ incidence of side-effects
CEPHALOSPORINS	H2 RECEPTOR BLOCKERS	↓ plasma concentrations and risk of treatment failure	↓ absorption of cephalosporin as ↑ gastric pH	Avoid concomitant use. If unable to avoid combination, take H2 antagonists at least 2–3 hours after the cephalosporin. Consider alternative antibiotic or separate the doses by at least 2 hours and give with an acidic drink, e.g. a carbonated drink; ↑ dose may be required
CEPHALOSPORINS	OESTROGENS	Reports of ↓ contraceptive effect	Possibly alteration of bacterial flora necessary for recycling of ethinylestradiol from the large bowel, although not certain in every case	Advise patients to use additional contraception for the period of antibiotic intake and for 1 month after stopping the antibiotic
CEPHALOSPORINS	PROTON PUMP INHIBITORS	Possible ↓ efficacy of cephalosporin	↓ absorption as ↑ gastric pH	Monitor for ↓ efficacy. Separate doses by at least 2 hours, and take cephalosporin with food
OTHER BETA-LACTAMS				
ERTAPENEM, MEROPENEM	ANTIEPILEPTICS – VALPROATE	↓ valproate levels	Induced metabolism	Monitor levels
MEROPENEM	ANTIGOUT DRUGS – PROBENECID	↑ meropenem levels	Uncertain	Manufacturers recommend avoiding co-administration
IMIPENEM WITH CILASTATIN	ANTIVIRALS – GANCICLOVIR/ VALGANCICLOVIR	↑ adverse effects (e.g. seizures)	Additive side-effects; these drugs can cause seizure activity	Avoid combination if possible; use only if benefit outweighs risk

ANTIBIOTICS – MACROLIDES				
MACROLIDES	DRUGS THAT PROLONG THE Q–T INTERVAL			
MACROLIDES (ESPECIALLY AZITHROMYCIN, CLARITHROMYCIN, PARENTERAL ERYTHROMYCIN, TELITHROMYCIN)	1. ANTIARRHYTHMICS – amiodarone, disopyramide, procainamide, propafenone 2. ANTIBIOTICS – quinolones (especially moxifloxacin), quinupristin/dalfopristin 3. ANTICANCER AND IMMUNOMODULATING DRUGS – arsenic trioxide 4. ANTIDEPRESSANTS – TCAs, venlafaxine 5. ANTIEMETICS – dolasetron 6. ANTIFUNGALS – fluconazole, posaconazole, voriconazole 7. ANTIHISTAMINES – terfenadine, hydroxyzine, mizolastine 8. ANTIMALARIALS – artemether with lumefantrine, chloroquine, hydroxychloroquine, mefloquine, quinine 9. ANTIPROTOZOALS – pentamidine isetionate 10. ANTIPSYCHOTICS – atypicals, phenothiazines, pimozide 11. BETA-BLOCKERS – sotalol 12. BRONCHODILATORS – parenteral bronchodilators 13. CNS STIMULANTS – atomoxetine	Risk of ventricular arrhythmias, particularly torsades de pointes	Additive effect; these drugs cause prolongation of the Q–T interval	Avoid co-administration

Primary drug	Secondary drug	Effect	Mechanism	Precautions
MACROLIDES	ANALGESICS – OPIOIDS	Effects of alfentanil ↑ by erythromycin	Erythromycin inhibits metabolism of alfentanil	Be aware that the effects of alfentanil (especially when given as an infusion) may be prolonged by erythromycin
AZITHROMYCIN	ANTACIDS	↓ levels of these antibiotics	↓ absorption	Take azithromycin at least 1 hour before or 2 hours after an antacid. Take these cephalosporins at least 2 hours after an antacid. Separate quinolones and antacids by 2–6 hours. Separate tetracyclines and antacids by 2–3 hours
MACROLIDES	**ANTIBIOTICS**			
MACROLIDES	RIFABUTIN	↑ rifabutin levels	Inhibition of CYP3A4-mediated metabolism of rifabutin	Watch for early features of toxicity of rifabutin (warn patients to report painful eyes)
CLARITHROMYCIN, TELITHROMYCIN	RIFAMPICIN	↓ levels of these macrolides	Rifampicins induce metabolism of these macrolides	Avoid co-administration for up to 2 weeks after stopping rifampicin
MACROLIDES	**ANTICANCER AND IMMUNOMODULATING DRUGS**			
MACROLIDES	**CYTOTOXICS**			
CLARITHROMYCIN, ERYTHROMYCIN	BUSULFAN	↑ plasma concentrations of busulfan and ↑ risk of toxicity of busulfan such as veno-occlusive disease and pulmonary fibrosis	Macrolides are inhibitors of CYP3A4. Busulfan clearance may be ↓ by 25%, and the AUC of busulfan may ↑ by 1500 μmol/L	Monitor clinically for veno-occlusive disease and pulmonary toxicity in transplant patients. Monitor busulfan blood levels as AUCs below 1500 μmol/L per minute tends to prevent toxicity
ERYTHROMYCIN	DOCETAXEL	↑ docetaxel levels	Inhibition of CYP3A4-mediated metabolism of docetaxel is metabolized by enzymes that are moderately inhibited by erythromycin, leading to ↑ levels and possible toxicity	Cautious use or consider use of azithromycin, which has little effect on CYP3A4 and therefore is not expected to interact with docetaxel

DRUGS TO TREAT INFECTIONS ANTIBIOTICS – MACROLIDES

CLARITHROMYCIN, ERYTHROMYCIN	DOXORUBICIN	↑ risk of myelosuppression due to ↑ plasma concentrations	Due to ↓ metabolism of doxorubicin by CYP3A4 isoenzymes due to inhibition of those enzymes	Monitor for ↑ myelosuppression, peripheral neuropathy, myalgias and fatigue
CLARITHROMYCIN, ERYTHROMYCIN	IFOSFAMIDE	↓ plasma concentrations of 4-hydroxyifosfamide, the active metabolite of ifosfamide, and risk of inadequate therapeutic response	Due to inhibition of the isoenzymatic conversion to active metabolites	Monitor clinically the efficacy of ifosfamide and ↑ dose accordingly
CLARITHROMYCIN, ERYTHROMYCIN	IMATINIB	↑ imatinib levels with ↑ risk of toxicity (e.g. abdominal pain, constipation, dyspnoea) and of neurotoxicity (e.g. taste disturbances, dizziness, headache, paraesthesia, peripheral neuropathy)	Due to inhibition of CYP3A4-mediated metabolism of imatinib	Monitor for clinical efficacy and for the signs of toxicity listed, along with convulsions, confusion, signs of oedema (including pulmonary oedema). Monitor electrolytes, liver function and for cardiotoxicity
CLARITHROMYCIN, ERYTHROMYCIN	IRINOTECAN	↑ plasma concentrations of SN-38 (>AUC by 100%) and ↑ toxicity of irinotecan, e.g. diarrhoea, acute cholinergic syndrome, interstitial pulmonary disease	Due to inhibition of the metabolism of irinotecan by CYP3A4 isoenzymes by macrolides	Peripheral blood counts should be checked before each course of treatment. Monitor lung function. Recommendation is to ↓ dose of irinotecan by 25%
CLARITHROMYCIN, ERYTHROMYCIN	VINCA ALKALOIDS – VINBLASTINE, VINCRISTINE, VINORELBINE	↑ adverse effects of vinblastine and vincristine	Inhibition of CYP3A4-mediated metabolism. Also inhibition of P-gp efflux of vinblastine	Monitor FBCs. Watch for early features of toxicity (pain, numbness, tingling in the fingers and toes, jaw pain, abdominal pain, constipation, ileus). Consider selecting an alternative drug
MACROLIDES	**HORMONES AND HORMONE ANTAGONISTS**			
CLARITHROMYCIN, ERYTHROMYCIN	TOREMIFENE	↑ plasma concentrations of toremifene with clarithromycin and erythromycin	Due to inhibition of metabolism of toremifene by the CYP3A4 isoenzymes	Clinical relevance is uncertain. Necessary to monitor for clinical toxicities

DRUGS TO TREAT INFECTIONS ANTIBIOTICS – MACROLIDES

Primary drug	Secondary drug	Effect	Mechanism	Precautions
MACROLIDES	**IMMUNOMODULATING DRUGS**			
CLARITHROMYCIN, ERYTHROMYCIN, TELITHROMYCIN	CICLOSPORIN	↑ plasma concentrations of ciclosporin, with risk of nephrotoxicity, myelosuppression, neurotoxicity and excessive immunosuppression, with risk of infection and post-transplant lymphoproliferative disease	Inhibition of CYP3A4-mediated metabolism of ciclosporin; these inhibitors vary in potency. Clarithromycin and telithromycin are classified as potent inhibitors	Avoid co-administration with clarithromycin and telithromycin. Consider alternative antibiotics but need to monitor plasma ciclosporin levels to prevent toxicity
CLARITHROMYCIN, ERYTHROMYCIN	CORTICOSTEROIDS	↑ adrenal suppressive effects of corticosteroids, which may ↑ risk of infections and produce an inadequate response to stress scenarios	Due to inhibition of metabolism of corticosteroids	Monitor cortisol levels and warn patients to report symptoms such as fever and sore throat
CLARITHROMYCIN, ERYTHROMYCIN	SIROLIMUS	↑ sirolimus levels	Inhibition of metabolism of sirolimus	Avoid co-administration
MACROLIDES	TACROLIMUS	↑ plasma concentrations of tacrolimus, with risk of toxic effect	Clarithromycin, erythromycin and telithromycin inhibit CYP3A4-mediated metabolism of tacrolimus. Azithromycin, if at all, mildly inhibits CYP3A4; a marked ↑ in tacrolimus levels is attributed to inhibition of P-gp	Be aware and monitor tacrolimus plasma concentrations
MACROLIDES	ANTICOAGULANTS – ORAL	Occasional episodes of ↑ anticoagulant effect	Uncertain at present	Monitor INR every 2–3 days
MACROLIDES	**ANTIDEPRESSANTS**			
ERYTHROMYCIN	MAOIs – PHENELZINE	Report of fainting and severe hypotension on initiation of erythromycin	Attributed to ↑ absorption of phenelzine due to rapid gastric emptying caused by erythromycin	Be aware

MACROLIDES	REBOXETINE	Risk of ↑ reboxetine levels	Possibly inhibition of CYP3A4-mediated metabolism of reboxetine	Avoid co-administration
TELITHROMYCIN	ST JOHN'S WORT	↓ telithromycin levels	Due to induction of CYP3A4-mediated metabolism of telithromycin	Avoid co-administration for up to 2 weeks after stopping St John's wort
ERYTHROMYCIN, CLARITHROMYCIN, TELITHROMYCIN	ANTIDIABETIC DRUGS – REPAGLINIDE	Likely to ↑ plasma concentrations of repaglinide and ↑ risk of hypoglycaemic episodes. ↑ risk of gastrointestinal side-effects with clarithromycin	Due to inhibition of CYP3A4 isoenzymes, which metabolize repaglinide. These drugs vary in potency as inhibitors (clarithromycin is a potent inhibitor) and ↑ plasma concentrations varies. Clarithromycin ↑ plasma concentrations by 60%. However, the alternative pathway – CYP2C8 – is unaffected by these inhibitors	Watch for and warn patients about hypoglycaemia ➢ ***For signs and symptoms of hypoglycaemia, see Clinical Features of Some Adverse Drug Interactions, Hypoglycaemia***
MACROLIDES	ANTIEMETICS – APREPITANT	↑ aprepitant levels	Inhibition of CYP3A4-mediated metabolism of aprepitant	Use with caution. Clinical significance unclear; monitor closely
MACROLIDES	**ANTIEPILEPTICS**			
TELITHROMYCIN	BARBITURATES	↓ levels of these drugs, with risk of therapeutic failure	Induction of hepatic metabolism	1. Avoid co-administration of telithromycin for up to 2 weeks after stopping phenobarbital 2. With the other drugs, monitor for ↓ clinical efficacy and ↑ dose as required
TELITHROMYCIN	CARBAMAZEPINE	↓ levels of these drugs, with risk of therapeutic failure	Induction of hepatic metabolism	1. Avoid co-administration of telithromycin for up to 2 weeks after stopping carbamazepine 2. With the other drugs, monitor for ↓ clinical efficacy and ↑ dose as required

DRUGS TO TREAT INFECTIONS ANTIBIOTICS – MACROLIDES

Primary drug	Secondary drug	Effect	Mechanism	Precautions
CLARITHROMYCIN, ERYTHROMYCIN	CARBAMAZEPINE	↑ carbamazepine levels	Inhibition of metabolism	Monitor carbamazepine levels
TELITHROMYCIN	PHENYTOIN	↓ levels of these drugs, with risk of therapeutic failure	Induction of hepatic metabolism	1. Avoid co-administration of telithromycin for up to 2 weeks after stopping phenytoin 2. With the other drugs, monitor for ↓ clinical efficacy and ↑ dose as required
CLARITHROMYCIN	PHENYTOIN	↑ phenytoin levels	Inhibited metabolism	Monitor phenytoin levels
ERYTHROMYCIN	VALPROATE	↑ valproate levels	Inhibited metabolism	Monitor levels
CLARITHROMYCIN, ERYTHROMYCIN, TELITHROMYCIN	ANTIFUNGALS – ITRACONAZOLE, KETOCONAZOLE, VORICONAZOLE	↑ plasma concentrations of itraconazole, ketoconazole and voriconazole, and risk of toxic effects	These antibiotics are inhibitors of metabolism of itraconazole by the CYP3A4. Erythromycin is a weaker inhibitor than clarithromycin. The role of clarithromycin and erythromycin as inhibitors of P-gp is not known with certainty. Ketoconazole is a potent inhibitor of P-gp	Monitor LFTs closely. Azithromycin does not cause this effect
ERYTHROMYCIN, CLARITHROMYCIN	ANTIGOUT DRUGS – COLCHICINE	Cases of colchicine toxicity when macrolides added	Uncertain; macrolides may inhibit hepatic metabolism of colchicine. Clarithromycin and erythromycin both inhibit intestinal P-gp, which may ↑ bioavailability of colchicine	Monitor FBC and renal function closely
MACROLIDES	**ANTIMIGRAINE DRUGS**			
MACROLIDES	ERGOT DERIVATIVES	↑ ergotamine/methysergide levels, with risk of toxicity	Inhibition of CYP3A4-mediated metabolism of the ergot derivatives	Avoid co-administration

DRUGS TO TREAT INFECTIONS ANTIBIOTICS – MACROLIDES

DRUGS TO TREAT INFECTIONS ANTIBIOTICS – MACROLIDES

CLARITHROMYCIN, ERYTHROMYCIN	ALMOTRIPTAN, ELETRIPTAN	↑ plasma concentrations of almotriptan and eletriptan, with risk of toxic effects, e.g. flushing, sensations of tingling, heat, heaviness, pressure or tightness of any part of body including the throat and chest, dizziness	Almotriptan is metabolized mainly by CYP3A4 isoenzymes. Most CYP isoenzymes are inhibited by clarithromycin to varying degrees, and since there is an alternative pathway of metabolism by MAOA, the toxicity responses will vary between individuals	Avoid co-administration
CLARITHROMYCIN, ERYTHROMYCIN	ANTIMUSCARINICS – TOLTERODINE	↑ tolterodine levels	Inhibition of CYP3A4-mediated metabolism	Avoid co-administration (manufacturers' recommendation)
ERYTHROMYCIN	ANTIPARKINSON'S DRUGS – BROMOCRIPTINE, CABERGOLINE	↑ bromocriptine and cabergoline levels	Inhibition of metabolism	Monitor BP closely and watch for early features of toxicity (nausea, headache, drowsiness)
ERYTHROMYCIN	ANTIPSYCHOTICS – CLOZAPINE	↑ clozapine levels, with risk of clozapine toxicity	Clozapine is metabolized by CYPIA2, which is moderately inhibited by erythromycin. Erythromycin is a potent inhibitor of CYP3A4, which has a minor role in the metabolism of clozapine. This may lead to ↓ clearance and therefore ↑ levels of clozapine	Cautious use advised
MACROLIDES	**ANTIVIRALS**			
CLARITHROMYCIN	NNRTIs	1. ↓ efficacy of clarithromycin but ↑ efficacy and adverse effects of the active metabolite 2. A rash occurs in 46% of patients when efavirenz is given with clarithromycin	1. Uncertain: possibly due to altered CYP3A4-mediated metabolism 2. Uncertain	1. Clinical significance unknown; no dose adjustment is recommended when clarithromycin is co-administered with nevirapine, but monitor LFTs and activity against *Mycobacterium avium intracellulare* complex closely 2. Consider alternatives to clarithromycin for patients on efavirenz

Primary drug	Secondary drug	Effect	Mechanism	Precautions
AZITHROMYCIN	PROTEASE INHIBITORS	Risk of ↑ adverse effects of azithromycin with nelfinavir	Possibly involves altered P-gp transport	Watch for signs of azithromycin toxicity
CLARITHROMYCIN, ERYTHROMYCIN	PROTEASE INHIBITORS	Possibly ↑ adverse effects of macrolide with atazanavir, ritonavir (with or without lopinavir) and saquinavir	Inhibition of CYP3A4- and possibly CYP1A2-mediated metabolism. Altered transport via P-gp may be involved. Amprenavir and indinavir are also possibly ↑ by erythromycin	Consider alternatives unless there is *Mycobacterium avium intracellulare* infection; if combined, ↓ dose by 50% (75% in the presence of renal failure with a creatinine clearance of <30 mL/min)
MACROLIDES	**ANXIOLYTICS AND HYPNOTICS**			
ERYTHROMYCIN, CLARITHROMYCIN, TELITHROMYCIN	MIDAZOLAM, TRIAZOLAM, POSSIBLY ALPRAZOLAM	↑ BZD levels	Inhibition of CYP3A4-mediated metabolism	↓ dose of BZD by 50%; warn patients not to perform skilled tasks such as driving for at least 10 hours after the dose of BZD
MACROLIDES	BUSPIRONE	↑ buspirone levels	Inhibition of CYP3A4-mediated metabolism	Warn patients to be aware of additional sedation
MACROLIDES	**BRONCHODILATORS**			
MACROLIDES	LEUKOTRIENE RECEPTOR ANTAGONISTS – ZAFIRLUKAST	↓ zafirlukast levels	Induction of metabolism	Watch for poor response to zafirlukast
AZITHROMYCIN, CLARITHROMYCIN, ERYTHROMYCIN	THEOPHYLLINE	1. ↑ theophylline levels 2. Possibly ↓ erythromycin levels when given orally	1. Inhibition of CYP2D6-mediated metabolism of theophylline (macrolides and quinolones – isoniazid not known) 2. ↓ bioavailability; uncertain mechanism	1. Monitor theophylline levels before, during and after co-administration 2. Consider an alternative macrolide

MACROLIDES	CALCIUM CHANNEL BLOCKERS	↑ plasma concentrations of felodipine when co-administered with erythromycin; cases of adverse effects of verapamil (bradycardia and ↓ BP) with both erythromycin and clarithromycin	Erythromycin inhibits CYP3A4-metabolism of felodipine and verapamil. Clarithromycin and erythromycin inhibit intestinal P-gp, which may ↑ bioavailability of verapamil	Monitor PR and BP closely; watch for bradycardia and ↓ BP. Consider ↓ dose of calcium channel blocker during macrolide therapy
MACROLIDES	CARDIAC GLYCOSIDES – DIGOXIN	Digoxin concentrations may be ↑ by the macrolides	Uncertain; postulated that macrolides inhibit P-gp in both the intestine (↑ bioavailability) and kidney (↓ clearance). It is possible that alterations in intestinal flora may also have a role	Monitor digoxin levels; watch for digoxin toxicity
CLARITHROMYCIN, TELITHROMYCIN	CNS STIMULANTS – MODAFINIL	↑ plasma concentrations of modafinil, with risk of adverse effects	Due to inhibition of CYP3A4, which has a partial role in the metabolism of modafinil	Be aware. Warn patients to report dose-related adverse effects, e.g. headache anxiety
ERYTHROMYCIN	DIURETICS – POTASSIUM-SPARING	↑ eplerenone results in ↑ risk of hypotension and hyperkalaemia	Eplerenone is primarily metabolized by CYP3A4; there are no active metabolites. Erythromycin moderately inhibits CYP3A4, leading to ↑ levels of eplerenone	Eplerenone dosage should not exceed 25 mg daily
ERYTHROMYCIN	H2 RECEPTOR BLOCKERS – CIMETIDINE	↑ efficacy and adverse effects of erythromycin, including hearing loss	↑ bioavailability	Consider an alternative antibiotic, e.g. clarithromycin. Deafness was reversible with cessation of erythromycin
MACROLIDES	IVABRADINE	1. Risk of arrhythmias with erythromycin 2. Possible ↑ levels with clarithromycin and telithromycin	1. Additive effect 2. Uncertain	Avoid co-administration

Primary drug	Secondary drug	Effect	Mechanism	Precautions
MACROLIDES	**LIPID-LOWERING DRUGS**			
MACROLIDES	ATORVASTATIN, SIMVASTATIN	Macrolides may ↑ levels of atorvastatin and simvastatin; the risk of myopathy ↑ >10x when erythromycin is co-administered with a statin	Macrolides inhibit CYP3A4-mediated metabolism of atorvastatin and simvastatin. Also, erythromycin and clarithromycin inhibit intestinal P-gp, which may ↑ bioavailability of statins	Avoid co-administration of macrolides with atorvastatin or simvastatin (temporarily stop the statin if the patient needs macrolide therapy). Manufacturers also recommend that patients are warned to look for the early signs of rhabdomyolysis when other statins are co-ingested with macrolides
ERYTHROMYCIN	ROSUVASTATIN	↓ rosuvastatin levels with erythromycin	Uncertain	Avoid chronic co-administration
ERYTHROMYCIN	OESTROGENS	Reports of ↓ contraceptive effect	Possibly alteration of the bacterial flora necessary for recycling ethinylestradiol from the large bowel, although not certain in every case	Advise patients to use additional contraception for the period of antibiotic intake and for 1 month after stopping the antibiotic
ERYTHROMYCIN	PARASYMPATHOMIMETICS – GALANTAMINE	↑ galantamine levels	Inhibition of CYP3A4-mediated metabolism of galantamine	Be aware; watch for ↑ side-effects from galantamine
ERYTHROMYCIN, CLARITHROMYCIN	PERIPHERAL VASODILATORS – CILOSTAZOL	Cilostazol levels ↑ by erythromycin and possibly clarithromycin	Erythromycin and clarithromycin inhibit CYP3A4-mediated metabolism of cilostazol	Avoid co-administration
MACROLIDES	PHOSPHODIESTERASE TYPE 5 INHIBITORS	↑ phosphodiesterase type 5 inhibitor levels with erythromycin, and possibly clarithromycin and telithromycin	Inhibition of metabolism	↓ dose of these phosphodiesterase inhibitors (e.g. start vardenafil at 5 mg)
CLARITHROMYCIN	PROTON PUMP INHIBITORS – OMEPRAZOLE	↑ efficacy and adverse effects of both drugs	↑ plasma concentration of both drugs	No dose adjustment recommended. Interaction considered useful for *Helicobacter pylori* eradication

ANTIBIOTICS – PENICILLINS				
AMPICILLIN	ANAESTHETICS – LOCAL – LIDOCAINE SOLUTIONS	Precipitation of drugs, which may not be immediately apparent	A pharmaceutical interaction	Do not mix in the same infusion or syringe
PENICILLIN V	ANTIBIOTICS – NEOMYCIN	↓ levels of phenoxymethylpenicillin and possible therapeutic failure	↓ absorption of phenoxymethylpenicillin due to malabsorption syndrome caused by neomycin	Patients should be monitored for efficacy of phenoxymethylpenicillin
PENICILLINS	ANTICANCER AND IMMUNOMODULATING DRUGS – METHOTREXATE	↑ plasma concentrations of methotrexate and risk of toxic effects of methotrexate, e.g. myelosuppression, liver cirrhosis, pulmonary toxicity	Penicillins ↓ renal elimination of methotrexate by renal tubular secretion, which is the main route of elimination of methotrexate. Penicillins compete with methotrexate for renal elimination. Displacement from protein-binding sites may occur and is only a minor contribution to the interaction	Avoid concurrent use. If concurrent use is necessary, monitor clinically and biochemically for blood dyscrasias, liver toxicity and pulmonary toxicity. Do FBCs and LFTs prior to concurrent treatment
PENICILLINS	ANTICOAGULANTS – ORAL	Occasional episodes of ↑ anticoagulant effect	Uncertain at present	Monitor INR every 2–3 days
PENICILLINS	**ANTIGOUT DRUGS**			
PENICILLINS	ALLOPURINOL	Possible ↑ risk of rash with amoxycillin and ampicillin (over 20% incidence in one study)	Uncertain	Reassure patients that the rash is unlikely to have clinical significance
PENICILLINS	PROBENECID, SULFINPYRAZONE	↑ penicillin levels	Uncertain	Watch for ↑ incidence of side-effects
AMPICILLIN	BETA-BLOCKERS	Plasma concentrations of atenolol were halved by 1 g doses of ampicillin (but not smaller doses)	Uncertain	Monitor BP closely during initiation of therapy with ampicillin
PIPERACILLIN	MUSCLE RELAXANTS – DEPOLARIZING, NON-DEPOLARIZING	↑ effect of muscle relaxants	Piperacillin has some neuromuscular blocking activity	Monitor neuromuscular blockade carefully

DRUGS TO TREAT INFECTIONS ANTIBIOTICS – QUINOLONES

Primary drug	Secondary drug	Effect	Mechanism	Precautions
AMPICILLIN	OESTROGENS	Reports of ↓ contraceptive effect	Possibly alteration of bacterial flora necessary for recycling ethinylestradiol from the large bowel, although not certain in every case	Advise patients to use additional contraception for the period of antibiotic intake and for 1 month after stopping the antibiotic
ANTIBIOTICS – QUINOLONES				
QUINOLONES	DRUGS THAT PROLONG THE Q–T INTERVAL			
QUINOLONES (especially moxifloxacin)	1. ANTIARRHYTHMICS – amiodarone, disopyramide, procainamide, propafenone 2. ANTIBIOTICS – macrolides (especially azithromycin, clarithromycin, parenteral erythromycin, telithromycin), quinupristin/dalfopristin 3. ANTICANCER AND IMMUNOMODULATING DRUGS – arsenic trioxide 4. ANTIDEPRESSANTS – TCAs, venlafaxine 5. ANTIEMETICS – dolasetron 6. ANTIFUNGALS – fluconazole, posaconazole, voriconazole 7. ANTIHISTAMINES – terfenadine, hydroxyzine, mizolastine 8. ANTIMALARIALS – artemether with lumefantrine, chloroquine, hydroxychloroquine, mefloquine, quinine 9. ANTIPROTOZOALS – pentamidine isetionate 10. ANTIPSYCHOTICS – atypicals, phenothiazines, pimozide 11. BETA-BLOCKERS – sotalol 12. BRONCHODILATORS – parenteral bronchodilators 13. CNS STIMULANTS – atomoxetine	Risk of ventricular arrhythmias, particularly torsades de pointes	Additive effect; these drugs cause prolongation of the Q–T interval	Avoid co-administration

QUINOLONES	ANALGESICS			
QUINOLONES	NSAIDs	Reports of convulsions when NSAIDs were added to quinolones in those with epilepsy	Unknown	Care in co-administering antiepileptics and NSAIDs in patients with epilepsy
CIPROFLOXACIN	OPIOIDS	1. Effects of methadone ↑ by ciprofloxacin 2. ↓ levels of ciprofloxacin with opioids	1. Ciprofloxacin inhibits CYP1A2-, CYP2D6- and CYP3A4-mediated metabolism of methadone 2. Uncertain	1. Watch for ↑ effects of methadone 2. Avoid opioid premedication when ciprofloxacin is used as surgical prophylaxis
QUINOLONES	ANTACIDS	↓ levels of these antibiotics	↓ absorption	Separate quinolones and antacids by 2–6 hours. Separate tetracyclines and antacids by 2–3 hours
QUINOLONES	**ANTICANCER AND IMMUNOMODULATING DRUGS**			
QUINOLONES	**CYTOTOXICS**			
NALIDIXIC ACID	MELPHALAN	Risk of melphalan toxicity	Uncertain	Avoid co-administration
CIPROFLOXACIN	METHOTREXATE	↑ plasma concentrations of methotrexate, with risk of toxic effects of methotrexate, e.g. liver cirrhosis, blood dyscrasias which may be fatal, pulmonary toxicity, stomatitis. Haematopoietic suppression can occur abruptly. Other adverse effects include anorexia, dyspepsia, gastrointestinal ulceration and bleeding and pulmonary oedema	Ciprofloxacin ↓ renal elimination of methotrexate. Ciprofloxacin is known to cause renal failure and interstitial nephritis	Although the toxic effects of methotrexate are more frequent with high doses of methotrexate, it is necessary to do FBC, liver and renal function tests before starting treatment even with low doses, repeating these tests weekly until therapy is stabilized and thereafter every 2–3 months. Patients should be advised to report symptoms such as sore throat and fever immediately, and also any gastrointestinal discomfort. A profound drop in white cell or platelet counts warrants immediate stoppage of methotrexate therapy and initiation of supportive therapy. Consider a non-reacting antibiotic

DRUGS TO TREAT INFECTIONS ANTIBIOTICS – QUINOLONES

DRUGS TO TREAT INFECTIONS ANTIBIOTICS – QUINOLONES

Primary drug	Secondary drug	Effect	Mechanism	Precautions
CIPROFLOXACIN	PORFIMER	↑ risk of photosensitivity reactions	Attributed to additive effects	Avoid exposure of skin and eyes to direct sunlight for 30 days after porfimer therapy
QUINOLONES	**IMMUNOMODULATING DRUGS**			
CIPROFLOXACIN	CICLOSPORIN	Ciprofloxacin may ↓ immunosuppressive effect (pharmacodynamic interaction)	Ciprofloxacin ↓ inhibitory effect of ciclosporin on IL-2 production to ↓ immunosuppressive effect	Avoid co-administration
NORFLOXACIN	CICLOSPORIN	↑ plasma concentrations of ciclosporin, with risk of nephrotoxicity, myelosuppression, neurotoxicity and excessive immunosuppression, with risk of infection and post-transplant lymphoproliferative disease	Inhibition of CYP3A4-mediated metabolism of ciclosporin; these inhibitors vary in potency	Monitor plasma ciclosporin levels to prevent toxicity. Monitor renal function
NORFLOXACIN	MYCOPHENOLATE	Significant ↓ plasma mycophenolate concentrations (>60% with rifampicin)	Inhibition of metabolism of mycophenolate	Avoid co-administration
QUINOLONES	ANTICOAGULANTS – ORAL	Occasional episodes of ↑ anticoagulant effect	Uncertain at present	Monitor INR every 2–3 days
CIPROFLOXACIN	ANTIDEPRESSANTS – DULOXETINE	↑ duloxetine levels, with risk of side-effects, e.g. arrhythmias	Inhibition of metabolism of duloxetine	Avoid co-administration
QUINOLONES	**ANTIDIABETIC DRUGS**			
QUINOLONES	ACARBOSE, METFORMIN, NATEGLINIDE, REPAGLINIDE, PIOGLITAZONE, ROSIGLITAZONE, SULPHONYLUREAS	↑ risk of hypoglycaemic episodes	Mechanism uncertain. Ciprofloxacin is a potent inhibitor of CYP1A2. Norfloxacin is a weak inhibitor of CYP1A2, but these may inhibit other CYP isoenzymes to varying degrees	Watch for and warn patients about symptoms of hypoglycaemia ➢ ***For signs and symptoms of hypoglycaemia, see Clinical Features of Some Adverse Drug Interactions, Hypoglycaemia***

LEVOFLOXACIN	INSULIN	Altered insulin requirements	Both hyperglycaemia and hypoglycaemia	Altered glycaemic control requires frequent monitoring
OFLOXACIN	INSULIN	↑ risk of hypoglycaemic episodes	Mechanism for hypoglycaemia is not known	Watch for and warn patients about symptoms of hypoglycaemia ➣ ***For signs and symptoms of hypoglycaemia, see Clinical Features of Some Adverse Drug Interactions, Hypoglycaemia***
CIPROFLOXACIN	ANTIEPILEPTICS – PHENYTOIN	Variable effect on phenytoin levels	Unknown	Monitor phenytoin levels
CIPROFLOXACIN, LEVOFLOXACIN, NALIDIXIC ACID, NORFLOXACIN	ANTIGOUT DRUGS – PROBENECID	↑ ciprofloxacin, nalidixic acid and norfloxacin levels	Uncertain	Watch for ↑ incidence of side-effects. Moxifloxacin, ofloxacin and sparfloxacin do not seem to interact and could be used as alternative therapy
QUINOLONES	ANTIMIGRAINE DRUGS – ZOLMITRIPTAN	Possible ↓ plasma concentrations of zolmitriptan, with risk of inadequate therapeutic efficacy	Possibly induced metabolism of zolmitriptan	Be aware of possibility of ↓ response to triptan and consider ↑ dose if effect is considered to be due to interaction
CIPROFLOXACIN	ANTIPARKINSON'S DRUGS – ROPINIROLE	↑ ropinirole levels	Inhibition of CYP1A2-mediated metabolism	Watch for early features of toxicity (nausea, drowsiness)
CIPROFLOXACIN	ANTIPSYCHOTICS – CLOZAPINE, OLANZAPINE	↑ clozapine levels and possibly ↑ olanzapine levels	Ciprofloxacin inhibits CYP1A2; clozapine is primarily metabolized by CYP1A2, while olanzapine is partly metabolized by it	Watch for the early features of toxicity to these antipsychotics. ↓ dose of clozapine and olanzapine may be required
QUINOLONES	**ANTIVIRALS**			
QUINOLONES	DIDANOSINE	↓ efficacy of ciprofloxacin and possibly levofloxacin, moxifloxacin, norfloxacin and ofloxacin with buffered didanosine	Cations in the buffer of didanosine preparation chelate and adsorb ciprofloxacin. Absorption of the other quinolones may be ↓ by the buffered didanosine formulation, which raises gastric pH	Give the antibiotic 2 hours before or 6 hours after didanosine. Alternatively, consider using the enteric-coated formulation of didanosine, which does not have to be given separately

DRUGS TO TREAT INFECTIONS ANTIBIOTICS – QUINOLONES

Primary drug	Secondary drug	Effect	Mechanism	Precautions
QUINOLONES	FOSCARNET SODIUM	Risk of seizures	Unknown; possibly additive side-effect	Avoid combination in patients with past medical history of epilepsy. Consider an alternative antibiotic
QUINOLONES	BRONCHODILATORS – THEOPHYLLINE	1. ↑ theophylline levels 2. Possibly ↓ erythromycin levels when given orally	1. Inhibition of CYP2D6-mediated metabolism of theophylline (macrolides and quinolones – isoniazid not known) 2. ↓ bioavailability; uncertain mechanism	1. Monitor theophylline levels before, during and after co-administration 2. Consider an alternative macrolide
CIPROFLOXACIN	CALCIUM	↓ antibiotic levels	↓ absorption	Separate doses by at least 2 hours
CIPROFLOXACIN, NORFLOXACIN	DAIRY PRODUCTS	↓ norfloxacin levels, with risk of therapeutic failure	The calcium from dairy products is thought to form an insoluble chelate with norfloxacin, leading to ↓ absorption from the gut	Dairy products should be avoided for 1–2 hours before and after taking norfloxacin. Alternatively, moxifloxacin, enoxacin, lomefloxacin and ofloxacin can be used as alternative therapies as they show minimal interaction
QUINOLONES	DRUG DEPENDENCE THERAPIES – BUPROPION	↑ risk of seizures. This risk is marked in elderly people, in patients with a history of seizures, with addiction to opiates/cocaine/stimulants, and in diabetics treated with oral hypoglycaemics or insulin	Bupropion is associated with a dose-related risk of seizures. These drugs, which lower seizure threshold, are individually epileptogenic. Additive effects occur when they are combined	Extreme caution. The dose of bupropion should not exceed 450 mg/day (or 150 mg/day in those with severe hepatic cirrhosis)
QUINOLONES	IRON – ORAL	↓ plasma concentrations of these drugs, with risk of therapeutic failure	Iron chelates with and ↓ their absorption	Separate doses of other drugs as much as possible and monitor their effects

DRUGS TO TREAT INFECTIONS ANTIBIOTICS – QUINOLONES

CIPROFLOXACIN	MUSCLE RELAXANTS – TIZANIDINE	↑ tizanidine levels	Tizanidine is a substrate for CYP1A2. Ciprofloxacin is a potent inhibitor of CYP1A2 and is thought to inhibit the presystemic metabolism, resulting in ↑ absorption and levels of tizanidine	Avoid co-administration
CIPROFLOXACIN	PERIPHERAL VASODILATORS – PENTOXIFYLLINE	Ciprofloxacin may ↑ pentoxifylline levels	Uncertain; likely to be due to inhibition of hepatic metabolism	Warn patients of the possibility of adverse effects of pentoxifylline
CIPROFLOXACIN	SEVELAMER	↓ plasma concentrations of ciprofloxacin	↓ absorption	Separate doses as much as possible
CIPROFLOXACIN	SODIUM BICARBONATE	↓ solubility of ciprofloxacin in the urine, leading to ↑ risk of crystalluria and renal damage	↑ urinary pH caused by sodium bicarbonate can result in ↓ ciprofloxacin solubility in the urine	If both drugs are used concomitantly, the patient should be well hydrated and be monitored for signs of renal toxicity
QUINOLONES	STRONTIUM RANELATE	↓ levels of these antibiotics	↓ absorption	Avoid co-administration
QUINOLONES	SUCRALFATE	↓ levels of these antibiotics	↓ absorption of these antibiotics	Give the antibiotics at least 2 hours before sucralfate
CIPROFLOXACIN	THYROID HORMONES – LEVOTHYROXINE	↓ levels of levothyroxine and possible therapeutic failure	The mechanism has not been elucidated, the concurrent administration of ciprofloxacin with levothyroxine may interfere with the absorption of levothyroxine and result in lower than expected levels	The interaction may be minimized by separating dosing of the two agents; ciprofloxacin should be taken several hours before or after taking levothyroxine
CIPROFLOXACIN	ZINC	↓ antibiotic levels	↓ absorption	Separate doses by at least 2 hours

DRUGS TO TREAT INFECTIONS ANTIBIOTICS – QUINOLONES

Primary drug	Secondary drug	Effect	Mechanism	Precautions
ANTIBIOTICS – RIFAMYCINS				
RIFAMYCINS	ANALGESICS			
RIFAMPICIN	NSAIDs	Rifampicin ↓ diclofenac celecoxib, etoricoxib, and parecoxib levels	Rifampicin ↑ CYP2C9-mediated metabolism of these NSAIDs	Monitor analgesic effects; consider using alternative NSAIDs
RIFAMPICIN	OPIOIDS	↓ effect of alfentanil, codeine, methadone and morphine	Rifampicin ↑ the hepatic metabolism of these opioids (alfentanil by CYP3A4, codeine by CYP2D6, morphine unknown). Rifampicin is also known to induce intestinal P-gp, which may ↓ bioavailability of oral morphine	Be aware that alfentanil, codeine, methadone and morphine doses may need to be ↑
RIFAMPICIN	PARACETAMOL	Rifampicin ↓ paracetamol levels	Rifampicin ↑ glucuronidation of paracetamol	Warn patients that paracetamol may be less effective
RIFAMYCINS	ANTACIDS	↓ rifamycin levels	↓ absorption	Separate doses by 2–3 hours
RIFAMYCINS	ANTIARRHYTHMICS			
RIFAMPICIN	AMIODARONE	↓ levels of amiodarone	Uncertain, but rifampicin is a known enzyme inducer and may therefore ↑ metabolism of amiodarone	Watch for a poor response to amiodarone
RIFAMPICIN	DISOPYRAMIDE	Disopyramide levels are ↓ by rifampicin	Rifampicin induces hepatic metabolism of disopyramide	Watch for poor response to disopyramide; check serum levels if necessary
RIFAMPICIN	MEXILETINE	Rifampicin ↓ mexiletine levels	Uncertain; postulated that rifampicin may ↑ mexiletine metabolism	Watch for poor response to mexiletine
RIFAMPICIN	PROPAFENONE	Rifampicin may ↓ propafenone levels	Rifampicin may inhibit CYP3A4/1A2-mediated metabolism of propafenone	Watch for poor response to propafenone

RIFAMYCINS	ANTIBIOTICS			
RIFAMYCINS	DAPSONE	↓ levels of dapsone	Rifamycins induce metabolism of dapsone	Watch for poor response to dapsone
RIFAMYCINS	MACROLIDES	1. ↓ levels of clarithromycin and telithromycin with rifampicin 2. ↑ rifabutin levels with macrolides	1. Rifampicins induce metabolism of these macrolides 2. Inhibition of CYP3A4-mediated metabolism of rifabutin	1. Watch for poor response to clarithromycin and telithromycin, which may last up to 2 weeks after stopping rifampicin 2. Watch for early features of toxicity of rifabutin; in particular, warn patients to report painful eyes
RIFAMPICIN	QUINUPRISTIN/ DALFOPRISTIN	Risk of hepatic toxicity	Additive effect	Monitor LFTs closely
RIFAMYCINS	**ANTICANCER AND IMMUNOMODULATING DRUGS**			
RIFAMYCINS	**CYTOTOXICS**			
RIFAMPICIN	DASATINIB	↓ dasatinib levels	Rifampicin ↑ metabolism of dasatinib	Avoid co-administration
RIFAMPICIN	ERLOTINIB	↓ erlotinib levels	Rifampicin ↑ metabolism of erlotinib	Avoid co-administration
RIFAMPICIN	IFOSFAMIDE	↑ rate of biotransformation to 4-hydroxyifosfamide, the active metabolite, but no change in AUC of 4-hydroxyifosfamide	Due to ↑ rate of metabolism and of clearance due to induction of CYP3A4 and CYP2D6	Be aware – clinical significance may be minimal or none
RIFAMPICIN	IMATINIB	↓ imatinib levels	Due to induction of CYP3A4-mediated metabolism of imatinib	Dose adjustments are necessary if concomitant administration is considered absolutely necessary; best, however, to avoid concomitant use

DRUGS TO TREAT INFECTIONS ANTIBIOTICS – RIFAMYCINS

Primary drug	Secondary drug	Effect	Mechanism	Precautions
RIFAMPICIN	IRINOTECAN	↓ plasma concentrations of irinotecan and risk of ↓ therapeutic efficacy. The effects may last for 3 weeks after discontinuation of CYP-inducer therapy	Due to induction of CYP3A4-mediated metabolism of irinotecan	Avoid concomitant use whenever possible; if not, ↑ dose of irinotecan by 50%
RIFAMPICIN	PACLITAXEL	↓ plasma concentration of paclitaxel and ↓ efficacy of paclitaxel	Due to induction of hepatic metabolism of paclitaxel by the CYP isoenzymes	Monitor for clinical efficacy, and need to ↑ dose if inadequate response is due to interaction
RIFAMPICIN	SUNITINIB	↓ sunitinib levels	Rifampicin ↑ metabolism of sunitinib	Avoid co-administration
RIFAMPICIN	VINCA ALKALOIDS – VINBLASTINE, VINCRISTINE	↓ of plasma concentrations of vinblastine and vincristine, with risk of inadequate therapeutic response. Reports of ↓ AUC by 40% and elimination half-life by 35%, and ↑ clearance by 63%, in patients with brain tumours taking vincristine, which could lead to dangerously inadequate therapeutic responses	Due to induction of CYP3A4-mediated metabolism	Monitor for clinical efficacy and ↑ dose of vinblastine and vincristine as clinically indicated; in the latter case, monitor clinically and radiologically for clinical efficacy in patients with brain tumours and ↑ dose to obtain the desired response
RIFAMYCINS	**HORMONES AND HORMONE ANTAGONISTS**			
RIFAMPICIN	TAMOXIFEN	↓ plasma concentrations of tamoxifen and risk of inadequate therapeutic response	Due to induction of metabolism of tamoxifen by the CYP3A isoenzymes by rifampicin	Avoid concurrent use if possible. Otherwise monitor for clinical efficacy of tamoxifen and ↑ dose of tamoxifen if required

DRUGS TO TREAT INFECTIONS ANTIBIOTICS – RIFAMYCINS

RIFAMYCINS	IMMUNOMODULATING DRUGS			
RIFAMYCINS	CICLOSPORIN	↓ plasma concentrations of ciclosporin, with risk of transplant rejection	Due to induction of CYP3A4-mediated metabolism of ciclosporin by these drugs. The potency of induction varies	Monitor for signs of rejection of transplants. Monitor ciclosporin levels to ensure adequate therapeutic concentrations and ↑ dose when necessary
RIFAMPICIN	CORTICOSTEROIDS	↓ plasma concentrations of corticosteroids and risk of poor or inadequate therapeutic response, which would be undesirable if used for e.g. cerebral oedema	Due to induction of the hepatic metabolism by the CYP3A4 isoenzymes	Monitor therapeutic response closely – clinically, with ophthalmoscopy and radiologically – and ↑ dose of corticosteroids for desired therapeutic effect
RIFAMPICIN	MYCOPHENOLATE	Significant ↓ plasma mycophenolate concentrations (>60% with rifampicin)	Attributed to induction of glucuronyl transferase	Avoid co-administration
RIFAMPICIN	SIROLIMUS	↓ sirolimus levels	Induction of CYP3A4-mediated metabolism of sirolimus	Avoid co-administration
RIFAMPICIN	TACROLIMUS	↓ tacrolimus levels	Induction of CYP3A4-mediated metabolism of tacrolimus	Avoid co-administration
RIFAMPICIN	ANTICOAGULANTS – ORAL	↓ anticoagulant effect	Rifampicin induces CYP2C9-mediated metabolism of warfarin	Monitor INR closely for at least 1 week after starting rifampicin and up to 5 weeks after stopping it. During co-administration, the warfarin dose may need to be markedly ↑
RIFAMPICIN	**ANTIDIABETIC DRUGS**			
RIFAMPICIN	PIOGLITAZONE, ROSIGLITAZONE	Significant ↓ blood levels of rosiglitazone. Metabolism and clearance is ↑, the latter threefold	Rosiglitazone is metabolized primarily by CYP2C8 with a minor contribution from CYP2C9. Rifampicin is a potent inducer of CYP2C8 and CYP2C9, and ↑ formation of *N*-desmethylrosiglitazone by about 40%	May need to use an alternative drug or ↑ dose of rosiglitazone

DRUGS TO TREAT INFECTIONS ANTIBIOTICS – RIFAMYCINS

Primary drug	Secondary drug	Effect	Mechanism	Precautions
RIFAMPICIN	REPAGLINIDE	↓ plasma concentrations of repaglinide likely. Rifampicin ↓ AUC of repaglinide by 25%	Due to inducing CYP3A4 isoenzymes that metabolize repaglinide. However, the alternative pathway – CYP2C8 – is unaffected by these inducers except by rifampicin	The interaction is likely to be most severe with rifampicin. Be aware and monitor for hypoglycaemia ➢ ***For signs and symptoms of hypoglycaemia, see Clinical Features of Some Adverse Drug Interactions, Hypoglycaemia***
RIFAMPICIN	SULPHONYLUREAS	↓ hypoglycaemic efficacy	Plasma levels of sulphonylureas are ↓ by induction of CYP-mediated metabolism	Watch for and warn patients about symptoms of hypoglycaemia ➢ ***For signs and symptoms of hypoglycaemia, see Clinical Features of Some Adverse Drug Interactions, Hypoglycaemia***
RIFAMPICIN	**ANTIEMETIC**			
RIFAMPICIN	APREPITANT	↓ aprepitant levels	Induction of CYP3A4-mediated metabolism of aprepitant	Watch for poor response to aprepitant
RIFAMPICIN	5-HT3 ANTAGONISTS – ONDANSETRON, TROPISETRON	↓ levels of these drugs	Induction of metabolism	Watch for poor response to ondansetron and tropisetron; consider using an alternative antiemetic
RIFAMYCINS	**ANTIEPILEPTICS**			
RIFAMPICIN	BARBITURATES	↓ levels of these drugs, with risk of therapeutic failure	Induction of hepatic metabolism	Monitor for ↓ clinical efficacy and ↑ their dose as required
RIFABUTIN	CARBAMAZEPINE	↓ carbamazepine levels	Induction of metabolism	Monitor carbamazepine levels
RIFAMPICIN	LAMOTRIGINE	↓ lamotrigine levels	↑ metabolism	Monitor levels
RIFAMPICIN, RIFABUTIN	PHENYTOIN	↓ phenytoin levels	Induced metabolism	Monitor phenytoin levels

DRUGS TO TREAT INFECTIONS ANTIBIOTICS – RIFAMYCINS

RIFAMYCINS	ANTIFUNGALS			
RIFAMPICIN, RIFABUTIN, RIFAPENTINE	ITRACONAZOLE, KETOCONAZOLE, POSACONAZOLE, VORICONAZOLE	↓ levels of these azoles, with significant risk of therapeutic failure. Rifampicin is a very potent inducer that can produce undetectable concentrations of ketoconazole	Rifampicin is a powerful inducer of CYP3A4 and other CYP isoenzymes. Rifabutin is a less powerful inducer but more potent than rifapentine. Rifapentine is an inducer of CYP3A4 and CYP2C8/9. Rifampicin is also a powerful inducer of P-gp, thus ↓ bioavailability of itraconazole	Avoid co-administration of ketoconazole or voriconazole with these drugs. Watch for inadequate therapeutic effects of itraconazole. Higher doses of itraconazole may not overcome this interaction, so consider the use of less lipophilic fluconazole, which is less dependent on CYP metabolism. Avoid co-administration of posaconazole with rifabutin
RIFABUTIN	VORICONAZOLE	↑ plasma concentrations of rifabutin, with risk of toxic effects of rifabutin (nausea, vomiting). Dangerous toxic effects such as leukopenia and thrombocytopenia may occur	Due to inhibition of metabolism of rifabutin by the CYP3A4 isoenzymes by voriconazole	Avoid concomitant use. If absolutely necessary, close monitoring of FBC and liver enzymes and examination of eyes for uveitis and corneal opacities is necessary
RIFAMPICIN	CASPOFUNGIN	↓ caspofungin levels, with risk of therapeutic failure	Induction of caspofungin metabolism	↑ dose of caspofungin to 70 mg daily
RIFAMPICIN	TERBINAFINE	↓ terbinafine levels	Induction of metabolism	Watch for poor response to terbinafine
RIFAMPICINS	**ANTIHYPERTENSIVES AND HEART FAILURE DRUGS**			
RIFAMPICIN	ACE INHIBITORS	↓ plasma concentrations and efficacy of imidapril and enalapril	Uncertain. ↓ production of active metabolites has been noted despite rifampicin being an enzyme inducer	Monitor BP at least weekly until stable

DRUGS TO TREAT INFECTIONS ANTIBIOTICS – RIFAMYCINS

Primary drug	Secondary drug	Effect	Mechanism	Precautions
RIFAMPICIN	ANGIOTENSIN II RECEPTOR ANTAGONISTS – LOSARTAN	↓ antihypertensive effect of losartan	Rifampicin induces CYP2C9	Monitor BP at least weekly until stable
RIFAMPICIN	VASODILATOR ANTIHYPERTENSIVES	↓ bosentan levels	Induction of metabolism	Avoid co-administration
RIFAMYCINS	ANTIMALARIALS – ATOVAQUONE	Both rifampicin and rifabutin ↓ atovaquone levels, although the effect is greater with rifampicin (↓ AUC 50% cf. with 34% rifabutin)	Uncertain because atovaquone is predominantly excreted unchanged via the gastrointestinal route	Avoid co-administration with rifampicin. Take care with rifabutin and watch for poor response to atovaquone
RIFAMPICIN	ANTIMIGRAINE DRUGS – ALMOTRIPTAN	Possible ↓ plasma concentrations of almotriptan, with risk of inadequate therapeutic efficacy	One of the major metabolizing enzymes of almotriptan – CYP3A4 isoenzymes – are induced by rifampicin. As there are alternative metabolic pathways, the effect may not be significant and could vary from individual to individual	Be aware of possibility of ↓ response to triptan and consider ↑ dose if the effect is considered to be due to interaction
RIFAMPICIN	ANTIPROTOZOALS – LEVAMISOLE	↓ therapeutic efficacy of rifampicin	Levamisole displaces rifampicin from protein-binding sites and ↑ free fraction nearly three times and thus ↑ clearance of rifampicin	Avoid co-administration if possible
RIFABUTIN, RIFAMPICIN	ANTIPSYCHOTICS – ARIPIPRAZOLE, CLOZAPINE, HALOPERIDOL	↓ levels of these antipsychotics	↑ metabolism	Watch for poor response to these antipsychotics; consider ↑ dose
RIFAMYCINS	**ANTIVIRALS**			
RIFABUTIN	EFAVIRENZ	Possible ↓ efficacy of rifabutin	↓ bioavailability	↑ rifabutin dose by 50% for daily treatment, or double the dose if the patient is on treatment two or three times a week

DRUGS TO TREAT INFECTIONS ANTIBIOTICS – RIFAMYCINS

RIFABUTIN	PROTEASE INHIBITORS	↑ efficacy and ↑ adverse effects of rifabutin	Inhibition of CYP3A4-mediated metabolism. Nelfinavir also competitively inhibits 2C19	↓ rifabutin dose by at least 50% when given with amprenavir, indinavir or nelfinavir, and by 75% with atazanavir, ritonavir (with or without lopinavir) or tipranavir
RIFABUTIN	SAQUINAVIR	↓ efficacy of saquinavir	Uncertain; probably via altered CYP3A4 metabolism	Avoid co-administration
RIFAMPICIN	EFAVIRENZ	Possible ↓ efficacy of efavirenz	Uncertain	↑ dose of efavirenz from 600 mg to 800 mg
RIFAMPICIN	NEVIRAPINE	↓ efficacy of nevirapine	Uncertain; probable ↑ metabolism of nevirapine	Avoid concomitant use. FDA recommend use only if clearly indicated and monitored closely
RIFAMPICIN	PROTEASE INHIBITORS	↓ levels of protease inhibitor. Risk of hepatotoxicity with saquinavir	Induction of metabolism	Avoid co-administration
RIFAMPICIN	ZIDOVUDINE	Unclear	Unclear	Avoid co-administration
RIFAMYCINS	**ANXIOLYTICS AND HYPNOTICS**			
RIFAMPICIN	BZDs, NOT LORAZEPAM, OXAZEPAM, TEMAZEPAM	↓ BZD levels	Induction of CYP3A4-mediated metabolism	Watch for poor response to these BZDs; consider ↑ dose, e.g. diazepam or nitrazepam 2–3-fold
RIFAMPICIN	BUSPIRONE	↓ buspirone levels	Induction of CYP3A4-mediated metabolism	Watch for poor response to buspirone; consider ↑ dose
RIFAMPICIN	ZALEPLON, ZOLPIDEM, ZOPICLONE	↓ levels of these hypnotics	Induction of CYP3A4-mediated metabolism	Watch for poor response to these agents
RIFAMPICIN	BETA-BLOCKERS	↓ plasma concentrations and efficacy of bisoprolol, carvedilol, celiprolol, metoprolol and propanolol	Rifampicin induces hepatic enzymes (e.g. CYP2C19), which ↑ metabolism of the beta-blockers; in addition, it may also ↑ P-gp expression	Monitor PR and BP; watch for poor response to beta-blockers

DRUGS TO TREAT INFECTIONS ANTIBIOTICS – RIFAMYCINS

Primary drug	Secondary drug	Effect	Mechanism	Precautions
RIFAMPICIN	BRONCHODILATORS – THEOPHYLLINE	↓ plasma concentrations of theophylline and risk of therapeutic failure	Due to induction of CYP1A2 and CYP3A3	May need to ↑ dose of theophylline by 25%
RIFAMPICIN	CALCIUM CHANNEL BLOCKERS	Plasma concentrations of calcium channel blockers may be ↓ by rifampicin	Rifampicin induces CYP3A4-mediated metabolism of calcium channel blockers. It also induces CYP2C9-mediated metabolism of verapamil and induces intestinal P-gp, which may ↓ bioavailability of verapamil	Monitor BP closely; watch for ↓ effect of calcium channel blockers
RIFAMYCINS	**CARDIAC GLYCOSIDES**			
RIFAMPICIN	DIGOXIN	Plasma concentrations of digoxin may be ↓ by rifampicin	Rifampicin seems to induce P-gp-mediated excretion of digoxin in the kidneys	Watch for ↓ response to digoxin, check plasma levels and ↑ dose as necessary
RIFAMPICIN	DIGITOXIN	Plasma concentrations of digitoxin may be halved by rifampicin	Due to ↑ hepatic metabolism	Watch for poor response to digitoxin
RIFAMPICIN, RIFABUTIN	CNS STIMULANTS – MODAFINIL	↓ plasma concentrations of modafinil, with possibility of ↓ therapeutic effect	Induction of CYP3A4, which has a partial role in the metabolism of modafinil	Be aware
RIFAMPICIN	DIURETICS – POTASSIUM-SPARING	↓ eplerenone levels	Induction of metabolism	Avoid co-administration
RIFAMPICIN	DRUG DEPENDENCE THERAPIES – BUPROPION	↓ plasma concentrations of bupropion and lack of therapeutic effect	Induction of CYP2B6	↑ dose of bupropion cautiously
RIFAMPICIN	GESTRINONE	↓ gestrinone levels	Induction of metabolism	Watch for poor response to gestrinone
RIFAMPICIN	H2 RECEPTOR BLOCKERS – CIMETIDINE	↓ efficacy of cimetidine	↑ metabolism	Change to alternative acid suppression, e.g. rabeprazole, or ↑ dose and/or frequency

DRUGS TO TREAT INFECTIONS ANTIBIOTICS – RIFAMYCINS

RIFAMPICIN	LIPID-LOWERING DRUGS – STATINS	Rifampicin may lower fluvastatin and simvastatin levels	Uncertain	Monitor lipid profile closely; look for poor response to fluvastatin and simvastatin
RIFAMPICIN, RIFABUTIN	OESTROGENS	Marked ↓ contraceptive effect	Induction of metabolism of oestrogens	Advise patients to use additional contraception for the period of intake and for 1 month after stopping co-administration of these drugs (4–8 weeks after stopping rifabutin or rifampicin)
RIFAMPICIN, RIFABUTIN	PROGESTOGENS	↓ progesterone levels, which may lead to a failure of contraception or poor response to treatment of menorrhagia	Possibly induction of metabolism of progestogens	Advise patients to use additional contraception for the period of intake and 1 month after stopping co-administration of these drugs
RIFAMPICIN	TADALAFIL	↓ tadalafil levels	Probable induction of metabolism	Watch for poor response
RIFAMPICIN	THYROID HORMONES	↓ levothyroxine levels	Induction of metabolism	Monitor TFTs regularly and consider ↑ dose of levothyroxine
RIFAMPICIN	TIBOLONE	↓ tibolone levels	Induction of metabolism of tibolone	Watch for poor response to tibolone; consider ↑ dose
ANTIBIOTICS – SULPHONAMIDES				
SULPHONAMIDES	ANAESTHETICS – GENERAL	↑ effect of thiopentone but duration of action shortened	Uncertain; possibly displacement from protein-binding sites	Be aware that a smaller dose may be needed
SULPHONAMIDES	**ANAESTHETICS – LOCAL**			
SULFADIAZINE	LIDOCAINE SOLUTIONS	Precipitation of drugs, which may not be immediately apparent	A pharmaceutical interaction	Do not mix in the same infusion or syringe
SULPHONAMIDES	PRILOCAINE	Risk of methaemoglobinaemia; there is a case report of methaemoglobinaemia with topical prilocaine in a patient taking sulphonamides	Additive effect	Avoid co-administration

DRUGS TO TREAT INFECTIONS ANTIBIOTICS – SULPHONAMIDES

Primary drug	Secondary drug	Effect	Mechanism	Precautions
SULPHONAMIDES	**ANTIARRHYTHMICS**			
CO-TRIMOXAZOLE	AMIODARONE	Risk of ventricular arrhythmias	Uncertain	Avoid co-administration
ANTIBIOTICS – TRIMETHOPRIM	PROCAINAMIDE	Procainamide levels are ↑ by trimethoprim	Trimethoprim is a potent inhibitor of organic cation transport in the kidney, and the elimination of procainamide is impaired	Watch for signs of procainamide toxicity; ↓ dose of procainamide, particularly in elderly patients
SULPHONAMIDES	**ANTIBIOTICS**			
TRIMETHOPRIM	DAPSONE	↑ levels of both drugs	Mutual inhibition of metabolism	Be aware – watch for ↑ incidence of side-effects
SULPHONAMIDES	METHENAMINE	Risk of crystalluria	Methenamine is only effective at a low pH, and this is achieved by acidifiers in the formulation. Sulfadiazine crystallizes in an acid environment	Avoid co-administration
SULPHONAMIDES	**ANTICANCER AND IMMUNOMODULATING DRUGS**			
SULPHONAMIDES	**CYTOTOXICS**			
CO-TRIMOXAZOLE	MERCAPTOPURINE	↑ risk of bone marrow toxicity	Additive effect	Avoid co-administration
SULFAMETHOXAZOLE/ TRIMETHOPRIM	METHOTREXATE	↑ plasma concentrations of methotrexate and risk of toxic effects of methotrexate, e.g. myelosuppression, liver cirrhosis, pulmonary toxicity	Sulfamethoxazole displaces methotrexate from plasma protein-binding sites and also ↓ renal elimination of methotrexate. Trimethoprim inhibits dihydrofolate reductase, which leads to additive toxic effects of methotrexate	Avoid concurrent use. If concurrent use is necessary, monitor clinically and biochemically for blood dyscrasias, liver toxicity, renal toxicity and pulmonary toxicity

DRUGS TO TREAT INFECTIONS ANTIBIOTICS – SULPHONAMIDES

SULPHONAMIDES	METHOTREXATE	↑ plasma concentrations of methotrexate, with risk of toxic effects of methotrexate, e.g. liver cirrhosis, blood dyscrasias that may be fatal, pulmonary toxicity, stomatitis. Haematopoietic suppression can occur abruptly. Other adverse effects include anorexia, dyspepsia, gastrointestinal ulceration and bleeding, pulmonary oedema	The mechanism differs from that caused by sulfamethoxazole–trimethoprim. Sulphonamides such as co-trimoxazole and sulfadiazine are known to cause renal dysfunction – interstitial nephritis, renal failure, which may ↓ excretion of methotrexate. Sulphonamides are also known to compete with methotrexate for renal elimination. Displacement from protein-binding sites of methotrexate is a minor contribution to the interaction	Although the toxic effects of methotrexate are more frequent with high doses of methotrexate, it is necessary to do FBC, liver and renal function tests before starting treatment even with low doses, repeating these tests weekly until therapy is stabilized and thereafter every 2–3 months. Patients should be advised to report symptoms such as sore throat and fever immediately, and also any gastrointestinal discomfort. A profound drop in white cell or platelet counts warrants immediate stoppage of methotrexate therapy and initiation of supportive therapy
SULPHONAMIDES	PORFIMER	↑ risk of photosensitivity reactions	Attributed to additive effects	Avoid exposure of skin and eyes to direct sunlight for 30 days after porfimer therapy
SULPHONAMIDES	**ANTICANCER AND IMMUNOMODULATING DRUGS**			
ANTIBIOTICS – CO-TRIMOXAZOLE	AZATHIOPRINE	↑ risk of leukopenia	Additive effects, as co-trimoxazole inhibits white cell production	Caution ➢ ***For signs and symptoms of leukopenia, see Clinical Features of Some Adverse Drug Interactions, Immunosuppression and blood dyscrasias***
CO-TRIMOXAZOLE	CICLOSPORIN	Exacerbates hyperkalaemia induced by ciclosporin	Additive effect	Monitor serum potassium levels during co-administration ➢ ***For signs and symptoms of hyperkalaemia, see Clinical Features of Some Adverse Drug Interactions, Hyperkalaemia***

DRUGS TO TREAT INFECTIONS ANTIBIOTICS – SULPHONAMIDES

DRUGS TO TREAT INFECTIONS ANTIBIOTICS – SULPHONAMIDES

Primary drug	Secondary drug	Effect	Mechanism	Precautions
CO-TRIMOXAZOLE	MYCOPHENOLATE	Exacerbates neutropenia caused by mycophenolate	Additive effect	Monitor blood count closely ➢ ***For signs and symptoms of neutropenia, see Clinical Features of Some Adverse Drug Interactions, Immunosuppression and blood dyscrasias***
CO-TRIMOXAZOLE	SIROLIMUS	Exacerbates neutropenia caused by sirolimus	Additive effect	Monitor blood count closely ➢ ***For signs and symptoms of neutropenia, see Clinical Features of Some Adverse Drug Interactions, Immunosuppression and blood dyscrasias***
CO-TRIMOXAZOLE	TACROLIMUS	Exacerbates hyperkalaemia induced by tacrolimus	Additive hyperkalaemic effects	Monitor electrolytes closely ➢ ***For signs and symptoms of hyperkalaemia, see Clinical Features of Some Adverse Drug Interactions, Hyperkalaemia***
SULPHONAMIDES, TRIMETHOPRIM	ANTICOAGULANTS – ORAL	↑ anticoagulant effect	Inhibition of CYP2C9-mediated metabolism of oral anticoagulants	Monitor INR every 2–3 days
SULPHONAMIDES	**ANTIDIABETIC DRUGS**			
TRIMETHOPRIM	PIOGLITAZONE, ROSIGLITAZONE	↑ in blood levels of rosiglitazone by nearly 40%	Trimethoprim is a relatively selective inhibitor of CYP2C8	Watch for hypoglycaemic events and ↓ dose of rosiglitazone after repeated blood sugar measurements. Warn patients about hypoglycaemia ➢ ***For signs and symptoms of hypoglycaemia, see Clinical Features of Some Adverse Drug Interactions, Hypoglycaemia***
TRIMETHOPRIM	REPAGLINIDE	↑ repaglinide levels (by approximately 40%); risk of hypoglycaemia	Hepatic metabolism inhibited	Manufacturers do not recommend concurrent use

SULPHONAMIDES, TRIMETHOPRIM	ANTIEPILEPTICS – PHENYTOIN	↑ phenytoin levels	Inhibited metabolism	Monitor phenytoin levels
TRIMETHOPRIM	ANTIHYPERTENSIVES AND HEART FAILURE DRUGS – ACE INHIBITORS	Risk of hyperkalaemia when trimethoprim is co-administered with ACE inhibitors in the presence of renal failure	Uncertain at present	Avoid concurrent use in the presence of severe renal failure
ANTIBIOTICS – SULPHONAMIDES, TRIMETHOPRIM	ANTIMALARIALS – PYRIMETHAMINE	↑ antifolate effect	Additive effect	Monitor FBC closely; the effect may take a number of weeks to occur
SULPHONAMIDES	ANTIPSYCHOTICS – CLOZAPINE	↑ risk of bone marrow toxicity	Additive effect	Avoid co-administration
SULPHONAMIDES	**ANTIVIRALS**			
TRIMETHOPRIM	GANCICLOVIR/ VALGANCICLOVIR	Possibly ↑ adverse effects (e.g. myelosuppression) when trimethoprim is co-administered with ganciclovir or valganciclovir	Small ↑ in bioavailability; possible additive toxicity	Well tolerated in a study. For patients at risk of additive toxicities, use only if benefits outweigh risks, and monitor FBC closely
CO-TRIMOXAZOLE	NUCLEOSIDE REVERSE TRANSCRIPTASE INHIBITORS	↑ adverse effects	Additive toxicity	↓ doses as necessary; monitor FBC and renal function closely. Doses of co-trimoxazole used for prophylaxis seem to be tolerated
TRIMETHOPRIM	NUCLEOSIDE REVERSE TRANSCRIPTASE INHIBITORS	Possibly ↑ haematological toxicity	Competition for renal excretion	Monitor FBC and renal function closely
TRIMETHOPRIM, CO-TRIMOXAZOLE	CARDIAC GLYCOSIDES – DIGOXIN	Trimethoprim may ↑ plasma concentrations of digoxin, particularly in elderly people	Uncertain; postulated that trimethoprim ↓ renal clearance of digoxin	Monitor digoxin levels; watch for digoxin toxicity
TRIMETHOPRIM	DIURETICS – POTASSIUM-SPARING	Risk of hyperkalaemia when trimethoprim is co-administered with eplerenone	Additive effect	Monitor potassium levels closely

DRUGS TO TREAT INFECTIONS ANTIBIOTICS – SULPHONAMIDES

Primary drug	Secondary drug	Effect	Mechanism	Precautions
ANTIBIOTICS – CO-TRIMOXAZOLE	LOPERAMIDE	↑ loperamide levels but no evidence of toxicity	Inhibition of metabolism	Be aware
SULPHONAMIDES	OESTROGENS	Reports of ↓ contraceptive effect	Possibly alteration of the bacterial flora necessary for recycling ethinylestradiol from the large bowel, although not certain in every case	Advise patients to use additional contraception for the period of antibiotic intake and for 1 month after stopping the antibiotic
ANTIBIOTICS – TETRACYCLINES				
TETRACYCLINES	ANTACIDS	↓ levels of these antibiotics	↓ absorption	Separate tetracyclines and antacids by 2–3 hours
TETRACYCLINES	**ANTICANCER AND IMMUNOMODULATING DRUGS**			
DOXYCYCLINE	CICLOSPORIN	↑ levels of ciclosporin leading to risk of nephrotoxicity, hepatotoxicity and possibly neurotoxicity such as hallucinations, convulsions and coma	The mechanism is not known, but doxycycline is thought to ↑ ciclosporin levels	Concomitant use in transplant patients should be well monitored with frequent ciclosporin levels. In non-transplant patients, renal function should be monitored closely and patients warned about potential side-effects such as back pain, flushing and gastrointestinal upset. The dose of ciclosporin should be ↓ appropriately
DOXYCYCLINE, TETRACYCLINE	METHOTREXATE	↑ plasma concentrations of methotrexate, with a risk of toxic effects of methotrexate, e.g. liver cirrhosis, blood dyscrasias that may be fatal, pulmonary toxicity, stomatitis. Haematopoietic suppression can occur abruptly. Other adverse effects include anorexia, dyspepsia, gastrointestinal ulceration and bleeding, and pulmonary oedema	Tetracyclines destroy the bacterial flora necessary for the breakdown of methotrexate. This results in ↑ free methotrexate concentrations. Tetracyclines are also considered to inhibit the elimination of methotrexate and allow a build-up of methotrexate in the bladder. The effects of the interaction is often delayed	Although the toxic effects of methotrexate are more frequent with high doses of methotrexate, it is necessary to do FBC, liver and renal function tests before starting treatment even with low doses, repeating these tests weekly until therapy is stabilized and thereafter every 2–3 months. The patients should be advised to report symptoms such as sore throat and fever immediately, and also any gastrointestinal discomfort. A profound drop in white cell or platelet counts warrants immediate stoppage of methotrexate therapy and initiation of supportive therapy

TETRACYCLINES	PORFIMER	↑ risk of photosensitivity reactions	Attributed to additive effects	Avoid exposure of skin and eyes to direct sunlight for 30 days after porfimer therapy
TETRACYCLINE	RETINOIDS	Risk of benign intracranial hypertension with tetracycline	Unknown	Avoid co-administration
TETRACYCLINES	ANTICOAGULANTS – ORAL	Additive effects of warfarin and oxytetracycline, leading to prolongation of the prothrombin time or INR and bleeding	Tetracyclines have been associated with ↓ prothrombin activity, causing hypoprothrombinaemia and bleeding. Tetracyclines may also ↓ intestinal flora of the gut, depleting the body of vitamin K2; this may only be significant if the patient's diet is low in vitamin K1	Monitor INR closely and adjust the dose of warfarin accordingly. Patients should be alert for signs of overanticoagulation, bleeding from the gums when brushing their teeth, nosebleeds, unusual bruising and weakness
DOXYCYCLINE	ANTIEPILEPTICS – BARBITURATES, CARBAMAZEPINE, PHENYTOIN	↓ doxycycline levels, with risk of therapeutic failure	Induction of hepatic metabolism	Monitor for ↓ clinical efficacy and ↑ dose as required
TETRACYCLINES	ANTIHYPERTENSIVES AND HEART FAILURE DRUGS – ACE INHIBITORS	↓ plasma concentrations and efficacy of tetracyclines with quinapril	Magnesium carbonate (found in a formulation of quinapril) chelates with tetracyclines in the gut to form a less soluble substance that ↓ absorption of tetracycline	For short-term antibiotic use, consider stopping quinapril for the duration of the course. For long-term use, consider an alternative ACE inhibitor
TETRACYCLINE	ANTIMALARIALS – ATOVAQUONE	↓ atovaquone levels (40%)	Uncertain	Not clinically significant; combination therapy has been used effectively
TETRACYCLINES	ANTIMIGRAINE DRUGS – ERGOT DERIVATIVES	Cases of ergotism with tetracyclines and ergotamine	Uncertain	Avoid co-administration. If absolutely necessary, advise patients to discontinue treatment immediately if numbness and tingling of the extremities are felt

DRUGS TO TREAT INFECTIONS ANTIBIOTICS – TETRACYCLINES

Primary drug	Secondary drug	Effect	Mechanism	Precautions
TETRACYCLINES	ANTIVIRALS – DIDANOSINE	↓ efficacy of tetracycline, and possibly demeclocycline, doxycycline, lymecycline, minocycline and oxytetracycline, with buffered didanosine	Absorption may be affected by the buffered didanosine formulation, which ↑ gastric pH	Avoid co-administration with buffered didanosine preparations. Consider changing to enteric-coated didanosine tablets
TETRACYCLINES	CALCIUM	↓ antibiotic levels	↓ absorption	Separate doses by at least 2 hours
TETRACYCLINES	DAIRY PRODUCTS	↓ antibiotic levels	↓ absorption (due to the calcium content of dairy produce)	Separate doses by at least 2 hours
TETRACYCLINES	DIURETICS	Possible risk of renal toxicity	Additive effect	Some recommend avoiding co-administration; others advise monitoring renal function closely. Doxycycline is likely to be less of a problem
DOXYCYCLINE	H2 RECEPTOR BLOCKERS	↓ plasma concentrations and risk of treatment failure	↓ absorption of cephalosporin as ↑ gastric pH	Avoid concomitant use. If unable to avoid combination, take H2 antagonists at least 2–3 hours after cephalosporin. Consider an alternative antibiotic or separate the doses by at least 2 hours and give with an acidic drink, e.g. carbonated drink; ↑ dose may be required
TETRACYCLINES	IRON – ORAL	1. ↓ iron levels when iron given orally 2. ↓ plasma concentrations of these drugs, with risk of therapeutic failure	1. ↓ absorption 2. Iron chelates with tetracyclines and ↓ their absorption	1. Separate doses as much as possible – monitor FBC closely 2. Separate doses of other drugs as much as possible and monitor their effect
TETRACYCLINES	KAOLIN	↓ tetracycline levels	↓ absorption	Separate doses by at least 2 hours
TETRACYCLINE	LIPID-LOWERING DRUGS – ANION EXCHANGE RESINS	↓ levels of tetracycline and possible therapeutic failure	Tetracycline binds with colestipol and colestyramine in the gut therefore ↓ its absorption	Dosing should be as separate as possible

DRUGS TO TREAT INFECTIONS ANTIBIOTICS – TETRACYCLINES

TETRACYCLINES	OESTROGENS	Reports of ↓ contraceptive effect	Possibly alteration of the bacterial flora necessary for recycling ethinylestradiol from the large bowel, although not certain in every case	Advise patients to use additional contraception for the period of antibiotic intake and for 1 month after stopping the antibiotic
TETRACYCLINE	SODIUM BICARBONATE	↓ tetracycline levels and possible therapeutic failure	It is suggested that when sodium bicarbonate alkalinizes the urine, the renal excretion of tetracycline is ↑	The interaction can be minimized by separating their dosing by 3–4 hours
TETRACYCLINES	STRONTIUM RANELATE	↓ levels of these antibiotics	↓ absorption	Avoid co-administration
TETRACYCLINES	SUCRALFATE	↓ levels of these antibiotics	↓ absorption of these antibiotics	Give the antibiotics at least 2 hours before sucralfate
TETRACYCLINES	TRIPOTASSIUM DICITRATOBISMUTHATE	↓ levels of tetracyclines	↓ absorption of tetracyclines	Separate doses by 2–3 hours
TETRACYCLINES	ZINC	↓ antibiotic levels; less of a problem with doxycycline	↓ absorption	Separate doses by at least 2 hours; alternatively, consider giving doxycycline
OTHER ANTIBIOTICS				
CHLORAMPHENICOL				
CHLORAMPHENICOL	ANTICANCER AND IMMUNOMODULATING DRUGS – TACROLIMUS	Toxic blood levels of tacrolimus, usually on the second day of starting chloramphenicol	Attributed to impaired clearance of tacrolimus by chloramphenicol	↓ dose of nearly 80% of tacrolimus may be required to prevent toxicity. Watch for adverse effects (see below). Monitor tacrolimus plasma concentrations
CHLORAMPHENICOL	ANTICOAGULANTS – ORAL	Occasional episodes of ↑ anticoagulant effect	Uncertain at present	Monitor INR every 2–3 days
CHLORAMPHENICOL	ANTIDIABETIC DRUGS – SULPHONYLUREAS	Possibly ↓ hypoglycaemic effect of sulphonylureas	Mechanism uncertain. Chloramphenicol is an inhibitor of CYP3A4	Be aware

Primary drug	Secondary drug	Effect	Mechanism	Precautions
CHLORAMPHENICOL	ANTIEPILEPTICS			
CHLORAMPHENICOL	BARBITURATES	↓ levels of these drugs, with risk of therapeutic failure	Induction of hepatic metabolism	1. Avoid co-administration of telithromycin for up to 2 weeks after stopping phenobarbital 2. With the other drugs, monitor for ↓ clinical efficacy, and ↑ their dose as required
CHLORAMPHENICOL	PHENYTOIN	↑ phenytoin levels	Inhibited metabolism	Monitor phenytoin levels
CHLORAMPHENICOL	ANTIPSYCHOTICS – CLOZAPINE	↑ risk of bone marrow toxicity	Additive effect	Avoid co-administration
CHLORAMPHENICOL	ANTIVIRALS – STAVUDINE, ZIDOVUDINE	Possible ↑ adverse effects when co-administered with stavudine or zidovudine	Uncertain	Use an alternative antibiotic if possible; otherwise monitor closely for peripheral neuropathy and check FBC regularly
CHLORAMPHENICOL	CNS STIMULANTS – MODAFINIL	May cause moderate ↑ plasma concentrations of these substrates	Modafinil is a reversible inhibitor of CYP2C19 when used in therapeutic doses	Be aware
CHLORAMPHENICOL	H2 RECEPTOR BLOCKERS – CIMETIDINE	↑ adverse effects of chloramphenicol, e.g. bone marrow depression	Additive toxicity	Use with caution, monitor FBC regularly
CHLORAMPHENICOL	IRON	↓ efficacy of iron	Chloramphenicol depresses the bone marrow; this opposes the action of iron	Be aware; monitor FBC and ferritin levels closely
CHLORAMPHENICOL	OESTROGENS	Reports of ↓ contraceptive effect	Possibly alteration of the bacterial flora necessary for recycling ethinylestradiol from the large bowel, although not certain in every case	Advise patients to use additional contraception for the period of antibiotic intake and for 1 month after stopping the antibiotic
CHLORAMPHENICOL	VITAMIN B12	↓ efficacy of hydroxycobalamin	Chloramphenicol depresses the bone marrow; this opposes the action of vitamin B12	Be aware; monitor FBC and vitamin B12 levels closely

DRUGS TO TREAT INFECTIONS OTHER ANTIBIOTICS

CLINDAMYCIN				
CLINDAMYCIN	MUSCLE RELAXANTS – DEPOLARIZING, NON-DEPOLARIZING	↑ efficacy of these muscle relaxants	Clindamycin has some neuromuscular blocking activity	Monitor neuromuscular blockade carefully
CLINDAMYCIN	OESTROGENS	Reports of ↓ contraceptive effect	Possibly alteration of the bacterial flora necessary for recycling ethinylestradiol from the large bowel, although not certain in every case	Advise patients to use additional contraception for the period of antibiotic intake and for 1 month after stopping the antibiotic
CLINDAMYCIN	PARASYMPATHOMIMETICS – NEOSTIGMINE, PYRIDOSTIGMINE	↓ efficacy of neostigmine and pyridostigmine	Uncertain	Watch for poor response to these parasympathomimetics and ↑ dose accordingly
COLISTIN				
COLISTIN	**ANTIBIOTICS**			
COLISTIN	AMINOGLYCOSIDES	↑ risk of nephrotoxicity	Additive effect	Renal function should be carefully monitored
COLISTIN	TEICOPLANIN, VANCOMYCIN	↑ risk of nephrotoxicity and ototoxicity	Additive effect	Hearing and renal function should be carefully monitored
COLISTIN	**ANTICANCER AND IMMUNOMODULATING DRUGS**			
COLISTIN	CICLOSPORIN	↑ risk of nephrotoxicity	Additive nephrotoxic effects	Monitor renal function
COLISTIN	PLATINUM COMPOUNDS	↑ risk of additive renal and ototoxicity. The ototoxicity tends to occur when cisplatin is administered early during the course of aminoglycoside therapy	Additive toxic effects	Monitor renal function and hearing prior to and during therapy, and ensure the intake of at least 2 L of fluid daily. Monitor serum potassium and magnesium and correct any deficiencies. Most side-effects of aminoglycosides are dose related, and it is necessary to ↑ interval between doses and ↓ dose of aminoglycoside if there is impaired renal function

Primary drug	Secondary drug	Effect	Mechanism	Precautions
COLISTIN	ANTIFUNGALS – AMPHOTERICIN	Risk of renal failure	Additive effect	Monitor renal function closely
COLISTIN	DIURETICS – LOOP	↑ risk of ototoxicity and possible deafness as a result of concomitant use of furosemide and colistin	Additive effect	If used concurrently, patients should be monitored for any hearing impairment
COLISTIN	MUSCLE RELAXANTS – DEPOLARIZING, NON-DEPOLARIZING	↑ efficacy of these muscle relaxants	Colistin has some neuromuscular blocking activity	Monitor neuromuscular blockade carefully
COLISTIN	PARASYMPATHOMIMETICS – NEOSTIGMINE, PYRIDOSTIGMINE	↓ efficacy of neostigmine and pyridostigmine	Uncertain	Watch for poor response to these parasympathomimetics and ↑ dose accordingly
CYCLOSERINE				
CYCLOSERINE	ALCOHOL	Risk of fits	Additive effect; cycloserine can cause fits	Warn patients to drink alcohol minimally while taking cycloserine
CYCLOSERINE	ISONIAZID	Risk of drowsiness and dizziness	Uncertain	Be aware; watch for ↑ sedation
DAPSONE				
DAPSONE	ANTIBIOTICS			
DAPSONE	RIFAMYCINS	↓ levels of dapsone	Rifamycins induce metabolism of dapsone	Watch for poor response to dapsone
DAPSONE	TRIMETHOPRIM	↑ levels of both drugs	Mutual inhibition of metabolism	Be aware – watch for ↑ incidence of side-effects
DAPSONE	ANTICANCER DRUGS – PORFIMER	↑ risk of photosensitivity reactions	Attributed to additive effects	Avoid exposure of skin and eyes to direct sunlight for 30 days after porfimer therapy
DAPSONE	ANTIGOUT DRUGS – PROBENECID	↑ dapsone levels, with risk of bone marrow suppression	Uncertain	Monitor FBC closely

DRUGS TO TREAT INFECTIONS OTHER ANTIBIOTICS

DAPSONE	ANTIVIRALS – ZIDOVUDINE	Possible ↑ adverse effects when co-administered with zidovudine	Uncertain; possible ↑ bioavailability of zidovudine	Use with caution; monitor for peripheral neuropathy
DAPTOMYCIN				
DAPTOMYCIN	ANTICANCER DRUGS – CICLOSPORIN	Risk of myopathy	Additive effect	Avoid co-administration
DAPTOMYCIN	LIPID-LOWERING DRUGS – FIBRATES, STATINS	Risk of myopathy	Additive effect	Avoid co-administration
ETHAMBUTOL				
ETHAMBUTOL	ANTIVIRALS – DIDANOSINE	Possibly ↑ adverse effects (e.g. peripheral neuropathy) with didanosine	Additive side-effects	Monitor closely for development of peripheral neuropathy but no dose adjustment is required
FUSIDIC ACID				
FUSIDIC ACID	ANTIVIRALS – PROTEASE INHIBITORS	Possibly ↑ adverse effects	Inhibition of CYP3A4-mediated metabolism of fusidic acid	Avoid co-administration
FUSIDIC ACID	LIPID-LOWERING DRUGS – STATINS	Cases of rhabdomyolysis reported when fusidic acid was co-administered with atorvastatin or simvastatin	Uncertain at present	Monitor LFTs and CK closely; warn patients to report any features of rhabdomyolysis
ISONIAZID				
ISONIAZID	ANALGESICS – PARACETAMOL	Risk of paracetamol toxicity at regular therapeutic doses when co-administered with isoniazid	Uncertain; it seems that the formation of toxic metabolites is ↑ in fast acetylators when isoniazid levels ↓ (i.e. at the end of a dosing period)	There have been cases of hepatic pathology; regular paracetamol should be avoided in those taking isoniazid
ISONIAZID	ANTACIDS	↓ levels of these antibiotics	↓ absorption	Separate isoniazid and antacids by 2–3 hours
ISONIAZID	ANTIBIOTICS – CYCLOSERINE	Risk of drowsiness and dizziness	Uncertain	Be aware; watch for ↑ sedation

Primary drug	Secondary drug	Effect	Mechanism	Precautions
ISONIAZID	ANTIDIABETIC DRUGS	↓ efficacy of antidiabetic drugs	Isoniazid causes hyperglycaemia, the mechanism being uncertain at present	Monitor capillary blood glucose levels closely; ↑ doses of antidiabetic drugs may be needed
ISONIAZID	**ANTIEPILEPTICS**			
ISONIAZID	CARBAMAZEPINE	↑ carbamazepine levels	Inhibited metabolism	Monitor carbamazepine levels
ISONIAZID	ETHOSUXIMIDE	Case of ↑ ethosuximide levels with toxicity	Inhibition of metabolism	Watch for early features of ethosuximide toxicity
ISONIAZID	PHENYTOIN	↑ phenytoin levels	Inhibited metabolism	Monitor phenytoin levels
ISONIAZID	ANTIFUNGALS – ITRACONAZOLE, KETOCONAZOLE, POSACONAZOLE, VORICONAZOLE	↓ levels of these azoles, with significant risk of therapeutic failure	Isoniazid is a known inhibitor of CYP2E1 and is likely to induce other CYP isoenzymes to varying degrees, usually in a time-dependent manner	Avoid co-administration of ketoconazole or voriconazole with isoniazid. Watch for inadequate therapeutic effects of itraconazole. Higher doses of itraconazole may not overcome this interaction, so consider the use of less lipophilic fluconazole, which is less dependent on CYP metabolism
ISONIAZID	ANTIVIRALS – NUCLEOSIDE REVERSE TRANSCRIPTASE INHIBITORS	↑ adverse effects with didanosine and possibly stavudine	Additive side-effects	Monitor closely for the development of peripheral neuropathy, but no dose adjustment is required
ISONIAZID	ANXIOLYTICS AND HYPNOTICS – DIAZEPAM	↑ diazepam levels	Inhibited metabolism	Watch for excessive sedation; consider ↓ dose of diazepam
ISONIAZID	BRONCHODILATORS – THEOPHYLLINE	↑ theophylline levels	Uncertain	Monitor theophylline levels before, during and after co-administration

LINEZOLID ➢ *Drugs Acting on the Nervous System, Antidepressants, Monoamine oxidase inhibitors*

DRUGS TO TREAT INFECTIONS OTHER ANTIBIOTICS

METHENAMINE				
METHENAMINE	ANTIBIOTICS – SULPHONAMIDES – SULFADIAZINE	Risk of crystalluria	Methenamine is only effective at a low pH, and this is achieved by acidifiers in the formulation. Sulfadiazine crystallizes in an acid environment	Avoid co-administration
METHENAMINE	DIURETICS – CARBONIC ANHYDRASE INHIBITORS	↓ efficacy of methenamine	Methenamine is only effective at a low pH; raising the urinary pH ↓ its effect	Avoid co-administration
METHENAMINE	POTASSIUM CITRATE	↓ efficacy of methenamine	Methenamine is only effective at a low pH; raising the urinary pH ↓ its effect	Avoid co-administration
METHENAMINE	SODIUM BICARBONATE	↓ efficacy of methenamine	Methenamine is only effective at a low pH; raising the urinary pH ↓ its effect	Avoid co-administration
METRONIDAZOLE				
METRONIDAZOLE	ALCOHOL	Disulfiram-like reaction	Metronidazole inhibits aldehyde dehydrogenase	Avoid co-ingestion
METRONIDAZOLE	ANTICANCER AND IMMUNOMODULATING DRUGS			
METRONIDAZOLE	BUSULFAN	↑ busulfan levels	Uncertain	Watch for early features of toxicity
METRONIDAZOLE	FLUOROURACIL	↑ risk of toxic effects of fluorouracil (>27%), e.g. bone marrow suppression, oral ulceration, nausea and vomiting due to ↑ plasma concentrations of fluorouracil	Metronidazole ↓ clearance of fluorouracil	Avoid co-administration

Primary drug	Secondary drug	Effect	Mechanism	Precautions
METRONIDAZOLE	MYCOPHENOLATE	Likely ↓ in plasma concentration of mycophenolate	Theoretically, drugs that alter gastrointestinal flora may ↓ oral bioavailability of mycophenolic acid products by ↓ bacterial hydrolytic enzymes that are responsible for regenerating mycophenolic acid from its glucuronide metabolites following first-pass metabolism	Avoid co-administration
METRONIDAZOLE	ANTICOAGULANTS – ORAL	↑ anticoagulant effect	Inhibition of CYP2C9-mediated metabolism of oral anticoagulants	Monitor INR every 2–3 days
METRONIDAZOLE	ANTIDEPRESSANTS – LITHIUM	↑ plasma concentrations of lithium, with risk of toxicity	Uncertain	Monitor clinically and by measuring blood lithium levels for lithium toxicity
METRONIDAZOLE	**ANTIEPILEPTICS**			
METRONIDAZOLE	BARBITURATES	↓ levels of these drugs, with risk of therapeutic failure	Induction of hepatic metabolism. Unlikely with topical metronidazole	1. Avoid co-administration of telithromycin for up to 2 weeks after stopping phenobarbital
METRONIDAZOLE	PHENYTOIN	↑ phenytoin levels	Inhibited metabolism	Monitor phenytoin levels
METRONIDAZOLE	**ANTIVIRALS**			
METRONIDAZOLE	DIDANOSINE, STAVUDINE	↑ adverse effects (e.g. peripheral neuropathy) with didanosine and possibly stavudine	Additive effect	Monitor closely for peripheral neuropathy during intensive or prolonged combination

METRONIDAZOLE	PROTEASE INHIBITORS	↑ adverse effects, e.g. disulfiram-like reaction, flushing, with ritonavir (with or without lopinavir)	Ritonavir and lopinavir oral solutions contain alcohol	Warn patient and give alternative preparation if possible
METRONIDAZOLE	DRUG DEPENDENCE THERAPIES – DISULFIRAM	Report of psychosis	Additive effect; both drugs may cause neurological/psychiatric side-effects (disulfiram by inhibiting metabolism of dopamine, metronidazole by an unknown mechanism)	Caution with co-administration. Warn patients and carers to watch for early features
METRONIDAZOLE	H2 RECEPTOR BLOCKERS – CIMETIDINE	↑ metronidazole levels	Inhibited metabolism	Watch for ↑ side-effects of metronidazole
METRONIDAZOLE	OESTROGENS	Reports of ↓ contraceptive effect	Possibly alteration of the bacterial flora necessary for recycling ethinylestradiol from the large bowel, although not certain in every case	Advise patients to use additional contraception for the period of antibiotic intake and for 1 month after stopping the antibiotic
NITROFURANTOIN				
NITROFURANTOIN	ANTACIDS	↓ levels of these antibiotics	↓ absorption	Separate nitrofurantoin and antacids by 2–3 hours
NITROFURANTOIN	ANTIGOUT DRUGS – PROBENECID, SULFINPYRAZONE	↓ efficacy of nitrofurantoin in urinary tract infections	↓ urinary excretion	Watch for poor response to nitrofurantoin
PYRAZINAMIDE				
PYRAZINAMIDE	ANTIGOUT DRUGS	↓ efficacy of antigout drugs	Pyrazinamide can induce hyperuricaemia	Pyrazinamide should not be used in patients with gout

Primary drug	Secondary drug	Effect	Mechanism	Precautions
QUINUPRISTIN/DALFOPRISTIN				
QUINUPRISTIN/ DALFOPRISTIN	DRUGS THAT PROLONG THE Q–T INTERVAL			
QUINUPRISTIN/ DALFOPRISTIN	1. ANTIARRHYTHMICS – amiodarone, disopyramide, procainamide, propafenone 2. ANTIBIOTICS – macrolides (especially azithromycin, clarithromycin, parenteral erythromycin, telithromycin), quinolones (especially moxifloxacin) 3. ANTICANCER AND IMMUNOMODULATING DRUGS – arsenic trioxide 4. ANTIDEPRESSANTS – TCAs, venlafaxine 5. ANTIEMETICS – dolasetron 6. ANTIFUNGALS – fluconazole, posaconazole, voriconazole 7. ANTIHISTAMINES – terfenadine, hydroxyzine, mizolastine 8. ANTIMALARIALS – artemether with lumefantrine, chloroquine, hydroxychloroquine, mefloquine, quinine 9. ANTIPROTOZOALS – pentamidine isetionate 10. ANTIPSYCHOTICS – atypicals, phenothiazines, pimozide 11. BETA-BLOCKERS – sotalol 12. BRONCHODILATORS – parenteral bronchodilators 13. CNS STIMULANTS – atomoxetine	Risk of ventricular arrhythmias, particularly torsades de pointes	Additive effect; these drugs cause prolongation of the Q–T interval	Avoid co-administration

QUINUPRISTIN/ DALFOPRISTIN	ANAESTHETICS – LOCAL – LIDOCAINE	Risk of arrhythmias	Additive effect when lidocaine given intravenously	Avoid co-administration of quinupristin/dalfopristin with intravenous lidocaine
QUINUPRISTIN/ DALFOPRISTIN	ANTIBIOTICS – RIFAMPICIN	Risk of hepatic toxicity	Additive effect	Monitor LFTs closely
QUINUPRISTIN/ DALFOPRISTIN	ANTICANCER AND IMMUNOMODULATING DRUGS – CICLOSPORIN	↑ plasma concentrations of immunosuppressants. ↑ risk of infections and toxic effects of ciclosporin	Due to inhibition of CYP3A4-mediated metabolism of ciclosporin	Monitor renal function prior to concurrent therapy, and blood count and ciclosporin levels during therapy. Warn patients to report symptoms (fever, sore throat) immediately
QUINUPRISTIN/ DALFOPRISTIN	ANTIMIGRAINE DRUGS – ERGOT DERIVATIVES	↑ ergotamine/methysergide levels, with risk of toxicity	Inhibition of CYP3A4-mediated metabolism of the ergot derivatives	Avoid co-administration
QUINUPRISTIN/ DALFOPRISTIN	ANXIOLYTICS AND HYPNOTICS – MIDAZOLAM	↑ midazolam levels	Inhibited metabolism	Watch for excessive sedation; consider ↓ dose of midazolam
QUINUPRISTIN/ DALFOPRISTIN	CALCIUM CHANNEL BLOCKERS	Plasma levels of nifedipine may be ↑ by quinupristin/ dalfopristin	Quinupristin inhibits CYP3A4-mediated metabolism of calcium channel blockers	Monitor BP closely; watch for ↓ BP
TEICOPLANIN				
TEICOPLANIN	ANTIBIOTICS – AMINOGLYCOSIDES, COLISTIN, VANCOMYCIN	↑ risk of nephrotoxicity and ototoxicity	Additive effect	Hearing and renal function should be carefully monitored
VANCOMYCIN				
VANCOMYCIN	ANTIBIOTICS – AMINOGLYCOSIDES, COLISTIN, TEICOPLANIN	↑ risk of nephrotoxicity and ototoxicity	Additive effect	Hearing and renal function should be carefully monitored

Primary drug	Secondary drug	Effect	Mechanism	Precautions
VANCOMYCIN	ANTICANCER AND IMMUNOMODULATING DRUGS			
VANCOMYCIN	CICLOSPORIN	Risk of renal toxicity and ototoxicity	Additive toxic effects	Monitor renal function closely
VANCOMYCIN	PLATINUM COMPOUNDS	↑ risk of renal toxicity and renal failure, and of ototoxicity	Additive renal toxicity	Monitor renal function and hearing prior to and during therapy, and ensure the intake of at least 2 L of fluid daily. Monitor serum potassium and magnesium, and correct any deficiencies
VANCOMYCIN	TACROLIMUS	Risk of renal toxicity	Additive effect	Monitor renal function closely
VANCOMYCIN	ANTIFUNGALS – AMPHOTERICIN	Risk of renal failure	Additive effect	Monitor renal function closely
VANCOMYCIN	ANTIVIRALS			
VANCOMYCIN	ADEFOVIR DIPIVOXIL	Possible ↑ efficacy and side-effects	Competition for renal excretion	Monitor renal function weekly
VANCOMYCIN	NUCLEOSIDE REVERSE TRANSCRIPTASE INHIBITORS – TENOFOVIR, ZIDOVUDINE	↑ adverse effects with zidovudine and possibly tenofovir	Additive toxicity	Monitor FBC and renal function closely (at least weekly)
VANCOMYCIN	DIURETICS – LOOP	Risk of renal toxicity	Additive effect	Monitor renal function closely
VANCOMYCIN (ORAL)	LIPID-LOWERING DRUGS – ANION EXCHANGE RESINS	↓ vancomycin levels	Inhibition of absorption	Separate doses as much as possible

VANCOMYCIN	MUSCLE RELAXANTS – DEPOLARIZING, NON-DEPOLARIZING	1. ↑ efficacy of these muscle relaxants 2. Possible risk of hypersensitivity reactions	1. Vancomycin has some neuromuscular blocking activity 2. Animal studies suggest an additive effect on histamine release	1. Monitor neuromuscular blockade carefully 2. Be aware
VANCOMYCIN	SYMPATHOMIMETICS	Vancomycin levels are ↓ by dobutamine or dopamine	Uncertain at present	Monitor vancomycin levels closely
ANTIFUNGAL DRUGS				
AMPHOTERICIN				
AMPHOTERICIN	ANAESTHETICS – LOCAL – LIDOCAINE AND PROCAINE SOLUTIONS	Precipitation of drugs, which may not be immediately apparent	A pharmaceutical interaction	Do not mix in the same infusion or syringe
AMPHOTERICIN	ANTIBIOTICS – AMINOGLYCOSIDES, COLISTIN, VANCOMYCIN	Risk of renal failure	Additive effect	Monitor renal function closely
AMPHOTERICIN	**ANTICANCER AND IMMUNOMODULATING DRUGS**			
AMPHOTERICIN	CYTOTOXICS – PLATINUM COMPOUNDS	↑ risk of renal toxicity and renal failure	Additive renal toxicity	Monitor renal function prior to and during therapy, and ensure the intake of at least 2 L of fluid daily. Monitor serum potassium and magnesium, and correct any deficiencies
AMPHOTERICIN	**IMMUNOMODULATING DRUGS**			
AMPHOTERICIN	CICLOSPORIN	↑ risk of nephrotoxicity	Additive nephrotoxic effects	Monitor renal function
AMPHOTERICIN	CORTICOSTEROIDS	Risk of hyperkalaemia	Additive effect	Avoid co-administration

DRUGS TO TREAT INFECTIONS ANTIFUNGAL DRUGS

Primary drug	Secondary drug	Effect	Mechanism	Precautions
AMPHOTERICIN	TACROLIMUS	Risk of renal toxicity	Additive effect	Monitor renal function closely
AMPHOTERICIN	ANTIFUNGALS – FLUCYTOSINE	↑ flucytosine levels, with risk of toxic effects	Amphotericin causes ↓ renal excretion of flucytosine and ↑ cellular uptake	The combination of flucytosine and amphotericin may be used therapeutically. Watch for early features of flucytosine toxicity (gastrointestinal upset); monitor renal and liver function closely
AMPHOTERICIN	ANTIPROTOZOALS – PENTAMIDINE ISETIONATE	Risk of arrhythmias	Additive effect	Monitor ECG closely
AMPHOTERICIN	**ANTIVIRALS**			
AMPHOTERICIN	ADEFOVIR DIPIVOXIL	Possible ↑ efficacy and side-effects	Competition for renal excretion	Monitor renal function weekly
AMPHOTERICIN	FOSCARNET SODIUM	Possible ↑ nephrotoxicity	Additive side-effect	Monitor renal function closely
AMPHOTERICIN	NUCLEOSIDE REVERSE TRANSCRIPTASE INHIBITORS – TENOFOVIR, ZIDOVUDINE	Possibly ↑ adverse effects with tenofovir and zidovudine	Additive toxicity	Avoid if possible; otherwise monitor FBC and renal function (weekly). ↓ doses as necessary
AMPHOTERICIN	CARDIAC GLYCOSIDES – DIGOXIN	Risk of digoxin toxicity due to hypokalaemia	Amphotericin may cause hypokalaemia	Monitor potassium levels closely. Monitor digoxin levels; watch for digoxin toxicity
AMPHOTERICIN	DIURETICS – LOOP DIURETICS AND THIAZIDES	Risk of hypokalaemia	Additive effect	Monitor potassium closely

AZOLES

AZOLES	DRUGS THAT PROLONG THE Q–T INTERVAL			
FLUCONAZOLE, POSACONAZOLE, VORICONAZOLE	1. ANTIARRHYTHMICS – amiodarone, disopyramide, procainamide, propafenone 2. ANTIBIOTICS – macrolides (especially azithromycin, clarithromycin, parenteral erythromycin, telithromycin), quinolones (especially moxifloxacin), quinupristin/dalfopristin 3. ANTICANCER AND IMMUNOMODULATING DRUGS – arsenic trioxide 4. ANTIDEPRESSANTS – TCAs, venlafaxine 5. ANTIEMETICS – dolasetron 6. ANTIHISTAMINES – terfenadine, hydroxyzine, mizolastine 7. ANTIMALARIALS – artemether with lumefantrine, chloroquine, hydroxychloroquine, mefloquine, quinine 8. ANTIPROTOZOALS – pentamidine isetionate 9. ANTIPSYCHOTICS – atypicals, phenothiazines, pimozide 10. BETA-BLOCKERS – sotalol 11. BRONCHODILATORS – parenteral bronchodilators 12. CNS STIMULANTS – atomoxetine	Risk of ventricular arrhythmias, particularly torsades de pointes	Additive effect; these drugs cause prolongation of the Q–T interval	Avoid co-administration
KETOCONAZOLE	ALISKIREN	Aliskiren levels ↑ by ketoconazole	Uncertain	Monitor BP and serum potassium at least weekly until stable

DRUGS TO TREAT INFECTIONS ANTIFUNGAL DRUGS

Primary drug	Secondary drug	Effect	Mechanism	Precautions
FLUCONAZOLE	ANALGESICS			
FLUCONAZOLE	NSAIDs	Fluconazole ↑ celecoxib and possibly parecoxib levels	Fluconazole inhibits CYP2C9-mediated metabolism of celecoxib and parecoxib	Halve the dose of celecoxib, and start parecoxib at the lowest dose
FLUCONAZOLE, ITRACONAZOLE, KETOCONAZOLE, VORICONAZOLE	OPIOIDS	1. Ketoconazole ↑ effect of buprenorphine 2. Fluconazole and itraconazole ↑ effect of alfentanil 3. Fluconazole and possibly voriconazole ↑ effect of methadone; recognized pharmacokinetic effect but uncertain clinical significance	1. Ketoconazole ↓ CYP3A4-mediated metabolism of buprenorphine 2. ↓ clearance of alfentanil 3. ↓ hepatic metabolism	1. The dose of buprenorphine needs to be ↓ (by up to 50%). 2. ↓ dose of alfentanil 3. Watch for ↑ effects of methadone
AZOLES	ANTACIDS	↓ plasma concentration of itraconazole and ketoconazole, with risk of therapeutic failure	Itraconazole absorption in capsule form requires an acidic gastric environment and thus absorption would ↓	Separate administration of agents that ↓ gastric acidity by 1–2 hours. However, absorption of itraconazole liquid solution does not require an acidic environment and could be used instead; it does not need to be given with food. Fluconazole absorption is not pH dependent, and this is a suitable alternative
ITRACONAZOLE	ANTIBIOTICS			
ITRACONAZOLE, KETOCONAZOLE, VORICONAZOLE	CLARITHROMYCIN, CLOTRIMAZOLE, ERYTHROMYCIN, TELITHROMYCIN	↑ plasma concentrations of itraconazole and ketoconazole, and risk of toxic effects	These antibiotics are inhibitors of metabolism of itraconazole by CYP3A4. Erythromycin is a weaker inhibitor than clarithromycin. The role of clarithromycin and erythromycin as inhibitors of P-gp is not known with certainty. Ketoconazole is a potent inhibitor of P-gp	Monitor LFTs closely. Azithromycin is not affected

ITRACONAZOLE, KETOCONAZOLE, POSACONAZOLE, VORICONAZOLE	ISONIAZID, RIFAMPICIN, RIFABUTIN, RIFAPENTINE	↓ levels of these azoles, with significant risk of therapeutic failure. Rifampicin is a very potent inducer that can produce undetectable concentrations of ketoconazole	Rifampicin is a powerful inducer of CYP3A4 and other CYP isoenzymes. Rifabutin is a less powerful inducer but more potent than rifapentine. Rifapentine is an inducer of CYP3A4 and CYP2C8/9. Isoniazid is a known inhibitor of CYP2E1 and is likely to induce other CYP isoenzymes to varying degrees, usually in a time-dependent manner. Rifampicin is also a powerful inducer of P-gp, thus ↓ bioavailability of itraconazole	Avoid co-administration of ketoconazole or voriconazole with these drugs. Watch for inadequate therapeutic effects of itraconazole. Higher doses of itraconazole may not overcome this interaction, so consider use of less lipophilic fluconazole, which is less dependent on CYP metabolism. Avoid co-administration of posaconazole with rifabutin
VORICONAZOLE	RIFABUTIN	↑ plasma concentrations of rifabutin, with risk of toxic effects of rifabutin (nausea, vomiting). Dangerous toxic effects such as leukopenia and thrombocytopenia may occur	Due to inhibition of metabolism of rifabutin by the CYP3A4 isoenzymes by voriconazole	Avoid concomitant use. If absolutely necessary, close monitoring of FBC, liver enzymes and examination of eyes for uveitis and corneal opacities are necessary
AZOLES	**ANTICANCER AND IMMUNOMODULATING DRUGS**			
AZOLES	**CYTOTOXICS**			
ITRACONAZOLE, KETOCONAZOLE	BUSULFAN	↑ busulfan levels, with risk of toxicity of busulfan, e.g. veno-occlusive disease and pulmonary fibrosis	Itraconazole is a potent inhibitor of CYP3A4. Busulfan clearance may be ↓ by 25% and the AUC of busulfan may ↑ by 1500 μmol/min	Dose adjustments are necessary if concomitant administration is considered absolutely necessary; best, however, to avoid concomitant use. Monitor clinically for veno-occlusive disease and pulmonary toxicity in transplant patients. Monitor busulfan blood levels as an AUC below 1500 μmol/min tends to prevent toxicity

Primary drug	Secondary drug	Effect	Mechanism	Precautions
FLUCONAZOLE, ITRACONAZOLE, KETOCONAZOLE, VORICONAZOLE	DOXORUBICIN	↑ risk of myelosuppression due to ↑ plasma concentration of doxorubicin	Due to ↓ metabolism of doxorubicin by CYP3A4 isoenzymes owing to inhibition of those enzymes	Monitor for ↑ myelosuppression, peripheral neuropathy, myalgias and fatigue
FLUCONAZOLE, ITRACONAZOLE, KETOCONAZOLE, VORICONAZOLE	ERLOTINIB	↑ erlotinib levels	↓ metabolism of erlotinib	Avoid co-administration
FLUCONAZOLE, ITRACONAZOLE, KETOCONAZOLE, VORICONAZOLE	IFOSFAMIDE	↓ plasma concentrations of 4-hydroxyifosfamide, the active metabolite of ifosfamide, and risk of inadequate therapeutic response	Due to inhibition of the isoenzymatic conversion to active metabolites	Monitor clinically the efficacy of ifosfamide, and ↑ dose accordingly
FLUCONAZOLE, ITRACONAZOLE, KETOCONAZOLE, VORICONAZOLE	IMATINIB	↑ plasma concentrations of imatinib, with ↑ risk of toxicity (e.g. abdominal pain, constipation, dyspnoea) and neurotoxicity (e.g. taste disturbances, dizziness, headache, paraesthesia, peripheral neuropathy)	Due to inhibition of CYP3A4-mediated metabolism of imatinib	Monitor for clinical efficacy and for the signs of toxicity listed, along with convulsions, confusion and signs of oedema (including pulmonary oedema). Monitor electrolytes, liver function and for cardiotoxicity
FLUCONAZOLE, ITRACONAZOLE, KETOCONAZOLE, VORICONAZOLE	IRINOTECAN	↑ plasma concentrations of SN-38 (>AUC by 100%) and ↑ toxicity of irinotecan, e.g. diarrhoea, acute cholinergic syndrome, interstitial pulmonary disease	Due to inhibition of the metabolism of irinotecan by CYP3A4 isoenzymes by ketoconazole	Peripheral blood counts should be checked before each course of treatment. Monitor lung function. Recommendation is to ↓ dose of irinotecan by 25%
FLUCONAZOLE, ITRACONAZOLE, KETOCONAZOLE, VORICONAZOLE (POSSIBLY POSACONAZOLE)	VINCA ALKALOIDS – VINBLASTINE, VINCRISTINE, VINORELBINE	↑ adverse effects of vinblastine and vincristine	Inhibition of CYP3A4-mediated metabolism. Also inhibition of P-gp efflux of vinblastine	Monitor FBCs and watch for early features of toxicity (pain, numbness, tingling in the fingers and toes, jaw pain, abdominal pain, constipation, ileus). Consider selecting an alternative drug

AZOLES	**HORMONES AND HORMONE ANTAGONISTS**			
AZOLES	TOREMIFENE	↑ plasma concentrations of toremifene	Due to inhibition of metabolism of toremifene by the CYP3A4 isoenzymes by ketoconazole	Clinical relevance is uncertain. Necessary to monitor for clinical toxicities
AZOLES	**IMMUNOMODULATING DRUGS**			
AZOLES – ITRACONAZOLE, KETOCONAZOLE, VORICONAZOLE	CICLOSPORIN	↑ plasma concentrations of ciclosporin, with risk of nephrotoxicity, myelosuppression, neurotoxicity and excessive immunosuppression, with risk of infection and post-transplant lymphoproliferative disease	Inhibition of CYP3A4-mediated metabolism of ciclosporin; these inhibitors vary in potency. Ketoconazole and itraconazole are classified as potent inhibitors. The effect is not clinically relevant with fluconazole	Avoid co-administration with itraconazole or ketoconazole. Consider an alternative azole but need to monitor plasma ciclosporin levels to prevent toxicity
AZOLES – FLUCONAZOLE, ITRACONAZOLE, KETOCONAZOLE, POSACONAZOLE, VORICONAZOLE	CORTICOSTEROIDS	↑ adrenal suppressive effects of corticosteroids, which may ↑ risk of infections and produce an inadequate response to stress scenarios	Due to inhibition of CYP3A4-mediated metabolism of corticosteroids and inhibition of P-gp (↑ bioavailability of corticosteroids)	Monitor cortisol levels and warn patients to report symptoms such as fever and sore throat
AZOLES	SIROLIMUS	↑ sirolimus levels	Inhibition of metabolism of sirolimus	Avoid co-administration
AZOLES	TACROLIMUS	↑ tacrolimus levels	Inhibition of CYP3A4-mediated metabolism of tacrolimus	Monitor clinical effects closely; check levels
FLUCONAZOLE, ITRACONAZOLE, KETOCONAZOLE, MICONAZOLE, VORICONAZOLE	ANTICOAGULANTS – WARFARIN	↑ anticoagulant effect with azole antifungals. There have been cases of bleeding when topical miconazole (oral gel or pessaries) was used by patients on warfarin. Posaconazole may be a safer alternative	Itraconazole potently inhibits CYP3A4, which metabolizes both *R*-warfarin (also metabolized by CYP1A2) and the more active *S*-warfarin (also metabolized by CYP2C9)	Necessary to monitor the effects of warfarin closely (weekly INR) and to warn patients to report any symptoms of bleeding ➢ ***For signs and symptoms of overanticoagulation, see Clinical Features of Some Adverse Drug Interactions, Bleeding disorders***

Primary drug	Secondary drug	Effect	Mechanism	Precautions
AZOLES	**ANTIDEPRESSANTS**			
KETOCONAZOLE	MIRTAZAPINE	↑ mirtazapine levels	Inhibition of metabolism via CYP1A2, CYP2D6 and CYP3A4	Consider alternative antifungals
AZOLES	REBOXETINE	Risk of ↑ reboxetine levels	Possibly inhibition of CYP3A4-mediated metabolism of reboxetine	Avoid co-administration
ITRACONAZOLE, KETOCONAZOLE, MICONAZOLE, FLUCONAZOLE, VORICONAZOLE	TCAs	Possible ↑ plasma concentrations of TCAs	All TCAs are metabolized primarily by CYP2D6. Other pathways include CYP1A2 (e.g. amitriptyline, clomipramine, imipramine), CYP2C9 and CYP2C19 (e.g. clomipramine, imipramine). Ketoconazole and voriconazole are documented inhibitors of CYP2C19. Fluconazole and voriconazole are reported to inhibit CYP2C9	Warn patients to report ↑ side-effects of TCAs such as dry mouth, blurred vision and constipation, which may be an early sign of ↑ TCA levels. In this case, consider ↓ dose of TCA
AZOLES	**ANTIDIABETIC DRUGS**			
KETOCONAZOLE, FLUCONAZOLE, ITRACONAZOLE, VORICONAZOLE	NATEGLINIDE, REPAGLINIDE	Likely to ↑ plasma concentrations of repaglinide and ↑ risk of hypoglycaemic episodes	Due to inhibition of CYP3A4-mediated metabolism. These drugs vary in potency as inhibitors (ketoconazole, itraconazole are potent inhibitors) and ↑ plasma concentrations will vary	Watch for and warn patients about symptoms of hypoglycaemia ➢ ***For signs and symptoms of hypoglycaemia, see Clinical Features of Some Adverse Drug Interactions, Hypoglycaemia***
ITRACONAZOLE, FLUCONAZOLE, MICONAZOLE, VORICONAZOLE	SULPHONYLUREAS	↑ risk of hypoglycaemic episodes	Inhibition of CYP2C9-mediated metabolism of these sulphonylureas	Watch for and warn patients about symptoms of hypoglycaemia ➢ ***For signs and symptoms of hypoglycaemia, see Clinical Features of Some Adverse Drug Interactions, Hypoglycaemia***

KETOCONAZOLE	ANTIEMETICS – APREPITANT	↑ aprepitant levels	Inhibition of CYP3A4-mediated metabolism of aprepitant	Use with caution. Clinical significance unclear; monitor closely
AZOLES	**ANTIEPILEPTICS**			
FLUCONAZOLE, ITRACONAZOLE, KETOCONAZOLE, VORICONAZOLE	BARBITURATES	↓ azole levels, with risk of therapeutic failure	Barbiturates induce CYP3A4, which metabolizes itraconazole and the active metabolite of itraconazole. Primidone is metabolized to phenobarbitone	Watch for inadequate therapeutic effects, and ↑ dose of azole if due to interaction
MICONAZOLE	BARBITURATES	↑ phenobarbital levels	Inhibition of metabolism	Be aware; watch for early features of toxicity (e.g. ↑ sedation)
ITRACONAZOLE, KETOCONAZOLE, MICONAZOLE, POSACONAZOLE, VORICONAZOLE	CARBAMAZEPINE, PHENYTOIN	↓ plasma concentrations of itraconazole and of its active metabolite, ketoconazole, posaconazole and voriconazole, with risk of therapeutic failure. ↑ phenytoin levels, but clinical significance uncertain. Carbamazepine plasma concentrations are also ↑	These azoles are highly lipophilic, and clearance is heavily dependent upon metabolism by CYP isoenzymes. Phenytoin and carbamazepine are powerful inducers of CYP3A4 and other CYP isoenzymes (CYP2C18/19, CYP1A2); the result is very low or undetectable plasma levels. Phenytoin extensively ↓ AUC of itraconazole by more than 90%. Inhibition of P-gp ↑ bioavailability of carbamazepine	Avoid co-administration of posaconazole or voriconazole with carbamazepine. Watch for inadequate therapeutic effects and ↑ dose of itraconazole. Higher doses of itraconazole may not overcome this interaction. Consider the use of less lipophilic fluconazole, which is less dependent on CYP metabolism. Necessary to monitor phenytoin and carbamazepine levels
ITRACONAZOLE	**ANTIFUNGALS**			
ITRACONAZOLE	KETOCONAZOLE	↑ itraconazole levels, with risk of toxic effects	Ketoconazole is a potent inhibitor of the metabolism of itraconazole by the CYP3A4 and a potent inhibitor of P-gp, which is considered to ↑ bioavailability of itraconazole	Warn patients about toxic effects such as swelling around the ankles (peripheral oedema), shortness of breath, loss of appetite (anorexia) and yellow discoloration of the urine and eyes (jaundice). ↓ dose if due to interaction

Primary drug	Secondary drug	Effect	Mechanism	Precautions
ITRACONAZOLE	VORICONAZOLE	↓ levels of itraconazole and of its active metabolite, and significant risk of therapeutic failure	Voriconazole is an inducer of CYP3A4	Watch for inadequate therapeutic effects, and ↑ dose of itraconazole if due to interaction. Higher doses of itraconazole may not overcome this interaction, so consider the use of less lipophilic fluconazole, which is less dependent on CYP metabolism
AZOLES	**ANTIHISTAMINES**			
AZOLES	MIZOLASTINE	↑ mizolastine levels	Inhibition of metabolism of mizolastine	Avoid co-administration
KETOCONAZOLE, POSACONAZOLE	LORATIDINE	↑ loratidine levels	Inhibition of cytochrome P450, P-gp or both	Avoid co-administration
AZOLES – ITRACONAZOLE	ANTIHYPERTENSIVES AND HEART FAILURE DRUGS – VASODILATOR ANTIHYPERTENSIVES – bosentan	Azole antifungals ↑ bosentan levels	Azoles inhibit CYP3A4 and CYP2C9	Monitor LFTs closely
AZOLES	ANTIMIGRAINE DRUGS – 5-HT1 AGONISTS	↑ levels of almotriptan and eletriptan	Inhibited metabolism	Avoid co-administration
ITRACONAZOLE, KETOCONAZOLE	ANTIMUSCARINICS	1. ↓ ketoconazole levels 2. ↑ darifenacin, solifenacin and tolterodine levels	1. ↓ absorption 2. Inhibited metabolism	1. Watch for poor response to ketoconazole 2. Avoid co-administration of ketoconazole and these antimuscarinics
KETOCONAZOLE	ANTIOBESITY DRUGS – RIMONABANT	↑ rimonabant levels	Ketoconazole inhibits CYP3A4-mediated metabolism of rimonabant	Avoid co-administration

DRUGS TO TREAT INFECTIONS ANTIFUNGAL DRUGS

AZOLES	ANTIVIRALS			
ITRACONAZOLE, KETOCONAZOLE	PROTEASE INHIBITORS	Possibly ↑ levels of ketoconazole by amprenavir, indinavir and ritonavir (with or without lopinavir). Conversely, indinavir, ritonavir and saquinavir levels ↑ by itraconazole and ketoconazole	Inhibition of, or competition for, CYP3A4-mediated metabolism	Use itraconazole with caution and monitor for adverse effects. No dose adjustment is recommended for doses <400 mg/day of ketoconazole
VORICONAZOLE	RITONAVIR	↓ efficacy of voriconazole	↓ plasma levels	Avoid co-administration if the dose of ritonavir is 400 mg twice a day or greater. Avoid combining low-dose ritonavir (100 mg twice a day) unless benefits outweigh risks
FLUCONAZOLE, VORICONAZOLE	NNRTIs	Possible ↓ efficacy of azole	↑ CYP3A4-mediated metabolism	Avoid co-administration
AZOLES	**NUCLEOSIDE REVERSE TRANSCRIPTASE INHIBITORS**			
ITRACONAZOLE, KETOCONAZOLE	DIDANOSINE	Possibly ↓ efficacy of ketoconazole and itraconazole with buffered didanosine	Absorption of the ketoconazole and itraconazole may be ↓ by the buffered didanosine formulation, which raises gastric pH	Give the ketoconazole and itraconazole 2 hours before or 6 hours after didanosine. Alternatively, consider using the enteric-coated formulation of didanosine, which does not have to be given separately
FLUCONAZOLE	ZIDOVUDINE	↑ zidovudine levels	Inhibition of metabolism	Avoid co-administration

DRUGS TO TREAT INFECTIONS ANTIFUNGAL DRUGS

Primary drug	Secondary drug	Effect	Mechanism	Precautions
ITRACONAZOLE	ANXIOLYTICS AND HYPNOTICS			
ITRACONAZOLE, KETOCONAZOLE, VORICONAZOLE	BZDs – ALPRAZOLAM, CHLORDIAZEPOXIDE, DIAZEPAM, LORAZEPAM, MIDAZOLAM, OXAZEPAM, TEMAZEPAM	↑ plasma concentrations of these BZDs, with ↑, with risk of adverse effects. These risks are greater following intravenous administration of midazolam compared with oral midazolam	Itraconazole and ketoconazole are potent inhibitors of phase I metabolism (oxidation and functionalization) of these BZDs by CYP3A4. In addition, the more significant ↑ in plasma concentrations following oral midazolam (15 times compared with five times following intravenous use) indicates that the inhibition of P-gp by ketoconazole is important following oral administration	Aim to avoid co-administration. If co-administration is necessary, always start with a low dose and monitor effects closely. Consider use of alternative BZDs that undergo predominantly phase II metabolism by glucuronidation, e.g. flurazepam, quazepam. Fluconazole and posaconazole are unlikely to cause this interaction
ITRACONAZOLE	BUSPIRONE	↑ buspirone levels	Inhibition of CYP3A4-mediated metabolism	Warn patients to be aware of additional sedation
KETOCONAZOLE	ZALEPLON, ZOLPIDEM, ZOPICLONE	↑ zolpidem levels reported; likely to occur with zaleplon and zopiclone	Inhibition of CYP3A4-mediated metabolism	Warn patients of the risk of ↑ sedation
ITRACONAZOLE, KETOCONAZOLE, POSACONAZOLE	BRONCHODILATORS – THEOPHYLLINE	↑ theophylline levels, with risk of toxicity, with itraconazole. Unpredictable effect on theophylline levels with ketoconazole	Theophylline is primarily metabolized by CYP1A2. Although azoles are best known as inhibitors of CYP3A4, they also inhibit other CYP isoenzymes to varying degrees	If concurrent use is necessary, monitor theophylline levels at the initiation of itraconazole therapy or on discontinuing therapy. Terbinafine may be a safer alternative

FLUCONAZOLE, ITRACONAZOLE, KETOCONAZOLE, POSACONAZOLE, VORICONAZOLE	CALCIUM CHANNEL BLOCKERS	Plasma concentrations of dihydropyridine calcium channel blockers are ↑ by fluconazole, itraconazole and ketoconazole. Risk of ↑ verapamil levels with ketoconazole and itraconazole. Itraconazole and possibly posaconazole may ↑ diltiazem levels	The azoles are potent inhibitors of CYP3A4 isoenzymes, which metabolize calcium channel blockers. They also inhibit CYP2C9-mediated metabolism of verapamil. Ketoconazole and itraconazole both inhibit intestinal P-gp, which may ↑ bioavailability of verapamil. Diltiazem is mainly a substrate of CYP3A5 and CYP3A5P1, which are inhibited by itraconazole. 75% of the metabolism of diltiazem occurs in the liver and the rest in the intestine. Diltiazem is a substrate of P-gp (also an inhibitor but unlikely to be significant at therapeutic doses), which is inhibited by itraconazole, resulting in ↑ bioavailability of diltiazem	Monitor PR, BP and ECG, and warn patents to watch for symptoms/signs of heart failure
ITRACONAZOLE	CARDIAC GLYCOSIDES – DIGOXIN	Itraconazole may cause ↑ plasma levels of digoxin; cases of digoxin toxicity have been reported	Itraconazole inhibits P-gp-mediated renal clearance and ↑ intestinal absorption of digoxin	Monitor digoxin levels; watch for digoxin toxicity
ITRACONAZOLE, KETOCONAZOLE	CNS STIMULANTS – MODAFINIL	↑ plasma concentrations of modafinil, with risk of adverse effects	Due to inhibition of CYP3A4, which has a partial role in the metabolism of modafinil	Be aware. Warn patients to report dose-related adverse effects, e.g. headache, anxiety
KETOCONAZOLE	DIURETICS – POTASSIUM-SPARING DIURETICS AND ALDOSTERONE ANTAGONISTS	↑ eplerenone levels	Inhibition of metabolism	Avoid co-administration

Primary drug	Secondary drug	Effect	Mechanism	Precautions
VORICONAZOLE	ERGOT ALKALOIDS – ERGOTAMINE	↑ ergotamine/methysergide levels, with risk of toxicity	Inhibition of metabolism of the ergot derivatives	Avoid co-administration. If absolutely necessary, advise patients to discontinue treatment immediately if numbness and tingling of the extremities are felt
ITRACONAZOLE	GRAPEFRUIT JUICE	Possibly ↓ efficacy	↓ absorption possibly by inhibition of intestinal CYP3A4, affecting P-gp or lowering duodenal pH	Clinical significance is unknown. The effect of the interaction may vary between capsules and oral liquid preparations
ITRACONAZOLE, KETOCONAZOLE, MICONAZOLE, POSACONAZOLE	H2 RECEPTOR BLOCKERS	↓ plasma concentrations and risk of treatment failure	↓ absorption of these antifungals as ↑ gastric pH	Avoid concomitant use. If unable to avoid combination, take H2 blockers at least 2–3 hours after the antifungal. Use an alternative antifungal or separate doses by at least 2 hours and give with an acidic drink, e.g. a carbonated drink; ↑ dose of antifungal may be required
FLUCONAZOLE, ITRACONAZOLE, KETOCONAZOLE	IVABRADINE	↑ levels with ketoconazole and possibly fluconazole and itraconazole	Uncertain	Avoid co-administration
FLUCONAZOLE, ITRACONAZOLE, KETOCONAZOLE, POSACONAZOLE	LIPID-LOWERING DRUGS – STATINS	Azoles markedly ↑ atorvastatin, simvastatin (both with cases of myopathy reported) and possibly pravastatin. These effects are less likely with fluvastatin and rosuvastatin, although fluconazole may cause moderate rises in their levels	Itraconazole and ketoconazole inhibit CYP3A4-mediated metabolism of these statins; they also inhibit intestinal P-gp, which ↑ bioavailability of statins. Itraconazole may block the transport of atorvastatin due to inhibition of the OATP1B1 enzyme system. Some manufacturers suggest that the small ↑ in plasma levels of pravastatin may be due to ↑ absorption. Voriconazole is an inhibitor of CYP2C9. Fluconazole inhibits CYP2C9 and CYP3A4	Avoid co-administration of simvastatin and atorvastatin with azole antifungals. Care should be taken with co-administration of other statins and azoles. Although fluvastatin and rosuvastatin may be considered as alternatives, consider ↓ dose of statin and warn patients to report any features of rhabdomyolysis. Check LFTs and CK regularly

FLUCONAZOLE, ITRACONAZOLE, KETOCONAZOLE, POSACONAZOLE, VORICONAZOLE	OESTROGENS – ORAL CONTRACEPTIVES	The Netherlands Pharmacovigilance Foundation has received reports of pill cycle disturbances 2–3 weeks after the start of the pill cycle, delayed bleeding and pregnancy. Effects of either or both of oestrogen excess and progestogen excess may occur (migraine headaches, thromboembolic episodes, breast tenderness, bloating, weight gain)	The metabolism of oral contraceptives is complex, dependent on composition, constituents and doses. Ethylenestradiol, a common constituent, as well as progestogens are substrates of CYP3A4 that are inhibited by itraconazole. The inhibition of ethinylestradiol and progestogens could lead to effects of oestrogen and progestogens excess. Triazole antifungals inhibit biotransformation of steroids, and such an ↑ may cause a delay of withdrawal bleeding	Due to the complex metabolic pathways of oral contraceptives, dependent on constituents, doses and the reported adverse effects during concomitant use, it is advisable to avoid use of azole antifungals or advise alternative methods of contraception
KETOCONAZOLE	PARASYMPATHOMIMETICS – GALANTAMINE	↑ galantamine levels	Inhibition of CYP3A4-mediated metabolism of galantamine	Monitor PR and BP closely, watching for bradycardia and hypotension
FLUCONAZOLE, ITRACONAZOLE, KETOCONAZOLE, MICONAZOLE	PERIPHERAL VASODILATORS – CILOSTAZOL	Fluconazole, itraconazole, ketoconazole and miconazole ↑ cilostazol levels	These azoles inhibit CYP3A4-mediated metabolism of cilostazol	Avoid co-administration
AZOLES	PHOSPHODIESTERASE TYPE 5 INHIBITORS	↑ sildenafil, tadalafil, and vardenafil levels	Inhibition of metabolism	↓ dose of these phosphodiesterase inhibitors
AZOLES	**PROTON PUMP INHIBITORS**			
ITRACONAZOLE, KETOCONAZOLE	PROTON PUMP INHIBITORS	Possible ↓ efficacy of the antifungal	↓ absorption	Monitor for ↓ efficacy; ↑ dose may be required. Separate doses by at least 2 hours and give ketoconazole with a cola drink
VORICONAZOLE	OMEPRAZOLE	Possible ↑ efficacy and adverse effects of both drugs	1. Inhibition of voriconazole metabolism via CYP2C19 and CYP3A4 2. Inhibition of metabolism of omeprazole	1. No dose adjustment of voriconazole is recommended 2. Halve the omeprazole dose

Primary drug	Secondary drug	Effect	Mechanism	Precautions
ITRACONAZOLE	TOLTERODINE	↑ tolterodine level. Supratherapeutic levels may cause prolongation of the Q–T interval	CYP3A4 is the major enzyme involved in the elimination of tolterodine in individuals with deficient CYP2D6 activity (poor metabolizers). Inhibition of CYP3A4 by triazoles in such individuals could cause dangerous ↑ tolterodine levels	Avoid co-administration
CASPOFUNGIN				
CASPOFUNGIN	ANTIBIOTICS – RIFAMPICIN	↓ caspofungin levels, with risk of therapeutic failure	Induction of caspofungin metabolism	↑ dose of caspofungin to 70 mg daily
CASPOFUNGIN	ANTICANCER AND IMMUNOMODULATING DRUGS			
CASPOFUNGIN	CICLOSPORIN	1. ↓ plasma concentrations of ciclosporin, with risk of transplant rejection 2. Enhanced toxic effects of caspofungin and ↑ alanine transaminase levels	1. Due to induction of metabolism of ciclosporin by these drugs. The potency of induction varies 2. Uncertain	1. Monitor for signs of rejection of transplants. Monitor ciclosporin levels to ensure adequate therapeutic concentrations and ↑ dose when necessary 2. Monitor LFTs
CASPOFUNGIN	DEXAMETHASONE	↓ caspofungin levels, with risk of therapeutic failure	Induction of caspofungin metabolism	↑ dose of caspofungin to 70 mg daily
CASPOFUNGIN	TACROLIMUS	↓ tacrolimus levels	Induction of CYP3A4-mediated metabolism of tacrolimus	Avoid co-administration
CASPOFUNGIN	ANTIEPILEPTICS – CARBAMAZEPINE, PHENYTOIN	↓ caspofungin levels, with risk of therapeutic failure	Induction of caspofungin metabolism	↑ dose of caspofungin to 70 mg daily
CASPOFUNGIN	ANTIVIRALS – EFAVIRENZ, NEVIRAPINE	↓ caspofungin levels, with risk of therapeutic failure	Induction of caspofungin metabolism	↑ dose of caspofungin to 70 mg daily

FLUCYTOSINE				
FLUCYTOSINE	ANTICANCER AND IMMUNOMODULATING DRUGS – CYTARABINE	↓ flucytosine levels	Uncertain	Watch for poor response to flucytosine
FLUCYTOSINE	ANTIFUNGALS – AMPHOTERICIN	↑ flucytosine levels, with risk of toxic effects	Amphotericin causes ↓ renal excretion of flucytosine and ↑ cellular uptake	The combination of flucytosine and amphotericin may be used therapeutically. Watch for early features of flucytosine toxicity (gastrointestinal upset); monitor renal and liver function closely
FLUCYTOSINE	ANTIVIRALS – ZIDOVUDINE	Possibly ↑ adverse effects with zidovudine	Additive toxicity	Avoid if possible; otherwise monitor FBC and renal function (weekly). ↓ doses as necessary
GRISEOFULVIN				
GRISEOFULVIN	ALCOHOL	Disulfiram-like reaction can occur	Uncertain	Warn patients not to drink alcohol while taking griseofulvin
GRISEOFULVIN	ANTICANCER AND IMMUNOMODULATING DRUGS – CICLOSPORIN	↓ plasma concentrations of ciclosporin (may be as much as 40%) and risk of rejection in patients who have received transplants	Induction of ciclosporin metabolism	Monitor ciclosporin levels closely
GRISEOFULVIN	ANTICOAGULANTS – ORAL	Possible ↓ anticoagulant effect coumarins and phenindione	Unknown	Necessary to monitor the effects of warfarin closely (weekly INR) and to warn patients to report any symptoms of bleeding ➢ ***For signs and symptoms of overanticoagulation, see Clinical Features of Some Adverse Drug Interactions, Bleeding disorders***

Primary drug	Secondary drug	Effect	Mechanism	Precautions
GRISEOFULVIN	ANTIDEPRESSANTS – TCAs	Possible ↑ plasma concentrations of TCAs	Inhibition of metabolism	Warn patients to report any ↑ side-effects of TCAs such as dry mouth, blurred vision and constipation, which may be an early sign of ↑ TCA levels. In this case, consider ↓ dose of TCA
GRISEOFULVIN	ANTIDIABETIC DRUGS – REPAGLINIDE	↓ repaglinide levels	Hepatic metabolism induced	Watch for and warn patients about hypoglycaemia ➢ ***For signs and symptoms of hypoglycaemia, see Clinical Features of Some Adverse Drug Interactions, Hypoglycaemia***
GRISEOFULVIN	ANTIEPILEPTICS – PHENOBARBITONE, PRIMIDONE	↓ griseofulvin levels	↓ absorption	Although the effect of ↓ plasma concentrations on therapeutic effect has not been established, concurrent use is preferably avoided
GRISEOFULVIN	BRONCHODILATORS – THEOPHYLLINE	↑ theophylline levels	Inhibition of metabolism of theophylline	Uncertain clinical significance. Watch for early features of theophylline toxicity
GRISEOFULVIN	OESTROGENS	↓ oestrogen levels, which may lead to failure of contraception	Induction of metabolism of oestrogens	Long-term use of griseofulvin is likely to ↓ effectiveness of oral contraceptives. Patients should be advised to use an alternative method of contraception during griseofulvin therapy and for 1 month after its discontinuation

GRISEOFULVIN	PROGESTOGENS	↓ progesterone levels, which may lead to a failure of contraception or a poor response to treatment of menorrhagia	Induction of the CYP-mediated metabolism of oestrogens	Long-term use of griseofulvin is likely to ↓ effectiveness of oral contraceptives. Patients should be advised to use an alternative method of contraception during griseofulvin therapy and for 1 month after its discontinuation
TERBINAFINE				
TERBINAFINE	ANTIBIOTICS – RIFAMPICIN	↓ terbinafine levels	Induction of metabolism	Watch for poor response to terbinafine
TERBINAFINE	ANTIDEPRESSANTS – IMIPRAMINE, NORTRIPTYLINE	Possible ↑ plasma concentrations of TCAs	Terbinafine strongly inhibits CYP2D6-mediated metabolism of nortriptyline	Warn patients to report ↑ side-effects of TCAs such as dry mouth, blurred vision and constipation, which may be an early sign of ↑ TCA levels. In this case, consider ↓ dose of TCA
TERBINAFINE	H2 RECEPTOR BLOCKERS – CIMETIDINE	↑ efficacy and adverse effects of terbinafine	↑ bioavailability	Consider alternative acid suppression or monitor more closely and consider ↓ dose
TERBINAFINE	OESTROGENS	↓ oestrogen levels, which may lead to failure of contraception	Alteration of the bacterial flora necessary for recycling ethinylestradiol from the large bowel	Patients should be advised to use an alternative method of contraception during terbinafine therapy and for 1 month after its discontinuation
TERBINAFINE	PROGESTOGENS	↓ progestogen levels, which may lead to a failure of contraception or poor response to treatment of menorrhagia	Induction of the CYP-mediated metabolism of oestrogens	Patients should be advised to use an alternative method of contraception during terbinafine therapy and for 1 month after its discontinuation

Primary drug	Secondary drug	Effect	Mechanism	Precautions
ANTIMALARIALS				
ARTEMETHER WITH LUMEFANTRINE				
ARTEMETHER WITH LUMEFANTRINE	DRUGS THAT PROLONG THE Q–T INTERVAL			
ARTEMETHER WITH LUMEFANTRINE	1. ANTIARRHYTHMICS – amiodarone, disopyramide, procainamide, propafenone 2. ANTIBIOTICS – macrolides (especially azithromycin, clarithromycin, parenteral erythromycin, telithromycin), quinolones (especially moxifloxacin), quinupristin/dalfopristin 3. ANTICANCER AND IMMUNOMODULATING DRUGS – arsenic trioxide 4. ANTIDEPRESSANTS – TCAs, venlafaxine 5. ANTIEMETICS – dolasetron 6. ANTIFUNGALS – fluconazole, posaconazole, voriconazole 7. ANTIHISTAMINES – terfenadine, hydroxyzine, mizolastine 8. ANTIMALARIALS – chloroquine, hydroxychloroquine, mefloquine, quinine 9. ANTIPROTOZOALS – pentamidine isetionate 10. ANTIPSYCHOTICS – atypicals, phenothiazines, pimozide 11. BETA-BLOCKERS – sotalol 12. BRONCHODILATORS – parenteral bronchodilators 13. CNS STIMULANTS – atomoxetine	Risk of ventricular arrhythmias, particularly torsades de pointes	Additive effect; these drugs cause prolongation of the Q–T interval	Avoid co-administration

ARTEMETHER WITH LUMEFANTRINE	ANTIARRHYTHMICS – FLECAINIDE	Risk of arrhythmias	Additive effect	Avoid co-administration
ARTEMETHER WITH LUMEFANTRINE	**ANTIDEPRESSANTS**			
ARTEMETHER WITH LUMEFANTRINE	REBOXETINE, SNRIs, TRYPTOPHAN	↑ artemether/lumefantrine levels, with risk of toxicity, including arrhythmias	Uncertain	Avoid co-administration
ARTEMETHER WITH LUMEFANTRINE	ST JOHN'S WORT	This antimalarial may cause dose-related dangerous arrhythmias	A substrate mainly of CYP3A4, which may be inhibited by St John's wort	Manufacturers recommend avoidance of antidepressants
ARTEMETHER WITH LUMEFANTRINE	SSRIs	This antimalarial may cause dose-related dangerous arrhythmias	A substrate mainly of CYP3A4, which may be inhibited by high doses of fluvoxamine and to a lesser degree by fluoxetine	Manufacturers recommend avoidance of antidepressants
ARTEMETHER WITH LUMEFANTRINE	ANTIMALARIALS	Risk of arrhythmias	Additive effect	Avoid co-administration
ARTEMETHER WITH LUMEFANTRINE	ANTIVIRALS – PROTEASE INHIBITORS	↑ artemether levels	Uncertain; possibly inhibited metabolism	Avoid co-administration
ARTEMETHER WITH LUMEFANTRINE	BETA-BLOCKERS – METOPROLOL	↑ risk of toxicity	Uncertain	Avoid co-administration
ARTEMETHER WITH LUMEFANTRINE	GRAPEFRUIT JUICE	Possibly ↑ efficacy and adverse effects	↑ bioavailability; ↓ presystemic metabolism. Constituents of grapefruit juice irreversibly inhibit intestinal cytochrome CYP3A4	Monitor more closely. No ECG changes were seen in the study
ARTEMETHER WITH LUMEFANTRINE	H2 RECEPTOR BLOCKERS – CIMETIDINE	↑ efficacy and adverse effects of antimalarials	Inhibition of metabolism, some definitely via CYP3A4	Avoid co-administration

Primary drug	Secondary drug	Effect	Mechanism	Precautions
ATOVAQUONE				
ATOVAQUONE	ANTIBIOTICS			
ATOVAQUONE	RIFAMPICINS	Both rifampicin and rifabutin ↓ atovaquone levels, although the effect is greater with rifampicin (↓ AUC by 50% cf. 34% for rifabutin)	Uncertain because atovaquone is predominantly excreted unchanged via the gastrointestinal route	Avoid co-administration with rifampicin. Take care with rifabutin and watch for poor response to atovaquone
ATOVAQUONE	TETRACYCLINE	↓ atovaquone levels (40%)	Uncertain	Not clinically significant; combination therapy has been used effectively
ATOVAQUONE	ANTIEMETICS – METOCLOPRAMIDE	↓ atovaquone levels	Uncertain	Avoid; consider an alternative antiemetic
ATOVAQUONE	ANTIVIRALS – ZIDOVUDINE	Atovaquone ↑ zidovudine levels	Atovaquone inhibits the glucuronidation of zidovudine	Uncertain clinical significance. Monitor FBC, LFTs and lactate closely during co-administration
ATOVAQUONE	H2 RECEPTOR BLOCKERS – CIMETIDINE	↑ efficacy and adverse effects of antimalarials	Inhibition of metabolism, some definitely via CYP3A4	Avoid co-administration

CHLOROQUINE/HYDROXYCHLOROQUINE				
CHLOROQUINE/ HYDROXYCHLOROQUINE	**DRUGS THAT PROLONG THE Q–T INTERVAL**			
CHLOROQUINE/ HYDROXYCHLOROQUINE	1. ANTIARRHYTHMICS – amiodarone, disopyramide, procainamide, propafenone 2. ANTIBIOTICS – macrolides (especially azithromycin, clarithromycin, parenteral erythromycin, telithromycin), quinolones (especially moxifloxacin), quinupristin/ dalfopristin 3. ANTICANCER AND IMMUNOMODULATING DRUGS – arsenic trioxide 4. ANTIDEPRESSANTS – TCAs, venlafaxine 5. ANTIEMETICS – dolasetron 6. ANTIFUNGALS – fluconazole, posaconazole, voriconazole 7. ANTIHISTAMINES – terfenadine, hydroxyzine, mizolastine 8. ANTIMALARIALS – artemether with lumefantrine, mefloquine, quinine 9. ANTIPROTOZOALS – pentamidine isetionate 10. ANTIPSYCHOTICS – atypicals, phenothiazines, pimozide 11. BETA-BLOCKERS – sotalol 12. BRONCHODILATORS – parenteral bronchodilators 13. CNS STIMULANTS – atomoxetine	Risk of ventricular arrhythmias, particularly torsades de pointes	Additive effect; these drugs cause prolongation of the Q–T interval	Avoid co-administration
CHLOROQUINE	AGALSIDASE BETA	↓ efficacy of agalsidase beta	Inhibition of intracellular activity of agalsidase beta	Avoid co-administration – manufacturers' recommendation
CHLOROQUINE	ANTACIDS	↓ chloroquine levels	↓ absorption	Separate doses by at least 4 hours

Primary drug	Secondary drug	Effect	Mechanism	Precautions
CHLOROQUINE	ANTICANCER AND IMMUNOMODULATING DRUGS			
CHLOROQUINE	CICLOSPORIN	↑ plasma concentrations of ciclosporin	Likely inhibition of ciclosporin	Monitor renal function weekly
HYDROXYCHLOROQUINE	PORFIMER	↑ risk of photosensitivity reactions	Attributed to additive effects	Avoid exposure of skin and eyes to direct sunlight for 30 days after porfimer therapy
CHLOROQUINE	ANTIDIARRHOEAL DRUGS – KAOLIN	↓ chloroquine levels	↓ absorption	Separate doses by at least 4 hours
CHLOROQUINE	ANTIEPILEPTICS	Risk of seizures	Chloroquine can ↓ seizure threshold	Care with co-administration; ↑ dose of antiepileptic if ↑ incidence of fits
CHLOROQUINE	ANTIMALARIALS – MEFLOQUINE	Risk of seizures	Additive effect	Warn patient of the risk; patients should be advised to avoid driving while taking these drugs in combination
CHLOROQUINE	CARDIAC GLYCOSIDES – DIGOXIN	Chloroquine may ↑ plasma concentrations of digoxin	Uncertain at present	Monitor digoxin levels; watch for digoxin toxicity
CHLOROQUINE	DRUG DEPENDENCE THERAPIES – BUPROPION	↑ risk of seizures. This risk is marked in elderly people, in patients with a history of seizures, with addiction to opiates/cocaine/stimulants, and in diabetics treated with oral hypoglycaemics or insulin	Bupropion is associated with a dose-related risk of seizures. These drugs, which lower seizure threshold, are individually epileptogenic. Additive effects occur when they are combined	Extreme caution. The dose of bupropion should not exceed 450 mg/day (or 150 mg/day in patients with severe hepatic cirrhosis)
CHLOROQUINE	H2 RECEPTOR BLOCKERS – CIMETIDINE	↑ efficacy and adverse effects of chloroquine	Inhibition of metabolism and excretion	Consider ranitidine as an alternative or take cimetidine at least 2 hours after chloroquine
CHLOROQUINE	LARONIDASE	↓ efficacy of laronidase	Uncertain	Avoid co-administration

CHLOROQUINE	PARASYMPATHOMIMETICS	↓ efficacy of parasympathomimetics	These antimalarials occasionally cause muscle weakness, which may exacerbate the symptoms of myasthenia gravis	Watch for poor response to these parasympathomimetics and ↑ dose accordingly
MEFLOQUINE				
MEFLOQUINE	**DRUGS THAT PROLONG THE Q–T INTERVAL**			
MEFLOQUINE	1. ANTIARRHYTHMICS – amiodarone, disopyramide, procainamide, propafenone 2. ANTIBIOTICS – macrolides (especially azithromycin, clarithromycin, parenteral erythromycin, telithromycin), quinolones (especially moxifloxacin), quinupristin/dalfopristin 3. ANTICANCER AND IMMUNOMODULATING DRUGS – arsenic trioxide 4. ANTIDEPRESSANTS – TCAs, venlafaxine 5. ANTIEMETICS – dolasetron 6. ANTIFUNGALS – fluconazole, posaconazole, voriconazole 7. ANTIHISTAMINES – terfenadine, hydroxyzine, mizolastine 8. ANTIMALARIALS – artemether with lumefantrine, chloroquine, hydroxychloroquine, quinine 9. ANTIPROTOZOALS – pentamidine isetionate 10. ANTIPSYCHOTICS – atypicals, phenothiazines, pimozide 11. BETA-BLOCKERS – sotalol 12. BRONCHODILATORS – parenteral bronchodilators 13. CNS STIMULANTS – atomoxetine	Risk of ventricular arrhythmias, particularly torsades de pointes	Additive effect; these drugs cause prolongation of the Q–T interval	Avoid co-administration

Primary drug	Secondary drug	Effect	Mechanism	Precautions
MEFLOQUINE	ANTIEPILEPTICS	↓ efficacy of antiepileptics	Mefloquine can ↓ seizure threshold	Care with co-administration; ↑ dose of antiepileptic if ↑ incidence of fits
MEFLOQUINE	ANTIMALARIALS – CHLOROQUINE, QUININE	Risk of seizures	Additive effect	Warn patients of the risk; patients should be advised to avoid driving while taking these drugs in combination
MEFLOQUINE	BETA-BLOCKERS	↑ risk of bradycardia	Mefloquine can cause cardiac conduction disorders, e.g. bradycardia. Additive bradycardic effect. Single case report of cardiac arrest with co-administration of mefloquine and propanolol possibly caused by Q–T prolongation	Monitor PR closely
MEFLOQUINE	CALCIUM CHANNEL BLOCKERS	Risk of bradycardia	Additive bradycardic effect; mefloquine can cause cardiac conduction disorders, e.g. bradycardia. There is also a theoretical risk of Q–T prolongation with co-administration of mefloquine and calcium channel blockers	Monitor PR closely
MEFLOQUINE	CARDIAC GLYCOSIDES – DIGOXIN	Risk of bradycardia	Uncertain; probably additive effect; mefloquine can cause AV block	Monitor PR and ECG closely
MEFLOQUINE	DRUG DEPENDENCE THERAPIES – BUPROPION	↑ risk of seizures. This risk marked in elderly people, in patients with history of seizures, with addiction to opiates/cocaine/stimulants, and in diabetics treated with oral hypoglycaemics or insulin	Bupropion is associated with a dose-related risk of seizures. These drugs, which lower seizure threshold, are individually epileptogenic. Additive effects occur when they are combined	Extreme caution. The dose of bupropion should not exceed 450 mg/day (or 150 mg/day in patients with severe hepatic cirrhosis)

MEFLOQUINE	H2 RECEPTOR BLOCKERS – CIMETIDINE	↑ efficacy and adverse effects of antimalarials	Inhibition of metabolism, some definitely via CYP3A4	Avoid co-administration
MEFLOQUINE	IVABRADINE	Risk of arrhythmias with mefloquine	Additive effect	Monitor ECG closely
PRIMAQUINE				
PRIMAQUINE	ANTIMALARIALS – ARTEMETHER WITH LUMEFANTRINE	Risk of arrhythmias	Additive effect	Avoid co-administration
PRIMAQUINE	H2 RECEPTOR BLOCKERS – CIMETIDINE	↑ efficacy and adverse effects of antimalarials	Inhibition of metabolism, some definitely via CYP3A4	Avoid co-administration
PRIMAQUINE	MEPACRINE	↑ primaquine levels	Inhibition of metabolism	Warn patients to report the early features of primaquine toxicity (e.g. gastrointestinal disturbance). Monitor FBC closely
PROGUANIL				
PROGUANIL	ANTACIDS	↓ proguanil levels	↓ absorption	Separate doses by at least 4 hours
PROGUANIL	ANTIDEPRESSANTS – TCAs	Possible ↑ plasma concentrations of proguanil	Inhibition of CYP2C19-mediated metabolism of proguanil. The clinical significance of this depends upon whether proguanil's alternative pathways of metabolism are also inhibited by co-administered drugs	Warn patient to report any evidence of excessive side-effects such as a change in bowel habit or stomatitis

DRUGS TO TREAT INFECTIONS ANTIMALARIALS

Primary drug	Secondary drug	Effect	Mechanism	Precautions
PROGUANIL	ANTIMALARIALS			
PROGUANIL	ARTEMETHER WITH LUMEFANTRINE	Risk of arrhythmias	Additive effect	Avoid co-administration
PROGUANIL	PYRIMETHAMINE	↑ antifolate effect	Additive effect	Monitor FBC closely; the effect may take a number of weeks to occur
PROGUANIL	CNS STIMULANTS – MODAFINIL	May cause moderate ↑ plasma concentrations of these substrates	Modafinil is a reversible inhibitor of CYP2C19 when used in therapeutic doses	Be aware
PROGUANIL	H2 RECEPTOR BLOCKERS – CIMETIDINE	↓ efficacy of proguanil	↓ absorption and ↓ formation of active metabolite	Avoid concomitant use. Clinical significance is not established; effectiveness of malarial prophylaxis may be ↓
PYRIMETHAMINE				
PYRIMETHAMINE	ANTIBIOTICS – SULPHONAMIDES, TRIMETHOPRIM	↑ antifolate effect	Additive effect	Monitor FBC closely; the effect may take a number of weeks to occur
PYRIMETHAMINE	ANTIEPILEPTICS – PHENYTOIN	1. ↓ efficacy of phenytoin 2. ↑ antifolate effect	1. Uncertain 2. Additive effect	1. Care with co-administration; ↑ dose of antiepileptic if ↑ incidence of fits 2. Monitor FBC closely; the effect may take a number of weeks to occur
PYRIMETHAMINE	ANTIMALARIALS			
PYRIMETHAMINE	ARTEMETHER WITH LUMEFANTRINE	Risk of arrhythmias	Additive effect	Avoid co-administration
PYRIMETHAMINE	PROGUANIL	↑ antifolate effect	Additive effect	Monitor FBC closely; the effect may take a number of weeks to occur

PYRIMETHAMINE	ANTICANCER AND IMMUNOMODULATING DRUGS – METHOTREXATE	↑ antifolate effect	Pyrimethamine should not be used alone and is combined with sulfadoxine. Pyrimethamine and methotrexate synergistically induce folate deficiency	Although the toxic effects of methotrexate are more frequent with high doses of methotrexate, it is necessary to do FBC, liver and renal function tests before starting treatment even with low doses, repeating these tests weekly until therapy is stabilized and thereafter every 2–3 months. Patients should be advised to report symptoms such as sore throat and fever immediately, and also any gastrointestinal discomfort. A profound drop in white cell or platelet counts warrants immediate stoppage of methotrexate therapy and initiation of supportive therapy
PYRIMETHAMINE	ANTIVIRALS – ZIDOVUDINE	Possibly ↑ adverse effects with zidovudine	Additive toxicity	Monitor FBC and renal function closely. ↓ doses as necessary. Use of pyrimethamine as prophylaxis seems to be tolerated
PYRIMETHAMINE	H2 RECEPTOR BLOCKERS – CIMETIDINE	↑ efficacy and adverse effects of antimalarials	Inhibition of metabolism, some definitely via CYP3A4	Avoid co-administration

Primary drug	Secondary drug	Effect	Mechanism	Precautions
QUININE				
QUININE	DRUGS THAT PROLONG THE Q–T INTERVAL			
QUININE	1. ANTIARRHYTHMICS – amiodarone, disopyramide, procainamide, propafenone 2. ANTIBIOTICS – macrolides (especially azithromycin, clarithromycin, parenteral erythromycin, telithromycin), quinolones (especially moxifloxacin), quinupristin/dalfopristin 3. ANTICANCER AND IMMUNOMODULATING DRUGS – arsenic trioxide 4. ANTIDEPRESSANTS – TCAs, venlafaxine 5. ANTIEMETICS – dolasetron 6. ANTIFUNGALS – fluconazole, posaconazole, voriconazole 7. ANTIHISTAMINES – terfenadine, hydroxyzine, mizolastine 8. ANTIMALARIALS – artemether with lumefantrine, chloroquine, hydroxychloroquine, mefloquine 9. ANTIPROTOZOALS – pentamidine isetionate 10. ANTIPSYCHOTICS – atypicals, phenothiazines, pimozide 11. BETA-BLOCKERS – sotalol 12. BRONCHODILATORS – parenteral bronchodilators 13. CNS STIMULANTS – atomoxetine	Risk of ventricular arrhythmias, particularly torsades de pointes	Additive effect; these drugs prolong the Q–T interval. In addition, quinine inhibits CYP2D6-mediated metabolism of procainamide	Avoid co-administration

QUININE	ANALGESICS – OPIOIDS	↑ codeine, fentanyl, pethidine and tramadol levels	Quinine inhibits CYP2D6	Watch for excessive narcotization
QUININE	**ANTIARRHYTHMICS**			
QUININE	FLECAINIDE	Quinine may ↑ flecainide levels	Quinine inhibits CYP2D6-mediated metabolism of flecainide	The effect seems to be slight, but watch for flecainide toxicity; monitor PR and BP closely
QUININE	MEXILETINE	Quinine may ↑ mexiletine levels	Quinine inhibits CYP2D6-mediated metabolism of mexiletine	Monitor PR and BP closely
QUININE	ANTICANCER AND IMMUNOMODULATING DRUGS – PORFIMER	↑ risk of photosensitivity reactions	Attributed to additive effects	Avoid exposure of skin and eyes to direct sunlight for 30 days after porfimer therapy
QUININE	ANTIMALARIALS – MEFLOQUINE	Risk of seizures	Additive effect	Warn patients of the risk; patients should be advised to avoid driving while taking these drugs in combination
QUININE	ANTIPARKINSON'S DRUGS – AMANTADINE	↑ side-effects	↓ renal excretion	Monitor closely for confusion, disorientation, headache, dizziness and nausea
QUININE	BETA-BLOCKERS	Risk of ↑ plasma concentrations and effects of labetalol, metoprolol and propranolol; ↑ systemic effects of timolol eye drops	Quinine inhibits CYP2D6, which metabolizes these beta-blockers	Monitor BP at least weekly until stable
QUININE	CARDIAC GLYCOSIDES – DIGOXIN	Plasma concentrations of digoxin may ↑ when it is co-administered with quinine	Uncertain, but seems to be due to ↓ non-renal (possibly biliary) excretion of digoxin	Monitor digoxin levels; watch for digoxin toxicity
QUININE	H2 RECEPTOR BLOCKERS – CIMETIDINE	↑ efficacy and adverse effects of antimalarials	Inhibition of metabolism, some definitely via CYP3A4	Avoid co-administration

Primary drug	Secondary drug	Effect	Mechanism	Precautions
QUININE	PARASYMPATHOMIMETICS	↓ efficacy of parasympathomimetics	These antimalarials occasionally cause muscle weakness, which may exacerbate the symptoms of myasthenia gravis	Watch for poor response to these parasympathomimetics and ↑ dose accordingly
OTHER ANTIPROTOZOALS				
This section consists of antiprotozoal drugs. Note that antimalarials are also antiprotozoals but have been described in a separate section				
Antibiotics with antiprotozoal activity are not included in this chapter. These include clindamycin, co-trimoxazole/trimethoprim, dapsone, doxycycline and metronidazole				
LEVAMISOLE				
LEVAMISOLE	ALCOHOL	Risk of a disulfiram-like reaction	Uncertain	Warn patients not to drink while taking levamisole
LEVAMISOLE	ANTIBIOTICS – RIFAMPICIN	↓ therapeutic efficacy of rifampicin	Levamisole displaces rifampicin from protein-binding sites, ↑ free fraction nearly three times and thus ↑ clearance of rifampicin	Avoid co-administration if possible
LEVAMISOLE	ANTICANCER AND IMMUNOMODULATING DRUGS – FLUOROURACIL	↑ risk of hepatotoxicity and neurotoxicity despite ↑ cytotoxic effects	Antiphosphatase activity of levamisole may ↑ fluorouracil cytotoxicity	This combination has been used successfully in the treatment of colon cancer. Monitor FBC and LFTs regularly. Advise patients to report symptoms such as diarrhoea, numbness and tingling and peeling of the skin of the hands and feet (hand–foot syndrome)

LEVAMISOLE	ANTICOAGULANTS – WARFARIN	Possible ↑ anticoagulant effect	Uncertain	Monitor INR closely
LEVAMISOLE	ANTIEPILEPTICS – PHENYTOIN	Possible ↑ phenytoin levels	Uncertain; case report of this interaction when levamisole and fluorouracil were co-administered with phenytoin	Monitor phenytoin levels and ↓ phenytoin dose as necessary
MEBENDAZOLE				
MEBENDAZOLE	ANTIEPILEPTICS – CARBAMAZEPINE, PHENYTOIN	↓ mebendazole levels	Induction of metabolism	Watch for poor response to mebendazole
MEBENDAZOLE	H2 RECEPTOR BLOCKERS – CIMETIDINE	↑ mebendazole levels	Inhibition of metabolism	Be aware; cases where this interaction have been used therapeutically
MEPACRINE				
MEPACRINE	ANTIMALARIALS – PRIMAQUINE	↑ primaquine levels	Inhibition of metabolism	Warn patients to report the early features of primaquine toxicity (e.g. gastrointestinal disturbance). Monitor FBC closely

Primary drug	Secondary drug	Effect	Mechanism	Precautions
PENTAMIDINE ISETIONATE				
PENTAMIDINE ISETIONATE	DRUGS THAT PROLONG THE Q–T INTERVAL			
PENTAMIDINE ISETIONATE	1. ANTIARRHYTHMICS – amiodarone, disopyramide, procainamide, propafenone 2. ANTIBIOTICS – macrolides (especially azithromycin, clarithromycin, parenteral erythromycin, telithromycin), quinolones (especially moxifloxacin), quinupristin/dalfopristin 3. ANTICANCER AND IMMUNOMODULATING DRUGS – arsenic trioxide 4. ANTIDEPRESSANTS – TCAs, venlafaxine 5. ANTIEMETICS – dolasetron 6. ANTIFUNGALS – fluconazole, posaconazole, voriconazole 7. ANTIHISTAMINES – terfenadine, hydroxyzine, mizolastine 8. ANTIMALARIALS – artemether with lumefantrine, chloroquine, hydroxychloroquine, mefloquine, quinine 9. ANTIPSYCHOTICS – atypicals, phenothiazines, pimozide 10. BETA-BLOCKERS – sotalol 11. BRONCHODILATORS – parenteral bronchodilators 12. CNS STIMULANTS – atomoxetine	Risk of ventricular arrhythmias, particularly torsades de pointes	Additive effect; these drugs cause prolongation of the Q–T interval	Avoid co-administration

PENTAMIDINE	ANTIDIABETIC DRUGS – INSULIN, SULPHONAMIDES, NATEGLINIDE, REPAGLINIDE, ACARBOSE	Altered insulin requirement	Attributed to pancreatic beta cell toxicity	Altered glycaemic control; need to monitor blood sugar until stable and following withdrawal of pentamidine
PENTAMIDINE ISETIONATE	ANTIFUNGALS – AMPHOTERICIN	Risk of arrhythmias	Additive effect	Monitor ECG closely
PENTAMIDINE ISETIONATE	**ANTIVIRALS**			
PENTAMIDINE ISETIONATE	ADEFOVIR DIPIVOXIL	Possible ↑ efficacy and side-effects	Competition for renal excretion	Monitor renal function weekly
PENTAMIDINE ISETIONATE (INTRAVENOUS)	FOSCARNET SODIUM	Risk of hypocalcaemia	Unclear; possibly additive hypocalcaemic effects	Use extreme caution with intravenous pentamidine; monitor serum calcium (correct before the start of treatment), renal function and signs of tetany closely. Stop one drug if necessary
PENTAMIDINE ISETIONATE	NUCLEOSIDE REVERSE TRANSCRIPTASE INHIBITORS	↑ adverse effects with didanosine, tenofovir and zidovudine	Additive toxicity	Monitor FBC and renal function closely. Consider stopping didanosine while pentamidine is required for *Pneumocystis jiroveci* pneumonia
PENTAMIDINE ISETIONATE	IVABRADINE	Risk of arrhythmias	Additive effect	Monitor ECG closely
TINIDAZOLE				
TINIDAZOLE	ALCOHOL	Risk of a disulfiram-like reaction	Uncertain	Warn patients not to drink alcohol while taking levamisole
TINIDAZOLE	OESTROGENS – COMBINED ORAL CONTRACEPTIVE PILL	Possible ↓ contraceptive effect	Uncertain; possibly due to ↓ absorption resulting from alterations in gut flora	Warn patients to use barrier contraception during and up to one month after stopping tinidazole

Primary drug	Secondary drug	Effect	Mechanism	Precautions
ANTIVIRALS – ANTIRETROVIRALS				
NON-NUCLEOSIDE REVERSE TRANSCRIPTASE INHIBITORS (NNRTIs)				
NNRTIs	ANALGESICS – OPIOIDS	Methadone levels may be significantly ↓ by efavirenz and nevirapine	↑ CYP3A4- and CYP2B6-mediated metabolism of methadone	Monitor closely for opioid withdrawal, ↑ dose as necessary. Likely to need dose titration of methadone (mean 22% but up to 186% ↑)
NNRTIs	ANTIBIOTICS			
NNRTIs	MACROLIDES – CLARITHROMYCIN	1. ↓ efficacy of clarithromycin but ↑ efficacy and adverse effects of active metabolite 2. Rash occurs in 46% of patients when efavirenz is given with clarithromycin	1. Uncertain: possibly due to altered CYP3A4-mediated metabolism 2. Uncertain	1. Clinical significance unknown; no dose adjustment is recommended when clarithromycin is co-administered with nevirapine, but monitor LFTs and activity against *Mycobacterium avium intracellulare* complex closely 2. Consider alternatives to clarithromycin for patients on efavirenz
NNRTIs	RIFAMYCINS			
EFAVIRENZ	RIFABUTIN	Possible ↓ efficacy of rifabutin	↓ bioavailability	↑ rifabutin dose by 50% for daily treatment, or double the dose if patient is on two or three times a week treatment
EFAVIRENZ	RIFAMPICIN	Possible ↓ efficacy of efavirenz	Uncertain	↑ dose of efavirenz from 600 mg to 800 mg
NEVIRAPINE	RIFAMPICIN	↓ efficacy of nevirapine	Uncertain; probable ↑ metabolism of nevirapine	Avoid concomitant use. FDA recommend use only if clearly indicated and monitored closely

NNRTIs	ANTICANCER AND IMMUNOMODULATING DRUGS			
NNRTIs	CYTOTOXICS			
EFAVIRENZ	DOXORUBICIN	↑ risk of myelosuppression due to ↑ plasma concentrations	Due to ↓ metabolism of doxorubicin by CYP3A4 isoenzymes owing to inhibition of those enzymes	Monitor for ↑ myelosuppression, peripheral neuropathy, myalgias and fatigue
EFAVIRENZ	IFOSFAMIDE	↓ plasma concentrations of 4-hydroxyifosfamide, the active metabolite of ifosfamide, and risk of inadequate therapeutic response	Due to inhibition of the isoenzymatic conversion to active metabolites	Monitor clinically the efficacy of ifosfamide and ↑ dose accordingly
EFAVIRENZ	IMATINIB	↑ imatinib levels with ↑ risk of toxicity (e.g. abdominal pain, constipation, dyspnoea) and of neurotoxicity (e.g. taste disturbances, dizziness, headache, paraesthesia, peripheral neuropathy)	Due to inhibition of CYP3A4-mediated metabolism of imatinib	Monitor for clinical efficacy and for the signs of toxicity listed, along with convulsions, confusion and signs of oedema (including pulmonary oedema). Monitor electrolytes, liver function and for cardiotoxicity
EFAVIRENZ	IRINOTECAN	↑ plasma concentrations of SN-38 (>AUC by 100%) and ↑ toxicity of irinotecan, e.g. diarrhoea, acute cholinergic syndrome, interstitial pulmonary disease	Due to inhibition of the metabolism of irinotecan by CYP3A4 isoenzymes by efavirenz	Peripheral blood counts should be checked before each course of treatment. Monitor lung function. Recommendation is to ↓ dose of irinotecan by 25%
EFAVIRENZ	VINCA ALKALOIDS	↑ adverse effects of vinblastine and vincristine	Inhibition of CYP3A4-mediated metabolism. Also inhibition of P-gp efflux of vinblastine	Monitor FBCs and watch for early features of toxicity (pain, numbness, tingling in the fingers and toes, jaw pain, abdominal pain, constipation, ileus). Consider selecting an alternative drug

Primary drug	Secondary drug	Effect	Mechanism	Precautions
NNRTIs	**HORMONES AND HORMONE ANTAGONISTS**			
EFAVIRENZ	TOREMIFENE	↑ plasma concentrations of toremifene	Due to inhibition of metabolism of toremifene by the CYP3A4 isoenzymes by efavirenz	Clinical relevance is uncertain. Necessary to monitor for clinical toxicities
NNRTIs	**IMMUNOMODULATING DRUGS**			
NNRTIs	CICLOSPORIN	↓ efficacy of ciclosporin	Possibly ↑ CYP3A4-mediated metabolism of ciclosporin	Monitor more closely; check levels
EFAVIRENZ	CORTICOSTEROIDS	↑ adrenal suppressive effects of corticosteroids, which may ↑ risk of infections and produce an inadequate response to stress scenarios	Due to inhibition of metabolism of corticosteroids	Monitor cortisol levels and warn patients to report symptoms such as fever and sore throat
NEVIRAPINE	ANTICOAGULANTS – WARFARIN	↓ efficacy of warfarin with nevirapine	Altered metabolism. *S*-warfarin is metabolized by CYP2D6, *R*-warfarin by CYP3A4	Monitor INR every 3–7 days when starting or altering treatment and adjust dose by 10% as necessary. May need around twofold ↑ in dose
EFAVIRENZ	ANTIDEPRESSANTS – SSRIs	1. Possible ↑ efficacy and ↑ adverse effects, including serotonin syndrome, with fluoxetine 2. Possible ↓ efficacy with sertraline	1. Uncertain mechanism; possibly ↑ bioavailability 2. CYP2B6 contributes most to the demethylation of sertraline with lesser contributions from CYP2C19, CYP2C9, CYP3A4 and CYP2D6	1. Use with caution; consider ↓ dose of fluoxetine 2. Watch for therapeutic failure, and advise patients to report persistence or lack of improvement of symptoms of depression. ↑ dose of sertraline as required, titrating to clinical response
EFAVIRENZ	ANTIDIABETIC DRUGS – REPAGLINIDE	Likely to ↑ plasma concentrations of repaglinide and ↑ risk of hypoglycaemic episodes	Due to inhibition of CYP3A4 isoenzymes, which metabolize repaglinide	Watch for and warn patients about hypoglycaemia ➢ ***For signs and symptoms of hypoglycaemia, see Clinical Features of Some Adverse Drug Interactions, Hypoglycaemia***

DRUGS TO TREAT INFECTIONS ANTIVIRALS – ANTIRETROVIRALS

NNRTIs	ANTIEPILEPTICS	Possible ↓ efficacy of carbamazepine	Uncertain	Monitor carbamazepine levels and side-effects when initiating or changing treatment
NNRTIs	**ANTIFUNGALS**			
NNRTIs	AZOLES – KETOCONAZOLE, VORICONAZOLE	Possible ↓ efficacy of azole	↑ CYP3A4-mediated metabolism	Avoid co-administration
EFAVIRENZ, NEVIRAPINE	CASPOFUNGIN	↓ caspofungin levels, with risk of therapeutic failure	Induction of caspofungin metabolism	↑ dose of caspofungin to 70 mg daily
NNRTIs	ANTIGOUT DRUGS – PROBENECID	↑ levels of zidovudine with cases of toxicity	↓ hepatic metabolism of zidovudine	Avoid co-administration if possible; if not possible, ↓ dose of zidovudine
NNRTIs	**ANTIMIGRAINE DRUGS**			
NNRTIs	ERGOT DERIVATIVES	↑ ergotamine/methysergide levels, with risk of toxicity	↓ CYP3A4-mediated metabolism of ergot derivatives	Avoid co-administration
EFAVIRENZ	5-HT1 AGONISTS– ALMOTRIPTAN, ELETRIPTAN	↑ plasma concentrations of almotriptan and eletriptan, and risk of toxic effects, e.g. flushing, sensations of tingling, heat, heaviness, pressure or tightness of any part of body including the throat and chest, dizziness	Almotriptan and eletriptan are metabolized by CYP3A4 isoenzymes, which may be inhibited by efavirenz. However, since there is an alternative pathway of metabolism by MAOA, the toxicity responses will vary between individuals	The CSM has advised that if chest tightness or pressure is intense, the triptan should be discontinued immediately and the patient investigated for ischaemic heart disease by measuring cardiac enzymes and doing an ECG. Avoid concomitant use in patients with coronary artery disease and in those with severe or uncontrolled hypertension

Primary drug	Secondary drug	Effect	Mechanism	Precautions
NNRTIs	**ANTIPSYCHOTICS**			
NNRTIs	ATYPICAL	↓ efficacy of aripiprazole	↑ CYP3A4-mediated metabolism of aripiprazole	Monitor patient closely and ↑ dose of aripiprazole as necessary
NNRTIs	PIMOZIDE	Possible ↑ efficacy and ↑ adverse effects, e.g. ventricular arrhythmias of pimozide	↓ CYP-3A4-mediated metabolism of pimozide	Avoid co-administration
NNRTIs	**ANTIVIRALS**			
EFAVIRENZ	NNRTIs–NEVIRAPINE	↓ efficacy of efavirenz when co-administered with nevirapine	Uncertain mechanism: ↓ bio-availability	If co-administered, consider ↑ dose of efavirenz to 800 mg once daily
EFAVIRENZ	NUCLEOSIDE REVERSE TRANSCRIPTASE INHIBITORS – DIDANOSINE (ENTERIC-COATED), TENOFOVIR	A high treatment failure rate is reported when tenofovir, enteric-coated didanosine and efavirenz are co-administered	Unknown	Use this combination with caution
NNRTIs	**PROTEASE INHIBITORS**			
NNRTIs	INDINAVIR	Possible ↓ efficacy of indinavir	↑ CYP3A4-mediated metabolism of indinavir	Monitor viral load; consider ↑ dose indinavir to 1000 mg 8-hourly
NNRTIs	LOPINAVIR AND RITONAVIR	Possible ↓ efficacy of lopinavir/ritonavir	Uncertain; ↓ bioavailability	Consider ↑ lopinavir/ritonavir dose (by 33% with efavirenz and to 53 mg/133 mg twice daily, and monitor drug concentrations, with nevirapine). Monitor viral load closely as this dose ↑ may be insufficient. Monitor LFTs closely
EFAVIRENZ	AMPRENAVIR	Possible ↓ efficacy of amprenavir	Uncertain; ↓ bioavailability of amprenavir	Consider ↑ dose of amprenavir to 1200 mg three times a day, or combine amprenavir 600 mg twice a day with ritonavir 100 mg twice a day

EFAVIRENZ	ATAZANAVIR	↓ efficacy of efavirenz	↑ CYP3A4-mediated metabolism of efavirenz	Recommended dose of atazanavir is 400 mg when given with efavirenz 600 mg. Optimal suggested treatment is this combination plus ritonavir 100 mg daily
EFAVIRENZ	NELFINAVIR	Possible ↑ efficacy of nelfinavir, with theoretical risk of adverse effects	Small ↑ bioavailability of nelfinavir	No dose adjustment necessary
EFAVIRENZ	RITONAVIR	↑ efficacy and ↑ adverse effects of ritonavir, e.g. dizziness, nausea, paraesthesia and liver dysfunction	↑ bioavailability of ritonavir; competition for metabolism via CYP3A4	Combination not well tolerated. Monitor closely including LFTs. Low-dose ritonavir has not been studied
EFAVIRENZ	SAQUINAVIR	Possible ↓ efficacy of saquinavir, with risk of treatment failure	↑ CYP3A4-mediated metabolism of saquinavir	Combination not recommended if saquinavir is the sole protease inhibitor; always use saquinavir in combination with another agent, e.g. ritonavir, when co-administering with efavirenz
NEVIRAPINE	AMPRENAVIR	Efficacy of amprenavir predicted to be ↓	Uncertain; ↓ bioavailability of amprenavir	Monitor viral load
NEVIRAPINE	ATAZANAVIR	↓ efficacy of atazanavir	Atazanavir is a substrate and inhibitor of CYP3A4	Avoid concomitant use
NEVIRAPINE	NELFINAVIR	Possible ↓ efficacy of nelfinavir	Uncertain	Dose adjustment probably not required, although one study suggests ↑ dose may be required
NEVIRAPINE	SAQUINAVIR	Possible ↓ efficacy, risk of treatment failure of saquinavir	↑ CYP3A4-mediated metabolism of saquinavir	Clinical significance unclear. Different formulations of saquinavir may have different magnitudes of interaction

Primary drug	Secondary drug	Effect	Mechanism	Precautions
EFAVIRENZ	ANXIOLYTICS AND HYPNOTICS – DIAZEPAM, MIDAZOLAM	↑ efficacy and ↑ adverse effects, e.g. prolonged sedation	↓ CYP3A4-mediated metabolism of diazepam and midazolam	With all anxiolytics, monitor more closely, especially sedation levels. May need ↓ dose of diazepam or alteration of timing of dose. Avoid co-administration with midazolam
EFAVIRENZ, NEVIRAPINE	CNS STIMULANTS – MODAFINIL	May ↓ modafinil levels	Induction of CYP3A4, which has a partial role in the metabolism of modafinil	Be aware
EFAVIRENZ	DRUG DEPENDENCE THERAPIES – BUPROPION	↑ plasma concentrations of bupropion and risk of adverse effects	Inhibition of CYP2B6	Warn patients about adverse effects, and use alternatives when possible. Co-administer efavirenz and bupropion with caution. A retrospective study showed that two patients received the combination without reported adverse effects. Potential ↑ risk of seizures
EFAVIRENZ	GRAPEFRUIT JUICE	Possibly ↑ efficacy and ↑ adverse effects	Unclear	Monitor more closely
EFAVIRENZ	LIPID-LOWERING DRUGS – STATINS	↓ levels of atorvastatin, pravastatin and simvastatin with efavirenz	Uncertain; efavirenz is known to induce intestinal P-gp, which may ↓ bioavailability of some statins (including atorvastatin)	Monitor lipid profile closely
NEVIRAPINE	OESTROGENS – ETHINYLESTRADIOL	Marked ↓ contraceptive effect with nevirapine	Induction of metabolism of oestrogens	Avoid co-administration, recommend alternative non-hormonal contraceptives – barrier methods are necessary to prevent transmission of infection

NEVIRAPINE	PROGESTOGENS – NORETHISTERONE	↓ efficacy of contraceptives, with risk of contraceptive failure	Uncertain	Avoid co-administration; recommend alternative non-hormonal contraceptives – barrier methods are necessary to prevent transmission of infection
NUCLEOSIDE REVERSE TRANSCRIPTASE INHIBITORS				
NUCLEOSIDE REVERSE TRANSCRIPTASE INHIBITORS	**ANALGESICS**			
ZIDOVUDINE	NSAIDs	Risk of haematological effects of zidovudine with NSAIDs	Unknown	Avoid co-administration
ABACAVIR	OPIOIDS	↓ efficacy of methadone when co-administered with abacavir	Uncertain; possibly enzyme induction	Monitor for opioid withdrawal and consider ↑ dose
DIDANOSINE, ZIDOVUDINE	PARACETAMOL	Cases of hepatotoxicity reported when paracetamol was added to either didanosine or zidovudine	Uncertain; possible additive hepatotoxic effect	Monitor liver function regularly during co-administration
NUCLEOSIDE REVERSE TRANSCRIPTASE INHIBITORS	**ANTIBIOTICS**			
NUCLEOSIDE REVERSE TRANSCRIPTASE INHIBITORS	AMINOGLYCOSIDES	Possibly ↑ risk of nephrotoxicity	Additive effect	Avoid co-administration if possible; otherwise monitor renal function weekly
DIDANOSINE	ETHAMBUTOL	Possibly ↑ adverse effects (e.g. peripheral neuropathy) with didanosine	Additive side-effects	Monitor closely for development of peripheral neuropathy, but no dose adjustment required
STAVUDINE, ZIDOVUDINE	CHLORAMPHENICOL	Possible ↑ adverse effects when co-administered with stavudine or zidovudine	Uncertain	Use an alternative antibiotic, if possible; otherwise monitor closely for peripheral neuropathy and check FBC regularly

Primary drug	Secondary drug	Effect	Mechanism	Precautions
NUCLEOSIDE REVERSE TRANSCRIPTASE INHIBITORS	CO-TRIMOXAZOLE	↑ adverse effects	Additive toxicity	↓ doses as necessary; monitor FBC and renal function closely. Doses of co-trimoxazole used for prophylaxis seem to be tolerated
ZIDOVUDINE	DAPSONE	Possible ↑ adverse effects when co-administered with zidovudine	Uncertain; possible ↑ bioavailability of zidovudine	Use with caution, monitor for peripheral neuropathy
NUCLEOSIDE REVERSE TRANSCRIPTASE INHIBITORS	ISONIAZID	↑ adverse effects with didanosine and possibly stavudine	Additive side-effects	Monitor closely for the development of peripheral neuropathy, but no dose adjustment required
DIDANOSINE, STAVUDINE	METRONIDAZOLE	↑ adverse effects (e.g. peripheral neuropathy) with didanosine and possibly stavudine	Additive effect	Monitor closely for peripheral neuropathy during intensive or prolonged combination
ZIDOVUDINE	RIFAMPICIN	Unclear	Unclear	Avoid co-administration
DIDANOSINE	QUINOLONES	↓ efficacy of ciprofloxacin and possibly levofloxacin, moxifloxacin, norfloxacin and ofloxacin with buffered didanosine	Cations in the buffer of didanosine preparation chelate and adsorb ciprofloxacin. Absorption of the other quinolones may be ↓ by the buffered didanosine formulation, which raises gastric pH	Give the antibiotic 2 hours before or 6 hours after didanosine. Alternatively, consider using the enteric-coated formulation of didanosine, which does not have to be given separately
DIDANOSINE	TETRACYCLINES	↓ efficacy of tetracycline, and possibly demeclocycline, doxycycline, lymecycline, minocycline and oxytetracycline with buffered didanosine	Absorption may be affected by the buffered didanosine formulation, which ↑ gastric pH	Avoid co-administration with buffered didanosine preparations. Consider changing to enteric-coated didanosine tablets
NUCLEOSIDE REVERSE TRANSCRIPTASE INHIBITORS	TRIMETHOPRIM	Possibly ↑ haematological toxicity	Competition for renal excretion	Monitor FBC and renal function closely

TENOFOVIR, ZIDOVUDINE	VANCOMYCIN	↑ adverse effects with zidovudine and possibly tenofovir	Additive toxicity	Monitor FBC and renal function closely (at least weekly)
NUCLEOSIDE REVERSE TRANSCRIPTASE INHIBITORS	**ANTICANCER AND IMMUNOMODULATING DRUGS**			
NUCLEOSIDE REVERSE TRANSCRIPTASE INHIBITORS	**CYTOTOXICS**			
ZIDOVUDINE	DOXORUBICIN	↑ adverse effects when doxorubicin is co-administered with zidovudine	Additive toxicity	Monitor FBC and renal function closely. ↓ doses as necessary
DIDANOSINE, ZIDOVUDINE	HYDROXYCARBAMIDE	↑ adverse effects with didanosine and possibly zidovudine	Additive effects, enhanced antiretroviral activity via ↓ intra-cellular deoxynucleotides	Avoid co-administration
ZIDOVUDINE	VINCA ALKALOIDS	↑ adverse effects when vincristine and possibly vinblastine are co-administered with zidovudine	Additive toxicity	Use with caution. Monitor FBC and renal function closely. ↓ doses as necessary
NUCLEOSIDE REVERSE TRANSCRIPTASE INHIBITORS	**IMMUNOMODULATING DRUGS**			
LAMIVUDINE	AZATHIOPRINE	↑ adverse effects with lamivudine	Unclear	Monitor closely
TENOFOVIR	IL-2	↑ adverse effects with tenofovir	Uncertain	Avoid if possible, otherwise monitor renal function weekly
ZIDOVUDINE	INTERFERON	↑ adverse effects with zidovudine	Additive toxicity	Monitor FBC and renal function closely. ↓ doses as necessary. Use of pyrimethamine as prophylaxis seems to be tolerated

Primary drug	Secondary drug	Effect	Mechanism	Precautions
NUCLEOSIDE REVERSE TRANSCRIPTASE INHIBITORS	**ANTIEPILEPTICS**			
DIDANOSINE, STAVUDINE, ZIDOVUDINE	PHENYTOIN	Possibly ↑ adverse effects (e.g. peripheral neuropathy) with didanosine, stavudine and zidovudine	Additive effect	Monitor closely for peripheral neuropathy during prolonged combination
ZIDOVUDINE	VALPROATE	↑ zidovudine levels	Inhibition of metabolism	Watch for early features of toxicity of zidovudine
NUCLEOSIDE REVERSE TRANSCRIPTASE INHIBITORS	**ANTIFUNGALS**			
TENOFOVIR, ZIDOVUDINE	AMPHOTERICIN	Possibly ↑ adverse effects with tenofovir and zidovudine	Additive toxicity	Avoid if possible, otherwise monitor FBC and renal function (weekly). ↓ doses as necessary
ZIDOVUDINE	AZOLES – FLUCONAZOLE	↑ zidovudine levels	Inhibition of metabolism	Avoid co-administration
DIDANOSINE	AZOLES – ITRACONAZOLE, KETOCONAZOLE	Possibly ↓ efficacy of ketoconazole and itraconazole with buffered didanosine	Absorption of ketoconazole and itraconazole may be ↓ by the buffered didanosine formulation, which raises gastric pH	Give the ketoconazole and itraconazole 2 hours before or 6 hours after didanosine. Alternatively, consider using the enteric-coated formulation of didanosine, which does not have to be given separately
ZIDOVUDINE	FLUCYTOSINE	Possibly ↑ adverse effects with zidovudine	Additive toxicity	Avoid if possible; otherwise monitor FBC and renal function (weekly). ↓ doses as necessary

NUCLEOSIDE REVERSE TRANSCRIPTASE INHIBITORS	ANTIGOUT DRUGS			
DIDANOSINE	ALLOPURINOL	Didanosine levels may be ↑	Uncertain	Watch for early signs of toxicity
ZIDOVUDINE	PROBENECID	↑ levels of zidovudine, with cases of toxicity	↓ hepatic metabolism of zidovudine	Avoid co-administration if possible; if not possible, ↓ dose of zidovudine
NUCLEOSIDE REVERSE TRANSCRIPTASE INHIBITORS	ANTIHYPERTENSIVES AND HEART FAILURE DRUGS – VASODILATOR ANTIHYPERTENSIVES	Risk of peripheral neuropathy when hydralazine is co-administered with didanosine, stavudine or zalcitabine	Additive effect; both drugs can cause peripheral neuropathy	Warn patients to report early features of peripheral neuropathy; if this occurs, the nucleoside reverse transcriptase inhibitor should be stopped
NUCLEOSIDE REVERSE TRANSCRIPTASE INHIBITORS	**ANTIMALARIALS**			
ZIDOVUDINE	ATOVAQUONE	Atovaquone ↑ zidovudine levels	Atovaquone inhibits glucuronidation of zidovudine	Uncertain clinical significance. Monitor FBC, LFTs and lactate closely during co-administration
ZIDOVUDINE	PYRIMETHAMINE	Possibly ↑ adverse effects with zidovudine	Additive toxicity	Monitor FBC and renal function closely. ↓ doses as necessary. Use of pyrimethamine as prophylaxis seems to be tolerated
NUCLEOSIDE REVERSE TRANSCRIPTASE INHIBITORS	ANTIPROTOZOALS – PENTAMIDINE ISETIONATE	↑ adverse effects with didanosine, tenofovir and zidovudine	Additive toxicity	Monitor FBC and renal function closely. Consider stopping didanosine while pentamidine is required for *Pneumocystis jiroveci* pneumonia

Primary drug	Secondary drug	Effect	Mechanism	Precautions
NUCLEOSIDE REVERSE TRANSCRIPTASE INHIBITORS	ANTIVIRALS			
NUCLEOSIDE REVERSE TRANSCRIPTASE INHIBITORS	ANTIVIRALS – OTHER			
TENOFOVIR	ADEFOVIR, CIDOFOVIR	↑ adverse effects	↑ plasma levels, competition for renal excretion via organic anion transporter	Monitor renal function weekly
LAMIVUDINE, TENOFOVIR, ZALCITABINE	FOSCARNET SODIUM	↑ adverse effects with tenofovir and possibly lamivudine and zalcitabine	Uncertain; possibly additive toxicity via competition for renal excretion	Avoid if possible; otherwise monitor FBC and renal function weekly
NUCLEOSIDE REVERSE TRANSCRIPTASE INHIBITORS	GANCICLOVIR/VALGANCICLOVIR	1. ↑ adverse effects with tenofovir, zidovudine and possibly didanosine, lamivudine and zalcitabine 2. Possibly ↓ efficacy of ganciclovir	1. Uncertain; possibly additive toxicity. Lamivudine may compete for active tubular secretion in the kidneys 2. Uncertain; ↓ bioavailability	1. Avoid if possible; otherwise monitor FBC and renal function weekly. It has been suggested that the dose of zidovudine should be halved from 600 mg to 300 mg daily. Monitor for peripheral neuropathy, particularly with zalcitabine 2. Uncertain clinical significance; if in doubt, consider alternative cytomegalovirus prophylaxis
NUCLEOSIDE REVERSE TRANSCRIPTASE INHIBITORS	RIBAVIRIN	1. ↑ side-effects, risk of lactic acidosis, peripheral neuropathy, pancreatitis, hepatic decompensation, mitochondrial toxicity and anaemia with didanosine and stavudine 2. ↓ efficacy of lamivudine	1. Additive side-effects; ↑ intracellular activation of didanosine and stavudine 2. ↓ intracellular activation of lamivudine	1. Not recommended. Use with extreme caution; monitor lactate, LFTs and amylase closely. Stop co-administration if peripheral neuropathy occurs. Stavudine and didanosine carry a higher risk 2. Monitor HIV RNA levels; if they ↑, review treatment combination

NUCLEOSIDE REVERSE TRANSCRIPTASE INHIBITORS	NNRTIs			
DIDANOSINE (ENTERIC-COATED), TENOFOVIR	EFAVIRENZ	A high treatment failure rate is reported when tenofovir, enteric-coated didanosine and efavirenz are co-administered	Unknown	Use this combination with caution
NUCLEOSIDE REVERSE TRANSCRIPTASE INHIBITORS	**NUCLEOSIDE REVERSE TRANSCRIPTASE INHIBITORS**			
EMTRICITABINE	LAMIVUDINE	Unknown	Unknown	Combination not recommended. No clinical experience of co-administration
DIDANOSINE	STAVUDINE	↑ adverse effects, including pancreatitis and neuropathy	Additive effect	Monitor more closely, especially for pancreatitis and peripheral neuropathy. Relative risk of neuropathy: stavudine alone 1.39 compared with didanosine; combined use 3.5. Sometimes fatal lactic acidosis is reported in pregnancy
DIDANOSINE	TENOFOVIR	Possibly ↑ adverse effects, including pancreatitis, lactic acidosis and neuropathy	↑ plasma levels of didanosine ± additive effects	Co-administration not recommended. Monitor closely for antiviral efficacy and side-effects (pancreatitis, neuropathy, lactic acidosis, renal failure). Not recommended in patients with a high viral load and low CD4 count (enteric-coated and buffered tablets). ↓ dose of didanosine to 250 mg has been tried. Do not use in combination as triple therapy with lamivudine as there is a high level of treatment failure

Primary drug	Secondary drug	Effect	Mechanism	Precautions
DIDANOSINE	ZIDOVUDINE	Possibly ↑ adverse effects	Uncertain	Monitor more closely, especially for haematological toxicity
EMTRICITABINE	ZIDOVUDINE	Possibly ↑ adverse effects	↑ bioavailability of zidovudine	Watch for adverse effects of zidovudine
LAMIVUDINE	ZIDOVUDINE	Possibly ↑ adverse effects	Additive side-effects	Monitor closely, especially for blood dyscrasias. Check FBC prior to concomitant use and then every month for 3 months
STAVUDINE	ZIDOVUDINE	Possibly ↓ efficacy	↓ cellular activation of stavudine and antagonism in vivo. Both are phosphorylated to the active form by thymidine kinase, which preferentially phosphorylates zidovudine; therefore causes ↓ phosphorylation of stavudine	Avoid co-administration
NUCLEOSIDE REVERSE TRANSCRIPTASE INHIBITORS	**PROTEASE INHIBITORS**			
TENOFOVIR	ATAZANAVIR	↓ efficacy of atazanavir	Uncertain; ↓ plasma levels of atazanavir	Use with caution, and consider using in combination with ritonavir
STAVUDINE	NELFINAVIR	Possibly ↑ adverse effects	Uncertain	Warn patient that diarrhoea may occur
ZIDOVUDINE	LOPINAVIR + RITONAVIR	↓ efficacy of zidovudine	↓ plasma levels by ↑ glucu-ronidation	Avoid co-administration
DIDANOSINE (BUFFERED)	PROTEASE INHIBITORS	↓ efficacy of amprenavir, atazanavir and indinavir	Absorption of these protease inhibitors may be affected by the buffered didanosine formulation, which ↑ gastric pH	Separate doses by at least 1 hour. Alternatively, consider using the enteric-coated formulation of didanosine

ABACAVIR	TIPRANAVIR + RITONAVIR	Possible ↓ efficacy; risk of treatment failure of abacavir	↓ plasma concentrations	Not recommended unless there are no other available nucleoside reverse transcriptase inhibitors
DIDANOSINE (ENTERIC-COATED)	TIPRANAVIR + RITONAVIR	Possible ↓ efficacy of didanosine	↓ absorption	Separate doses by at least 2 hours
ZIDOVUDINE	TIPRANAVIR + RITONAVIR	Possible ↓ efficacy; risk of treatment failure of zidovudine	↓ plasma concentrations	Not recommended unless there are no other available nucleoside reverse transcriptase inhibitors
ZIDOVUDINE	ANXIOLYTICS AND HYPNOTICS – BZDs	↑ adverse effects, including ↑ incidence of headaches when oxazepam is co-administered with zidovudine	Uncertain	Monitor closely
ZALCITABINE	H2 RECEPTOR BLOCKERS – CIMETIDINE	↑ efficacy and adverse effects of zalcitabine	↓ excretion via inhibition of tubular secretion	Clinical significance unclear. Monitor more closely
PROTEASE INHIBITORS				
PROTEASE INHIBITORS	ANAESTHETICS – LOCAL	↑ adverse effects of lidocaine with lopinavir and ritonavir	Uncertain; ↑ bioavailability	Caution; consider using an alternative local anaesthetic
PROTEASE INHIBITORS	**ANALGESICS**			
PROTEASE INHIBITORS	NSAIDs – PIROXICAM	Ritonavir ↑ piroxicam levels	Uncertain; ritonavir is known to inhibit CYP2C9, for which NSAIDs are substrates	Avoid co-administration
PROTEASE INHIBITORS	**OPIOIDS**			
PROTEASE INHIBITORS	ALFENTANIL, BUPRENORPHINE, FENTANYL, TRAMADOL	Possibly ↑ adverse effects when buprenorphine is co-administered with indinavir, ritonavir (with or without lopinavir) or saquinavir	Inhibition of CYP3A4 (CYP2D6 in the case of tramadol)	Halve the starting dose and titrate to effect. For fentanyl, give a single injection – monitor sedation and respiratory function closely. If continued use of fentanyl is needed, ↓ dose may be required. Concomitant use of ritonavir and transdermal fentanyl is not recommended

Primary drug	Secondary drug	Effect	Mechanism	Precautions
PROTEASE INHIBITORS	CODEINE, DIHYDROCODEINE	↓ efficacy of codeine and dihydrocodeine when given with ritonavir	Inhibition of CYP2D6-mediated metabolism of codeine to its active metabolites	Use an alternative opioid
PROTEASE INHIBITORS	METHADONE, PETHIDINE	↓ efficacy of methadone, with risk of withdrawal, when co-administered with amprenavir, nelfinavir, ritonavir (with or without lopinavir) or saquinavir	Uncertain; possibly due to induction of CYP3A4 and CYP2D6	Monitor closely for opioid withdrawal, and ↑ dose of methadone as necessary, This advice includes co-administration of methadone with low-dose ritonavir. Short-term use of pethidine is unlikely to cause a problem
PROTEASE INHIBITORS	**ANTIARRHYTHMICS**			
PROTEASE INHIBITORS	AMIODARONE	Amiodarone levels may be ↑ by protease inhibitors	Uncertain but postulated to be due to ↓ metabolism of amiodarone	Watch closely for amiodarone toxicity; for patients taking high doses of amiodarone, consider ↓ dose when starting protease inhibitor anti-HIV therapy
PROTEASE INHIBITORS	DISOPYRAMIDE	Disopyramide levels may be ↑ by protease inhibitors	Inhibition of CYP3A4-mediated metabolism of disopyramide	Watch closely for disopyramide toxicity
PROTEASE INHIBITORS	FLECAINIDE	Amprenavir, ritonavir and possibly saquinavir and tipranavir with ritonavir ↑ flecainide levels, with risk of ventricular arrhythmias	Uncertain; possibly inhibition of CYP3A4- and CYP2D6-mediated metabolism of flecainide	Manufacturers recommend avoiding co-administration of flecainide with amprenavir, ritonavir or saquinavir
PROTEASE INHIBITORS	MEXILETINE	Mexiletine levels may be ↑ by ritonavir	Inhibition of metabolism via CYP2D6, particularly in rapid metabolizers (90% of the population)	Monitor PR, BP and ECG closely
PROTEASE INHIBITORS	PROPAFENONE	Amprenavir, ritonavir and possibly saquinavir and tipranavir with ritonavir ↑ propafenone levels, with risk of ventricular arrhythmias	Uncertain	Manufacturers recommend avoiding co-administration of propafenone with amprenavir, ritonavir or tipranavir

PROTEASE INHIBITORS	ANTIBIOTICS			
PROTEASE INHIBITORS	FUSIDIC ACID	Possibly ↑ adverse effects	Inhibition of CYP3A4-mediated metabolism of fusidic acid	Avoid co-administration
PROTEASE INHIBITORS	MACROLIDES – AZITHROMYCIN	Risk of ↑ adverse effects of azithromycin with nelfinavir	Possibly involves altered P-gp transport	Watch for signs of azithromycin toxicity
PROTEASE INHIBITORS	MACROLIDES – CLARITHROMYCIN, ERYTHROMYCIN	Possibly ↑ adverse effects of macrolide with atazanavir, ritonavir (with or without lopinavir) or saquinavir	Inhibition of CYP3A4- and possibly CYP1A2-mediated metabolism. Altered transport via P-gp may be involved. Amprenavir and indinavir are also possibly ↑ by erythromycin	Consider alternatives unless *Mycobacterium avium intracellulare* infection; if combined, ↓ dose by 50% (75% in the presence of renal failure with a creatinine clearance of <30 mL/min)
PROTEASE INHIBITORS	METRONIDAZOLE	↑ adverse effects, e.g. a disulfiram-like reaction and flushing, with ritonavir (with or without lopinavir)	Ritonavir and lopinavir oral solutions contain alcohol	Warn patients, and give alternative preparations if possible
PROTEASE INHIBITORS	RIFABUTIN	↑ efficacy and ↑ adverse effects of rifabutin	Inhibition of CYP3A4-mediated metabolism. Nelfinavir also competitively inhibits CYP2C19	↓ rifabutin dose by at least 50% when given with amprenavir, indinavir or nelfinavir, and by 75% with atazanavir, ritonavir (with or without lopinavir) or tipranavir
SAQUINAVIR	RIFABUTIN	↓ efficacy of saquinavir	Uncertain; probably via altered CYP3A4 metabolism	Avoid co-administration
PROTEASE INHIBITORS	RIFAMPICIN	↓ levels of the protease inhibitor. Risk of hepatotoxicity with saquinavir	Induction of metabolism	Avoid co-administration

Primary drug	Secondary drug	Effect	Mechanism	Precautions
PROTEASE INHIBITORS	ANTICANCER AND IMMUNOMODULATING DRUGS			
PROTEASE INHIBITORS	CYTOTOXICS			
RITONAVIR	IFOSFAMIDE	↓ plasma concentrations of 4-hydroxyifosfamide, the active metabolite of ifosfamide, and risk of inadequate therapeutic response	Due to inhibition of the isoenzymatic conversion to active metabolites	Monitor clinically the efficacy of ifosfamide and ↑ dose accordingly
RITONAVIR	IMATINIB	↑ imatinib levels with ↑ risk of toxicity (e.g. abdominal pain, constipation, dyspnoea) and of neurotoxicity (e.g. taste disturbances, dizziness, headache, paraesthesia, peripheral neuropathy)	Due to inhibition of CYP3A4-mediated metabolism of imatinib	Monitor for clinical efficacy and for the signs of toxicity listed, along with convulsions, confusion and signs of oedema (including pulmonary oedema). Monitor electrolytes, liver function and for cardiotoxicity
RITONAVIR	IRINOTECAN	↑ plasma concentrations of SN-38 (>AUC by 100%) and ↑ toxicity of irinotecan, e.g. diarrhoea, acute cholinergic syndrome, interstitial pulmonary disease	Due to inhibition of the metabolism of irinotecan by CYP3A4 isoenzymes by ritonavir	Peripheral blood counts should be checked before each course of treatment. Monitor lung function. Recommendation is to ↓ dose of irinotecan by 25%
PROTEASE INHIBITORS	VINCA ALKALOIDS	↑ adverse effects of vinblastine and vincristine	Inhibition of CYP3A4-mediated metabolism of vinblastine	Monitor FBCs watch for early features of toxicity (pain, numbness, tingling in the fingers and toes, jaw pain, abdominal pain, constipation, ileus). Consider selecting an alternative drug
PROTEASE INHIBITORS	HORMONES AND HORMONE ANTAGONISTS			
RITONAVIR	TOREMIFENE	↑ plasma concentrations of toremifene	Due to inhibition of metabolism of toremifene by the CYP3A4 isoenzymes by ritonavir	Clinical relevance is uncertain. Necessary to monitor for clinical toxicities

PROTEASE INHIBITORS	**IMMUNOMODULATING DRUGS**			
PROTEASE INHIBITORS	CICLOSPORIN, SIROLIMUS, TACROLIMUS	↑ levels with protease inhibitors	Inhibition of CYP3A4-mediated metabolism of these immunomodulating drugs	Monitor clinical effects closely and check levels
PROTEASE INHIBITORS	CORTICOSTEROIDS	↑ plasma levels of betamethasone, dexamethasone, hydrocortisone, prednisolone and both inhaled and intranasal budesonide and fluticasone with ritonavir (with or without lopinavir)	Inhibition of CYP3A4-mediated metabolism	Monitor closely for signs of corticosteroid toxicity and immunosupression, and ↓ dose as necessary. Consider using inhaled beclometasone
PROTEASE INHIBITORS	DOCETAXEL, PACLITAXEL	↑ risk of adverse effects of docetaxel and paclitaxel	Inhibition of CYP3A4-mediated metabolism. Also inhibition of P-gp efflux of vinblastine	Use with caution. Additional monitoring is required. Monitor FBC weekly
PROTEASE INHIBITORS	DOXORUBICIN	↑ risk of myelosuppression due to ↑ plasma concentrations	Due to ↓ metabolism of doxorubicin by CYP3A4 isoenzymes owing to inhibition of those enzymes	Monitor for ↑ myelosuppression, peripheral neuropathy, myalgias and fatigue
PROTEASE INHIBITORS	IL-2	↑ protease inhibitor levels, with risk of toxicity	Aldesleukin induces the formation of IL-6, which inhibits the metabolism of protease inhibitors by the CYP3A4 isoenzymes	Warn patients to report symptoms such as nausea, vomiting , flatulence, dizziness and rashes. Monitor blood sugar on initiating and discontinuing treatment
PROTEASE INHIBITORS	ANTICOAGULANTS – ORAL	1. Anticoagulant effect may be altered (cases of both ↑ and ↓) when ritonavir and possibly saquinavir are given with warfarin 2. Possibly ↓ anticoagulant effect when ritonavir and nelfinavir are given with acenocoumarol	Uncertain. Ritonavir inhibits CYP3A4 and CYP2C9 while inducing CYP1A2	Monitor INR closely

DRUGS TO TREAT INFECTIONS ANTIVIRALS – ANTIRETROVIRALS

Primary drug	Secondary drug	Effect	Mechanism	Precautions
PROTEASE INHIBITORS	**ANTIDEPRESSANTS**			
PROTEASE INHIBITORS	SSRIs	↑ adverse effects of fluoxetine, paroxetine and sertraline when co-administered with ritonavir (with or without lopinavir). Cardiac and neurological events have been reported, including serotonin syndrome	Ritonavir is associated with the most significant interaction of the protease inhibitors due to potent inhibition of CYP3A, CYP2D6, CYP2C9 and CYP2C19 isoenzymes	Warn patients to watch for ↑ side-effects of SSRIs and consider ↓ dose of SSRI
PROTEASE INHIBITORS	**TCAs**			
PROTEASE INHIBITORS	AMITRIPTYLINE	↑ adverse effects when amitriptyline is co-administered with ritonavir (with or without lopinavir), and possibly atazanavir	Inhibition of CYP3A4-mediated metabolism. Note that SSRIs are metabolized by a number of enzymes, including CYP2C9, CYP2C19, CYP2D6 and CYP3A4; therefore, the effect of protease inhibitors is variable	Monitor closely
PROTEASE INHIBITORS	AMOXAPINE, CLOMIPRAMINE, DOXEPIN, IMIPRAMINE, NORTRIPTYLINE, TRIMIPRAMINE	Possibly ↑ adverse effects of amoxapine with atazanavir and ritonavir	Inhibition of CYP3A4-mediated metabolism of amoxapine, clomipramine and doxepin; inhibition of CYP3A4-, CYP2D6- and CYP2C9-mediated metabolism of imipramine; inhibition of CYP2D6-mediated metabolism of nortriptyline and trimipramine	Monitor closely
PROTEASE INHIBITORS	ST JOHN'S WORT	Markedly ↓ levels and efficacy of protease inhibitors by St John's wort	Possibly ↑ CYP3A4-mediated metabolism of protease inhibitors	Avoid co-administration

PROTEASE INHIBITORS	ANTIDIABETIC DRUGS			
PROTEASE INHIBITORS	INSULIN	↓ efficacy of insulin	Several mechanisms considered include insulin resistance, impaired insulin-stimulated glucose uptake by skeletal muscle cells, ↓ insulin binding to receptors and inhibition of intrinsic transport activity of glucose transporters in the body	Necessary to establish baseline values for blood sugar before initiating therapy with a protease inhibitor. Warn patients about hyperglycaemia. Atazanavir, darunavir, fosamprenavir or tipranavir may be safer ➢ ***For signs and symptoms of hyperglycaemia, see Clinical Features of Some Adverse Drug Interactions, Hyperglycaemia***
PROTEASE INHIBITORS	NATEGLINIDE, PIOGLITAZONE, REPAGLINIDE	↑ levels of these antidiabetic drugs	Inhibition of CYP2C9- and CYP3A4-mediated metabolism of nateglinide and CYP3A4-mediated metabolism of pioglitazone and repaglinide	Monitor blood sugar closely
PROTEASE INHIBITORS	SULPHONYLUREAS	↑ effect of tolbutamide with ritonavir	Ritonavir is a potent inhibitor of CYP2C9, which metabolizes many sulphonylureas	Watch for hypoglycaemia. Warn patients about hypoglycaemia ➢ ***For signs and symptoms of hypoglycaemia, see Clinical Features of Some Adverse Drug Reactions, Hypoglycaemia***
PROTEASE INHIBITORS	ANTIDIARRHOEAL DRUGS – LOPERAMIDE	↑ risk of adverse effects when loperamide is co-ingested with ritonavir	Ritonavir inhibits P-gp and CYP3A4	Monitor for clinical effect, and consider ↓ dose if necessary. Stop if there are signs of abdominal distension in HIV patients as toxic megacolon has been reported
PROTEASE INHIBITORS	ANTIEMETICS – APREPITANT	↑ adverse effects of aprepitant with nelfinavir and ritonavir (with or without lopinavir)	Inhibition of CYP3A4-mediated metabolism of aprepitant	Use with caution; clinical significance unclear; monitor closely

Primary drug	Secondary drug	Effect	Mechanism	Precautions
PROTEASE INHIBITORS	**ANTIEPILEPTICS**			
PROTEASE INHIBITORS	CARBAMAZEPINE	Possibly ↑ adverse effects of carbamazepine with protease inhibitors	Inhibition of CYP3A4-mediated metabolism of carbamazepine	Use with caution. Monitor carbamazepine levels and side-effects when initiating or changing treatment
PROTEASE INHIBITORS	PHENYTOIN	Possibly ↓ efficacy of phenytoin, with a risk of fits when it is co-administered with indinavir, nelfinavir or ritonavir (with or without lopinavir)	Uncertain; ↓ plasma levels of phenytoin	Use with caution. Monitor phenytoin levels weekly. Adjust doses at 7–10-day intervals. Maximum suggested dose adjustment each time is 25 mg
PROTEASE INHIBITORS	**ANTIFUNGALS – AZOLES**			
PROTEASE INHIBITORS	ITRACONAZOLE, KETOCONAZOLE	Possibly ↑ levels of ketoconazole by amprenavir, indinavir and ritonavir (with or without lopinavir). Conversely, indinavir, ritonavir and saquinavir levels are ↑ by itraconazole and ketoconazole	Inhibition of, or competition for, CYP3A4-mediated metabolism	Use itraconazole with caution and monitor for adverse effects. No dose adjustment is recommended for doses <400 mg/day of ketoconazole
PROTEASE INHIBITORS	VORICONAZOLE	↓ efficacy of voriconazole	↓ plasma levels	Avoid co-administration if the dose of ritonavir is 400 mg twice a day or greater. Avoid combining low-dose ritonavir (100 mg once a day) unless benefits outweigh risks
PROTEASE INHIBITORS	ANTIHISTAMINES – ASTEMIZOLE, CHLORPHENAMINE, TERFENADINE	Possibly ↑ adverse effects with amprenavir, atazanavir, indinavir, ritonavir (with or without lopinavir), saquinavir and tipranavir	Inhibition of CYP3A4-mediated metabolism of astemizole; the risk is greatest in patients who are slow CYP2D6 metabolizers because chlorphenamine and terfenadine are also metabolized by this route	Avoid co-administration

PROTEASE INHIBITORS	ANTIHYPERTENSIVES AND HEART FAILURE DRUGS			
PROTEASE INHIBITORS	ALPHA-BLOCKERS	Possible ↑ alfuzosin levels with ritonavir	Uncertain	Avoid co-administration
PROTEASE INHIBITORS	VASODILATOR ANTIHYPERTENSIVES	↑ adverse effects of bosentan by ritonavir	Inhibition of CYP3A4-mediated metabolism of bosentan	Co-administration not recommended
PROTEASE INHIBITORS	ANTIMALARIALS – ARTEMETHER WITH LUMEFANTRINE	↑ artemether levels	Uncertain; possibly inhibited metabolism	Avoid co-administration
PROTEASE INHIBITORS	**ANTIMIGRAINE DRUGS**			
PROTEASE INHIBITORS	ERGOT ALKALOIDS	↑ ergotamine/methysergide levels, with risk of toxicity	↓ CYP3A4-mediated metabolism of ergot derivatives	Avoid co-administration
PROTEASE INHIBITORS	5-HT1 AGONISTS – ALMOTRIPTAN, ELETRIPTAN	Possibly ↑ adverse effects when almotriptan or eletriptan is co-administered with indinavir, ritonavir (with or without lopinavir) or nelfinavir	Inhibition of CYP3A4- and possibly CYP2D6-mediated metabolism of eletriptan and CYP3A4-mediated metabolism of almotriptan	Avoid co-administration
PROTEASE INHIBITORS	**ANTIMUSCARINICS**			
PROTEASE INHIBITORS	SOLIFENACIN	↑ adverse effects with nelfinavir and ritonavir (with or without lopinavir)	Inhibition of CYP3A4-mediated metabolism of solifenacin	Limit maximum dose of solifenacin to 5 mg daily
PROTEASE INHIBITORS	TOLTERODINE	Possibly ↑ adverse effects, including arrythmias with protease inhibitors	Inhibition of CYP2D6- and CYP3A4-mediated metabolism of tolterodine	Avoid co-administration

Primary drug	Secondary drug	Effect	Mechanism	Precautions
PROTEASE INHIBITORS	ANTIPSYCHOTICS			
PROTEASE INHIBITORS	ARIPIPRAZOLE, HALOPERIDOL, CLOZAPINE, PIMOZIDE, RISPERIDONE, SERTINDOLE, THIORIDAZINE	Possibly ↑ levels of antipsychotic	Inhibition of CYP3A4- and/or CYP2D6-mediated metabolism	Avoid co-administration of clozapine with ritonavir, and pimozide or sertindole with protease inhibitors. Use other antipsychotics with caution; ↓ dose may be required. With risperidone, watch closely for extrapyramidal side-effects and neuroepileptic malignant syndrome
PROTEASE INHIBITORS	OLANZAPINE	Possibly ↓ efficacy of olanzapine when co-ingested with ritonavir (with or without lopinavir)	Possibly ↑ metabolism via CYP1A2 and glucuronyl transferases	Monitor clinical response; ↑ dose as necessary
PROTEASE INHIBITORS				
PROTEASE INHIBITORS	ANTIVIRALS – FOSCARNET SODIUM	↓ renal function when co-administered with ritonavir or saquinavir	Uncertain; possibly ↓ renal excretion of foscarnet	Monitor renal function closely
PROTEASE INHIBITORS	NNRTIs			
AMPRENAVIR	EFAVIRENZ	Possible ↓ efficacy of amprenavir	Uncertain; ↓ bioavailability of amprenavir	Consider ↑ dose of amprenavir to 1200 mg three times a day, or combine amprenavir 600 mg twice a day with ritonavir 100 mg twice a day
AMPRENAVIR	NEVIRAPINE	Efficacy of amprenavir predicted to be ↓	Uncertain; ↓ bioavailability of amprenavir	Monitor viral load
ATAZANAVIR	EFAVIRENZ	↓ efficacy of efavirenz	↑ CYP3A4-mediated metabolism of efavirenz	Recommended dose of atazanavir is 400 mg when given with efavirenz 600 mg. Optimal suggested treatment is this combination plus ritonavir 100 mg daily

ATAZANAVIR	NEVIRAPINE	↓ efficacy of atazanavir	Atazanavir is a substrate and inhibitor of CYP3A4	Avoid concomitant use
INDINAVIR	NNRTIs	Possible ↓ efficacy of indinavir	↑ CYP3A4-mediated metabolism of indinavir	Monitor viral load; consider ↑ dose of indinavir to 1000 mg 8-hourly
LOPINAVIR AND RITONAVIR	NNRTIs	Possible ↓ efficacy of lopinavir/ritonavir	Uncertain; ↓ bioavailability	Consider ↑ lopinavir/ritonavir dose (by 33% with efavirenz and to 53 mg/133 mg twice daily, and monitor drug concentrations, with nevirapine). Monitor viral load closely as this ↑ dose may be insufficient. Monitor LFTs closely
NELFINAVIR	EFAVIRENZ	Possible ↑ efficacy of nelfinavir, with theoretical risk of adverse effects	Small ↑ bioavailability of nelfinavir	No dose adjustment necessary
NELFINAVIR	NEVIRAPINE	Possible ↓ efficacy of nelfinavir	Uncertain	Dose adjustment probably not required, although one study suggests ↑ dose may be needed
RITONAVIR	EFAVIRENZ	↑ efficacy and ↑ adverse effects of ritonavir, e.g. dizziness, nausea, paraesthesia, liver dysfunction	↑ bioavailability of ritonavir; competition for metabolism via CYP3A4	Combination is not well tolerated. Monitor closely, including LFTs. Low-dose ritonavir has not been studied
SAQUINAVIR	EFAVIRENZ	Possible ↓ efficacy of saquinavir, with risk of treatment failure	↑ CYP3A4-mediated metabolism of saquinavir	Combination is not recommended if saquinavir is the sole protease inhibitor; always use saquinavir in combination with another agent, e.g. ritonavir, when co-administering with efavirenz
SAQUINAVIR	NEVIRAPINE	Possible ↓ efficacy; risk of treatment failure of saquinavir	↑ CYP3A4-mediated metabolism of saquinavir	Clinical significance unclear. Different formulations of saquinavir may have different magnitudes of interaction

DRUGS TO TREAT INFECTIONS ANTIVIRALS – ANTIRETROVIRALS

Primary drug	Secondary drug	Effect	Mechanism	Precautions
PROTEASE INHIBITORS	**NUCLEOSIDE REVERSE TRANSCRIPTASE INHIBITORS**			
PROTEASE INHIBITORS	DIDANOSINE (BUFFERED)	↓ efficacy of amprenavir, atazanavir and indinavir	Absorption of these protease inhibitors may be affected by the buffered didanosine formulation, which ↑ gastric pH	Separate doses by at least 1 hour. Alternatively, consider using the enteric-coated formulation of didanosine
ATAZANAVIR	TENOFOVIR	↓ efficacy of atazanavir	Uncertain; ↓ plasma levels of atazanavir	Use with caution and consider using in combination with ritonavir
LOPINAVIR + RITONAVIR	ZIDOVUDINE	↓ efficacy of zidovudine	↓ plasma levels by ↑ glucu-ronidation	Avoid co-administration
NELFINAVIR	STAVUDINE	Possibly ↑ adverse effects	Uncertain	Warn patients that diarrhoea may occur
TIPRANAVIR + RITONAVIR	ABACAVIR	Possible ↓ efficacy; risk of treatment failure of abacavir	↓ plasma concentrations	Not recommended unless there are no other available nucleoside reverse transcriptase inhibitors
TIPRANAVIR + RITONAVIR	DIDANOSINE (ENTERIC-COATED)	Possible ↓ efficacy of didanosine	↓ absorption	Separate doses by at least 2 hours
TIPRANAVIR + RITONAVIR	ZIDOVUDINE	Possible ↓ efficacy; risk of treatment failure of zidovudine	↓ plasma concentrations	Not recommended unless there are no other available nucleoside reverse transcriptase inhibitors
PROTEASE INHIBITORS	**PROTEASE INHIBITORS**			
AMPRENAVIR	RITONAVIR	↑ efficacy and ↑ adverse effects of both, e.g. ↑ triglycerides and creatine phosphokinase	Complex alterations in bioavailability. Ritonavir is a more potent CYP3A4 inhibitor than amprenavir, also inhibiting CYP2D6 and inducing CYP3A4, CYP1A2 and CYP2C9	Monitor closely. ↓ dose of both if used together; amprenavir 600 mg + ritonavir 100 mg twice a day is suggested

ATAZANAVIR	INDINAVIR	↑ efficacy and ↑ adverse effects of indinavir; ↑ adverse effects of atazanavir, e.g. hyperbilirubinaemia	↑ bioavailability. Inhibition of metabolism via CYP3A4 by atazanavir; inhibition of UDGPT by indinavir	Avoid co-administration
ATAZANAVIR	SAQUINAVIR	↑ efficacy and ↑ adverse effects of saquinavir	Inhibition of CYP3A4-mediated metabolism of saquinavir	Monitor more closely
INDINAVIR	NELFINAVIR	Possibly ↑ efficacy and ↑ adverse effects of both	Inhibition of CYP3A4-mediated metabolism	Uncertain if interaction is clinically significant; however, monitor more closely for adverse effects
INDINAVIR	RITONAVIR	↑ efficacy and ↑ adverse effects of indinavir. Risk of nephrolithiasis if the dose of indinavir exceeds 800 mg twice a day	Inhibition of CYP3A4-mediated metabolism of indinavir	Dose of indinavir can be ↓ from 800 mg three times a day to 600 mg twice daily. Adequate hydration and monitoring are essential. Adults must drink at least 1500 mL/24 hours
INDINAVIR	SAQUINAVIR	Possibly ↑ efficacy and ↑ adverse effects of both	Inhibition of CYP3A4-mediated metabolism	Safety of combination not established. The formulation may affect the interaction. Monitor closely
NELFINAVIR	RITONAVIR AND LOPINAVIR	Possibly ↓ efficacy of lopinavir and ritonavir, and ↑ efficacy of nelfinavir	↓ bioavailability of lopinavir and ritonavir, but ↑ minimum plasma levels of nelfinavir and its active metabolites	Monitor closely. May need to ↑ doses of lopinavir and ritonavir
NELFINAVIR	RITONAVIR	↑ efficacy and ↑ adverse effects of nelfinavir; unclear effects on ritonavir	Involves CYP450 inhibition and induction. ↑ concentration of nelfinavir and its active metabolite M8	Monitor closely if combination used
NELFINAVIR	SAQUINAVIR (SOFT GEL)	Possibly ↑ efficacy and ↑ adverse effects, e.g. diarrhoea	Additive toxicity; ↑ bioavailability. Inhibition of metabolism via CYP3A4	Warn patients of ↑ side-effects

Primary drug	Secondary drug	Effect	Mechanism	Precautions
SAQUINAVIR (SOFT GEL)	RITONAVIR AND LOPINAVIR	↑ efficacy of saquinavir	Inhibition of CYP3A4-mediated metabolism	Dose of saquinavir can be ↓ from 1.2 g three times a day to 800 mg twice daily
SAQUINAVIR	RITONAVIR	↑ efficacy and ↑ adverse effects of saquinavir; no clinically significant interaction for ritonavir	Large ↑ bioavailability of saquinavir via inhibition of CYP3A4 in gut wall and liver	Adjust dose and monitor closely. Saquinavir 1000 mg with ritonavir 100 mg twice a day is approximately equivalent to saquinavir 1200 mg three times a day on its own
TIPRANAVIR + RITONAVIR	AMPRENAVIR + RITONAVIR	Possibly ↓ efficacy	Significant ↓ bioavailability	Avoid co-administration
TIPRANAVIR + RITONAVIR	ATAZANAVIR	Possibly ↓ efficacy of atazanavir and ↑ toxicity of tipranavir + ritonavir	Significant ↓ bioavailability	Avoid co-administration
TIPRANAVIR + RITONAVIR	LOPINAVIR + RITONAVIR	Possibly ↓ efficacy	Significant ↓ bioavailability	Avoid co-administration
TIPRANAVIR + RITONAVIR	SAQUINAVIR + RITONAVIR	Possibly ↓ efficacy	Significant ↓ bioavailability	Avoid co-administration
PROTEASE INHIBITORS	ANXIOLYTICS AND HYPNOTICS – BZDs, BUSPIRONE	↑ adverse effects, e.g. prolonged sedation	Inhibition of CYP3A4-mediated metabolism of BZDs and buspirone	Watch closely for ↑ sedation; ↓ dose of sedative as necessary. Some recommend considering substituting long-acting for shorter-acting BZDs with less active metabolites (e.g. lorazepam for diazepam)
RITONAVIR, TIPRANAVIR	BETA-BLOCKERS	↑ adverse effects of carvedilol, metoprolol, propanolol and timolol	Inhibition of CYP2D6-mediated metabolism of these beta-blockers	Use an alternative beta-blocker if possible; if not, monitor closely. Avoid co-administration of metoprolol with ritonavir + tipranavir

DRUGS TO TREAT INFECTIONS ANTIVIRALS – ANTIRETROVIRALS

PROTEASE INHIBITORS	BRONCHODILATORS – THEOPHYLLINES			
INDINAVIR	THEOPHYLLINE	Possibly ↑ efficacy	Inhibition of metabolism via CYP3A4 but mainly metabolized via CYP1A2, which is not inhibited	Not thought to be clinically significant; however, monitor levels more closely in unstable patients
RITONAVIR (± LOPINAVIR)	THEOPHYLLINE	↓ efficacy	↑ metabolism via induction of CYP1A2 also altered metabolism via CYP3A4	Monitor clinical response. Measure levels weekly after starting; ↑ doses may be required
PROTEASE INHIBITORS	CALCIUM CHANNEL BLOCKERS	Plasma concentrations of calcium channel blockers are ↑ by protease inhibitors	Protease inhibitors inhibit CYP3A4-mediated metabolism of calcium channel blockers	Monitor PR, BP and ECG closely; ↓ dose of calcium channel blocker if necessary (e.g. manufacturers of diltiazem suggest starting at 50% of the standard dose and titrating to effect)
RITONAVIR (WITH OR WITHOUT LOPINAVIR)	CARDIAC GLYCOSIDES – DIGOXIN	Plasma digoxin concentrations may be ↑ by ritonavir	Uncertain; probably due to inhibition of P-gp-mediated renal excretion of digoxin and ↑ intestinal absorption	Monitor digoxin levels; watch for digoxin toxicity
INDINAVIR, NELFINAVIR, RITONAVIR, SAQUINAVIR	CNS STIMULANTS – MODAFINIL	↑ plasma concentrations of modafinil, with risk of adverse effects	Due to inhibition of CYP3A4, which has a partial role in the metabolism of modafinil	Be aware. Warn patients to report dose-related adverse effects, e.g. headache, anxiety
PROTEASE INHIBITORS	DIURETICS – POTASSIUM-SPARING	Possibly ↑ adverse effects of eplerenone with nelfinavir, ritonavir (with or without lopinavir) and saquinavir	Inhibition of CYP3A4-mediated metabolism of eplerenone	Avoid concomitant use
PROTEASE INHIBITORS	**DRUG DEPENDENCE THERAPIES**			
PROTEASE INHIBITORS	BUPROPION	↑ adverse effects of bupropion with nelfinavir and ritonavir (with or without lopinavir)	Possibly inhibition of CYP2B6-mediated metabolism of bupropion	Avoid co-administration

Primary drug	Secondary drug	Effect	Mechanism	Precautions
PROTEASE INHIBITORS	DISULFIRAM	↑ risk of disulfiram reaction with ritonavir (with or without lopinavir)	Ritonavir and lopinavir/ritonavir oral solutions contain 43% alcohol	Warn patients. Consider using capsule preparation as an alternative
PROTEASE INHIBITORS	DUTASTERIDE	Possibly ↑ adverse effects of dutasteride with indinavir or ritonavir (with or without lopinavir)	Inhibition of CYP3A4-mediated metabolism of dutasteride	Monitor closely; ↓ dosing frequency if side-effects occur
SAQUINAVIR (INVIRASE HARD CAPSULES)	GRAPEFRUIT JUICE	Possibly ↑ efficacy	Possibly ↑ bioavailability; ↓ presystemic metabolism. Constituents of grapefruit irreversibly inhibit intestinal cytochrome CYP3A4. Transport via P-gp and MRP-2 efflux pumps is also inhibited	No dose adjustment is advised. Oral bioavailability is very low and is enhanced beneficially with grapefruit juice or grapefruit. Soft gel capsules have greater bioavailability so may interact to a lesser degree
AMPRENAVIR, ATAZANAVIR	H2 RECEPTOR BLOCKERS – CIMETIDINE	↓ efficacy of amprenavir; possible ↑ levels of cimetidine	↓ absorption of amprenavir and atazanavir. Uncertain mechanism of action on cimetidine	Amprenavir: separate doses by at least 1 hour. Take atazanavir at least 2 hours before or 10 hours after the H2 blocker. In both cases, monitor viral load closely
PROTEASE INHIBITORS	IVABRADINE	↑ levels with nelfinavir and ritonavir	Uncertain	Avoid co-administration
PROTEASE INHIBITORS	**LIPID-LOWERING DRUGS – STATINS**			
PROTEASE INHIBITORS	ATORVASTATIN	↑ efficacy and ↑ risk of adverse effects of atorvastatin	Inhibition of CYP3A4-mediated metabolism of atorvastatin	Use with caution. Monitor for atorvastatin toxicity, and monitor CK. Inform patients and ↓ dose if necessary or start with 10 mg once daily. Use the lowest dose possible to attain the target low-density lipoprotein ↓. Alternatives are pravastatin and fluvastatin

PROTEASE INHIBITORS	LOVASTATIN, SIMVASTATIN	↑ risk of adverse effects	Inhibition of CYP3A4-mediated metabolism of these statins	Avoid co-administration
PROTEASE INHIBITORS	OESTROGENS	Marked ↓ contraceptive effect with nelfinavir and ritonavir	Induction of metabolism of oestrogens	Advise patients to use additional contraception for the period of intake and for 1 month after stopping co-administration with nelfinavir and ritonavir. Barrier methods are necessary to prevent transmission of infection from patients with HIV
PROTEASE INHIBITORS	PERIPHERAL VASODILATORS	Amprenavir, indinavir, lopinavir, nelfinavir, ritonavir and saquinavir ↑ cilostazol levels	These protease inhibitors inhibit CYP3A4-mediated metabolism of cilostazol	Avoid co-administration
PROTEASE INHIBITORS	PHOSPHODIESTERASE TYPE 5 INHIBITORS – SILDENAFIL, TADALAFIL, VARDENAFIL	↑ sildenafil, tadalafil and vardenafil levels	Inhibition of CYP3A4- and possibly CYP2C9-mediated metabolism of sildenafil	Use with caution; monitor BP closely. UK manufacturers recommend avoiding co-administration of vardenafil with protease inhibitors in patients >75 years. US manufacturers recommend using with caution, starting with a daily dose of 2.5 mg
PROTEASE INHIBITORS	PROGESTOGENS – NORETHISTERONE	↑ adverse effects with amprenavir and atazanavir. Possibly ↓ efficacy and risk of contraceptive failure with nelfinavir and ritonavir (with or without lopinavir)	Uncertain	Advise patients to use additional contraception for the period of intake and for 1 month after stopping co-administration with these drugs. Barrier methods are necessary to prevent transmission of infection from patients with HIV. Watch for early features of toxicity of amprenavir and atazanavir, and adjust the dose accordingly

Primary drug	Secondary drug	Effect	Mechanism	Precautions
PROTEASE INHIBITORS	PROTON PUMP INHIBITORS			
ATAZANAVIR	PROTON PUMP INHIBITORS	Possibly ↓ efficacy of atazanavir	↓ plasma concentration; uncertain cause	Avoid co-administration
INDINAVIR	OMEPRAZOLE	Possibly ↓ efficacy of indinavir	↓ plasma concentration; uncertain cause	↑ dose of indinavir from 800 mg three times a day to 1 g three times a day, or preferably add ritonavir 200 mg once daily
PROTEASE INHIBITORS	SYMPATHOMIMETICS	1. Risk of serotonin syndrome when dexamfetamine is administered with ritonavir 2. Indinavir may ↑ phenylpropanolamine levels	1. Protease inhibitors inhibit CYP2D6-mediated metabolism 2. Likely inhibition of phenylpropanolamine metabolism	1. Avoid co-administration 2. Monitor BP closely; watch for marked ↑ BP
PROTEASE INHIBITORS	THYROID HORMONES	↓ efficacy of levothyroxine by ritonavir (with or without lopinavir) and possibly indinavir and nelfinavir	Uncertain; possibly ↑ metabolism via induction of glucuronosyl transferases	Monitor thyroid function closely
ANTIVIRALS – OTHER				
AMANTADINE is used to treat Parkinson's disease as well as having antiviral activity. It has been included in the antiparkinson's drugs section				
ACICLOVIR, VALACICLOVIR				
ACICLOVIR/ VALACICLOVIR	ANTICANCER AND IMMUNOMODULATING DRUGS – 1. CICLOSPORIN 2. MYCOPHENOLATE 3. TACROLIMUS	1. ↑ nephrotoxicity 2. Possible ↑ efficacy 3. ↑ levels with protease inhibitors	1. Additive side-effect 2. Competition for renal excretion 3. Inhibition of CYP3A4-mediated metabolism of tacrolimus	1. Monitor renal function prior to concomitant therapy and monitor ciclosporin levels 2. Monitor renal function particularly if on >4 g valaciclovir; ↓ dose of aciclovir if there is a background of renal failure 3. Monitor clinical effects closely; check levels

ACICLOVIR/ VALACICLOVIR	ANTIDEPRESSANTS – LITHIUM	↑ lithium levels, with risk of toxicity	Possible ↓ renal excretion	Ensure adequate hydration; monitor lithium levels if intravenous aciclovir or >4 g/day valaciclovir is required
ACICLOVIR/ VALACICLOVIR	ANTIEPILEPTICS – PHENYTOIN, VALPROATE	↓ efficacy of phenytoin	Unclear	Warn patients and monitor seizure frequency
ACICLOVIR/ VALACICLOVIR	ANTIGOUT DRUGS – PROBENECID	↑ levels of aciclovir, valaciclovir and ganciclovir	Competitive inhibition of renal excretion	Care with co-administering probenecid with high-dose antivirals
ACICLOVIR/ VALACICLOVIR	BRONCHODILATORS – THEOPHYLLINES	↑ theophylline levels	Uncertain	Monitor for signs of toxicity and check levels
ACICLOVIR/ VALACICLOVIR	H2 RECEPTOR BLOCKERS – CIMETIDINE	↑ efficacy and adverse effects of antivirals	Competition for renal excretion	Use doses >4 g/day valaciclovir with caution or consider alternative acid suppression. For doses <1 g/day, interaction is not thought to be clinically significant. Studies available only for valaciclovir
GANCICLOVIR, VALGANCICLOVIR				
GANCICLOVIR/ VALGANCICLOVIR	ANTIBIOTICS – 1. IMIPENEM WITH CILASTATIN 2. TRIMETHOPRIM	1. ↑ adverse effects (e.g. seizures) 2. Possibly ↑ adverse effects (e.g. myelosuppression) when trimethoprim is co-administered with ganciclovir or valganciclovir	1. Additive side-effects; these drugs can cause seizure activity 2. Small ↑ bioavailability; possible additive toxicity	1. Avoid combination if possible; use only if benefit outweighs risk 2. Well tolerated in one study. For patients at risk of additive toxicities, use only if benefits outweigh risks and monitor FBC closely
GANCICLOVIR/ VALGANCICLOVIR	ANTICANCER AND IMMUNOMODULATING DRUGS –1. CICLOSPORIN 2. MYCOPHENOLATE 3. TACROLIMUS	1. ↑ risk of nephrotoxicity 2. Possible ↑ efficacy 3. Possible ↑ nephrotoxicity/neurotoxicity	1. Additive nephrotoxic effects 2. Competition for renal excretion 3. Additive side-effects	1.Monitor renal function 2. Monitor renal function particularly if on >4 g valaciclovir; ↓ dose of aciclovir if there is a background of renal failure 3. Monitor more closely; check tacrolimus levels

Primary drug	Secondary drug	Effect	Mechanism	Precautions
GANCICLOVIR/ VALGANCICLOVIR	ANTIGOUT DRUGS – PROBENECID	↑ levels of ganciclovir/ valganciclovir	Competitive inhibition of renal excretion	Care with co-administering probenecid with high-dose antivirals
GANCICLOVIR/ VALGANCICLOVIR	ANTIVIRALS – NUCLEOSIDE REVERSE TRANSCRIPTASE INHIBITORS	1. ↑ adverse effects with tenofovir, zidovudine and possibly didanosine, lamivudine and zalcitabine 2. Possibly ↓ efficacy of ganciclovir	1. Uncertain; possibly additive toxicity. Lamivudine may compete for active tubular secretion in the kidneys 2. Uncertain; ↓ bioavailability	1. Avoid if possible, otherwise monitor FBC and renal function weekly. It has been suggested that the dose of zidovudine should be halved from 600 mg to 300 mg daily. Monitor for peripheral neuropathy, particularly with zalcitabine 2. Uncertain clinical significance; if in doubt, consider alternative cytomegalovirus prophylaxis
ADEFOVIR DIPIVOXIL				
ADEFOVIR DIPIVOXIL	1. ANTIBIOTICS – aminoglycosides, vancomycin 2. ANTICANCER AND IMMUNOMODULATING DRUGS – ciclosporin, tacrolimus 3. ANTIFUNGALS – amphotericin, 4. ANTIPROTOZOALS – pentamidine 5. ANTIVIRALS – cidofovir, foscarnet sodium, tenofovir	Possible ↑ efficacy and side-effects	Competition for renal excretion	Monitor renal function weekly

CIDOFOVIR				
CIDOFOVIR	ANTIDIABETIC DRUGS – METFORMIN	↑ risk of lactic acidosis	↓ renal excretion of metformin	Watch for lactic acidosis. The onset of lactic acidosis is often subtle, with symptoms of malaise, myalgia, respiratory distress and ↑ non-specific abdominal distress. There may be hypothermia and resistant bradyarrhythmias
CIDOFOVIR	**ANTIVIRALS**			
CIDOFOVIR	ADEFOVIR DIPIVOXIL	Possible ↑ efficacy and side-effects	Competition for renal excretion	Monitor renal function weekly
CIDOFOVIR	TENOFOVIR	↑ adverse effects	↑ plasma levels; competition for renal excretion via organic anion transporter	Monitor renal function weekly
FOSCARNET SODIUM				
FOSCARNET SODIUM	**ANTIBIOTICS**			
FOSCARNET SODIUM	AMINOGLYCOSIDES	Possible ↑ nephrotoxicity	Additive side-effect	Monitor renal function closely
FOSCARNET SODIUM	QUINOLONES	Risk of seizures	Unknown; possibly additive side-effect	Avoid combination in patients with past medical history of epilepsy. Consider an alternative antibiotic
FOSCARNET SODIUM	ANTICANCER AND IMMUNOMODULATING DRUGS – CICLOSPORIN	↑ risk of renal failure	Additive nephrotoxic effects	Monitor renal function
FOSCARNET SODIUM	ANTIFUNGALS – AMPHOTERICIN	Possible ↑ nephrotoxicity	Additive side-effect	Monitor renal function closely

Primary drug	Secondary drug	Effect	Mechanism	Precautions
FOSCARNET SODIUM	ANTIPROTOZOALS – PENTAMIDINE (INTRAVENOUS)	Risk of hypocalcaemia	Unclear; possibly additive hypocalcaemic effects	Use extreme caution with intravenous pentamidine; monitor serum calcium (correct before the start of treatment), renal function and for signs of tetany closely. Stop one drug if necessary
FOSCARNET SODIUM	**ANTIVIRALS**			
FOSCARNET SODIUM	ADEFOVIR DIPIVOXIL	Possible ↑ efficacy and side-effects	Competition for renal excretion	Monitor renal function weekly
FOSCARNET SODIUM	NUCLEOSIDE REVERSE TRANSCRIPTASE INHIBITORS – LAMIVUDINE, TENOFOVIR, ZALCITABINE	↑ adverse effects with tenofovir and possibly lamivudine and zalcitabine	Uncertain; possibly additive toxicity via competition for renal excretion	Avoid if possible; otherwise monitor FBC and renal function weekly
FOSCARNET SODIUM	PROTEASE INHIBITORS	↓ renal function when co-administered with ritonavir or saquinavir	Uncertain; possibly ↓ renal excretion of foscarnet	Monitor renal function closely
OSELTAMIVIR	METHOTREXATE	Possible ↑ efficacy/toxicity	Competition for renal excretion	Monitor more closely for signs of immunosupression. Predicted interaction
RIBAVIRIN				
RIBAVIRIN	ANTIVIRALS – NUCLEOSIDE REVERSE TRANSCRIPTASE INHIBITORS	1. ↑ side-effects; risk of lactic acidosis, peripheral neuropathy, pancreatitis, hepatic decompensation, mitochondrial toxicity and anaemia with didanosine and stavudine 2. ↓ efficacy of lamivudine	1. Additive side-effects; ↑ intracellular activation of didanosine and stavudine. 2. ↓ intracellular activation of lamivudine	1. Not recommended; use with extreme caution. Monitor lactate, LFTs and amylase closely. Stop co-administration if peripheral neuropathy occurs. Stavudine and didanosine carry a higher risk 2. Monitor HIV RNA levels; if they ↑, review treatment combination
TELBIVUDINE	INTERFERON	Peripheral neuropathy	Unclear	Use with caution

DRUGS TO TREAT INFECTIONS ANTIVIRALS – OTHER

Part 11 DRUGS ACTING ON THE GASTROINTESTINAL TRACT

Antacids

Antacids are gastric-acid neutralizing or adsorbing medications, usually containing aluminium and/or magnesium salts (e.g. aluminium hydroxide, magnesium carbonate, hydroxide or trisilicate), which have the ability to decrease the absorption of several medications that are co-administered (often due to the formation of chelates/insoluble unabsorbable complexes).

H2 receptor blockers

The potential for adverse drug interactions is considerable with cimetidine, which inhibits CYP1A2, CYP2C9, CYP2C19, CYP2D6, CYP2E and CYP3A4. Ranitidine has a lower potential for clinically significant interactions, while nizatidine and famotidine do not seem to be associated with significant adverse drug interactions.

Proton pump inhibitors

Generally, only a few of the adverse drug interactions involving proton pump inhibitors are of clinical significance, but an awareness of all interactions is necessary as individual variations do occur. Metabolism involves CYP2C19 and CYP3A4. Individual proton pump inhibitors differ considerably in their potential for adverse drug interactions, which are due to:

- elevation of gastric pH, which decreases the intragastric release of co-administered drugs (e.g. ketoconazole, itraconazole);
- interaction with P-gp interfering with the efflux of co-administered drugs such as digoxin;
- interference with CYP450 isoenzymes, for example inhibition of the metabolism of simvastatin.

Omeprazole carries a higher risk for interactions as it has a high affinity for CYP2C19 and a somewhat lower affinity for CYP3A4. Pantoprazole (which is further metabolized by non-saturable phase II reactions after initial metabolism by CYP isoenzymes) has a lower potential for interaction associated with CYP450 inhibition. It is also likely that, despite the limited information, esomeprazole, lansoprazole and rabeprazole also have weaker potential for interaction compared with omeprazole. Pantoprazole has been reported to be used without dose adjustments in critical care patients with organ dysfunction.

DRUGS ACTING ON THE GASTROINTESTINAL TRACT ANTACIDS

Primary drug	Secondary drug	Effect	Mechanism	Precautions
ANTACIDS				
ANTACIDS	ANALGESICS – NSAIDs	1. Magnesium hydroxide ↑ absorption of ibuprofen, flurbiprofen, mefenamic acid and tolfenamic acid 2. Aluminium-containing antacids ↓ absorption of these NSAIDs	Uncertain	These effects are ↓ by taking these drugs with food
ANTACIDS	ANTIBIOTICS – AZITHROMYCIN, CEFPODOXIME, CEFUROXIME, ISONIAZID, NITROFURANTOIN, QUINOLONES, RIFAMYCINS, TETRACYCLINES	↓ levels of these antibiotics	↓ absorption	Take azithromycin at least 1 hour before or 2 hours after an antacid. Take these cephalosporins at least 2 hours after an antacid. Separate quinolones and antacids by 2–6 hours. Separate nitrofurantoin, rifamycins or tetracyclines and antacids by 2–3 hours
ANTACIDS	**ANTICANCER AND IMMUNOMODULATING DRUGS**			
ANTACIDS	MYCOPHENOLATE	↓ plasma concentrations of mycophenolate (may be 30%)	↓ absorption	Do not co-administer simultaneously – separate by at least 4 hours
ANTACIDS	PENICILLAMINE	↓ penicillamine levels	↓ absorption of penicillamine	Avoid co-administration
ANTACIDS	ANTIEPILEPTICS – GABAPENTIN, PHENYTOIN	↓ levels of these antiepileptics	↓ absorption	Separate by at least 3 hours
ANTACIDS	ANTIFUNGALS – AZOLES	↓ plasma concentration of itraconazole and ketoconazole, with risk of therapeutic failure	Itraconazole absorption in capsule form requires an acidic gastric environment, and thus absorption would be ↓	Separate administration of agents that ↓ gastric acidity by 1–2 hours. However, absorption of itraconazole liquid solution does not require an acidic environment; it could be used instead and does not need to be given with food. Fluconazole absorption is not pH-dependent, so this is a suitable alternative

ANTACIDS	ANTIHISTAMINES – FEXOFENADINE	↓ fexofenadine levels	↓ absorption	Be aware
ANTACIDS	ANTIHYPERTENSIVES AND HEART FAILURE DRUGS – ACE INHIBITORS	↓ effect, particularly of captopril, fosinopril and enalapril	↓ absorption due to ↑ gastric pH	Watch for poor response to ACE inhibitors
ANTACIDS	ANTIMALARIALS – PROGUANIL, CHLOROQUINE	↓ chloroquine and proguanil levels	↓ absorption	Separate doses by at least 4 hours
ANTACIDS	ANTIPLATELET AGENTS – DIPYRIDAMOLE	Possible ↓ bioavailability of dipyridamole	Dipyridamole tablets require an acidic environment for adequate dissolution; ↑ pH of the stomach impairs dissolution and therefore may ↓ absorption of drug	↑ dose of dipyridamole or consider using an alternative antiplatelet drug
ANTACIDS	ANTIPSYCHOTICS – PHENOTHIAZINES, SULPIRIDE	↓ levels of these antipsychotics	↓ absorption	Separate doses by 2 hours (in the case of sulpiride, give sulpiride 2 hours after but not before the antacid)
ANTACIDS CONTAINING MAGNESIUM AND ALUMINIUM	BETA-BLOCKERS	↑ bioavailability of metoprolol and atenolol, which may produce a mild variation in response to both drugs	Variations in absorption of the respective beta-blockers	Clinical significance may be minimal but be aware. Monitor BP at least weekly until stable when initiating antacid therapy. Warn patients to report symptoms of hypotension (light-headedness, dizziness on standing, etc.)
ANTACIDS	BISPHOSPHONATES	↓ bisphosphonate levels	↓ absorption	Separate doses by at least 30 minutes
ANTACIDS CONTAINING ALUMINIUM	DEFERASIROX	↓ levels of deferasirox	↓ absorption	Avoid co-administration (manufacturers' recommendation)

DRUGS ACTING ON THE GASTROINTESTINAL TRACT ANTACIDS

Primary drug	Secondary drug	Effect	Mechanism	Precautions
ANTACIDS CONTAINING MAGNESIUM	IRON	↓ iron levels when iron given orally	↓ absorption	Separate doses as much as possible – monitor FBC closely
ANTACIDS	LIPID-LOWERING DRUGS – FIBRATES	Gemfibrozil levels may be ↓ by antacids	Uncertain	Give gemfibrozil 1–2 hours before the antacid
ANTACIDS	PROTON PUMP INHIBITORS – LANSOPRAZOLE	Possible ↓ efficacy of lansoprazole	↓ absorption	Separate doses by at least 1 hour
ANTACIDS – MAGNESIUM-CONTAINING	SODIUM POLYSTYRENE SULPHONATE	Cases of metabolic alkalosis	Uncertain; possibly absorption of bicarbonate due to its abnormal neutralization in the stomach	Consider an alternative antacid or administer sodium polystyrene sulphonate as an enema. If both need to be co-administered orally, monitor U&Es and blood gases closely
ANTACIDS – CALCIUM- AND MAGNESIUM-CONTAINING	TRIENTINE	Possibly ↓ trientine levels	↓ absorption	Separate doses as much as possible; take antacids after trientine
ANTACIDS CONTAINING ALUMINIUM	VITAMIN C	↑ aluminium levels, with risk of encephalopathy in patients with renal failure	Uncertain; possibly ↑ absorption due to ascorbic acid in the presence of ↓ renal excretion	Avoid co-ingestion in patients with renal failure
ANTIDIARRHOEALS				
CODEINE, DIPHENOXYLATE, MORPHINE ➢ *Analgesics, Opioids*				
KAOLIN				
KAOLIN	ANTIBIOTICS – TETRACYCLINES	↓ tetracycline levels	↓ absorption	Separate doses by at least 2 hours
KAOLIN	ANTIMALARIALS – CHLOROQUINE	↓ chloroquine levels	↓ absorption	Separate doses by at least 4 hours
KAOLIN	BETA-BLOCKERS	Possibly ↓ levels of atenolol, propranolol and sotalol	↓ absorption	Separate doses by at least 2 hours
KAOLIN	CARDIAC GLYCOSIDES – DIGOXIN	Possibly ↓ levels of digoxin	↓ absorption	Separate doses by at least 2 hours

LOPERAMIDE				
LOPERAMIDE	ANTIBIOTICS – CO-TRIMOXAZOLE	↑ loperamide levels but no evidence of toxicity	Inhibition of metabolism	Be aware
LOPERAMIDE	ANTIVIRALS – PROTEASE INHIBITORS	↑ risk of adverse effects when loperamide is co-ingested with ritonavir	Ritonavir inhibits P-gp and CYP3A4	Monitor for clinical effect; consider ↓ dose if necessary. Stop if there are signs of abdominal distension in patients with HIV as toxic megacolon has been reported
LOPERAMIDE	DESMOPRESSIN	↑ desmopressin levels when given orally	Delayed intestinal transit time ↑ absorption of desmopressin	Watch for early features of desmopressin toxicity (e.g. abdominal pain, headaches)
ANTIEMETICS ➢ *Drugs Acting on the Nervous System, Antiemetics*				
ANTIMUSCARINICS ➢ *Drugs Acting on the Nervous System, Antiparkinson's drugs*				
DRUGS AFFECTING BILE				
URSODEOXYCHOLIC ACID				
URSODEOXYCHOLIC ACID	ANTICANCER AND IMMUNOMODULATING DRUGS – CICLOSPORIN	↑ ciclosporin levels	↑ absorption	Watch for early features of ciclosporin toxicity; monitor FBC closely
COLESTYRAMINE ➢ *Cardiovascular Drugs, Lipid-lowering drugs*				
DRUGS USED TO TREAT INFLAMMATORY BOWEL DISEASE				
AMINOSALICYLATES ➢ *Anticancer and Immunomodulating Drugs, Other immunomodulating drugs*				
CORTICOSTEROIDS ➢ *Anticancer and Immunomodulating Drugs, Other immunomodulating drugs*				
INFLIXIMAB ➢ *Anticancer and Immunomodulating Drugs, Other immunomodulating drugs*				

Primary drug	Secondary drug	Effect	Mechanism	Precautions
H2 RECEPTOR BLOCKERS				
CIMETIDINE, RANITIDINE	ANAESTHETICS – LOCAL – LIDOCAINE	↑ efficacy and adverse effects of local anaesthetic, e.g. light-headedness, paraesthesia	Unknown for most local anaesthetics. Lidocaine ↑ bioavailability	Uncertain. Monitor more closely. No toxicity reported to date with bupivacaine. If using intravenous lidocaine, monitor closely for symptoms of toxicity; ↓ dose may be required
H2 RECEPTOR BLOCKERS	**ANALGESICS – OPIOIDS**			
CIMETIDINE	ALFENTANIL, FENTANYL, PETHIDINE, TRAMADOL	Cimetidine may ↑ fentanyl, pethidine and tramadol levels	Cimetidine inhibits CYP2D6-mediated metabolism of these opioids. Ranitidine weakly inhibits CYP2D6	Watch for excessive narcotization
CIMETIDINE	CODEINE	Cimetidine may ↓ efficacy of codeine	Due to initiation of enzymatic conversion to active metabolite	Watch for poor response to codeine. Consider using an alternative opioid or acid suppression therapy
CIMETIDINE, RANITIDINE	ANTIARRHYTHMICS – AMIODARONE, FLECAINIDE, MEXILETINE, PROCAINAMIDE, PROPAFENONE	Likely ↑ plasma concentrations of these antiarrhythmics and risk of adverse effects	Cimetidine inhibits CYP2D6-mediated metabolism of flecainide, mexiletine, procainamide and propafenone. Ranitidine is a much weaker CYP2D6 inhibitor. Cimetidine is a potent inhibitor of organic cation transport in the kidney, and the elimination of procainamide is impaired	Monitor PR and BP at least weekly until stable. Warn patients to report symptoms of hypotension (light-headedness, dizziness on standing, etc.). Consider alternative acid suppression therapy

H2 RECEPTOR BLOCKERS	ANTIBIOTICS			
H2 RECEPTOR BLOCKERS	CEPHALOSPORINS TETRACYCLINES – DOXYCYCLINE	↓ plasma concentrations and risk of treatment failure	↓ absorption of cephalosporin as ↑ gastric pH	Avoid concomitant use. If unable to avoid combination, take H2 antagonists at least 2–3 hours after cephalosporin. Consider an alternative antibiotic or separate the doses by at least 2 hours and give with an acidic drink, e.g. a carbonated drink; ↑ dose may be required
CIMETIDINE	CHLORAMPHENICOL	↑ adverse effects of chloramphenicol, e.g. bone marrow depression	Additive toxicity	Use with caution; monitor FBC regularly
CIMETIDINE	MACROLIDES – ERYTHROMYCIN	↑ efficacy and adverse effects of erythromycin, including hearing loss	↑ bioavailability	Consider an alternative antibiotic, e.g. clarithromycin. Deafness has been reversible with cessation of erythromycin
CIMETIDINE	METRONIDAZOLE	↑ metronidazole levels	Inhibited metabolism	Watch for ↑ side-effects of metronidazole
CIMETIDINE	RIFAMPICIN	↓ efficacy of cimetidine	↑ metabolism	Change to alternative acid suppression, e.g. rabeprazole, or ↑ dose and/or frequency
H2 RECEPTOR BLOCKERS	**ANTICANCER AND IMMUNOMODULATING DRUGS**			
H2 RECEPTOR BLOCKERS	**CYTOTOXICS**			
CIMETIDINE	BUSULFAN, CARMUSTINE, CHLORAMBUCIL, CYCLOPHOSPHAMIDE, ESTRAMUSTINE, IFOSFAMIDE, LOMUSTINE, THIOTEPA, TREOSULFAN	↑ adverse effects of cytotoxic, e.g. myelosuppression	Additive toxicity. Possible minor inhibition of cyclophosphamide metabolism via CYP2C9	Monitor more closely; monitor FBC regularly. Avoid co-administration of cimetidine with cyclophosphamide

DRUGS ACTING ON THE GASTROINTESTINAL TRACT H2 RECEPTOR BLOCKERS

Primary drug	Secondary drug	Effect	Mechanism	Precautions
FAMOTIDINE	DASATINIB	Possible ↓ dasatinib levels	Famotidine ↑ metabolism of dasatinib	Consider using alternative acid suppression therapy
CIMETIDINE	DOXORUBICIN	↑ risk of myelosuppression due to ↑ plasma concentrations	Due to ↓ metabolism of doxorubicin by CYP3A4 isoenzymes due to inhibition of those enzymes	Monitor for ↑ myelosuppression, peripheral neuropathy, myalgias and fatigue
CIMETIDINE	EPIRUBICIN	↑ epirubicin levels, with risk of toxicity	Attributed to inhibition of hepatic metabolism of epirubicin by cimetidine	Avoid concurrent treatment and consider using an alternative H2 receptor blocker, e.g. ranitidine, famotidine
CIMETIDINE	FLUOROURACIL	Altered efficacy of fluorouracil	Inhibition of metabolism and altered action	Monitor more closely. May be of clinical benefit. No additional toxicity was noted in one study
CIMETIDINE	IFOSFAMIDE	↓ plasma concentrations of 4-hydroxyifosfamide, the active metabolite of ifosfamide, and risk of inadequate therapeutic response	Due to inhibition of the isoenzymatic conversion to active metabolites	Monitor clinically the efficacy of ifosfamide, and ↑ dose accordingly
CIMETIDINE	IMATINIB	↑ imatinib levels with ↑ risk of toxicity (e.g. abdominal pain, constipation, dyspnoea) and of neurotoxicity (e.g. taste disturbances, dizziness, headache, paraesthesia, peripheral neuropathy)	Due to inhibition of CYP3A4-mediated metabolism of imatinib	Monitor for clinical efficacy and for the signs of toxicity listed, along with convulsions, confusion and signs of oedema (including pulmonary oedema). Monitor electrolytes, liver function and for cardiotoxicity
CIMETIDINE	IRINOTECAN	↑ plasma concentrations of SN-38 (active metabolite of irinotecan) and ↑ toxicity of irinotecan, e.g. diarrhoea, acute cholinergic syndrome, interstitial pulmonary disease	Due to inhibition of the metabolism of irinotecan by CYP3A4 isoenzymes by cimetidine	Peripheral blood counts should be checked before each course of treatment. Monitor lung function. Recommendation is to ↓ dose of irinotecan by 25%

CIMETIDINE	MELPHALAN	↓ plasma concentrations and bioavailability of melphalan by 30% and risk of poor therapeutic response to melphalan	Cimetidine causes a change in gastric pH, which ↓ absorption of melphalan	Avoid concurrent use
CIMETIDINE	VINCA ALKALOIDS	↑ adverse effects of vinblastine and vincristine	Inhibition of CYP3A4-mediated metabolism. Also inhibition of P-gp efflux of vinblastine	Monitor FBCs and watch for early features of toxicity (pain, numbness, tingling in the fingers and toes, jaw pain, abdominal pain, constipation, ileus). Consider selecting an alternative drug
H2 RECEPTOR BLOCKERS	**HORMONES AND HORMONE ANTAGONISTS**			
CIMETIDINE	TOREMIFENE	↑ plasma concentrations of toremifene	Due to inhibition of metabolism of toremifene by the CYP3A4 isoenzymes by cimetidine	Clinical relevance is uncertain. Need to monitor for clinical toxicities
H2 RECEPTOR BLOCKERS	**IMMUNOMODULATING DRUGS**			
CIMETIDINE	CICLOSPORIN	↑ plasma concentrations of ciclosporin, with risk of nephrotoxicity, myelosuppression, neurotoxicity and excessive immunosuppression, with risk of infection and post-transplant lymphoproliferative disease	Inhibition of CYP3A4-mediated metabolism of ciclosporin; these inhibitors vary in potency. Cimetidine is classified as a potent inhibitor	Avoid co-administration with cimetidine. Consider an alternative H2 blocker but need to monitor plasma ciclosporin levels to prevent toxicity
CIMETIDINE	CORTICOSTEROIDS	↑ adrenal suppressive effects of corticosteroids, which may ↑ risk of infections and produce an inadequate response to stress scenarios	Due to inhibition of metabolism of corticosteroids	Monitor cortisol levels and warn patients to report symptoms such as fever and sore throat

DRUGS ACTING ON THE GASTROINTESTINAL TRACT H2 RECEPTOR BLOCKERS

Primary drug	Secondary drug	Effect	Mechanism	Precautions
CIMETIDINE, FAMOTIDINE, RANITIDINE	SIROLIMUS, TACROLIMUS	↑ adverse effects of ciclosporin e.g. thrombocytopenia, hepatotoxicity	Ciclosporin, tacrolimus and sirolimus are metabolized primarily by CYP3A4 isoenzymes, which are inhibited by cimetidine. Cimetidine is also an inhibitor of CYP2D6, CYP2C19 and CYP1A2. Sirolimus has multiple pathways of metabolism, which would be inhibited by cimetidine. Ciclosporin is also a substrate of P-gp	Consider alternative acid suppression, e.g. alginate suspension or rabeprazole. Not thought to be clinically significant. Ensure close monitoring of immunosuppressant levels and renal function
CIMETIDINE, FAMOTIDINE	ANTICOAGULANTS – ORAL	↑ anticoagulant effect with cimetidine and possibly famotidine	Inhibition of metabolism via CYP1A2, CYP2C9 and CYP2C19	Use alternative acid suppression, e.g. another H2 antagonist or proton pump inhibitor (not esomeprazole, lansoprazole or omeprazole) or monitor INR more closely; ↓ dose may be required. Take acid suppression regularly and not PRN if affects INR control
H2 RECEPTOR BLOCKERS	**ANTIDEPRESSANTS**			
CIMETIDINE	MAOIs – MOCLOBEMIDE	↑ plasma concentrations of moclobemide (by up to 40%)	Due to cimetidine inhibiting metabolism	↓ dose of moclobemide to one-half to one-third of original and then alter as required
CIMETIDINE	MIRTAZAPINE	↑ efficacy and adverse effects of mirtazapine	Inhibition of metabolism via CYP1A2, CYP2D6 and CYP3A4	Consider alternative acid suppression, e.g. H2 antagonist (proton pump inhibitors will interact in poor CYP2D6 metabolizers) or monitor more closely for side-effects; ↓ dose as necessary

DRUGS ACTING ON THE GASTROINTESTINAL TRACT H2 RECEPTOR BLOCKERS

CIMETIDINE	SNRIs – VENLAFAXINE	↑ efficacy and adverse effects	Inhibition of metabolism	Not thought to be clinically significant, but take care in elderly people and patients with hepatic impairment
CIMETIDINE	SSRIs	↑ efficacy and adverse effects e.g. nausea, diarrhoea, dyspepsia, dizziness, sexual dysfunction	↑ bioavailability	Use with caution; monitor for ↑ side-effects. ↓ dose may be necessary
CIMETIDINE	TCAs	↑ efficacy and adverse effects, e.g. dry mouth, urinary retention, blurred vision, constipation	↓ metabolism	Use alternative acid suppression or monitor more closely and ↓ dose. Rapid hydroxylators may be at ↑ risk
H2 RECEPTOR BLOCKERS	**ANTIDIABETIC DRUGS**			
RANITIDINE	ACARBOSE	↓ blood levels of ranitidine	Possibly due to ↓ absorption of ranitidine	Be aware
H2 RECEPTOR BLOCKERS	METFORMIN	↑ level of metformin and risk of lactic acidosis. The onset of lactic acidosis is often subtle with symptoms of malaise, myalgia, respiratory distress and ↑ non-specific abdominal distress. There may be hypothermia and resistant bradyarrhythmias	Metformin is not metabolized in humans and is not protein bound. Competition for renal tubular excretion is the basis for ↑ activity or retention of metformin. Cimetidine competes for excretory pathway	Theoretical possibility. Requires ↓ metformin dose to be considered or to avoid co-administration. Warn patients about hypoglycaemia ➢ ***For signs and symptoms of hypoglycaemia, see Clinical Features of Some Adverse Drug Interactions, Hypoglycaemia***
CIMETIDINE	NATEGLINIDE, REPAGLINIDE	Likely to ↑ plasma concentrations of these antidiabetic drugs and ↑ risk of hypoglycaemic episodes	Due to inhibition of CYP3A4-mediated metabolism of nateglinide and repaglinide	Watch for and warn patients about hypoglycaemia ➢ ***For signs and symptoms of hypoglycaemia, see Clinical Features of Some Adverse Drug Interactions, Hypoglycaemia***

DRUGS ACTING ON THE GASTROINTESTINAL TRACT H2 RECEPTOR BLOCKERS

Primary drug	Secondary drug	Effect	Mechanism	Precautions
H2 RECEPTOR BLOCKERS	SULPHONYLUREAS – GLIMEPIRIDE	↑ plasma concentrations of glimepride and ↑ risk of hypoglycaemic episodes	Cimetidine and ranitidine ↓ renal elimination of glimepride and ↑ intestinal absorption of glimepride. Cimetidine is also an inhibitor of CYP2D6 and CYP3A4	Consider alternative acid suppression, e.g. a proton pump inhibitor (not omeprazole), and monitor more closely
CIMETIDINE, FAMOTIDINE, RANITIDINE	ANTIEPILEPTICS – CARBAMAZEPINE PHENYTOIN	↑ plasma concentrations of phenytoin and risk of adverse effects, including phenytoin toxicity, bone marrow depression and skin reactions	Inhibition of metabolism via CYP2C9 and CYP2C19	Use alternative acid suppression, e.g. ranitidine, or warn the patient that the effects last 1 week. Consider monitoring carbamazepine levels and adjust dose as necessary
H2 RECEPTOR BLOCKERS	**ANTIFUNGALS**			
H2 RECEPTOR BLOCKERS	ITRACONAZOLE, KETOCONAZOLE, MICONAZOLE	↓ plasma concentrations and risk of treatment failure	↓ absorption of these antifungals as ↑ gastric pH	Avoid concomitant use. If unable to avoid combination, take H2 blockers at least 2–3 hours after antifungals. Use an alternative antifungal or separate the doses by at least 2 hours and give with an acidic drink, e.g. a carbonated drink; ↑ dose of the antifungal may be required
CIMETIDINE	TERBINAFINE	↑ efficacy and adverse effects of terbinafine	↑ bioavailability	Consider alternative acid suppression or monitor more closely and consider ↓ dose
H2 RECEPTOR BLOCKERS	ANTIHISTAMINES – LORATIDINE	Possibly ↑ loratidine levels	Inhibition of metabolism	Be aware
H2 RECEPTOR BLOCKERS	ANTIHYPERTENSIVES AND HEART FAILURE DRUGS – ALPHA-BLOCKERS	↓ efficacy of tolazoline	Uncertain; possibly ↓ absorption	Watch for poor response to tolazoline

DRUGS ACTING ON THE GASTROINTESTINAL TRACT H2 RECEPTOR BLOCKERS

H2 RECEPTOR BLOCKERS	ANTIMALARIALS			
CIMETIDINE	CHLOROQUINE, HYDROXYCHLOROQUINE	↑ efficacy and adverse effects of chloroquine	Inhibition of metabolism and excretion	Consider ranitidine as alternative or take cimetidine at least 2 hours after chloroquine
CIMETIDINE	ANTIMALARIALS OTHER THAN PROGUANIL	↑ efficacy and adverse effects of antimalarials	Inhibition of metabolism, some definitely via CYP3A4	Avoid co-administration
CIMETIDINE	PROGUANIL	↓ efficacy of proguanil	↓ absorption and ↓ formation of active metabolite	Avoid concomitant use. Clinical significance not established; effectiveness of malarial prophylaxis may be ↓
CIMETIDINE	ANTIPARKINSON'S DRUGS – PRAMIPEXOLE, ROPINIROLE	↑ efficacy and adverse effects of pramipexole	↓ renal excretion of pramipexole by inhibition of cation transport system. Inhibition of CYP1A2-mediated metabolism of ropinirole	Monitor closely; ↓ dose of pramipexole may be required. Adjust the dose of ropinirole as necessary or use alternative acid suppression, e.g. H2 antagonist or proton pump inhibitor (not omeprazole or lansoprazole)
H2 RECEPTOR BLOCKERS	ANTIPLATELET AGENTS – DIPYRIDAMOLE	Possible ↓ bioavailability of dipyridamole	Dipyridamole tablets require an acidic environment for adequate dissolution; ↑ pH of the stomach impairs dissolution and may therefore ↓ absorption of drug	↑ dose of dipyridamole or consider using an alternative antiplatelet drug
CIMETIDINE	ANTIPROTOZOALS – MEBENDAZOLE	↑ mebendazole levels	Inhibition of metabolism	Be aware; case reports of where this interaction has been used therapeutically

DRUGS ACTING ON THE GASTROINTESTINAL TRACT H2 RECEPTOR BLOCKERS

DRUGS ACTING ON THE GASTROINTESTINAL TRACT H2 RECEPTOR BLOCKERS

Primary drug	Secondary drug	Effect	Mechanism	Precautions
CIMETIDINE	ANTIPSYCHOTICS – CHLORPROMAZINE, CLOZAPINE, HALOPERIDOL, OLANZAPINE, PERPHENAZINE, RISPERIDONE, SERTINDOLE, THIORIDAZINE, ZUCLOPENTHIXOL	↑ plasma concentrations of these antipsychotics, with risk of associated adverse effects ➢ ***Drugs Acting on the Nervous System, Antipsychotics***	Cimetidine is an inhibitor of CYP3A4 (sertindole, haloperidol, risperidone) CYP2D6 (chlorpromazine, risperidone, zuclopenthixol, thioridazine, perphenazine) and CYP1A2 (clozapine, olanzapine, sertindole, haloperidol)	Avoid concomitant use. Choose alternative acid suppression
H2 RECEPTOR BLOCKERS	**ANTIVIRALS**			
CIMETIDINE	ACICLOVIR/VALACICLOVIR	↑ efficacy and adverse effects of antivirals	Competition for renal excretion	Use doses of valaciclovir >4 g/day with caution or consider alternative acid suppression. For doses <1 g/day, interaction is not thought to be clinically significant. Studies only reported with valaciclovir
H2 RECEPTOR BLOCKERS	AMPRENAVIR, ATAZANAVIR	↓ efficacy of amprenavir; possible ↑ levels of cimetidine	↓ absorption of amprenavir and atazanavir. Uncertain mechanism of action on cimetidine	Amprenavir: separate doses by at least 1 hour. Take atazanavir at least 2 hours before or 10 hours after an H2 blocker. In both cases, monitor viral load closely
CIMETIDINE	ZALCITABINE	↑ efficacy and adverse effects of zalcitabine	↓ excretion via inhibition of tubular secretion	Clinical significance unclear. Monitor more closely
H2 RECEPTOR BLOCKERS	**ANXIOLYTICS AND HYPNOTICS**			
CIMETIDINE, RANITIDINE	BZDs (NOT LORAZEPAM OR TEMAZEPAM)	↑ efficacy and adverse effects of BZDs, e.g. sedation	Cimetidine is an inhibitor of CYP3A4, CYP2D6, CYP2C19 and CYP1A2	Not clinically significant for most patients. Conflicting information for some BZDs. Monitor more closely; ↓ dose if necessary
CIMETIDINE	CHLORMETHIAZOLE	↑ efficacy and adverse effects, e.g. sedation, 'hangover' effect	Inhibition of metabolism	Monitor closely; ↓ dose may be required

DRUGS ACTING ON THE GASTROINTESTINAL TRACT H2 RECEPTOR BLOCKERS

CIMETIDINE, RANITIDINE	BETA-BLOCKERS	↑ plasma concentrations and effects of labetalol, metoprolol and propranolol; possibly systemic effects of timolol eye drops	Cimetidine is an inhibitor of CYP3A4, CYP2D6, CYP2C19 and CYP1A2	Monitor BP and PR
NIZATIDINE	BETA-BLOCKERS	↑ bradycardia when nizatidine is added to atenolol. Other beta-blockers have not been studied	Uncertain	Monitor PR when administering nizatidine to patients on beta-blockers
CIMETIDINE FAMOTIDINE NIZATIDINE, RANITIDINE	BRONCHODILATORS – THEOPHYLLINE	↑ efficacy and adverse effects, including seizures. There is conflicting information associated with ranitidine, famotidine and nizatidine	Inhibition of metabolism via CYP1A2, cimetidine being the best known inhibitor	Use alternative acid suppression, e.g. a proton pump inhibitor (not omeprazole or lansoprazole) or monitor closely; considerable patient variation. Check levels on day 3 and then at 1 week. A 30–50% ↓ dose of theophylline may be required. For doses <400 mg/day, the interaction may not be clinically significant
CIMETIDINE	CALCIUM CHANNEL BLOCKERS	↑ levels of calcium channel blockers, especially diltiazem and nifedipine	Inhibition of CYP3A isoform-mediated metabolism	Monitor BP closely; be aware of possibility of significant ↓ BP. Consider ↓ dose of diltiazem and nifedipine by up to 50%
FAMOTIDINE	CALCIUM CHANNEL BLOCKERS	Reports of heart failure and ↓ BP when famotidine given with nifedipine	Additive negative inotropic effects	Caution with co-administering famotidine with calcium channel blockers, especially in elderly people
H2 RECEPTOR BLOCKERS	DRUG DEPENDENCE THERAPIES – BUPROPION	↑ plasma concentrations of cimetidine and ranitidine	Bupropion and its metabolite hydroxybupropion inhibit CYP2D6	Initiate therapy of these drugs at the lowest effective dose
CIMETIDINE	ERGOT ALKALOIDS	↑ ergotamine/methysergide levels, with risk of toxicity	Inhibition of metabolism via CYP3A4	Avoid co-administration

Primary drug	Secondary drug	Effect	Mechanism	Precautions
CIMETIDINE	5-HT1 AGONISTS – ZOLMITRIPTAN	↑ efficacy and adverse effects of zolmitriptan, e.g. flushing, sensations of tingling, heat, heaviness, pressure or tightness of any part of the body, including the throat and chest, dizziness	Inhibition of metabolism via CYP1A2	Consider alternative acid suppression e.g. a proton pump inhibitor (not omeprazole or lansoprazole), or monitor more closely and ↓ maximum dose of zolmitriptan to 5 mg/24 hours
CIMETIDINE	MUSCLE RELAXANTS – VECURONIUM	↑ efficacy of vecuronium	Unclear	Potential for slightly prolonged recovery time (minutes)
CIMETIDINE	PERIPHERAL VASODILATORS – CILOSTAZOL, PENTOXIFYLLINE	Cimetidine↑ cilostazol and pentoxifylline levels	Cimetidine inhibits CYP3A4-mediated metabolism of cilostazol. Uncertain mechanism for pentoxifylline	Avoid co-administration
CIMETIDINE	PHOSPHODIESTERASE TYPE 5 INHIBITORS – SILDENAFIL	↑ efficacy and adverse effects of sildenafil	Inhibition of metabolism via CYP3A4	Consider a starting dose of 25 mg of sildenafil
CIMETIDINE	SYMPATHOMIMETICS	↑ efficacy and adverse effects of sympathomimetics	Unclear	↑ hypertensive response; ↓ dose may be required. Monitor ECG for tachycardias
CIMETIDINE	THYROID HORMONES	↓ efficacy of levothyroxine	↓ absorption	Clinical significance unclear. Monitor requirement for ↑ levothyroxine dose
RANITIDINE	TRIPOTASSIUM DICITRATOBISMUTHATE	↑ adverse effects of tripotassium dicitratobismuthate	↑ absorption	Do not use together for more than 16 weeks. Bismuth salicylate and subnitrate do not interact
PANCREATIN				
PANCREATIN	ANTIDIABETIC DRUGS – ACARBOSE	Theoretical risk of ↓ efficacy of acarbose	↓ absorption	Watch for poor response to acarbose; monitor capillary blood glucose level closely
PANCREATIN	IRON	Possible ↓ iron levels when iron is taken orally	↓ absorption	Watch for poor response to oral iron; monitor FBC closely

PROTON PUMP INHIBITORS				
LANSOPRAZOLE	ANTACIDS	Possible ↓ efficacy of lansoprazole	↓ absorption	Separate doses by at least 1 hour
PROTON PUMP INHIBITORS	**ANTIBIOTICS**			
PROTON PUMP INHIBITORS	CEPHALOSPORINS	Possible ↓ efficacy of cephalosporin	↓ absorption as ↑ gastric pH	Monitor for ↓ efficacy. Separate doses by at least 2 hours; take cephalosporin with food
OMEPRAZOLE	MACROLIDES – CLARITHROMYCIN	↑ efficacy and adverse effects of both drugs	↑ plasma concentration of both drugs	No dose adjustment is recommended. Interaction is considered useful for *Helicobacter pylori* eradication
PROTON PUMP INHIBITORS	**ANTICANCER AND IMMUNOMODULATING DRUGS**			
PROTON PUMP INHIBITORS	**CYTOTOXICS**			
OMEPRAZOLE	IMATINIB	↑ plasma concentrations, with risk of toxic effects of these drugs	Imatinib is a potent inhibitor of CYP2C9 isoenzymes, which metabolize these drugs	Watch for the early toxic effects of these drugs. If necessary, consider using alternative drugs while the patient is being given imatinib
PROTON PUMP INHIBITORS	METHOTREXATE	Likely ↑ plasma concentrations of methotrexate and ↑ risk of toxic effects, e.g. blood dyscrasias, liver cirrhosis, pulmonary toxicity, renal toxicity	Attributed to omeprazole ↓ renal elimination of methotrexate	Monitor clinically and biochemically for blood dyscrasias, liver toxicity, renal toxicity and pulmonary toxicity
PROTON PUMP INHIBITORS	**IMMUNOMODULATING DRUGS**			
OMEPRAZOLE	CICLOSPORIN	Conflicting information. Possible altered efficacy of ciclosporin	Unclear	Monitor closely. Studies have reported combination use with no significant changes in ciclosporin levels

DRUGS ACTING ON THE GASTROINTESTINAL TRACT PROTON PUMP INHIBITORS

Primary drug	Secondary drug	Effect	Mechanism	Precautions
PROTON PUMP INHIBITORS	TACROLIMUS	Possible ↑ efficacy and adverse effects of immunosuppression	Altered metabolism from CYP2C19 to CYP3A4 in patients with low CYP2C19 levels	Monitor levels more closely
PROTON PUMP INHIBITORS	ANTICOAGULANTS – ORAL	Possibly ↑ anticoagulant effect when esomeprazole, lansoprazole or omeprazole is added to warfarin	Uncertain at present. Omeprazole and lansoprazole are known to induce CYP1A2, which plays a role in the activation of coumarins	Monitor INR more closely. ↓ dose may be required. If values are 10%, 20% or 30% over range, omit the dose for 1, 2 or 3 days respectively, and consider ↓ maintenance dose by 10%. Regular dosing of a proton pump inhibitor is preferable if it affects INR significantly. Not reported with pantoprazole or rabeprazole
PROTON PUMP INHIBITORS	**ANTIDEPRESSANTS**			
OMEPRAZOLE/ ESOMEPRAZOLE	MAOIs – MOCLOBEMIDE	Possible ↑ efficacy and adverse effects of moclobemide	Inhibition of CYP2C19	Monitor more closely. Effect is seen only in extensive CYP2C19 metabolizers. ↓ dose may be required
OMEPRAZOLE	SSRIs – FLUVOXAMINE	↓ fluvoxamine levels with loss of therapeutic efficacy	Inhibition of CYP1A2-mediated metabolism	Monitor for lack of therapeutic effect. When omeprazole is withdrawn, monitor for fluvoxamine toxicity
PROTON PUMP INHIBITORS	ANTIDIABETIC DRUGS – SULPHONYLUREAS	Possible ↑ efficacy and adverse effects of sulphonylurea, e.g. hypoglycaemia	Possible ↑ absorption	Monitor capillary blood glucose more closely; ↓ dose may be required
PROTON PUMP INHIBITORS	**ANTIEPILEPTICS**			
PROTON PUMP INHIBITORS	CARBAMAZEPINE	Possible altered efficacy of carbamazepine	Unclear; possibly via ↓ clearance	Use with caution. Monitor carbamazepine levels when starting or stopping therapy, and use the proton pump inhibitor regularly, not PRN. Not reported with pantoprazole or rabeprazole

DRUGS ACTING ON THE GASTROINTESTINAL TRACT PROTON PUMP INHIBITORS

PROTON PUMP INHIBITORS	PHENYTOIN	Possible ↑ efficacy and adverse effects of phenytoin	Unclear; possible altered metabolism via CYP2C19	↓ dose may be required. Use the proton pump inhibitor regularly, not PRN. Monitor phenytoin levels when starting or stopping treatment. Patients have received omeprazole for 3–5 weeks without altered phenytoin levels. Not reported with pantoprazole or rabeprazole
PROTON PUMP INHIBITORS	**ANTIFUNGALS**			
PROTON PUMP INHIBITORS	ITRACONAZOLE, KETOCONAZOLE	Possible ↓ efficacy of antifungal	↓ absorption	Monitor for ↓ efficacy; ↑ dose may be required. Separate doses by at least 2 hours and give ketoconazole with a carbonated drink
OMEPRAZOLE	VORICONAZOLE	Possible ↑ efficacy and adverse effects of both drugs	1. Inhibition of voriconazole metabolism via CYP2C19 and CYP3A4 2. Inhibition of metabolism of omeprazole	1. No dose adjustment of voriconazole recommended 2. Half omeprazole dose
PROTON PUMP INHIBITORS	**ANTIPLATELET AGENTS**			
PROTON PUMP INHIBITORS	DIPYRIDAMOLE	Possible ↓ bioavailability of dipyridamole	Dipyridamole tablets require an acidic environment for adequate dissolution; ↑ pH of the stomach impairs dissolution and may therefore ↓ absorption of the drug	↑ dose of dipyridamole or consider using an alternative antiplatelet drug

DRUGS ACTING ON THE GASTROINTESTINAL TRACT PROTON PUMP INHIBITORS

Primary drug	Secondary drug	Effect	Mechanism	Precautions
PROTON PUMP INHIBITORS	CLOPIDOGREL	Patients after myocardial infarction on clopidogrel were more likely to suffer reinfarction with concomitant proton pump inhibitor treatment	Proton pump inhibitors inhibit CYP2C19, which converts clopidogrel to the active metabolite	Pantoprazole is not known as yet to cause this effect. Consider using acid suppression therapy with H2 blockers when clopidogrel is used as secondary prevention of coronary heart disease
OMEPRAZOLE	ANTIPSYCHOTICS – CLOZAPINE	Possible ↓ efficacy of clozapine	↑ metabolism via CYP1A2	Clinical significance unclear; monitor more closely
PROTON PUMP INHIBITORS	**ANTIVIRALS – PROTEASE INHIBITORS**			
PROTON PUMP INHIBITORS	ATAZANAVIR, NELFINAVIR	↓ plasma levels of atazanavir and nelfinavir with esomeprazole, and ↑ risk of therapeutic failure of the antiviral agent	Uncertain; possibly due to enzyme induction	Avoid co-administration
PROTON PUMP INHIBITORS	SAQUINAVIR	Significantly ↑ plasma concentrations of saquinavir during concomitant treatment with esomeprazole. ↑ risk of toxic effects of saquinavir	Uncertain	FDA in April 2009 recommended that patients should be monitored for toxic effects of saquinavir and that ↓ dose of saquinavir may be required
OMEPRAZOLE	INDINAVIR	Possibly ↓ plasma concentrations and ↓ efficacy of indinavir	Uncertain	↑ dose of indinavir from 800 mg three times a day to 1 g three times a day, or preferably add ritonavir 200 mg once daily
OMEPRAZOLE/ ESOMEPRAZOLE	ANXIOLYTICS AND HYPNOTICS – BZDs	↑ efficacy and adverse effects, e.g. prolonged sedation	Inhibition of metabolism via CYP450 (some show competitive inhibition via CYP2C19)	Monitor for ↑ side-effects; ↓ dose as necessary. May take longer for patients to recover from interventions or surgical procedures, particularly when BZDs have been used. Consider an alternative proton pump inhibitor, e.g. lansoprazole or pantoprazole

DRUGS ACTING ON THE GASTROINTESTINAL TRACT PROTON PUMP INHIBITORS

PROTON PUMP INHIBITORS	BETA-BLOCKERS	Risk of ↑ plasma concentrations and effects of propranolol	Omeprazole inhibits CYP2D6- and CYP2C19-mediated metabolism of propanolol	Monitor BP at least weekly until stable
OMEPRAZOLE	CALCIUM CHANNEL BLOCKERS – NIFEDIPINE	Possible ↑ efficacy and adverse effects	Small ↑ bioavailability possible via ↑ intragastric pH	Unlikely to be clinically significant
PROTON PUMP INHIBITORS	CARDIAC GLYCOSIDES – DIGOXIN	Plasma concentrations of digoxin are possibly ↑ by proton pump inhibitors	Small ↑ bioavailability, possibly via ↑ intragastric pH or altered intestinal P-gp transport	Not thought to be clinically significant unless a poor CYP2C19 metabolizer. No specific recommendations. Different proton pump inhibitors may interact differently – monitor if changing therapy or doses
PROTON PUMP INHIBITORS	CNS STIMULANTS – MODAFINIL	May cause moderate ↑ plasma concentrations of these substrates	Modafinil is a reversible inhibitor of CYP2C19 when used in therapeutic doses	Be aware
OMEPRAZOLE	DRUG DEPENDENCE THERAPIES – DISULFIRAM	Possible ↑ adverse effects of disulfiram	Accumulation of metabolites	Monitor closely for ↑ side-effects, although patients have received the combination without reported problems
PROTON PUMP INHIBITORS	LIPID-LOWERING DRUGS – ATORVASTATIN	Possible ↑ efficacy and adverse effects of atorvastatin	Inhibition of P-gp; ↓ first pass clearance	Monitor closely
LANSOPRAZOLE	MUSCLE RELAXANTS – VECURONIUM	Possible ↑ efficacy and adverse effects of vecuronium	Unclear	Altered duration of action. May need ↑ recovery time
LANSOPRAZOLE	OESTROGENS – ORAL CONTRACEPTIVES	Possible altered efficacy of contraceptive	Unclear	Clinical significance is uncertain. It would seem to be wise to advise patients to use an alternative form of contraception during and for 1 month after stopping co-administration with lansoprazole

Primary drug	Secondary drug	Effect	Mechanism	Precautions
PROTON PUMP INHIBITORS	PERIPHERAL VASODILATORS – CILOSTAZOL	Cilostazol levels are ↑ by omeprazole and possibly lansoprazole	Omeprazole inhibits CYP2C19-mediated metabolism of cilostazol	Avoid concomitant use. US manufacturer advises halving the dose of cilostazol
LANSOPRAZOLE	SUCRALFATE	Possible ↓ efficacy of lansoprazole	Unclear	Separate doses by at least 1 hour
SUCRALFATE				
SUCRALFATE	ANTIBIOTICS – QUINOLONES, TETRACYCLINES	↓ levels of these antibiotics	↓ absorption of these antibiotics	Give the antibiotics at least 2 hours before sucralfate
SUCRALFATE	ANTICOAGULANTS – ORAL	Possible ↓ anticoagulant effect	↓ absorption of warfarin	Monitor INR at least weekly until stable
SUCRALFATE	ANTIDEPRESSANTS – AMITRIPTYLINE	Possible ↓ amitriptyline levels	↓ absorption of amitriptyline	Watch for poor response to amitriptyline
SUCRALFATE	ANTIEPILEPTICS – PHENYTOIN	↓ phenytoin levels	↓ absorption of phenytoin	Give phenytoin at least 2 hours after sucralfate
SUCRALFATE	ANTIFUNGALS – KETOCONAZOLE	↓ ketoconazole levels	↓ absorption of ketoconazole	Separate doses by at least 2–3 hours
SUCRALFATE	ANTIPSYCHOTICS – SULPIRIDE	↓ sulpiride levels	↓ absorption of sulpiride	Give sulpiride at least 2 hours after sucralfate
SUCRALFATE	BRONCHODILATORS – THEOPHYLLINE	Possibly ↓ theophylline levels (with modified-release preparations)	Possibly ↓ absorption	Watch for poor response to theophylline and monitor levels
SUCRALFATE	CARDIAC GLYCOSIDES – DIGOXIN	Plasma concentrations of digoxin may be ↓ by sucralfate	Uncertain; possibly sucralfate binds with digoxin and ↓ its absorption	Watch for poor response to digoxin
SUCRALFATE	PROTON PUMP INHIBITORS – LANSOPRAZOLE	Possible ↓ efficacy of lansoprazole	Unclear	Separate doses by at least 1 hour
SUCRALFATE	THYROID HORMONES	↓ thyroxine levels	↓ absorption	Give thyroxine 2–3 hours before sucralfate

DRUGS ACTING ON THE GASTROINTESTINAL TRACT SUCRALFATE

TRIPOTASSIUM DICITRATOBISMUTHATE				
TRIPOTASSIUM DICITRATOBISMUTHATE	ANTIBIOTICS – TETRACYCLINES	↓ levels of tetracyclines	↓ absorption of tetracyclines	Separate doses by 2–3 hours
TRIPOTASSIUM DICITRATOBISMUTHATE	H2 RECEPTOR BLOCKERS – RANITIDINE	↑ adverse effects of tripotassium dicitratobismuthate	↑ absorption	Do not use together for more than 16 weeks. Bismuth salicylate and subnitrate do not interact
TRIPOTASSIUM DICITRATOBISMUTHATE	PROTON PUMP INHIBITORS – OMEPRAZOLE	↑ adverse effects of tripotassium dicitratobismuthate	↑ absorption	Do not use together for more than 16 weeks. Bismuth salicylate and subnitrate do not interact

Part 12 RESPIRATORY DRUGS

Antihistamines

The term 'antihistamines' refers to antagonists of H1 histamine receptors rather than drugs that block other histamine receptors.

Antihistamines are to varying degrees sedative, the more sedating members ('older antihistamines') of the class interacting with other sedating drugs (antipsychotics, BZDs, opioids, barbiturates).

Some antihistamines are associated with prolongation of the Q–T interval, and it is important to avoid co-administering these with other drugs that also prolong the Q–T interval.

Bronchodilators

Antimuscarinics

Antimuscarinic agents act by blocking the vagal acetylcholine, which causes bronchoconstriction. Two antimuscarinic agents are in use: short-acting ipratropium bromide and longer-acting tiotropium. No interactions have been reported with inhaled formulations, and drug interactions are rare with nebulized preparations.

For interactions involving antimuscarinic agents, see Drugs Acting on the Nervous System, Antimuscarinics.

Beta-2 agonists

These act on beta-2 adrenergic receptors, which relax bronchial smooth muscle. The primary side-effects are tachyarrhythmias and hypokalaemia, both of which tend to become clinically significant at high doses (i.e. when they are given in nebulized form or are intravenously administered, compared with the inhalation of aerosol or dry powder).

Non-selective beta-agonists (ephedrine, orciprenaline) are now rarely used because of the higher incidence of cardiovascular side-effects by their action on beta-1 receptors

Theophylline

Theophylline produces bronchodilation possibly by inhibiting phosphodiesterase isomers, has some anti-inflammatory effect and reduces muscle tone in the diaphragm. Theophylline is a positive inotrope and chronotrope, and is associated with hypokalaemia. It is both a substrate for, and an inhibitor of, CYP1A2. The toxic dose of theophylline is close to the therapeutic dose, i.e. there is a narrow therapeutic index.

Corticosteroids

Many corticosteroids undergo metabolism via CYP3A4 and are substrates of P-gp. They are used to suppress inflammation in the respiratory tract, reducing mucosal oedema and decreasing bronchial secretions. They are employed both to prevent acute exacerbations of chronic airways disease and to treat acute flare-ups. They may be subject to interactions when administered orally, but interactions with high-dose inhaled formulations are thought to occur due to steroid that is deposited in the oropharynx, swallowed and absorbed via the gastrointestinal tract.

For interactions with corticosteroids, see Anticancer and Immunomodulating Drugs, Other immunomodulating drugs.

Leukotriene receptor antagonists

These block the cysteinyl leukotriene type 1 receptor, which mediates the bronchoconstriction and anti-inflammatory actions of leukotrienes; the latter do not seem to be reduced by corticosteroids. Therefore leukotriene receptor antagonists are used to complement steroids when the latter do not effectively control symptoms.

Respiratory stimulants

Doxapram increases the tidal volume and respiratory rate by stimulating carotid chemoreceptors. Its use has been limited since the introduction of non-invasive ventilatory techniques for respiratory failure.

Primary drug	Secondary drug	Effect	Mechanism	Precautions
ANTIHISTAMINES				
ANTIHISTAMINES	DRUGS THAT PROLONG THE Q–T INTERVAL			
ANTIHISTAMINES – TERFENADINE, HYDROXYZINE, MIZOLASTINE	1. ANTIARRHYTHMICS – amiodarone, disopyramide, procainamide, propafenone 2. ANTIBIOTICS – macrolides (especially azithromycin, clarithromycin, parenteral erythromycin, telithromycin), quinolones (especially moxifloxacin), quinupristin/dalfopristin 3. ANTICANCER AND IMMUNOMODULATING DRUGS – arsenic trioxide 4. ANTIDEPRESSANTS – TCAs, venlafaxine 5. ANTIEMETICS – dolasetron 6. ANTIFUNGALS – fluconazole, posaconazole, voriconazole 7. ANTIMALARIALS – artemether with lumefantrine, chloroquine, hydroxychloroquine, mefloquine, quinine 8. ANTIPROTOZOALS – pentamidine isetionate 9. ANTIPSYCHOTICS – atypicals, phenothiazines, pimozide 10. BETA-BLOCKERS – sotalol 11. BRONCHODILATORS – parenteral bronchodilators 12. CNS STIMULANTS – atomoxetine	Risk of ventricular arrhythmias, particularly torsades de pointes	Additive effect; these drugs cause prolongation of the Q–T interval.	Avoid co-administration

ANTIHISTAMINES	DRUGS WITH ANTIMUSCARINIC EFFECTS			
ANTIHISTAMINES – CHLORPHENAMINE, CYPROHEPTADINE, HYDROXYZINE	1. ANALGESICS – nefopam 2. ANTIARRHYTHMICS – disopyramide, propafenone 3. ANTIDEPRESSANTS – TCAs 4. ANTIMUSCARINICS – atropine, benzatropine, cyclopentolate, dicycloverine, flavoxate, homatropine, hyoscine, orphenadrine, oxybutynin, procyclidine, propantheline, tolterodine, trihexyphenidyl, tropicamide 5. ANTIPARKINSON'S DRUGS – dopaminergics 6. ANTIPSYCHOTICS – phenothiazines, clozapine, pimozide 7. MUSCLE RELAXANTS – baclofen 8. NITRATES – isosorbide dinitrate	↑ risk of antimuscarinic side-effects. **NB ↓ efficacy of sublingual nitrate tablets**	Additive effect; both drugs cause antimuscarinic side-effects. **Antimuscarinic effects ↓ saliva production, which ↓ dissolution of the tablet**	Warn patients of this additive effect. **Consider changing the formulation to a sublingual nitrate spray**
ANTIHISTAMINES	ALCOHOL	↑ sedation with sedating antihistamines	Additive effect	Warn patients about this effect
ANTIHISTAMINES	**ANALGESICS**			
ANTIHISTAMINES	OPIOIDS	Promethazine ↑ analgesic and anaesthetic effects of opioids. However, it has an additive sedative effect	Unknown	Monitor vital signs closely during co-administration

RESPIRATORY DRUGS ANTIHISTAMINES

Primary drug	Secondary drug	Effect	Mechanism	Precautions
ANTIHISTAMINES	PARACETAMOL	Chlorphenamine, cyclizine, cyproheptadine and hydroxyzine may slow the onset of action of intermittent-dose paracetamol	Anticholinergic effects delay gastric emptying and absorption	Warn patients that the action of paracetamol may be delayed. This will not be the case when paracetamol is taken regularly
FEXOFENADINE	ANTACIDS	↓ fexofenadine levels	↓ absorption	Be aware
ANTIHISTAMINES	**ANTIARRHYTHMICS**			
TERFENADINE, HYDROXYZINE, MIZOLASTINE	FLECAINIDE	Risk of arrhythmias	Additive effect	Avoid co-administration
MIZOLASTINE	MEXILETINE	Risk of arrhythmias	Additive effect	Avoid co-administration
ALIMEMAZINE (TRIMEPRAZINE), CHLORPHENIRAMINE, PROMETHAZINE	ANTICANCER AND IMMUNOMODULATING DRUGS – PROCARBAZINE	1. The antimuscarinic effects (dry mouth, urinary retention, blurred vision, gastrointestinal disturbances) are ↑, as are the sedating effects of these older antihistamines 2. Excessive sedation may occur	1. MAOIs cause anticholinergic effects (including antimuscarinic effects), hence the additive effects of both antimuscarinic activity and CNS depression 2. Additive effects on the CNS, although on occasions chlorpheniramine may cause CNS stimulation	Concurrent use is not recommended. If used together, patients should be warned to report any gastrointestinal problems as paralytic ileus has been reported. Also, caution is required when performing activities needing alertness (e.g. driving, using sharp objects). Do not use OTC medications such as nasal decongestants, asthma and allergy remedies without consulting the pharmacist/doctor as these preparations may contain antihistamines
ANTIHISTAMINES	**ANTIDEPRESSANTS**			
ANTIHISTAMINES	MAOIs	↑ occurrence of antimuscarinic effects such as blurred vision, confusion (in the elderly), restlessness and constipation	Additive antimuscarinic effects	Warn patients and carers, particularly those managing elderly patients

ANTIHISTAMINES – SEDATIVE	MAOIs	Additive depression of CNS ranging from drowsiness to coma and respiratory depression	Synergistic depressant effects on CNS function	Necessary to warn patients, particularly regards activities that require attention, e.g. driving and using machinery and equipment that could cause self-harm
CYPROHEPTADINE	SSRIs	Antidepressant effect of SSRIs are possibly antagonized by cyproheptadine	Cyproheptadine is an antihistamine with antiserotonergic activity	Be aware
TERFENADINE	SSRIs	Possibility of ↑ plasma concentrations of these drugs and potential risk of dangerous arrhythmias	These drugs are metabolized mainly by CYP3A4. Fluvoxamine and fluoxetine are inhibitors of CYP3A4 but are relatively weak compared with ketoconazole, which is possibly 100 times more potent as an inhibitor	The interaction is unlikely to be of clinical significance but there is a need to be aware
KETOTIFEN	ANTIDIABETIC DRUGS – METFORMIN	↓ platelet count	Unknown	Avoid co-administration (manufacturers' recommendation)
ANTIHISTAMINES	**ANTIFUNGALS – AZOLES**			
MIZOLASTINE	AZOLES	↑ mizolastine levels	Inhibition of metabolism of mizolastine	Avoid co-administration
LORATADINE	KETOCONAZOLE, POSACONAZOLE	↑ loratadine levels	Inhibition of cytochrome P450, P-gp or both	Avoid co-administration
ASTEMIZOLE, CHLORPHENAMINE, TERFENADINE	ANTIVIRALS – PROTEASE INHIBITORS	Possibly ↑ adverse effects with amprenavir, atazanavir, indinavir, ritonavir (with or without lopinavir), saquinavir and tipranavir	Inhibition of CYP3A4-mediated metabolism of astemizole; risk is greatest in those who are slow CYP2D6 metabolizers because chlorphenamine and terfenadine are also metabolized by this route	Avoid co-administration

Primary drug	Secondary drug	Effect	Mechanism	Precautions
ANTIHISTAMINES	ANXIOLYTICS AND HYPNOTICS – SODIUM OXYBATE	Risk of CNS depression – coma, respiratory depression	Additive depression of CNS	Avoid co-administration. Caution even with relatively non-sedating antihistamines (cetrizine, desloratadine, fexofenadine, levocetirizine, loratadine, mizolastine) as they can impair the performance of skilled tasks
ANTIHISTAMINES	**GRAPEFRUIT JUICE**			
FEXOFENADINE	GRAPEFRUIT JUICE	Possibly ↓ efficacy	↓ absorption possibly by affecting P-gp and direct inhibition of uptake by intestinal OATP-1A2	Clinical significance unclear. No clinically significant changes in ECG parameters were observed in one study
TERFENADINE	GRAPEFRUIT JUICE	Possibly ↑ efficacy and ↑ adverse effects, e.g. torsade de points	Altered metabolism so parent drug accumulates	Avoid concomitant intake
LORATADINE	H2 RECEPTOR BLOCKERS	Possibly ↑ loratadine levels	Inhibition of metabolism	Be aware
BRONCHODILATORS				
ANTIMUSCARINICS (IPRATROPIUM, TIOTROPIUM) ➢ ***Drugs Acting on the Nervous System, Antiparkinson's drugs***				
BETA-2 AGONISTS				
TERBUTALINE	ANAESTHETICS GENERAL – HALOTHANE	Cases of arrhythmias when terbutaline co-administered with halothane	Possibly due to sensitization of the myocardium to circulating catecholamines	Risk of cardiac events is higher with halothane. Desflurane is irritant to the upper respiratory tract, and ↑ secretions can occur; it is best avoided in patients with bronchial asthma. Sevoflurane is non-irritant and unlikely to cause serious adverse effects
BETA-2 AGONISTS	ANALGESICS – NSAIDs	Etoricoxib may ↑ oral salbutamol levels	Etoricoxib inhibits sulphotransferase activity	Monitor PR and BP closely
BETA-2 AGONISTS	ANTIBIOTICS – LINEZOLID	Theoretical risk of hypertensive reactions	Linezolid has weak MAOI properties	Monitor BP closely during co-administration

BETA-2 AGONISTS	ANTICANCER AND IMMUNOMODULATING DRUGS – CORTICOSTEROIDS	Risk of hypokalaemia	Additive effect. The CSM notes that this effect occurs with beta-2 agonists, theophyllines and corticosteroids, all of which may be given during severe asthma; hypoxia exacerbates this effect	Monitor blood potassium levels prior to concomitant administration and during therapy (monitor 1–2-hourly during parenteral administration). Administer potassium supplements to prevent hypokalaemia, which may also be worsened by hypoxia during severe attacks of asthma
BETA-2 AGONISTS	ANTIDEPRESSANTS – MAOIs	↑ occurrence of headache and hypertensive episodes. Unlikely to occur with moclobemide and selegiline	Due to impaired metabolism of these sympathomimetic amines due to inhibition of MAO. Moclobemide is involved in the breakdown of serotonin, while selegiline is mainly involved in the breakdown of dopamine	Be aware. Monitor BP closely
BETA AGONISTS	ANTIDIABETIC DRUGS	↑ risk of hyperglycaemia. If administered during pregnancy, there is a risk of hypoglycaemia in the fetus, independent of maternal blood glucose levels. ↑ risk of ketoacidosis when administered intravenously	By inducing glycogenolysis, beta-adrenergic agonists cause elevation of blood sugar in adults. In the fetus, these agents cause a depletion of fetal glycogen stores	Monitor blood sugar closely during concomitant administration until blood sugar levels are stable. Be cautious during use in pregnancy. Formoterol and salmeterol are long-acting beta-agonists
BETA-2 AGONISTS	ANTIHYPERTENSIVE AND HEART FAILURE DRUGS – CENTRALLY ACTING ANTIHYPERTENSIVES	Cases of ↓ BP when intravenous salbutamol is given with methyldopa	Uncertain at present	Monitor BP closely
BETA-2 AGONISTS	BETA-BLOCKERS	Non-selective beta-blockers (e.g. propanolol) ↓ or prevent the bronchodilator effect of beta-2 agonists	Non-selective beta-blockers antagonize the effect of beta-2 agonists on bronchial smooth muscle	Avoid co-administration

Primary drug	Secondary drug	Effect	Mechanism	Precautions
SALBUTAMOL	BETAHISTINE	↓ or prevents the bronchodilator effect	Betahistine causes bronchoconstriction	Avoid co-administration
BETA-2 AGONISTS	**BRONCHODILATORS**			
BETA-2 AGONISTS	THEOPHYLLINE	Risk of hypokalaemia	Additive effect. The CSM notes that this effect occurs with beta-2 agonists, theophyllines and corticosteroids, all of which may be given during severe asthma; hypoxia exacerbates this effect	Co-administration is useful for the management of severe asthma. Monitor blood potassium levels prior to concomitant administration and during therapy (monitor 1–2-hourly during parenteral administration). Administer potassium supplements to prevent hypokalaemia, which may also be worsened by hypoxia during severe asthma attacks
SALBUTAMOL	IPRATROPIUM BROMIDE	A few reports of acute closed-angle glaucoma when nebulized ipratropium and salbutamol were co-administered	Ipratropium dilates the pupil, which ↓ drainage of aqueous humour, while salbutamol ↑ production of aqueous humour	Warn patients to prevent the solution/mist entering the eye. Use extreme caution in co-administering these bronchodilators by the nebulized route in patients with a history of acute closed-angle glaucoma
BETA-2 AGONISTS	CARDIAC GLYCOSIDES – DIGOXIN	1. Hypokalaemia may exacerbate digoxin toxicity 2. Salbutamol may ↓ digoxin levels (by 16–22%) after 10 days of concurrent therapy	1. Beta-2 agonists may cause hypokalaemia 2. Uncertain	1. Monitor potassium levels closely 2. Clinical significance is uncertain. Useful to monitor digoxin levels if there is a clinical indication of ↓ response to digoxin
SALBUTAMOL	CNS STIMULANTS – ATOMOXETINE	↑ risk of arrhythmias with parenteral salbutamol	Additive effect	Avoid co-administration of atomoxetine with parenteral salbutamol

BETA-2 AGONISTS	DIURETICS – CARBONIC ANHYDRASE INHIBITORS, LOOP AND THIAZIDES	Risk of hypokalaemia	Additive effects	Monitor blood potassium levels prior to concomitant administration and during therapy. Administer potassium supplements to prevent hypokalaemia
SALBUTAMOL	EPHEDRA	Risk of marked ↑ heart rate and of BP	Additive effect; ephedra causes vasoconstriction	The US FDA has banned products containing ephedra. Warn patients on salbutamol to avoid traditional remedies containing ephedra
BAMBUTEROL	MUSCLE RELAXANTS – SUXAMETHONIUM	↑ effect of suxamethonium	Bambuterol is an inhibitor of pseudocholinesterase, which hydrolyses suxamethonium	Be cautious of prolonged periods of respiratory muscle paralysis, and monitor respiration closely until complete recovery
SALBUTAMOL	YOHIMBINE	↑ risk of CNS stimulation	Uncertain; yohimbine may cause ↑ dopamine levels	Warn patients taking salbutamol to avoid remedies containing yohimbine
NON-SELECTIVE BETA-AGONISTS ➢ *Sympathomimetics section – CVS Chapter*				
THEOPHYLLINES				
THEOPHYLLINE	**ANAESTHETICS – GENERAL**			
THEOPHYLLINE	HALOTHANE	Case reports of arrhythmias	Possibly due to sensitization of the myocardium to circulating catecholamines	Risk of cardiac events is higher with halothane. Desflurane is irritant to the upper respiratory tract, and ↑ secretions can occur; it is best avoided in patients with bronchial asthma. Sevoflurane is non-irritant and unlikely to cause serious adverse effects

Primary drug	Secondary drug	Effect	Mechanism	Precautions
THEOPHYLLINE	KETAMINE	Risk of fits	Uncertain	A careful risk–benefit assessment should be made before using ketamine. However, there are significant benefits for the use of ketamine to anaesthetize patients for the emergency management of life-threatening asthma
AMINOPHYLLINE	PROCAINE SOLUTIONS	Precipitation of drugs, which may not be immediately apparent	A pharmaceutical interaction	Do not mix in the same infusion or syringe
THEOPHYLLINE	**ANTIARRHYTHMICS**			
THEOPHYLLINE	ADENOSINE	↓ efficacy of adenosine	Theophylline and other xanthines are adenosine receptor antagonists	Watch for poor response to adenosine; higher doses may be required
THEOPHYLLINE	AMIODARONE	Theophylline levels may be ↑ by amiodarone (single case report of theophylline levels doubling)	Uncertain; amiodarone probably inhibits the metabolism of theophylline	Watch for theophylline toxicity; monitor levels regularly until stable
THEOPHYLLINE	MEXILETINE	Theophylline levels may be ↑ by mexiletine; cases of theophylline toxicity have been reported	Mexiletine inhibits CYP1A2-mediated metabolism of theophylline	↓ theophylline dose (by up to 50%). Monitor theophylline levels and watch for toxicity
THEOPHYLLINE	MORACIZINE	↓ plasma concentrations of theophylline and risk of therapeutic failure	Due to induction of microsomal enzyme activity	May need to ↑ dose of theophylline by 25%
THEOPHYLLINE	PROPAFENONE	Case reports of ↑ theophylline levels with toxicity when propafenone was added	Uncertain at present	Watch for signs of theophylline toxicity

THEOPHYLLINE	ANTIBIOTICS			
THEOPHYLLINE	ISONIAZID, MACROLIDES (azithromycin, clarithromycin, erythromycin, telithromycin), QUINOLONES	1. ↑ theophylline levels 2. Possibly ↓ erythromycin levels when given orally	1. Inhibition of CYP2D6-mediated metabolism of theophylline (macrolides and quinolones – isoniazid not known) 2. ↓ bioavailability; uncertain mechanism	1. Monitor theophylline levels before, during and after co-administration 2. Consider alternative macrolide
THEOPHYLLINE	RIFAMPICIN	↓ plasma concentrations of theophylline and risk of therapeutic failure	Due to induction of CYP1A2 and CYP3A3	May need to ↑ dose of theophylline by 25%
THEOPHYLLINE	**ANTICANCER AND IMMUNOMODULATING DRUGS**			
THEOPHYLLINE	CORTICOSTEROIDS	Risk of hypokalaemia	Additive effect. The CSM notes that this effect occurs with beta-2 agonists, theophyllines and corticosteroids, all of which may be given during severe asthma; hypoxia exacerbates this effect	Monitor blood potassium levels prior to concomitant administration and during therapy (monitor 1–2-hourly during parenteral administration). Administer potassium supplements to prevent hypokalaemia, which may also be worsened by hypoxia during severe attacks of asthma
THEOPHYLLINE	INTERFERON ALFA	↑ theophylline levels	Inhibition of theophylline metabolism	Monitor theophylline levels before, during and after co-administration
THEOPHYLLINE	METHOTREXATE	Possible ↑ theophylline levels	Possibly inhibition of CYP2D6-mediated metabolism of theophylline	Monitor clinically for toxic effects, and advise patients to seek medical attention if they have symptoms suggestive of theophylline toxicity. Measure theophylline levels before, during and after co-administration

Primary drug	Secondary drug	Effect	Mechanism	Precautions
THEOPHYLLINE	**ANTIDEPRESSANTS**			
THEOPHYLLINE	LITHIUM	↓ plasma levels of lithium and risk of therapeutic failure	Theophylline ↑ renal clearance of lithium	May need to ↑ dose of lithium by 60%
THEOPHYLLINE	ST JOHN'S WORT	↓ theophylline levels	Inhibition of CYP1A2-mediated metabolism of theophylline	Avoid co-administration
THEOPHYLLINE	SSRIs – FLUVOXAMINE	↑ theophylline levels	Fluvoxamine is potent inhibitor of CYP1A2	Consider an alternative antidepressant
THEOPHYLLINE	TCAs	Possible ↑ theophylline levels	Inhibition of CYP1A2- and CYP2D6-mediated metabolism of theophylline. The clinical significance of this depends upon whether theophylline's alternative pathways of metabolism are also inhibited by co-administered drugs	Warn patients to report any ↑ side-effects of theophylline, and monitor PR and ECG carefully
THEOPHYLLINE	ANTIEPILEPTICS – BARBITURATES, CARBAMAZEPINE, PHENYTOIN	↓ theophylline levels. Possibly ↓ carbamazepine and phenytoin levels	Due to induction of microsomal enzyme activity. Theophylline ↓ absorption of phenytoin	May need to ↑ dose of theophylline by 25%. Monitor for inadequate therapeutic response to carbamazepine and phenytoin. Measure levels of these drugs
THEOPHYLLINE	**ANTIFUNGALS**			
THEOPHYLLINE	AZOLES – ITRACONAZOLE, KETOCONAZOLE	↑ theophylline levels, with risk of toxicity with itraconazole. Unpredictable effect on theophylline levels with ketoconazole	Theophylline is primarily metabolized by CYP1A2. Although azoles are best known as inhibitors of CYP3A4, they also inhibit other CYP isoenzymes to varying degrees	If concurrent use is necessary, monitor theophylline levels on initiation and discontinuation of itraconazole therapy. Other azoles or terbinafine may be a safer alternative
THEOPHYLLINE	GRISEOFULVIN	↑ theophylline levels	Inhibition of metabolism of theophylline	Uncertain clinical significance. Watch for early features of theophylline toxicity

THEOPHYLLINE	ANTIGOUT DRUGS			
THEOPHYLLINE	ALLOPURINOL	↑ theophylline levels	Allopurinol inhibits xanthine oxidase	Watch for early features of toxicity of theophylline (headache and nausea)
THEOPHYLLINE	SULFINPYRAZONE	↓ theophylline levels	Due to ↑ demethylation and hydroxylation, and thus ↑ clearance of theophylline	May need to ↑ dose of theophylline by 25%
THEOPHYLLINE	**ANTIVIRALS**			
THEOPHYLLINE	ACICLOVIR/VALACICLOVIR	↑ theophylline levels	Uncertain	Monitor for signs of toxicity and check levels
THEOPHYLLINE	INDINAVIR	Possibly ↑ efficacy	Inhibition of metabolism via CYP3A4, but mainly metabolized via CYP1A2, which is not inhibited	Not thought to be clinically significant; however, monitor levels more closely in unstable patients
THEOPHYLLINE	RITONAVIR (± LOPINAVIR)	↓ efficacy	↑ metabolism via induction of CYP1A2; also altered metabolism via CYP3A4	Monitor clinical response; measure levels weekly after starting. ↑ doses may be required
THEOPHYLLINE	ANXIOLYTICS AND HYPNOTICS – BZDs	↓ therapeutic effect of BZDs	BZDs ↑ CNS concentrations of adenosine, a potent CNS depressant, while theophylline blocks adenosine receptors	Larger doses of diazepam are required to produce desired therapeutic effects such as sedation. Discontinuation of theophylline without ↓ dose of BZDs ↑ risk of sedation and of respiratory depression
THEOPHYLLINE	BETA-BLOCKERS – PROPRANOLOL	↑ plasma levels of theophylline with propranolol	Propranolol exerts a dose-dependent inhibitory effect on the metabolism of theophylline	Monitor theophylline levels during propranolol co-administration

Primary drug	Secondary drug	Effect	Mechanism	Precautions
THEOPHYLLINE	BRONCHODILATORS – BETA-2 AGONISTS	Risk of hypokalaemia	Additive effect. The CSM notes that this effect occurs with beta-2 agonists, theophyllines and corticosteroids, all of which may be given during severe asthma; hypoxia exacerbates this effect	Co-administration is useful for the management of severe asthma. Monitor blood potassium levels prior to concomitant administration and during therapy (monitor 1–2-hourly during parenteral administration). Administer potassium supplements to prevent hypokalaemia, which may also be worsened by hypoxia during severe attacks of asthma
THEOPHYLLINE	**CALCIUM CHANNEL BLOCKERS**			
THEOPHYLLINE	DILTIAZEM, VERAPAMIL	↑ theophylline levels with diltiazem and verapamil. Mostly not clinically significant but two case reports of theophylline toxicity with verapamil	Uncertain but thought to be due to inhibition of CYP1A2-mediated metabolism of theophylline	Be aware of the small possibility of theophylline toxicity when commencing calcium channel blockers; check levels if any problems occur, and consider either ↓ dose of theophylline or using an alternative calcium channel blocker
THEOPHYLLINE	NIFEDIPINE	Clinically non-significant ↓ theophylline levels with nifedipine, but case reports of theophylline toxicity after starting nifedipine	Uncertain; probably due to alterations in either the metabolism or volume of distribution of theophylline	Be aware of the small possibility of theophylline toxicity when commencing calcium channel blockers; check levels if any problems occur, and consider either ↓ dose of theophylline or using an alternative calcium channel blocker
THEOPHYLLINE	CNS STIMULANTS – MODAFINIL	May cause ↓ theophylline levels	Modafinil is a moderate inducer of CYP1A2 in a concentration-dependent manner	Be aware; watch for poor response to theophylline and measure levels

THEOPHYLLINE	DIURETICS – CARBONIC ANHYDRASE INHIBITORS, LOOP AND THIAZIDES	Risk of hypokalaemia	Additive effects	Monitor blood potassium levels prior to concomitant administration and during therapy. Administer potassium supplements to prevent hypokalaemia
THEOPHYLLINE	DOXAPRAM	Reports of ↑ muscle tone and CNS excitation	Uncertain	Be aware
THEOPHYLLINE	**DRUG DEPENDENCE THERAPIES**			
THEOPHYLLINE	BUPROPION	1. ↑ theophylline levels 2. ↑ risk of seizures. This risk is marked in elderly people, patients with a history of seizures, with addiction to opiates/cocaine/stimulants, and in diabetics treated with oral hypoglycaemics or insulin	1. Smoking induces mainly CYP1A2 and CYP2E1. Thus, de-induction takes place following the cessation of smoking 2. Bupropion is associated with a dose-related risk of seizures. These drugs, which lower seizure threshold, are individually epileptogenic. Additive effects occur when they are combined	1. Be aware , particularly with drugs with a narrow therapeutic index (see section). Monitor clinically and biochemically (e.g. INR, plasma theophylline levels) 2. Extreme caution. The dose of bupropion should not exceed 450 mg/day (or 150 mg/day in patients with severe hepatic cirrhosis)
THEOPHYLLINE	DISULFIRAM	↑ theophylline levels	Disulfiram ↓ theophylline clearance by inhibiting hydroxylation and demethylation	Monitor theophylline levels before, during and after co-administration
THEOPHYLLINE	GRAPEFRUIT JUICE	Possibly ↓ efficacy	Unclear. ↓ bioavailability (significant from 1–4 hours)	Avoid concomitant intake if slow-release theophylline preparations are used. Monitor levels and clinical state weekly if the intake of grapefruit is altered

Primary drug	Secondary drug	Effect	Mechanism	Precautions
THEOPHYLLINE	H2 RECEPTOR BLOCKERS – CIMETIDINE, FAMOTIDINE, NIZATIDINE, RANITIDINE	↑ efficacy and adverse effects, including seizures. There is conflicting information associated with ranitidine, famotidine and nizatidine	Inhibition of metabolism via CYP1A2, cimetidine being the best known inhibitor	Use alternative acid suppression, e.g. an H2 antagonist or proton pump inhibitor (not omeprazole or lansoprazole), or monitor closely; there is considerable patient variation. Check levels on day 3 and then at 1 week. A 30–50% ↓ dose of theophylline may be required. For doses <400 mg/day, the interaction may not be clinically significant
THEOPHYLLINE	LEUKOTRIENE RECEPTOR ANTAGONISTS – ZAFIRLUKAST	Possibly ↑ theophylline levels. Also possibly ↓ zafirlukast levels	Mutual alteration of metabolism	Be aware; watch for features of theophylline toxicity and measure levels
THEOPHYLLINE	MUSCLE RELAXANTS – PANCURONIUM	Antagonism of neuromuscular block	Uncertain	Larger doses of pancuronium may be needed to obtain the desired muscle relaxation during anaesthesia; other non-depolarizing muscle relaxants do not seem to be affected
THEOPHYLLINE	OESTROGENS	↑ theophylline levels	↓ clearance of theophylline in a dose-dependent manner	Be aware; watch for features of theophylline toxicity and measure levels
THEOPHYLLINE	PERIPHERAL VASODILATORS – PENTOXIFYLLINE	Possibly ↑ theophylline levels	Uncertain; possibly competitive inhibition of theophylline metabolism (pentoxifylline is also a xanthine derivative)	Warn patients of the possibility of adverse effects of theophylline; monitor levels if necessary
THEOPHYLLINE	PHOSPHODIESTERASE INHIBITORS – ENOXIMONE	Theophylline may ↓ efficacy of enoximone	Possibly competitive inhibition of phosphodiesterases	Be aware; watch for poor response to enoximone
THEOPHYLLINE	SUCRALFATE	Possibly ↓ theophylline levels (with modified-release preparations)	Possibly ↓ absorption	Watch for poor response to theophylline and monitor levels

THEOPHYLLINE	**SYMPATHOMIMETICS**			
THEOPHYLLINE	INDIRECTLY ACTING SYMPATHOMIMETICS	↑ incidence of side-effects of theophylline (without a change in its serum concentrations) when co-administered with ephedrine	Uncertain	Avoid co-administration. Warn patients to avoid OTC remedies containing ephedrine
THEOPHYLLINE	DIRECTLY ACTING SYMPATHOMIMETICS	Case report of marked tachycardia when dobutamine was given to a patient already taking theophylline	Uncertain	Carefully titrate the dose of dobutamine in patients taking theophylline therapy
THEOPHYLLINE	THYROID HORMONES	Altered theophylline levels (↑ or ↓) when thyroid status is altered therapeutically	Uncertain	Monitor theophylline levels closely during changes in treatment of abnormal thyroid function. Watch for early features of theophylline toxicity
DOXAPRAM				
DOXAPRAM	BRONCHODILATORS – THEOPHYLLINE	Reports of ↑ muscle tone and CNS excitation	Uncertain	Be aware
DOXAPRAM	SYMPATHOMIMETICS	Risk of ↑ BP	Uncertain at present	Monitor BP closely
LEUKOTRIENE RECEPTOR ANTAGONISTS				
ZAFIRLUKAST	ANTIPLATELET AGENTS – ASPIRIN	↑ levels of zafirlukast	Uncertain	Watch for early features of zafirlukast toxicity. Monitor FBC and liver function closely
ZAFIRLUKAST	ANTIBIOTICS – MACROLIDES	↓ zafirlukast levels	Induction of metabolism	Watch for poor response to zafirlukast
ZAFIRLUKAST	ANTICOAGULANTS – ORAL	Zafirlukast ↑ anticoagulant effect	Zafirlukast inhibits CYP2C9-mediated metabolism of warfarin	Monitor INR at least weekly until stable

RESPIRATORY DRUGS LEUKOTRIENE RECEPTOR ANTAGONISTS

Primary drug	Secondary drug	Effect	Mechanism	Precautions
ZAFIRLUKAST	ANTIDEPRESSANTS – TCAs	Possible ↑ plasma concentrations of zafirlukast	Inhibition of CYP2C9-mediated metabolism of zafirlukast. The clinical significance of this depends upon whether alternative pathways of metabolism are also inhibited by co-administered drugs	Warn patients to report ↑ side-effects
MONTELUKAST	ANTIDIABETIC DRUGS – REPAGLINIDE	↑ repaglinide levels, risk of hypoglycaemia	Hepatic metabolism inhibited	Watch for and warn patients about hypoglycaemia ➢ ***For signs and symptoms of hypoglycaemia, see Clinical Features of Some Adverse Drug Interactions, Hypoglycaemia***
MONTELUKAST	ANTIEPILEPTICS – BARBITURATES	↓ montelukast levels	Induction of metabolism	Watch for poor response to montelukast
ZAFIRLUKAST	BRONCHODILATORS – THEOPHYLLINE	Possibly ↑ theophylline levels. Also possibly ↓ zafirlukast levels	Mutual alteration of metabolism	Be aware; watch for features of theophylline toxicity and measure levels

RESPIRATORY DRUGS LEUKOTRIENE RECEPTOR ANTAGONISTS

Part 13 METABOLIC DRUGS

Primary drug	Secondary drug	Effect	Mechanism	Precautions
AGALSIDASE				
AGALSIDASE BETA	ANTIARRHYTHMICS – AMIODARONE	↓ clinical effect of agalsidase beta	Uncertain	Avoid co-administration
AGALSIDASE BETA	ANTIBIOTICS – GENTAMICIN	Possibly ↓ clinical effect of agalsidase beta	Uncertain	Avoid co-administration
AGALSIDASE BETA	ANTIMALARIALS – CHLOROQUINE	↓ efficacy of agalsidase beta	Inhibition of intracellular activity of agalsidase beta	Avoid co-administration – manufacturers' recommendation
LARONIDASE				
LARONIDASE	ANAESTHETICS – LOCAL – procaine	Possibly ↓ efficacy of laronidase	Uncertain	Avoid co-administration
LARONIDASE	ANTIMALARIALS – CHLOROQUINE	↓ efficacy of laronidase	Uncertain	Avoid co-administration
PENICILLAMINE ➢ *Anticancer and Immunomodulating Drugs, Other immunomodulating drugs*				
SODIUM PHENYLBUTYRATE				
SODIUM PHENYLBUTYRATE	ANTIGOUT DRUGS – PROBENECID	Possibly ↑ sodium phenylbutyrate levels	Possibly ↓ excretion of sodium phenylbutyrate	Watch for signs of sodium phenylbutyrate toxicity. Monitor FBC, U&Es and ECG
SODIUM PHENYLBUTYRATE	CORTICOSTEROIDS, HALOPERIDOL, VALPROATE	Possibly ↓ efficacy of sodium phenylbutyrate	These drugs are associated with ↑ ammonia levels	Avoid co-administration
TRIENTINE				
TRIENTINE	ANTACIDS – CALCIUM AND MAGNESIUM-CONTAINING	Possibly ↓ trientine levels	↓ absorption	Separate doses as much as possible; take antacids after trientine
TRIENTINE	IRON – ORAL	↓ iron levels when iron is given orally	↓ absorption	Separate doses by at least 2 hours – monitor FBC closely
TRIENTINE	ZINC	↓ zinc and trientine levels	Mutually ↓ absorption	Separate doses by at least 2 hours

Part 14 DRUGS USED IN OBSTETRICS AND GYNAECOLOGY

Primary drug	Secondary drug	Effect	Mechanism	Precautions
DANAZOL				
DANAZOL	**ANTICANCER AND IMMUNOMODULATING DRUGS**			
DANAZOL	CICLOSPORIN	↑ plasma concentrations of ciclosporin, with risk of toxic effects	Inhibition of ciclosporin metabolism	Watch for toxic effects of ciclosporin
DANAZOL	TACROLIMUS	Cases of ↑ tacrolimus levels	Uncertain	Watch for early features of tacrolimus toxicity
DANAZOL	ANTICOAGULANTS – ORAL	Possible ↓ anticoagulant effect	Uncertain	Monitor INR at least weekly until stable
DANAZOL	ANTIEPILEPTICS – CARBAMAZEPINE	↑ plasma concentrations of carbamazepine, with risk of toxic effects	Inhibition of carbamazepine metabolism	Watch for toxic effects of carbamazepine
DANAZOL	OESTROGENS	↓ efficacy of both danazol and oestrogen contraceptives	Uncertain; possibly competition for same receptors	Use alternative forms of contraception
ERGOMETRINE ➢ *Drugs Acting on the Nervous System, Antimigraine drugs*				
FEMALE HORMONES				
OESTROGENS				
OESTROGENS	**REDUCED EFFICACY OF OESTROGENS**			
OESTROGENS	1. ANTIBIOTICS – ampicillin, cephalosporins, chloramphenicol, clindamycin, erythromycin, metronidazole, sulphonamides, tetracyclines 2. ANTIPROTOZOALS – tinidazole	Reports of ↓ contraceptive effect	Possibly alteration of the bacterial flora necessary for recycling ethinylestradiol from the large bowel, although not certain in every case	Advise patients to use additional contraception for the period of antibiotic intake and for 1 month after stopping the antibiotic

OESTROGENS	1. ANTIBIOTICS – rifabutin, rifampicin 2. ANTIDEPRESSANTS – St John's wort 3. ANTIEPILEPTICS – barbiturates, carbamazepine, oxcarbazepine, phenytoin, topiramate 4. ANTIFUNGALS – griseofulvin, terbinafine 5. ANTIVIRALS – nelfinavir, nevirapine, ritonavir 6. CNS STIMULANTS – modafinil	Marked ↓ contraceptive effect	Induction of metabolism of oestrogens. Modafinil is moderate inducer of CYP1A2 in a concentration-dependent manner	Advise patients to use additional contraception for the period of intake and for 1 month after stopping co-administration of these drugs (4–8 weeks after stopping rifabutin or rifampicin). Barrier methods are necessary to prevent transmission of infection from patients with HIV. Avoid co-administration of oestrogens with St John's wort
OESTROGENS	1. ANTICANCER AND IMMUNOMODULATING DRUGS – mycophenolate 2. ANTIEMETICS – aprepitant 3. ANXIOLYTICS AND HYPNOTICS – BZDs, meprobamate 4. PROTON PUMP INHIBITORS – lansoprazole	Possible altered efficacy of contraceptive; reports of breakthrough bleeding when BZDs or meprobamate were co-administered with oral contraceptives	Unclear	Clinical significance uncertain. It would seem to be wise to advise patients to use an alternative form of contraception during and for 1 month after stopping co-administration of these drugs

Primary drug	Secondary drug	Effect	Mechanism	Precautions
OESTROGENS – ORAL CONTRACEPTIVES	FLUCONAZOLE, ITRACONAZOLE, KETOCONAZOLE, POSACONAZOLE, VORICONAZOLE	The Netherlands Pharmacovigilance Foundation received reports of pill cycle disturbances 2–3 weeks after the start of the pill cycle, delayed bleeding and pregnancy. Effects of either or both of oestrogen excess and progestogen excess may occur (migraine headaches, thromboembolic episodes, breast tenderness, bloating, weight gain)	The metabolism of oral contraceptives is complex, dependent on composition, constituents and doses. Ethylene oestradiol (EE), a common constituent, as well as progestogens are substrates of CYP3A4, which is inhibited by itraconazole. The inhibition of ethinylestradiol and progestogens could lead to effects of oestrogen and progestogen excess. Triazole antifungals inhibit the biotransformation of steroids, and such an ↑ may cause delay of withdrawal bleeding	Due to the complex metabolic pathways of oral contraceptives, dependent on constituents, doses and the reported adverse effects during concomitant use, it is advisable to avoid the use of azole antifungals and advise alternative methods of contraception
OESTROGENS	**INCREASED EFFICACY OF OESTROGENS**			
OESTROGENS	1. ANTICANCER AND IMMUNOMODULATING DRUGS – ciclosporin, tacrolimus 2. CALCIUM CHANNEL BLOCKERS – nicardipine, nisoldipine, verapamil 3. DIURETICS – spironolactone	Risk of gynaecomastia	Inhibition of 2-hydroxylation or 17-oxidation of oestradiol in the liver, causing ↑ oestradiol pool in the body	Watch for gynaecomastia and warn patients
OESTROGENS – ESTRADIOL, POSSIBLY ETHINYLESTRADIOL	GRAPEFRUIT JUICE	↑ efficacy and ↑ adverse effects of oestrogens	Oral administration only. ↑ bioavailability and ↓ presystemic metabolism. Constituents of grapefruit juice irreversibly inhibit intestinal cytochrome CYP3A4. Transport via P-gp and MRP-2 efflux pumps is also inhibited	Monitor for ↑ side-effects

OESTROGENS	ANALGESICS			
OESTROGENS	NSAIDs	Etoricoxib may ↑ ethinylestradiol levels	Etoricoxib inhibits sulphotransferase activity	Consider using a formulation with a lower dose of ethinylestradiol
OESTROGENS	OPIOIDS	Effect of morphine may be ↓ by combined oral contraceptives	↑ hepatic metabolism of morphine	Be aware that the morphine dose may need to be ↑. Consider using an alternative opioid such as pethidine
OESTROGENS	ANTICANCER AND IMMUNOMODULATING DRUGS – ciclosporin, corticosteroids, tacrolimus	Possibly ↑ plasma concentrations of these immunomodulating drugs	Inhibition of metabolism	Monitor blood levels of these drugs; warn patients to report symptoms such as fever and sore throat
OESTROGENS	ANTICOAGULANTS – ORAL	↑ anticoagulant effect	Uncertain at present	Oestrogens are usually not recommended in patients with a history of thromboembolism; if they are used, monitor INR closely
OESTROGENS	ANTIDIABETIC DRUGS	Altered glycaemic control	Uncertain at present	Monitor blood glucose closely
OESTROGENS	1. ANTIHYPERTENSIVES AND HEART FAILURE DRUGS 2. BETA-BLOCKERS 3. CALCIUM CHANNEL BLOCKERS 4. NITRATES	↓ hypotensive effect	Oestrogens cause sodium and fluid retention	Monitor BP at least weekly until stable; the routine prescription of oestrogens in patients with ↑ BP is not advisable
OESTROGENS	ANTIEPILEPTICS – LAMOTRIGINE	↓ lamotrigine levels	↑ metabolism	Monitor levels
OESTROGENS	ANTIPARKINSON'S DRUGS – ROPINIROLE, SELEGILINE	↑ levels of ropinirole and selegiline	Inhibition of metabolism (possibly *N*-demethylation)	Watch for early features of toxicity (nausea, drowsiness) when starting oestrogens in a patient stabilized on these dopaminergics. Conversely, watch for a poor response to them if oestrogens are stopped

Primary drug	Secondary drug	Effect	Mechanism	Precautions
OESTROGENS	BRONCHODILATORS – THEOPHYLLINE	↑ theophylline levels	↓ clearance of theophylline in a dose-dependent manner	Be aware; watch for features of theophylline toxicity and measure levels
OESTROGENS	DANAZOL	↓ efficacy of both danazol and oestrogen contraceptives	Uncertain; possibly competition for the same receptors	Use alternative forms of contraception
OESTROGENS	SOMATROPIN	Possible ↓ efficacy of somatropin	Uncertain	↑ dose of somatropin may be needed
OESTROGENS	VASODILATOR ANTIHYPERTENSIVES	Risk of hyperglycaemia when diazoxide is co-administered with combined oral contraceptives	Additive effect; both drugs have a hyperglycaemic effect	Monitor blood glucose closely, particularly with diabetics
PROGESTOGENS				
PROGESTOGENS	**REDUCED EFFICACY OF PROGESTOGENS**			
PROGESTOGENS	1. ANTIBIOTICS – rifabutin, rifampicin 2. ANTIDEPRESSANTS – St John's wort 3. ANTIEPILEPTICS – barbiturates, carbamazepine, oxcarbazepine, phenytoin, topiramate 4. ANTIFUNGALS – griseofulvin, terbinafine 5. ANTIVIRALS – amprenavir, nelfinavir, nevirapine, ritonavir 6. VASODILATOR ANTIHYPERTENSIVES – bosentan	↓ progesterone levels, which may lead to failure of contraception or poor response to treatment of menorrhagia	Possibly induction of metabolism of progestogens	Advise patients to use additional contraception for the period of intake and for 1 month after stopping co-administration with these drugs. Barrier methods are necessary to prevent transmission of infection from patients with HIV. Avoid co-administration of progestogens with St John's wort
PROGESTOGENS	ANTIEMETICS – APREPITANT	↓ progestogen levels, with risk of contraceptive failure	Uncertain	Advise patients to use an alternative form of contraception during and for 1 month after discontinuing the aprepitant

PROGESTOGENS	RISK OF HYPERKALAEMIA			
PROGESTOGENS	1. ANALGESICS – NSAIDs 2. ANTIHYPERTENSIVES AND HEART FAILURE DRUGS – ACE inhibitors, angiotensin II receptor antagonists 3. DIURETICS – potassium-sparing	↑ risk of hyperkalaemia	Drospirenone (component of the Yasmin brand of combined contraceptive pill) is a progestogen derived from spironolactone that can cause potassium retention	Monitor serum potassium weekly until stable and then every 6 months
PROGESTOGENS	ANALGESICS – OPIOIDS	Gestodene ↑ effect of buprenorphine	Gestodene ↓ CYP3A4-mediated metabolism of buprenorphine	The dose of buprenorphine needs to be ↓ (by up to 50%)
PROGESTOGENS	ANTICANCER AND IMMUNOMODULATING DRUGS – CICLOSPORIN	↑ plasma concentrations of ciclosporin	Inhibition of metabolism of ciclosporin	Monitor blood ciclosporin concentrations. Monitor renal function prior to concurrent therapy. Be aware that infections in immunocompromised patients carry a serious threat to life
PROGESTOGENS	ANTICOAGULANTS – ORAL	↓ anticoagulant effect	Uncertain at present	Monitor INR closely
PROGESTOGENS	ANTIDIABETIC DRUGS	Altered glycaemic control	Uncertain at present	Monitor blood glucose closely
PROGESTOGENS	ANTIEPILEPTICS – LAMOTRIGINE	↓ lamotrigine levels	↑ metabolism	Monitor level
PROGESTOGENS	ANTIPARKINSON'S DRUGS – SELEGILINE	↑ selegiline levels	Inhibition of metabolism	Watch for early features of toxicity (nausea, drowsiness) when starting progestogens in a patient stabilized on these dopaminergics. Conversely, watch for a poor response to them if progestogens are stopped
NORETHISTERONE	ANTIVIRALS – PROTEASE INHIBITORS	↑ adverse effects with amprenavir and atazanavir	Uncertain	Watch for early features of toxicity of amprenavir and atazanavir, and adjust the dose accordingly

Primary drug	Secondary drug	Effect	Mechanism	Precautions
GESTRINONE				
GESTRINONE	1. ANTIBIOTICS – rifampicin 2. ANTIEPILEPTICS – barbiturates, carbamazepine, phenytoin	↓ gestrinone levels	Induction of metabolism	Watch for poor response to gestrinone
MIFEPRISTONE				
MIFEPRISTONE	ANTIPLATELET AGENTS – ASPIRIN	↓ efficacy of mifepristone	Antiprostaglandin effect of aspirin antagonizes the action of mifepristone	Avoid co-administration
MIFEPRISTONE	NSAIDs	↓ efficacy of mifepristone	NSAIDs have an antiprostaglandin effect	Avoid co-administration
OXYTOCICS				
OXYTOCICS	ANAESTHETICS – GENERAL	Report of arrhythmias and cardiovascular collapse when halothane was given to patients taking oxytocin	Uncertain; possibly an additive effect. High-dose oxytocin may cause hypotension and arrhythmias	Monitor PR, BP and ECG closely; give oxytocin in the lowest possible dose. Otherwise consider using an alternative inhalational anaesthetic
OXYTOCICS	SYMPATHOMIMETICS	Risk of ↑ BP when oxytocin is co-administered with ephedrine, metaraminol, norepinephrine or pseudoephedrine	Additive vasoconstriction	Monitor PR, BP and ECG closely; start inotropes at a lower dose
PROSTAGLANDINS				
PROSTAGLANDINS – ALPROSTADIL	ANTIHYPERTENSIVES AND HEART FAILURE DRUGS, BETA-BLOCKERS, CALCIUM CHANNEL BLOCKERS, NITRATES	↑ hypotensive effect	Additive hypotensive effect	Monitor BP at least weekly until stable. Warn patients to report symptoms of hypotension (light-headedness, dizziness on standing, etc.)
PROSTAGLANDINS – ALPROSTADIL	PERIPHERAL VASODILATORS – MOXISYLYTE	Risk of priapism if intracavernous alprostadil is given with moxisylyte	Additive effect	Avoid co-administration

OBSTETRICS AND GYNAECOLOGY PROSTAGLANDINS

RALOXIFENE				
RALOXIFENE	ANTICOAGULANTS – ORAL	Possible ↓ anticoagulant, effect which may take several weeks to develop	Uncertain at present	Monitor INR closely for several weeks
RALOXIFENE	LIPID-LOWERING DRUGS – ANION EXCHANGE RESINS	Raloxifene levels may be ↓ by colestyramine	Colestyramine interrupts the enterohepatic circulation of raloxifene	Avoid co-administration
TIBOLONE				
TIBOLONE	ANTIBIOTICS – RIFAMPICIN	↓ tibolone levels	Induction of metabolism of tibolone	Watch for poor response to tibolone; consider ↑ dose
TIBOLONE	ANTIEPILEPTICS – BARBITURATES, CARBAMAZEPINE, PHENYTOIN	↓ tibolone levels	Induction of metabolism of tibolone	Watch for poor response to tibolone; consider ↑ dose

OBSTETRICS AND GYNAECOLOGY TIBOLONE

Part 15 UROLOGICAL DRUGS

Primary drug	Secondary drug	Effect	Mechanism	Precautions
URINARY RETENTION				
ALPHA-BLOCKERS ➢ *Cardiovascular Drugs, Antihypertensives and heart failure drugs*				
PARASYMPATHOMIMETICS ➢ *Drugs Acting on the Nervous System, Drugs used to treat neuromuscular diseases and movement disorders*				
DUTASTERIDE				
DUTASTERIDE	ANTIVIRALS – PROTEASE INHIBITORS	Possibly ↑ adverse effects of dutasteride with indinavir or ritonavir (with or without lopinavir)	Inhibition of CYP3A4-mediated metabolism of dutasteride	Monitor closely; ↓ dosing frequency if side-effects occur
DUTASTERIDE	CALCIUM CHANNEL BLOCKERS	Plasma concentrations of dutasteride may ↑ when it is co-administered with diltiazem or verapamil	Uncertain but postulated that it may be due to inhibition of CYP3A4-mediated metabolism of dutasteride	Watch for side-effects of dutasteride
URINARY INCONTINENCE				
DULOXETINE ➢ *Drugs Acting on the Nervous System, Antidepressants*				
ANTIMUSCARINICS (DARIFENACIN, FLAVOXATE, OXYBUTYNIN, PROPANTHELINE, PROPIVERINE, SOLIFENACIN, TOLTERODINE, TROSPIUM) ➢ *Drugs Acting on the Nervous System, Antiparkinson's drugs*				
TOLTERODINE				
TOLTERODINE	ANTIFUNGALS – ITRACONAZOLE	↑ tolterodine level. Supratherapeutic levels may cause prolongation of the Q–T interval	CYP3A4 is the major enzyme involved in the elimination of tolterodine in individuals with deficient CYP2D6 activity (poor metabolizers). Inhibition of CYP3A4 by triazoles in such individuals could cause a dangerous ↑ in tolterodine levels	Avoid co-administration

Primary drug	Secondary drug	Effect	Mechanism	Precautions
ERECTILE DYSFUNCTION				
ALPROSTADIL ➢ *Drugs Used in Obstetrics and Gynaecology, Prostaglandins*				
PHOSPHODIESTERASE TYPE 5 INHIBITORS				
PHOSPHODIESTERASE TYPE 5 INHIBITORS	ANTIBIOTICS			
PHOSPHODIESTERASE TYPE 5 INHIBITORS	MACROLIDES	↑ phosphodiesterase type 5 inhibitor levels with erythromycin, and possibly clarithromycin and telithromycin	Inhibition of metabolism.	↓ dose of these phosphodiesterase type 5 inhibitors (e.g. start vardenafil at 5 mg)
TADALAFIL	RIFAMPICIN	↓ tadalafil levels	Probable induction of metabolism	Watch for poor response
PHOSPHODIESTERASE TYPE 5 INHIBITORS – SILDENAFIL	ANTICANCER AND IMMUNOMODULATING DRUGS – CICLOSPORIN	↑ plasma concentrations of ciclosporin, with risk of adverse effects	Competitive inhibition of CYP3A4-mediated metabolism of ciclosporin	Be aware. Sildenafil is taken intermittently and is unlikely to be of clinical significance unless concomitant therapy is long term
PHOSPHODIESTERASE TYPE 5 INHIBITORS	ANTIFUNGALS – AZOLES	↑ sildenafil, tadalafil and vardenafil levels	Inhibition of metabolism	↓ dose of these phosphodiesterase type 5 inhibitors
PHOSPHODIESTERASE TYPE 5 INHIBITORS	ANTIHYPERTENSIVES AND HEART FAILURE DRUGS			
PHOSPHODIESTERASE TYPE 5 INHIBITORS	ALPHA-ADRENERGIC BLOCKERS	Risk of marked ↓ BP	Additive hypotensive effect	Avoid co-administration. Avoid alpha-blockers for 4 hours after intake of sildenafil (6 hours after vardenafil)
SILDENAFIL	VASODILATOR ANTIHYPERTENSIVES – BOSENTAN	↓ sildenafil levels	Probable induction of metabolism	Watch for poor response

PHOSPHODIESTERASE TYPE 5 INHIBITORS	ANTIVIRALS – PROTEASE INHIBITORS	↑ sildenafil, tadalafil and vardenafil levels	Inhibition of CYP3A4- and possibly CYP2C9-mediated metabolism of sildenafil	Use with caution; monitor BP closely. UK manufacturers recommend avoiding co-administration of vardenafil with protease inhibitors in people >75 years. US manufacturers recommend using with caution, starting with a daily dose of 2.5 mg
PHOSPHODIESTERASE TYPE 5 INHIBITORS	CALCIUM CHANNEL BLOCKERS	↑ hypotensive action, particularly with sildenafil and vardenafil	Additive effect; phosphodiesterase type 5 inhibitors cause vasodilatation	Warn patients of the small risk of postural ↓ BP
PHOSPHODIESTERASE TYPE 5 INHIBITORS (e.g. sildenafil, tadalafil, vardenafil)	GRAPEFRUIT JUICE	Possibly ↑ efficacy and ↑ adverse effects, e.g. hypotension	Small ↑ in bioavailability. ↑ variability in pharmacokinetics, i.e. interindividual variations in metabolism	Safest to advise against intake of grapefruit juice for at least 48 hours prior to intending to take any of these preparations. When necessary, the starting dose of sildenafil should not exceed 25–50 mg and that of tadalafil 10 mg. Avoid co-administration with vardenafil
PHOSPHODIESTERASE TYPE 5 INHIBITORS – SILDENAFIL	H2 RECEPTOR BLOCKERS – CIMETIDINE	↑ efficacy and adverse effects of sildenafil	Inhibition of metabolism via CYP3A4	Consider a starting dose of 25 mg of sildenafil
PHOSPHODIESTERASE TYPE 5 INHIBITORS	NICORANDIL	Risk of severe ↓ BP	Additive effect	Avoid co-administration
PHOSPHODIESTERASE TYPE 5 INHIBITORS	NITRATES	Risk of severe ↓ BP and precipitation of myocardial infarction	Additive effect	Avoid co-administration
PHOSPHODIESTERASE TYPE 5 INHIBITORS	POTASSIUM CHANNEL ACTIVATORS	↑ hypotensive effect	Both drugs have vasodilating properties	Monitor BP closely

UROLOGICAL DRUGS URINARY ALKALINIZATION

Primary drug	Secondary drug	Effect	Mechanism	Precautions
URINARY ALKALINIZATION				
SODIUM BICARBONATE	ANAESTHETICS – LOCAL – procaine solutions	Precipitation of drugs, which may not be immediately apparent	A pharmaceutical interaction	Do not mix in the same infusion or syringe
AMMONIUM CHLORIDE, SODIUM BICARBONATE	ANTIARRHYTHMICS – FLECAINIDE	Urinary alkalinization ↑ flecainide levels	Flecainide excretion ↓ in the presence of an alkaline urine; flecainide exists in predominantly non-ionic form, which is more readily reabsorbed from the renal tubules	Monitor PR and BP closely
SODIUM BICARBONATE	**ANTIBIOTICS**			
SODIUM BICARBONATE	CIPROFLOXACIN	↓ solubility of ciprofloxacin in the urine, leading to ↑ risk of crystalluria and renal damage	Any ↑ urinary pH caused by sodium bicarbonate can result in ↓ ciprofloxacin solubility in the urine	If both drugs are used concomitantly, the patient should be well hydrated and be monitored for signs of renal toxicity
SODIUM BICARBONATE	TETRACYCLINE	↓ tetracycline levels and possible therapeutic failure	It is suggested that when sodium bicarbonate alkalinizes the urine, the renal excretion of tetracycline ↑	The interaction can be minimised by administering the doses 3–4 hours apart
SODIUM BICARBONATE	ANTIDEMENTIA DRUGS – MEMANTINE	Possible ↑ memantine levels	↓ renal excretion	Watch for early features of memantine toxicity
SODIUM BICARBONATE	ANTIDEPRESSANTS – LITHIUM	↓ plasma concentrations of lithium, with risk of lack of therapeutic effect	Due to ↑ renal excretion of lithium	Monitor clinically and by measuring blood lithium levels to ensure adequate therapeutic efficacy
SODIUM BICARBONATE	SYMPATHOMIMETICS – EPHEDRINE, PSEUDOEPHEDRINE	Possibly ↑ ephedrine/ pseudoephedrine levels	Alkalinizing the urine ↓ excretion of these sympathomimetics	Watch for early features of toxicity (tremor, insomnia, tachycardia)

Part 16 DRUGS OF ABUSE

Primary drug	Secondary drug	Effect	Mechanism	Precautions
CANNABIS				
This is the most widely used illicit drug. The US FDA has approved it for chemotherapy-related nausea and vomiting, and for loss of appetite and weight loss associated with HIV/AIDS Buccal spray from the whole cannabis plant has been developed in Canada for the treatment of neuropathic pain associated with multiple sclerosis The active constituents – cannabinoids (there are others) – are highly protein-bound and are metabolized by CYP2C9 and CYP3A4 Any form of smoking induces CYP1A2. May cause inhibition/induction of CYP3A4				
CANNABIS	ANAESTHETICS – LOCAL – LIDOCAINE	Unpredictable changes in plasma concentrations. Risk of toxicity or therapeutic failure with intravenous lidocaine	Induction or inhibition of CYP3A4-mediated metabolism by cannabis. It is not yet known whether the effects are dependent on the degree of cannabis consumption	Be aware. Watch for signs of toxicity, especially when cannabis use abruptly changes
CANNABIS	ANALGESICS – OPIOIDS – alfentanil, fentanyl, methadone, codeine, dextromethorphan	Unpredictable changes in plasma concentration. Risk of toxicity or therapeutic failure, particularly of drugs with a narrow therapeutic index	Induction or inhibition of CYP3A4-mediated metabolism by cannabis. It is not yet known whether the effects are dependent on the degree of cannabis consumption	Be aware. Watch for signs of toxicity, especially when cannabis use abruptly changes
CANNABIS	**ANTIARRHYTHMICS**			
CANNABIS	AMIODARONE	Unpredictable changes in plasma concentration. Risk of toxicity or therapeutic failure, particularly of drugs with a narrow therapeutic index	Induction or inhibition of CYP3A4-mediated metabolism by cannabis. It is not yet known whether the effects are dependent on the degree of cannabis consumption	Be aware. Watch for signs of toxicity especially when cannabis use abruptly changes
CANNABIS	PROPAFENONE	Unpredictable changes in plasma concentration. Risk of toxicity or therapeutic failure, particularly of drugs with a narrow therapeutic index	Induction or inhibition of CYP3A4-mediated metabolism by cannabis. It is not yet known whether the effects are dependent on the degree of cannabis consumption	Be aware. Watch for signs of toxicity especially when cannabis use abruptly changes

CANNABIS	ANTIBIOTICS – MACROLIDES – erythromycin	Unpredictable changes in plasma concentration. Risk of toxicity or therapeutic failure, particularly of drugs with a narrow therapeutic index	Induction or inhibition of CYP3A4-mediated metabolism by cannabis. It is not yet known whether the effects are dependent on the degree of cannabis consumption	Be aware. Watch for signs of toxicity especially when cannabis use abruptly changes
CANNABIS	**ANTICANCER AND IMMUNOMODULATING DRUGS**			
CANNABIS	CYTOTOXICS – CYCLOPHOSPHAMIDE, DOXORUBICIN, IFOSFAMIDE, LOMUSTINE, VINCA ALKALOIDS	Unpredictable changes in plasma concentration. Risk of toxicity or therapeutic failure, particularly of drugs with a narrow therapeutic index	Induction or inhibition of CYP3A4-mediated metabolism by cannabis. It is not yet known whether the effects are dependent on the degree of cannabis consumption	Be aware. Watch for signs of toxicity, especially when cannabis use abruptly changes
CANNABIS	HORMONES AND HORMONE ANTAGONISTS – TAMOXIFEN	Unpredictable changes in plasma concentration. Risk of toxicity or therapeutic failure, particularly of drugs with a narrow therapeutic index	Induction or inhibition of CYP3A4-mediated metabolism by cannabis. It is not yet known whether the effects are dependent on the degree of cannabis consumption	Be aware. Watch for signs of toxicity, especially when cannabis use abruptly changes
CANNABIS	IMMUNOMODULATING DRUGS – CICLOSPORIN, CORTICOSTEROIDS	Unpredictable changes in plasma concentration. Risk of toxicity or therapeutic failure, particularly of drugs with a narrow therapeutic index	Induction or inhibition of CYP3A4-mediated metabolism by cannabis. It is not yet known whether the effects are dependent on the degree of cannabis consumption	Be aware. Watch for signs of toxicity, especially when cannabis use abruptly changes
CANNABIS	ANTICOAGULANTS – WARFARIN	Unpredictable changes in plasma concentration	1. Induction or inhibition of CYP3A4-mediated metabolism by cannabis. It is not yet known whether the effects are dependent on the degree of cannabis consumption 2. Induction of CYP1A2-mediated metabolism by any form of smoking. Foods (e.g. broccoli, cabbage, Brussels sprouts, chargrilled meat) also induce this isoenzyme	Be aware. Monitor INR closely, especially when cannabis use abruptly changes

DRUGS OF ABUSE CANNABIS

Primary drug	Secondary drug	Effect	Mechanism	Precautions
CANNABIS	**ANTIDEPRESSANTS**			
CANNABIS	LITHIUM	May ↑ plasma concentrations of lithium	Mechanism uncertain	Be aware and measure plasma lithium levels if indicated by clinical observations
CANNABIS	**SSRIs**			
CANNABIS	FLUOXETINE	Report of mania	Mechanism uncertain and may not be due to an interaction	Be aware
CANNABIS	FLUVOXAMINE	↓ levels, with risk of therapeutic failure	Induction of CYP1A2-mediated metabolism by any form of smoking. Foods (e.g. broccoli, cabbage, Brussels sprouts, chargrilled meat) also induce this isoenzyme	Watch for poor response to fluvoxamine; conversely, watch for toxic effects if a previously heavy cannabis user stops smoking
CANNABIS	SERTRALINE, VENLAFAXINE	Unpredictable changes in plasma concentration. Risk of toxicity or therapeutic failure, particularly of drugs with a narrow therapeutic index	Induction or inhibition of CYP3A4-mediated metabolism by cannabis. It is not yet known whether the effects are dependent on the degree of cannabis consumption	Be aware. Watch for signs of toxicity, especially when cannabis use abruptly changes
CANNABIS	**TCAs**			
CANNABIS	AMITRIPTYLINE, CLOMIPRAMINE, DESIPRAMINE, IMIPRAMINE, NORTRIPTYLINE	↑ risk of tachycardia. Heart rate may ↑ to 100–160 beats per minute, with some records of 300 beats per minute resistant to verapamil therapy	Additive antimuscarinic effect	Ask patients about cannabis use if they present with otherwise unexplained tachycardias while taking these drugs
CANNABIS	TCAs	Unpredictable changes in plasma concentration. Risk of toxicity or therapeutic failure, particularly of drugs with a narrow therapeutic index	Induction or inhibition of CYP3A4-mediated metabolism by cannabis. It is not yet known whether the effects are dependent on the degree of cannabis consumption	Be aware. Watch for signs of TCA toxicity, especially when cannabis use abruptly changes

CANNABIS	OTHER ANTIDEPRESSANTS			
CANNABIS	MIRTAZAPINE	↓ levels, with risk of therapeutic failure	Induction of CYP1A2-mediated metabolism by any form of smoking. Foods (e.g. broccoli, cabbage, Brussels sprouts, chargrilled meat) also induce this isoenzyme	Watch for poor response to mirtazapine; conversely, watch for toxic effects if a previously heavy cannabis user stops smoking
CANNABIS	ANTIEMETICS – ONDANSETRON	↓ levels, with risk of therapeutic failure	Induction of CYP1A2-mediated metabolism by any form of smoking. Foods (e.g. broccoli, cabbage, Brussels sprouts, chargrilled meat) also induce this isoenzyme	Watch for poor response to ondansetron; conversely, watch for toxic effects if a previously heavy cannabis user stops smoking
CANNABIS	ANTIHISTAMINES – BROMPHENIRAMINE, CHLORPHENIRAMINE	↑ risk of tachycardia. Heart rate may ↑ to 100–160 beats per minute, with some records of 300 beats per minute resistant to verapamil therapy	Additive antimuscarinic effect	Ask patients about cannabis use if they present with otherwise unexplained tachycardias while taking these drugs
CANNABIS	ANTIMUSCARINICS – ATROPINE, FLAVOXATE, HYOSCINE, OXYBUTYNIN, TOLTERODINE	↑ risk of tachycardia. Heart rate may ↑ to 100–160 beats per minute, with some records of 300 beats per minute resistant to verapamil therapy	Additive antimuscarinic effect	Ask patients about cannabis use if they present with otherwise unexplained tachycardias while taking these drugs
CANNABIS	ANTIOBESITY DRUGS – RIMONABANT	↓ most effects of cannabis that are due to its activity at central cannabinoid receptor	Rimonabant is a selective antagonist at central cannabinoid receptors, and thus the effects of either drug may be ↓	Be aware
CANNABIS	ANTIPARKINSON'S DRUGS – PROCYCLIDINE, TRIHEXYPHENIDYL (BENZHEXOL)	↑ risk of tachycardia. Heart rate may ↑ to 100–160 beats per minute, with some records of 300 beats per minute resistant to verapamil therapy	Additive antimuscarinic effect	Ask patients about cannabis use if they present with otherwise unexplained tachycardias while taking these drugs

DRUGS OF ABUSE CANNABIS

DRUGS OF ABUSE CANNABIS

Primary drug	Secondary drug	Effect	Mechanism	Precautions
CANNABIS	ANTIPSYCHOTICS – CLOZAPINE, OLANZAPINE, HALOPERIDOL	↓ plasma levels of these antipsychotics (plasma concentrations of clozapine may be halved), with the risk of therapeutic failure	Induction of CYP1A2-mediated metabolism by any form of smoking. Foods (e.g. broccoli, cabbage, Brussels sprouts, chargrilled meat) also induce this isoenzyme	Watch for poor response to these antipsychotics; conversely, watch for toxic effects of these antipsychotics if a previously heavy cannabis user stops smoking
CANNABIS	ANTIVIRALS – PROTEASE INHIBITORS – indinavir, nelfinavir, nevirapine, ritonavir, saquinavir	Cannabis may cause ↓ plasma concentrations of protease inhibitors, particularly indinavir and nelfinavir	Cannabis may cause inhibition or induction of CYP3A4 isoenzymes, which metabolize these protease inhibitors	Be aware. Regular monitoring of viral indicators is necessary
CANNABIS	ANXIOLYTICS AND HYPNOTICS – BZDs – alprazolam, diazepam, midazolam, triazolam	Unpredictable changes in plasma concentration. Risk of toxicity or therapeutic failure, particularly of drugs with a narrow therapeutic index	Induction or inhibition of CYP3A4-mediated metabolism by cannabis. It is not yet known whether the effects are dependent on the degree of cannabis consumption	Be aware. Watch for signs of toxicity, especially when cannabis use abruptly changes
CANNABIS	BETA-BLOCKERS – PROPRANOLOL	↓ levels, with risk of therapeutic failure	Induction of CYP1A2-mediated metabolism by any form of smoking. Foods (e.g. broccoli, cabbage, Brussels sprouts, chargrilled meat) also induce this isoenzyme	Watch for poor response to propanolol; conversely, watch for toxic effects if a previously heavy cannabis user stops smoking
CANNABIS	BRONCHODILATORS – THEOPHYLLINE	↓ theophylline levels, with risk of therapeutic failure (theophylline has a narrow therapeutic range)	Induction of CYP1A2-mediated metabolism by any form of smoking. Foods (e.g. broccoli, cabbage, Brussels sprouts, chargrilled meat) also induce this isoenzyme. Although cannabis is considered to cause bronchodilatation, regular smoking leads to poorer respiratory function	Watch for poor response to theophylline; consider monitoring theophylline levels if a previously heavy cannabis user stops smoking, because of the risk of toxic effects

CANNABIS	CALCIUM CHANNEL BLOCKERS			
CANNABIS	DILTIAZEM, FELODIPINE, NIFEDIPINE, NIMODIPINE, NISOLDIPINE	Unpredictable changes in plasma concentration. Risk of toxicity or therapeutic failure, particularly of drugs with a narrow therapeutic index	Induction or inhibition of CYP3A4-mediated metabolism by cannabis. It is not yet known whether the effects are dependent on the degree of cannabis consumption	Be aware. Watch for signs of toxicity, especially when cannabis use abruptly changes
CANNABIS	VERAPAMIL	Unpredictable changes in plasma concentration. Risk of toxicity or therapeutic failure, particularly of drugs with a narrow therapeutic index	1. Induction of CYP1A2-mediated metabolism by any form of smoking. Foods (e.g. broccoli, cabbage, Brussels sprouts, chargrilled meat) also induce this isoenzyme 2. Induction or inhibition of CYP3A4-mediated metabolism by cannabis. It is not yet known whether the effects are dependent on the degree of cannabis consumption	Watch for poor response to verapamil; conversely, watch for toxic effects if a previously heavy cannabis user stops smoking
CANNABIS	**DRUG DEPENDENCE THERAPIES**			
CANNABIS	BUPROPION	Unpredictable changes in plasma concentration. Risk of toxicity or therapeutic failure, particularly of drugs with a narrow therapeutic index	Induction or inhibition of CYP3A4-mediated metabolism by cannabis. It is not yet known whether the effects are dependent on the degree of cannabis consumption	Be aware. Watch for signs of toxicity, especially when cannabis use abruptly changes
CANNABIS	DISULFIRAM	Risk of hypomania	Mechanism uncertain and may be due to the presence of adulterants	Be aware

DRUGS OF ABUSE CANNABIS

Primary drug	Secondary drug	Effect	Mechanism	Precautions
CANNABIS	DRUGS OF ABUSE – COCAINE	Quickens the onset of effects of cocaine and ↑ bioavailability of cocaine, leading to enhanced subjective effects of cocaine (e.g. euphoria), and ↑ heart rate and other cardiac effects such as ischaemia	Attributed to cannabis-induced vasodilatation of the nasal mucosa, which leads to ↑ absorption of cocaine	Be aware. May be the cause of ischaemic cardiac pain in young adults
CANNABIS	ECHINACEA AND OTHER IMMUNOSTIMULANTS	May ↓ immunostimulant effects	The cannabinoid receptor is considered to mediate immunosuppressant effects and is currently being investigated in the development of novel immunosuppressants	Be aware
CANNABIS	OESTROGENS – ETHINYLESTRADIOL	Unpredictable changes in plasma concentration. Risk of toxicity or therapeutic failure, particularly of drugs with a narrow therapeutic index	Induction or inhibition of CYP3A4-mediated metabolism by cannabis. It is not yet known whether the effects are dependent on the degree of cannabis consumption	Be aware. Watch for signs of toxicity, especially when cannabis use abruptly changes
CANNABIS	PHOSPHODIESTERASE TYPE 5 INHIBITORS – SILDENAFIL	Report of myocardial infarction	Both drugs have been independently linked to myocardial infarction. However, the exact mechanism is uncertain	Be aware
CANNABIS	PROGESTOGENS	Unpredictable changes in plasma concentration. Risk of toxicity or therapeutic failure, particularly of drugs with a narrow therapeutic index	Induction or inhibition of CYP3A4-mediated metabolism by cannabis. It is not yet known whether the effects are dependent on the degree of cannabis consumption	Be aware. Watch for signs of toxicity, especially when cannabis use abruptly changes

CANNABIS	PROTON PUMP INHIBITORS – OMEPRAZOLE, LANSOPRAZOLE	Unpredictable changes in plasma concentration. Risk of toxicity or therapeutic failure, particularly of drugs with a narrow therapeutic index	Induction or inhibition of CYP3A4-mediated metabolism by cannabis. It is not yet known whether the effects are dependent on the degree of cannabis consumption	Be aware. Watch for signs of toxicity, especially when cannabis use abruptly changes
AMPHETAMINES				
Amphetamines are available in various forms. It is metabolized primarily by CYP2D6 There is a salt form – methylamphetamine ('speed') – and a free base form ('base'), which looks like a damp or oily paste Crystalloid form ('ice' or 'crystal meth') is taken orally or intranasally ('snorting'), or injected intravenously Primary mode of action is ↑ release of dopamine. Also inhibits dopamine metabolism and its reuptake, and ↑ release of norepinephrine and serotonin Toxic effects include restlessness, tremor, anxiety, irritability, insomnia, psychosis, aggression, sweating, palpitations, chest pain, ↑ blood pressure, shortness of breath and headache				
AMPHETAMINES	ALPHA-BLOCKERS	Antagonism of hypotensive effect	Due to ↑ release of norepinephrine	Be aware
AMPHETAMINES	ANALGESICS – OPIOIDS – alfentanil, fentanyl, propoxyphene	↑ plasma concentrations of amphetamine, with risk of toxic effects	Due to inhibition of CYP2D6-mediated metabolism of amphetamine	Avoid concurrent use
AMPHETAMINES	ANTIARRHYTHMICS – AMIODARONE	↑ plasma concentrations of amphetamine, with risk of toxic effects	Due to inhibition of CYP2D6-mediated metabolism of amphetamine	Avoid concurrent use
AMPHETAMINES	**ANTIDEPRESSANTS**			
AMPHETAMINES	MAOIs	Risk of severe and life-threatening hypertension. The risk is greatest with non-selective MAOIs	MAO is an enzyme that metabolizes dopamine, nor-epinephrine and other amines	Avoid concurrent use
AMPHETAMINES	**SSRIs**			
AMPHETAMINES	SSRIs	↑ plasma concentrations of amphetamine, with risk of toxic effects	Due to inhibition of CYP2D6-mediated metabolism of amphetamine	Avoid concurrent use

DRUGS OF ABUSE AMPHETAMINES

Primary drug	Secondary drug	Effect	Mechanism	Precautions
AMPHETAMINES	TCAs	Risk of severe and life-threatening hypertension and arrhythmias. May give false-positive urine tests for amphetamines	Additive effects on cardiovascular system due to enhanced noradrenergic activity	Avoid concurrent use
AMPHETAMINES	VENLAFAXINE	Risk of severe and life-threatening hypertension and arrhythmias	Additive effects on cardiovascular system due to enhanced noradrenergic activity	Avoid concurrent use
AMPHETAMINES	ANTIMIGRAINE DRUGS – ERGOT ALKALOIDS	↑ risk of ergotism, usually beginning as numbness and tingling of the extremities	Additive peripheral vasoconstriction	Avoid concurrent use
AMPHETAMINES	ANTIVIRALS – RITONAVIR	↑ plasma concentrations of amphetamine, with risk of toxic effects	Due to inhibition of CYP2D6-mediated metabolism of amphetamine	Avoid concurrent use
AMPHETAMINES	BRONCHODILATORS – BETA-2 AGONISTS	↑ risk of tachycardia, arrhythmias and hypertension	Additive effect on target organ receptors (myocardium, blood vessels)	Avoid concurrent use
AMPHETAMINES	H2 RECEPTOR BLOCKERS – CIMETIDINE	↑ plasma concentrations of amphetamine, with risk of toxic effects	Due to inhibition of CYP2D6-mediated metabolism of amphetamine	Avoid concurrent use
AMPHETAMINES	SYMPATHOMIMETICS	Risk of severe and life-threatening hypertension and arrhythmias	Additive effects on cardiovascular system due to enhanced noradrenergic activity	Avoid concurrent use

METHYLENEDIOXYMETHAMPHETAMINE (MDMA, ECSTASY)

This is 'ecstasy', which is structurally related to amphetamine and the hallucinogen mescaline. It is metabolized by a range of CYP isoenzymes, mainly CYP2D6

It produces a massive ↑ in serotonin release via its effects on the serotonin transporter. MDMA damages brain serotonergic neurones, and functional sequelae (verbal and visual memory problems) may persist even after long periods of abstinence

Adverse effects are related to excessive CNS and cardiovascular system stimulation (similar to amphetamines). Others are due to excess serotonin – jaw-clenching, tooth-grinding

Importantly, most MDMA tablets contain other potentially toxic substances, e.g. ephedrine, dextromethorphan

MDMA	ANALGESICS – OPIOIDS			
MDMA	CODEINE, FENTANYL, METHADONE, MEPERIDINE, PENTAZOCINE, D-PROPOXYPHENONE, TRAMADOL	↑ risk of serotonin syndrome	Tramadol produces analgesia by an opioid effect and by the enhancement of serotonergic and adrenergic pathways. The phenylpiperidine series of opioids (meperidine, tramadol, methadone, fentanyl, D-propoxyphene) are very weak serotonin reuptake inhibitors. Thus, additive serotonergic effects on the brain are likely with SSRIs that ↓ reuptake of serotonin. Codeine and pentazocine causes the release of stored serotonin, and codeine is also a substrate of CYP2D6	Avoid concomitant use ➢ ***For signs and symptoms of serotonin toxicity, see Clinical Features of Some Adverse Drug Interactions, Serotonin toxicity and serotonin syndrome***
MDMA	ALFENTANIL, FENTANYL, PROPOXYPHENE	↑ plasma concentrations of MDMA, with risk of toxic effects	Due to inhibition of CYP2D6-mediated metabolism of MDMA	Avoid concurrent use
MDMA	ANTIARRHYTHMICS – AMIODARONE	↑ plasma concentrations of MDMA, with risk of toxic effects	Due to inhibition of CYP2D6-mediated metabolism of MDMA	Avoid concurrent use

DRUGS OF ABUSE METHYLENEDIOXYMETHAMPHETAMINE (MDMA, ECSTASY)

DRUGS OF ABUSE METHYLENEDIOXYMETHAMPHETAMINE (MDMA, ECSTASY)

Primary drug	Secondary drug	Effect	Mechanism	Precautions
MDMA	**ANTIDEPRESSANTS**			
MDMA	ANTIDEPRESSANTS	Risk of hyponatraemia, particularly where dehydration may occur, such as long periods of dancing. The CSM has advised that hyponatraemia should be considered in all patients who develop drowsiness, confusion or convulsions while taking an antidepressant	Hyponatraemia (usually in elderly people and possibly due to inappropriate secretion of ADH) has been associated with all types of antidepressant, more frequently with SSRIs. Additive effect	Be aware and measure serum electrolytes when there is clinical suspicion
MDMA	DULOXETINE	↑ risk of serotonin syndrome	Duloxetine inhibits the reuptake of both serotonin and norepinephrine, and is metabolized by CYP1A2 and CYP2D6	Avoid concomitant use ➢ ***For signs and symptoms of serotonin toxicity, see Clinical Features of Some Adverse Drug Interactions, Serotonin toxicity and serotonin syndrome***
MDMA	MAOIs	Risk of severe and life-threatening hypertension. Risk is greatest with non-selective MAOIs. At least four deaths have been reported following the ingestion of MDMA and moclobemide. Another death was reported after phenelzine co-ingestion	MAO is an enzyme that metabolizes dopamine, norepinephrine and other amines	Avoid concurrent use
MDMA	SSRIs	↑ risk of serotonin syndrome	Due to ↑ brain concentrations of serotonin due to ↑ release by MDMA and inhibition of reuptake by SSRIs. Initial use of MDMA ↑ release of serotonin, and subsequent administration of an SSRI prevents its removal	Avoid concurrent use

MDMA	TRYPTOPHAN	Tryptophan administration produces poor therapeutic response and adverse effects as passage across the blood–brain barrier is impaired in users and ex-users	Tryptophan ↑ amount of precursors of serotonin	Avoid concomitant use ➢ ***For signs and symptoms of serotonin toxicity, see Clinical Features of Some Adverse Drug Interactions, Serotonin toxicity and serotonin syndrome***
MDMA	ANTIMIGRAINE DRUGS – 5-HT1 AGONISTS	↑ risk of serotonin syndrome	Triptans cause direct stimulation of 5-HT receptors, while MDMA causes ↑ release of serotonin	Avoid concomitant use ➢ ***For signs and symptoms of serotonin toxicity, see Clinical Features of Some Adverse Drug Interactions, Serotonin toxicity and serotonin syndrome***
MDMA	ANTIVIRALS – RITONAVIR	↑ plasma concentrations of MDMA, with risk of toxic effects	Due to inhibition of CYP2D6-mediated metabolism of MDMA	Avoid concurrent use
MDMA	DRUG DEPENDENCE THERAPIES – BUSPIRONE	Markedly ↑ risk of serotonin syndrome	Buspirone is a direct stimulant of 5-HT receptors (5-HT1A)	Avoid concomitant use ➢ ***For signs and symptoms of serotonin toxicity, see Clinical Features of Some Adverse Drug Interactions, Serotonin toxicity and serotonin syndrome***
MDMA	H2 RECEPTOR BLOCKERS – CIMETIDINE	↑ plasma concentrations of MDMA, with risk of toxic effects	Due to inhibition of CYP2D6-mediated metabolism of MDMA	Avoid concurrent use

COCAINE

Blocks sodium channels. Produces euphoria, mood elevation, energy, tremors, chest pain, agitation, paranoia and convulsions

It ↑ heart rate, BP and cardiac output, as well as enhancing platelet aggregation

COCAINE	**ANTIDEPRESSANTS**			
COCAINE	MAOIs	Hypertensive crisis	Due to ↓ metabolism of vasoactive amines	Avoid concurrent use

DRUGS OF ABUSE COCAINE

DRUGS OF ABUSE AMYL NITRITE

Primary drug	Secondary drug	Effect	Mechanism	Precautions
COCAINE	SSRIs – FLUOXETINE	↓ euphoria of cocaine	Mechanism uncertain	Be aware
COCAINE	BETA-BLOCKERS	Risk of hypertensive crisis	Cocaine produces both alpha- and beta-adrenergic agonist effects; selective beta-blockade leads to unopposed alpha agonism (vasoconstriction)	Avoid concurrent use
HEROIN ➢ *Analgesics, Opioids*				
HALLUCINOGENS				
LSD – 'acid'; psilocybin – magic mushrooms; mescaline – peyote cactus Most hallucinogens act on the serotonergic system				
HALLUCINOGENS	ANTIDEPRESSANTS – LITHIUM, MAOIs, SSRIs, TCAs	Chronic use is considered to ↑ subjective effects of LSD	Uncertain	Be aware
GAMMA HYDROXYBUTYRIC ACID ➢ *Drugs Acting on the Nervous System, Anxiolytics and Hypnotics*				
AMYL NITRITE				
AMYL NITRITE	SILDENAFIL	Risk of potentially fatal hypotension	Additive effects on blood vessels	Avoid concurrent use

Part 17 MISCELLANEOUS

This section considers other constituents that may cause adverse interactions when taken alongside drugs.

Alcohol

See pp. 713–719.

Food

It is known that foods have the potential to affect in particular the pharmacokinetics of some drugs (the way the body handles drugs). Similarly, drugs may affect the way the body handles food and therefore influence an individual's nutrition.

Some mechanisms by which foods affect the pharmacokinetics of drugs are:

- *Altering the motility of the gastrointestinal tract*. Several drugs are absorbed mainly from the small intestine, which provides the initial peak plasma concentration of the drug. Any increase in gastrointestinal motility provides less time for absorption, thus decreasing the peak plasma concentration, while a reduction in gastrointestinal motility tends to raise the peak plasma concentration.
- *Delaying gastric emptying*.
  - When food enters the stomach, some hormones, such as cholecystokinin, which tends to delay gastric emptying, are released. Solid foods, particularly those rich in fat and dietary fibre, delay gastric emptying, fatty foods being one of the most potent inducers of these hormones. This delays the absorption of the drug and thus the onset of the therapeutic effect.
  - Carbohydrates in the ileum tend to decrease gastric emptying. Therefore carbohydrates taken in an earlier meal could affect the absorption of a drug taken subsequently.
  - If the size of the particles of a drug is large (e.g. > 1.1 mm in diameter), these do not enter the main site of absorption – the small intestine – until the stomach contents have been completely emptied. This may occur with some enteric-coated tablets. Therefore, if there is insufficient time for gastric emptying (i.e. frequent meals), drug absorption may be delayed until night, when the stomach is emptied completely. Hence, some drugs should be taken on an empty stomach.

- In contrast, taking some drugs with water may result in the drug leaving the stomach rapidly, thus causing a reduction in gastrointestinal transit time, which may result in a decrease in the total amount of drug absorbed.
- Furthermore, some drugs (e.g. **NSAIDs, aspirin**) may, if taken on an empty stomach, cause irritation of the stomach mucosa, and food usually helps to lessen this adverse effect. However, drug intake with food may slow the rate of absorption of such drugs, for example **paracetamol** (acetaminophen), **aspirin, piroxicam, quinidine** (if it causes gastric irritation), **amoxicillin** and **ampicillin** (if it causes gastric discomfort). Food is considered to slow the absorption of drugs such as **atenolol, astemizole, avitriptan, cephalosporins, cimetidine, digoxin, demeclocycline, furosemide, glipizide, metronidazole, sulphonamides** and **valproic acid**.

Some drug–food interactions are listed below. It is necessary to be aware that drug–food interactions are generally unpredictable as individual factors such as age, sex (e.g. stage of the menstrual cycle in women) and presence of gastrointestinal disease can influence the effect of foods on drug absorption. At best, the following should be taken into consideration when providing advice to patients while prescribing and dispensing:

- Among drugs considered to be absorbed more quickly with food are **carbamazepine, phenytoin, diazepam, dicoumarol, erythromycin** (contentious), **griseofulvin, hydralazine, hydrochlorothiazide, lithium citrate, labetalol, propranolol, metoprolol, nitrofurantoin, propoxyphene** and **spironolactone**.
- Drugs that are considered to be absorbed to a lesser degree with food include antibiotics (**ampicillin, penicillins G and VK, isoniazid, rifampicin, lincomycin, nafcillin, tetracyclines**), **methyldopa** and **levodopa** (to be avoided with high-protein diets as amino acids compete for absorption with these drugs), and **penicillamine**.
- Milk and dairy foods decrease the absorption of some tetracyclines (**doxycycline** and **minocycline** are not affected), some quinolone antibiotics (absorption of **ciprofloxacin** and **norfloxacin** is decreased but **ofloxacin** is not affected), **penicillamine** and **alendronate**. Large volumes of milk can reduce the ulcer-healing properties of **bismuth tripotassium dicitratobismuthate** (bismuth chelate).
- Potassium-rich foods (e.g. bananas) can cause hyperkalaemia if the medication(s) used also tend to cause hyperkalaemia, for example potassium-sparing diuretics (**triamterene, spironolactone**), ACE inhibitors (**captopril, enalapril**, etc.), **angiotensin receptor blockers** and **indometacin**.
- High fat-containing foods reduce the absorption of protease inhibitors.
- High-protein diets decrease the bioavailability of **theophylline** (high-carbohydrate diets increasing the bioavailability of **theophylline**) and reduce the effects of **levodopa** and **methyldopa** (from competition of amino acids for absorption).

- Salt restriction may result in **lithium** toxicity.
- Several interactions of **grapefruit juice** are listed separately (see below).
- The effects of tyramine-containing foods on people taking, in particular, MAOI antidepressants are discussed in the section on MAOI interactions. Avocado contains tyramine and, although this is contentious, should be avoided by patients on **warfarin** treatment.

For interactions of MAOIs, see Drugs Acting on the Nervous System, Antidepressants

- Histamine-containing foods such as cheese and some fish may induce flushing reactions with headache, breathing difficulty, nausea and tachycardia in patients taking **isoniazid**.
- Large amounts (usually in excess of 500 g daily) of vegetables such as spinach, sprouts, broccoli and cabbage (these vegetables contain indoles, which stimulate drug-metabolizing enzymes) along with large amounts of soya bean products and large quantities of ice cream (in excess of 1 L at once) are known to decrease or even abolish the anticoagulant effect of **warfarin**. Several green vegetables contain vitamin K, which impairs the effect of **warfarin** as anticoagulants compete with vitamin K to reduce the production of blood-clotting factors.
- Caffeine (particularly more than five cups a day) increases the risk of insomnia (therefore avoid it in patients on **tranquillizers**, **hypnotics** and **antidepressants**) and may cause arrhythmias in susceptible patients, such as those with cardiac disease who are taking **antiarrhythmics**.
- Phytates found in cereals, legumes, nuts and oil seeds form complexes with minerals, the mineral–phytate complexes in decreasing order of stability being zinc > copper > nickel > cobalt > manganese > calcium. Thus, zinc is affected most. An increase in pH results in phytic acid becoming more ionized and initiates binding to cations.

Grapefruit Juice

The major effect of grapefruit juice appears to be to selectively decrease intestinal CYP3A4 activity, thus reducing first-pass metabolism. There is little or no effect on drug disposition after intravenous administration, and grapefruit juice does not affect liver CYP3A4 activity. Grapefruit juice also inhibits the efflux transporter P-gp, thus increasing the bioavailability of several drugs. Components that are most probable causes of interactions are the furanocoumarin derivatives and the flavonoid naringenin.

The onset of interaction can occur within 30 minutes of drinking a single glass of juice, and inhibition can last up to 3 days following the last administration of grapefruit juice. The interaction potential of even high amounts of grapefruit juice with CYP3A4 substrates is considered to dissipate within 3–7 days after last intake of juice.

See table of interactions on pp. 720–732.

Nutritional supplements

Drugs and nutrients share similar characteristics, including sites of absorption in the intestine, the ability to cause changes in the body's physiological processes and the ability to cause toxic effects in high doses.

Drugs in general influence nutrient intake by:

- causing nausea, vomiting, diarrhoea or other gastrointestinal side-effects that will impair the intake of nutrients;
- causing 'taste disturbances', for example **ACE inhibitors**, **allopurinol**, **metronidazole** and **penicillamine**;
- affecting appetite, for example **digoxin** and **fluoxetine**, which decrease appetite, and **TCAs** and **valproate**, which increase appetite.

Some examples can be given:

- *Antiepileptics*. Large doses of vitamin B6 can reduce serum levels of **phenytoin** and **phenobarbital**, and thus cause loss of control of epilepsy. Vitamin B6 in excess of 10 mg a day should be avoided. The antiepileptics **phenytoin**, **phenobarbital** and **primidone** can cause folate deficiency (resulting in a megaloblastic anaemia). However, folic acid supplements can reduce plasma concentrations of these antiepileptics, leading to loss of control of seizures. Therefore, folic acid supplements should be administered only to those patients who are 'folate-deficient' and can be monitored. Antiepileptics can also cause disturbances in vitamin D metabolism, leading to osteomalacia, hence the need to monitor patients on antiepileptics and provide vitamin D supplements when indicated. Drugs known to prevent or block folic acid production and/or absorption include **methotrexate**, **NSAIDs**, **H2 blockers**, **colestyramine** and **colestipol**.
- *Antibiotics*. Long-term administration of antibiotics could lead to vitamin B6 deficiency. If symptoms of peripheral neuropathy develop (numbness and tingling of the extremities), administer vitamin B6. **Sulfasalazine** can decrease the absorption of folic acid, and **trimethoprim** can cause folate deficiency, hence the need to administer folic acid if there is evidence of deficiency. **Rifampicin** can cause disturbances in vitamin D metabolism and lead to osteomalacia. The absorption of **tetracyclines** can be reduced by calcium, magnesium, iron and zinc, while this antibiotic could also decrease the absorption of these minerals. This effect is probably least with **minocycline** and is not confirmed with **doxycycline**. Doses of minerals and antibiotic should be separated by at least 2 hours. The absorption of quinolones is reduced by cationic and anionic supplements.

For more information on absorption of quinolones, see Drugs to Treat Infections, Antibiotics – quinolones; Drugs Acting on the Gastrointestinal Tract, Antacids.

- *Diuretics*. Hypercalcaemia may develop in patients administered **thiazide diuretics** with either calcium or vitamin D supplements, leading to a need to monitor plasma or serum calcium levels. The concurrent use of **potassium-sparing diuretics**, and other potassium supplements or potassium-containing salt substitutes, could lead to serious hyperkalaemia. Hyperkalaemia is known to interfere with the absorption of vitamin B12. There is a need to warn patients and monitor serum potassium levels. The risk of hypokalaemia is minimal with low doses of **thiazides**, for example 5 mg of bendroflumethiazide. Hypokalaemia is a concern in patients receiving treatment with drugs such as **digoxin, amiodarone, disopyramide** or **flecainide** (drugs used to treat cardiac disorders).
- *Laxatives*. Prolonged use of laxatives can cause hypokalaemia. Liquid paraffin reduces the absorption of vitamins A, D, E and K. The CSM has advised that prolonged use of liquid paraffin should be avoided. Deficiency of these vitamins is associated with the prolonged use of anion exchange resins such as **colestyramine** and **colestipol**.
- *Anticoagulants*. Anticoagulant effects could be increased by fish oils, so fish oil supplements should be avoided by people on, for example, **warfarin**. A large intake of vitamin K could reduce the anticoagulant effects of warfarin (see above). Large doses of vitamin E (e.g. > 100 IU daily) are known to increase the anticoagulant effects of warfarin and should be avoided by patients taking this drug.
- *Antiepileptic drugs*. These have caused bleeding in the newborn (usually during the first 2 days after birth). This has been attributed to their crossing the placenta and impairing vitamin K synthesis in the fetal liver. The advice has been to administer vitamin K in 10 mg doses daily during the last month of pregnancy if the mother is taking antiepileptic drugs.
- The long-term intake of **hydralazine** could lead to vitamin B6 deficiency, while the therapeutic effects of **verapamil** could be antagonized by calcium supplements.
- *Levodopa*. The absorption of **levodopa** is decreased by iron preparations, while the effects of levodopa may be reduced or abolished by vitamin B6 supplements providing more than 5 mg daily. If the intake of vitamin B6 supplements cannot be discontinued, substitute **co-careldopa** or **co-beneldopa** for levodopa.
- *Oral contraceptives*. Combined oral contraceptives reduce serum folic acid levels, while the administration of large doses of vitamin C (e.g. 1 g daily) can cause an increase in serum oestrogen levels. There is thus a need to consider folic acid supplements in people discontinuing the oral contraceptive pill and planning a pregnancy. For those on antiepileptic drugs during pregnancy (see above), there is a risk of producing a baby with a neural tube defect, so these mothers-to-be require folic acid supplements of 5 mg daily.

- *Evening primrose oil*. Evening primrose oil supplements can increase the risk of epileptogenic side-effects of **phenothiazines**.
- The absorption of **penicillamine** is decreased by mineral supplements, and vice versa.
- *Antacids*. See the relevant sections for the interactions of **antacids**. Antacids such as aluminium-, magnesium- and calcium-containing antacids and sodium bicarbonate reduce the absorption of iron and also of drugs that require an acidic pH in the stomach for their optimal uptake.

Minerals

Minerals (inorganic elements that act as co-factors for enzymes influencing all aspects of energy metabolism – not sources of energy) are affected by several drugs.

Mineral–mineral interactions

- The best known of these is the interference of copper absorption caused by zinc due to the induction of intestinal metallothionem; this binds to copper and prevents its entry into the bloodstream. The intestinal cells eventually slough, carrying the copper with them. The prolonged intake of zinc necessitates copper supplements except in patients with Wilson's disease.
- Copper absorption is decreased by iron, tin and molybdenum.
- Zinc also interferes with the absorption calcium and selenium. Zinc absorption is usually decreased by aluminium-, phosphate- and tin-containing compounds.
- Iron and calcium supplements should not be taken at the same time, as these minerals compete for absorption.
- Increased cadmium absorption takes place when blood/body levels of zinc are low.
- Magnesium-, aluminium- and calcium-containing medications can impair the absorption of phosphorus/phosphates.
- Calcium acetate and calcium carbonate are used as phosphate-binding agents in hyperphosphataemia.
- Aluminium may decrease the absorption of fluoride.

See pp. 710 and 734–737.

Herbal medicines

Reports of adverse interactions between St John's wort and drugs such as digoxin, warfarin, protease inhibitors and oral contraceptives sparked off an interest in herb–drug interactions. Reports of herb–drug interactions are rare compared with drug–drug interactions. However, herbal medicines are most often mixtures of more than one pharmacologically active ingredient, and thus the potential for interactions is far greater than with allopathic medicines, most of which contain only one active constituent.

Most reports of interactions remain speculative, unsubstantiated and considered minor or theoretical. However, most herbal preparations are self-prescribed and associated with a certain degree of anonymity as many of the common uses are related to slimming, fertility, impotence and mental stress. They are mostly used in the long term, thus increasing the potential for the induction or inhibition of metabolizing enzymes and drug transporters. As with adverse drug–drug interactions, the main dangers are associated with allopathic drugs used in the treatment of cardiovascular disease (including anticoagulants) and diseases of the CNS, for contraception and related to the immune system.

It is necessary to be aware that this surge in use of herbal medicines has resulted in new information about adverse interactions appearing even weekly. Therefore, there is a need to be cautious of herbal medicines with varying constituents and different concentrations of constituents, which may be from the same supplier. There is also a need for prescribers and dispensers to seek information of the use of such medications prior to their use by a consumer, who most likely has made an independent decision with limited information of the toxic effects and potential for adverse interactions with other medications.

It is important to be aware that many 'herbal' preparations may contain adulterants such as corticosteroids (e.g. eczema preparations), analgesics (even those banned in the UK, e.g. phenylbutazone, fenfluramine) and warfarin. For example, PC-SPES, a mixture of at least eight herbs taken for prostate cancer, was shown to contain baikal skullcap and warfarin.

Therapeutic drug monitoring is an essential component of safe prescribing. It is necessary to be aware that many herbal medicines can affect laboratory tests (e.g. chan su, dan shen, St John's wort, kava kava, chaparral, germander and allopathic medicines, which are adulterants of herbal preparations).

In 2006, a survey in Italy revealed that herbal products were taken in combination with drugs by nearly 45% of the population. The information provided was derived from a multitude of sources that described interactions in the form of case reports, animal studies and, rarely, human volunteer studies.

Interactions with St John's wort are included in the section on antidepressants.

See table of herbal/allopathic drug interactions on pp. 711 and 742–759.

Information sources

Bauer LA, Schumock G, Horn J, Opheim K. Verapamil inhibits ethanol elimination and prolongs the perception of intoxication. *Clin Pharmacol Ther* 1992; **52**: 6–10.

Bjornsson TD, Callaghan JT, Einolf HJ et al. The conduct of in vitro and in vivo drug-drug interaction studies: a PhRMA perspective. *J Clin Pharmacol* 2003; **43**: 443–69.

Dasgupta A, Bernard DW. Herbal remedies: effects on clinical laboratory tests. *Arch Pathol Lab Med* 2006; **130**: 521–8.

DiPadova C, Roine R, Frezza M, Gentry RT, Baraona E, Lieber CS. Effects of ranitidine on blood alcohol levels after ethanol ingestion. Comparison with other H2-receptor antagonists. *JAMA* 1992; **267**: 83–6. Erratum in: *JAMA* 1992; **268**: 2652.

Fraser AG, Hudson M, Sawyer AM et al. Ranitidine has no effect on postbreakfast ethanol absorption. *Am J Gastroenterol* 1993; **88**: 217–21.

Holistic online. Herbal Medicine. http:/www.holisticonline.com/Herbal-Med/hol

http:/www.Pharminfo.net/reviews/drug-interactions-grape fruit juice.

Izzo AA. *Herb–drug interactions: an overview of the clinical evidence. Fundam Clin Pharmacol* 2005; **19**: 1–16.

Karalliedde L, Gawarammana I. *Traditional Herbal Remedies: Guide to Safer Use*. London: Hammersmith Press, 2007.

McNeece J. Interactions between grape fruit juice and some drugs available in Australia. *Aust Prescriber* 2002; **25**: 37.

Mason P. Drug–food interactions – foods and medicines. *Pharm J* 2002; **269**: 571–3.

Mason P. Food–drug interactions – nutritional supplements and drugs. *Pharm J* 2002; **269**: 609–11.

Midell E, Hopkins V. *Health and Fitness*. Florida: University of Florida Centre for Food–Drug Interaction Research and Education, 2003.

Miller LG. Herbal medicinals. *Arch Intern Med* 1998; **158**: 2200–11.

Palmer RH, Frank WO, Nambi P, Wetherington JD, Fox MJ. Effects of various concomitant medications on gastric alcohol dehydrogenase and the first-pass metabolism of ethanol. *Am J Gastroenterol* 1991; **86**: 1749–55.

People's Pharmacy, Guide to Drug & Alcohol Interactions. Available at: www.peoplespharmacy.com/archives/indepth_guides/guide_to_drug_and_alcohol_interactions.php (accessed May 2009).

Roine R, Gentry RT, Hernández-Munõz R, Baraona E, Lieber CS. Aspirin increases blood alcohol concentrations in humans after ingestion of ethanol. *JAMA* 1990; **264**: 2406–8.

Snyman T, Stewart MJ, Grove A, Steenkamp V. Adulterations of South African traditional herbal remedies. *Ther Drug Monit* 2005; **27**: 86–9.

University of Florida Centre for Food–Drug Interaction Research.

Williamson EM. Drug interactions between herbal and prescription remedies. *Drug Saf* 2003; **26**: 1075–92.

Zaffani S, Cuzzolin L, Benoni G. Herbal products: behaviours and beliefs among Italian women. *Pharmacoepidemiol Drug Saf* 2006; **15**: 354–9.

MISCELLANEOUS ALCOHOL

Primary drug	Secondary drug	Effect	Mechanism	Precautions
ALCOHOL				
ALCOHOL	ANALGESICS			
ALCOHOL	ASPIRIN	Alleged ↑ effects of alcohol after relatively innocuous amounts of wine, beer, etc., which made it popular among users; the effects are, however, unproven. One study found that aspirin taken an hour before drinking a modest amount of alcohol (one and a half drinks) raised levels in the bloodstream by 26%. ↑ risk of gastric irritation	A study suggested the presence of alcohol dehydrogenase in the stomach of some men, which was inactivated by aspirin. Additive irritant effects on gastric mucosa	Be aware. The FDA has considered the probability of inactivation of stomach alcohol dehydrogenase as 'not dangerous'
ALCOHOL	OPIOIDS	↑ sedation. Report of hypotension with codeine	Additive effect	Warn patients
ALCOHOL	ANTIBIOTICS			
ALCOHOL	CEPHALOSPORINS	Disulfiram-like reaction, with flushing, wheezing, breathing difficulties, nausea and vomiting with some cephalosporins. This potentially dangerous interaction can come on right away, or it may be delayed by as much as a few days	It is considered that a reactive metabolite probably inactivates alcohol dehyrogenase	Do not consume alcohol for 3 days following stopping the antibiotic
ALCOHOL	CYCLOSERINE	Risk of fits	Additive effect; cycloserine can cause fits	Warn patients to drink alcohol only minimally while taking cycloserine

MISCELLANEOUS ALCOHOL

Primary drug	Secondary drug	Effect	Mechanism	Precautions
ALCOHOL	METRONIDAZOLE	Disulfiram-like reaction. Unsteadiness, and incoordination caused by metronidazole may be aggravated by alcohol	Metronidazole inhibits aldehyde dehydrogenase. Additive side-effects	Avoid co-ingestion
ALCOHOL	TETRACYCLINE	Likely ↓ efficacy of antibiotic	Uncertain	Be aware
ALCOHOL	**ANTICANCER AND IMMUNOMODULATING DRUGS**			
ALCOHOL	METHOTREXATE	↑ risk of liver damage/toxicity	Additive liver toxicity	Be aware; advocate abstinence. Monitor liver function
ALCOHOL	PROCARBAZINE	May cause a disulfiram-like reaction, additive depression of the CNS and postural hypotension	Some alcoholic beverages (beer, wine, ale) contain tyramine, which may induce hypertensive reactions	Avoid co-administration
ALCOHOL	ANTICOAGULANTS – ORAL	Fluctuations in anticoagulant effect in heavy drinkers or patients with liver disease who drink alcohol	Alcohol may reduce the half-life of oral anticoagulants by inducing hepatic enzymes. Also they may alter the hepatic synthesis of clotting factors	Caution should be taken when prescribing oral anticoagulants to alcoholics, particularly those who binge drink or have liver damage
ALCOHOL	**ANTIDEPRESSANTS**			
ALCOHOL	MAOIs	Additive depression of CNS ranging from drowsiness to coma and respiratory depression	Synergistic depressant effects on CNS function	Necessary to warn patients, particularly regards activities that require attention, e.g. driving or using machinery and equipment that could cause self-harm
ALCOHOL	SSRIs	↑ risk of sedation	Additive CNS depressant effects. Acute ingestion of alcohol inhibits CYP2D6 and CYP2C19, whereas chronic use induces CYP2E1 and CYP3A4	Be aware and caution against excessive alcohol intake

MISCELLANEOUS ALCOHOL

ALCOHOL	TCAs, MIRTAZAPINE	↑ sedation	Additive effect	Warn patients about this effect
ALCOHOL	**ANTIEPILEPTICS**			
ALCOHOL	BARBITURATES	↑ sedation	Additive sedative effect	Warn patients about this effect
ALCOHOL	TOPIRAMATE	↑ sedation	Additive sedative effect	Warn patients about this effect
ALCOHOL	**ANTIDIABETIC DRUGS**			
ALCOHOL	ANTIDIABETIC DRUGS	Tends to mask signs of hypoglycaemia and ↑ risk of hypoglycaemic episodes	Inhibits glucose production and release from many sources including the liver	Watch for and warn patients about symptoms of hypoglycaemia ➢ ***For signs and symptoms of hypoglycaemia, see Clinical Features of Some Adverse Drug Interactions, Hypoglycaemia***
ALCOHOL	METFORMIN	Enhanced effect of metformin and ↑ risk of lactic acidosis. May cause a disulfiram-like interaction	Alcohol is known to potentiate the effect of metformin on lactate metabolism. It inhibits glucose production and release from many sources including the liver	The onset of lactic acidosis is often subtle with symptoms of malaise, myalgia, respiratory distress and ↑ non-specific abdominal distress. There may be hypothermia and resistant bradyarrhythmias
ALCOHOL	**ANTIFUNGALS**			
ALCOHOL	GRISEOFULVIN	A disulfiram-like reaction can occur	Uncertain	Warn patients not to drink alcohol while taking griseofulvin
ALCOHOL	KETOCONAZOLE	May ↑ risk of liver damage. Symptoms of nausea, headache, flushing and discomfort (similar to a disulfiram-type reaction) may occur	Additive liver toxicity	Be aware

Primary drug	Secondary drug	Effect	Mechanism	Precautions
ALCOHOL	**ANTIHISTAMINES**			
ALCOHOL	ANTIHISTAMINES	↑ sedation with sedating antihistamines	Additive effect	Warn patients about this effect. Remember that cold medicines as well as allergy pills may well contain antihistamines
ALCOHOL	CIMETIDINE, RANITIDINE	Alleged ↑ effects of alcohol after relatively innocuous amounts of wine, beer, etc., which made it popular among users; the effect is, however, unproven	A study suggested the presence of alcohol dehydrogenase in the stomach of some men, which was inactivated by cimetidine and ranitidine	Be aware. The FDA has considered the probability of inactivation of stomach alcohol dehydrogenase as 'not dangerous'
ALCOHOL	**ANTIHYPERTENSIVES AND HEART FAILURE DRUGS**			
ALCOHOL	ANTIHYPERTENSIVES AND HEART FAILURE DRUGS, e.g. PRAZOSIN	1. Acute alcohol ingestion may ↑ hypotensive effects 2. Chronic moderate or heavy drinking ↓ hypotensive effects	1. Additive hypotensive effect 2. Chronic alcohol excess is associated with hypertension	Monitor BP closely as unpredictable responses can occur. Advise patients to drink alcohol only in moderation and to avoid large variations in the amount of alcohol drunk
ALCOHOL	ALPHA-BLOCKERS	↑ levels of both alcohol and indoramin occur with concurrent use	Uncertain	Warn patients about the risk of ↑ sedation
ALCOHOL	CENTRALLY ACTING ANTIHYPERTENSIVES	Clonidine and moxonidine may exacerbate the sedative effects of alcohol, particularly during initiation of therapy	Uncertain	Warn patients of this effect, and advise them to avoid driving or operating machinery if they suffer from sedation
ALCOHOL	RESERPINE	↑ effects of both reserpine and alcohol	Reserpine has CNS effects, while alcohol may act as a vasodilator-hypotensive	Avoid concomitant use
ALCOHOL	ANTIMUSCARINICS – ATROPINE, GLYCOPYRRONIUM	↑ sedation	Additive effect	Warn patients about this effect, and advise them not to drink while taking these antimuscarinics

ALCOHOL	**ANTIPROTOZOALS**			
ALCOHOL	LEVAMISOLE	Risk of a disulfiram-like reaction	Uncertain	Warn patients not to drink alcohol while taking levamisole
ALCOHOL	TINIDAZOLE	Risk of a disulfiram-like reaction	Uncertain	Warn patients not to drink alcohol while taking tinidazole
ALCOHOL	ANTIPSYCHOTICS	Risk of excessive sedation	Additive effect	Warn patients of this effect, and advise them to drink alcohol only in moderation
CNS DEPRESSANTS – INCLUDING ALCOHOL	ANXIOLYTICS AND HYPNOTICS	↑ sedation	Additive effect	Warn patients to be aware of this added effect
ALCOHOL	BETA-BLOCKERS	Acute alcohol ingestion may ↑ hypotensive effects. Chronic moderate or heavy drinking ↓ hypotensive effects. Might cause higher blood alcohol levels from modest amounts of alcohol	Additive hypotensive effect. Mechanism underlying the opposite effect with chronic intake is uncertain. A study suggested the presence of alcohol dehydrogenase in the stomach of some men, which was inactivated by propranolol	Monitor BP closely as unpredictable responses can occur. Advise patients to drink alcohol only in moderation and to avoid large variations in the amount of alcohol drunk. The FDA has considered the probability of inactivation of stomach alcohol dehydrogenase as 'not dangerous'
ALCOHOL	BETA-CAROTENE (a precursor to vitamin A and a popular antioxidant supplement)	↑ risk of liver damage	Alcohol combined with beta-carotene led to more liver damage than was produced by alcohol exposure alone	Be aware
ALCOHOL	BROMOCRIPTINE	↑ risk of severe side-effects if alcohol is taken at the same time. (e.g. nausea, stomach pain, dizziness)	Uncertain	Be aware

Primary drug	Secondary drug	Effect	Mechanism	Precautions
ALCOHOL	CALCIUM CHANNEL BLOCKERS	1. Acute alcohol ingestion may ↑ hypotensive effects. Chronic moderate or heavy drinking ↓ hypotensive effects 2. Verapamil may ↑ peaked serum concentration and prolong the effects of alcohol	1. Additive hypotensive effect with acute alcohol excess. Chronic alcohol excess is associated with hypertension 2. Uncertain at present, but presumed to be due to inhibition of the hepatic metabolism of alcohol, a mechanism similar to that with cimetidine, ranitidine and aspirin	1. Monitor BP closely as unpredictable responses can occur. Advise patients to drink alcohol only in moderation and to avoid large variations in the amount of alcohol drunk 2. Warn patients about potentiation of the effects of alcohol, particularly the risks to driving
ALCOHOL	DRUG DEPENDENCE THERAPIES			
ALCOHOL	BUPROPION	Rare reports of adverse neuropsychiatric events, including report of seizures. ↓ alcohol tolerance	Uncertain	Warn patients to avoid or minimize alcohol intake during bupropion treatment
ALCOHOL	DISULFIRAM	Disulfiram reaction	See Drugs Acting on the Nervous System	Do not co-administer. Disulfiram must not be given within 12 hours of ingestion of alcohol. This reaction could occur even with the small amounts of alcohol found in cough syrup or cold remedies
ALCOHOL, BZDs, BARBITURATES	LOFEXIDINE	↑ sedation	Additive effect	Warn patients of risk of excessive sedation
ALCOHOL	MINERALS	Regular intake of alcohol could cause depletion of iron, zinc, magnesium and selenium. Alcoholic drinks such as wine and whisky may have high or potentially toxic contents of the toxic element cadmium	Attributed to ↓ absorption or ↓ intake of nutrients	Be a ware. Monitor cadmium levels as well as plasma levels of other minerals

MISCELLANEOUS ALCOHOL

ALCOHOL	MUSCLE RELAXANTS – BACLOFEN, METHOCARBAMOL, TIZANIDINE	↑ sedation	Additive effect	Warn patients; advise them to drink alcohol only in moderation and not to drive if they have drunk any alcohol while taking these muscle relaxants
ALCOHOL	NITRATES, NITROGLYCERIN	↑ risk of postural ↓ BP when GTN is taken with alcohol	Additive effect; both are vasodilators	Warn patients about the risk of feeling faint. Advise them to drink alcohol only in moderation and to avoid binge drinking
ALCOHOL	PARACETAMOL	↑ risk of liver damage. Might cause higher blood alcohol levels from modest amounts of alcohol, as with aspirin, cimetidine, ranitidine, propranolol and verapamil	Paracetamol tends to cause greater toxicity in chronic alcoholics with malnutrition or diseased livers. A study suggested the presence of alcohol dehydrogenase in the stomach of some men, which could be inactivated by paracetamol	Be aware, particularly when toxic doses of paracetamol have been taken. The FDA has considered the probability of inactivation of stomach alcohol dehydrogenase as 'not dangerous'
ALCOHOL	POTASSIUM CHANNEL ACTIVATORS	Acute alcohol ingestion may ↑ hypotensive effects. Chronic moderate or heavy drinking ↓ hypotensive effects	Additive hypotensive effect. Mechanism underlying the opposite effect with chronic intake is uncertain	Monitor BP closely as unpredictable responses can occur. Advise patients to drink alcohol only in moderation and to avoid large variations in the amount of alcohol drunk
ALCOHOL	VITAMIN C (large doses, e.g. 1000 mg)	May ↑ elimination of alcohol, but this is unproven	Uncertain	Unlikely to be of clinical significance

NOTE: Alcohol is an ingredient in many OTC and even some prescription medicines. The amounts are modest in most cases, but a few reach concentrations of 40% or 50% proof. Cough and cold elixirs are the most likely sources, but some vitamin 'tonics' and laxatives also contain alcohol.

Primary drug	Secondary drug	Effect	Mechanism	Precautions
GRAPEFRUIT JUICE				
GRAPEFRUIT JUICE	**ANALGESICS**			
GRAPEFRUIT JUICE	PARACETAMOL	↑ half-life of paracetamol. White grapefruit juice ↑ plasma concentrations in 1 hour, while pink grapefruit juice caused the ↑ in 2 hours	Attributed to ↑ elimination half-life of paracetamol caused by grapefruit juice	Be aware
GRAPEFRUIT JUICE	DICLOFENAC	Although low doses (1mg/kg) of grapefruit juice did not potentiate the effect of diclofenac, higher doses ↑ anti-inflammatory effect (as assessed by an effect on rat's paw oedema)	Diclofenac undergoes phenyl hydroxylation catalysed by CYP2C9 and CYP3A4. High dose of grapefruit juice possibly ↑ effects by inhibiting CYP3A4	Be aware as all the effects of diclofenac, including toxic effects, may ↑
GRAPEFRUIT JUICE	METHADONE	↑ plasma concentrations and ↑ risk of adverse effects. Interaction is considered to be of rapid onset but of minor clinical significance	Methadone is metabolized by intestinal CYP3A4, which is inhibited by grapefruit juice	Prudent to be aware and warn users and carers
GRAPEFRUIT JUICE	MORPHINE	Grapefruit juice ↑ morphine antinociception. Gradually ↓ CSF and blood concentrations following repeated treatment with morphine	Grapefruit juice is considered to ↑ intestinal absorption of morphine due to inhibition of P-gp, which also probably contributes to ↓ CSF concentrations	This interaction is unlikely to be of clinical significance, but be aware
GRAPEFRUIT JUICE	**ANTHELMINTICS**			
GRAPEFRUIT JUICE	ALBENDAZOLE	↑ plasma levels of albendazole by nearly threefold. Risk of toxic effects of albendazole	Albendazole is metabolized by intestinal CYP3A4, which is inhibited by grapefruit juice	Monitor for toxic effects of albendazole

GRAPEFRUIT JUICE	PRAZIQUANTEL	Marked ↑ in plasma concentrations of praziquantel (AUC ↑ 2.5-fold, maximum concentration ↑ threefold). In human liver, maximum concentration ↑ 1.6-fold and AUC 1.9-fold	Possibly via a role of P-gp – inhibition of P-gp may ↑ plasma concentrations	Be aware and watch for toxic effects of praziquantel
GRAPEFRUIT JUICE	**ANTIARRHYTHMICS**			
GRAPEFRUIT JUICE	AMIODARONE	Markedly ↑ plasma concentrations of amiodarone (AUC >50%, maximum concentration >84%). Possibly ↓ effect of amiodarone (↓ in P–R and Q–Tc intervals). This could lead to ↓ therapeutic effect due to ↓ production of active metabolite	Due to inhibition of CYP3A4-mediated metabolism of amiodarone by grapefruit juice, which results in near-complete inhibition of the production of N-DEA (desethylamiodarone, the active and major metabolite of amiodarone)	Warn patients to avoid grapefruit juice; if amiodarone becomes less effective, ask the patient about grapefruit juice ingestion
GRAPEFRUIT JUICE	AMLODIPINE	↑ plasma amlodipine levels (AUC ↑ by 116%, maximum concentration ↑ by 115%) but no adverse haemodynamic (no changes in PR, heart rate) effects. Unlikely to be clinically significant	There is report of pharmacokinetic interaction between amlodipine and grapefruit in healthy volunteers (maximum concentration and AUC were significantly higher when amlodipine 5 mg was administered with grapefruit compared with water)	Considering the interindividual variation in the pharmacokinetics of amlodipine, the possible interaction between amlodipine and grapefruit juice cannot be negelcted in the clinical setting even though the interaction does not seem to be of great clinical significance in human volunteer studies
GRAPEFRUIT JUICE	DISOPYRAMIDE	Likely interaction with possibility of ↑ plasma concentrations and toxic effects of disopyramide. However, the clinical significance is not yet known as the interaction has not been scientifically tested	Unclear	Monitor ECG and side-effects more closely

Primary drug	Secondary drug	Effect	Mechanism	Precautions
GRAPEFRUIT JUICE	PROPAFENONE	Significantly ↑ plasma concentrations are likely in people with ↓ CYP2D6 activity – poor metabolizers	Propafenone is primarily metabolized by CYP2D6, the secondary metabolic pathways being CYP1A2 and CYP3A4. Lower CYP2D6 levels cause a shift of propafenone metabolism to CYP3A4 isoenzymes, which are inhibited by grapefruit juice	Be aware that there are significant numbers of CYP2D6 poor metabolizers in some communities. Therefore, there is a need to monitor for toxic effects of propafenone at least twice weekly on initiating treatment
GRAPEFRUIT JUICE	QUINIDINE	Absorption of quinidine is delayed (e.g. from 1.6 to 3.3 hours) by grapefruit juice in a dose-dependent manner	Possibly due to effects on intestinal CYP3A4	Be aware
GRAPEFRUIT JUICE	TALINOLOL	Significant risk of ↓ therapeutic effects	Talinolol is a substrate of P-gp, and less than 1% is metabolized in the liver. However, inhibition by grapefruit juice of an intestinal uptake process other than P-gp is considered likely	Do not co-administer
GRAPEFRUIT JUICE	ANTIBIOTICS – CLARITHROMYCIN, ERYTHROMYCIN	Significant delay in onset of action of clarithromycin (↑ from 82 to 148 minutes). ↑ plasma concentrations of erythromycin (maximum concentration ↑, AUC ↑ 1.5-fold)	Due to inhibition of absorption attributed to effect on P-gp	The interaction is unlikely to cause clinically relevant ↓ antimicrobial activity of clarithromycin Telithromycin is unlikely to be affected by grapefruit juice. Be aware
GRAPEFRUIT JUICE	**ANTICANCER AND IMMUNOMODULATING DRUGS**			
GRAPEFRUIT JUICE	**CYTOTOXICS**			
GRAPEFRUIT JUICE	BEXAROTENE	Possibly ↑ efficacy and ↑ adverse effects	Possibly via inhibition of intestinal CYP3A4	Clinical significance unknown. Monitor more closely

GRAPEFRUIT JUICE	DOXORUBICIN	↑ risk of myelosuppression due to ↑ in plasma concentrations	Due to ↓ metabolism of doxorubicin by CYP3A4 isoenzymes due to inhibition of those enzymes	Monitor for ↑ myelosuppression, peripheral neuropathy, myalgias and fatigue
GRAPEFRUIT JUICE	ERLOTINIB	Markedly ↑ plasma concentrations of erlotinib (↑ AUC, ↑ maximum concentration). Likely to cause toxic effects of erlotinib	Due to inhibition of metabolism of erlotinib by grapefruit juice as CYP3A4 inhibition is known to result in a 2.1-fold ↑ in erlotinib exposure	Monitor for toxic effects of erlotinib
GRAPEFRUIT JUICE	ETOPOSIDE	↓ in plasma concentrations of etoposide (AUC ↓ 1.32-fold). Clinical significance is uncertain. Possibly ↓ efficacy	↓ bioavailability. Unclear	Interindividual variability is considerable. Be aware. Advise patients to ↓ intake of foods and beverages containing bioflavonoids. Monitor therapeutic effects closely
GRAPEFRUIT JUICE	IFOSFAMIDE	↓ plasma concentrations of 4-hydroxyifosfamide, the active metabolite of ifosfamide, and risk of inadequate therapeutic response	Due to inhibition of the isoenzymatic conversion to active metabolites	Monitor clinically the efficacy of ifosfamide and ↑ dose accordingly
GRAPEFRUIT JUICE	IMATINIB	Likely interaction. ↑ imatinib levels with ↑ risk of toxicity (e.g. abdominal pain, constipation, dyspnoea) and of neurotoxicity (e.g. taste disturbances, dizziness, headache, paraesthesia, peripheral neuropathy)	Due to inhibition of CYP3A4-mediated metabolism of imatinib. Clinical significance is not yet known as the interaction has not been scientifically tested	Monitor for clinical efficacy and for the signs of toxicity listed, along with convulsions, confusion and signs of oedema (including pulmonary oedema). Monitor electrolytes, liver function and for cardiotoxicity
GRAPEFRUIT JUICE	IRINOTECAN	↑ plasma concentrations of SN-38 (active metabolite of irinotecan) and ↑ toxicity of irinotecan, e.g. diarrhoea, acute cholinergic syndrome, interstitial pulmonary disease	Due to inhibition of metabolism of irinotecan by CYP3A4 isoenzymes by grapefruit juice	Peripheral blood counts should be checked before each course of treatment. Monitor lung function. Recommendation is to ↓ dose of irinotecan by 25%

Primary drug	Secondary drug	Effect	Mechanism	Precautions
GRAPEFRUIT JUICE	NILOTINIB (tyrosine kinase inhibitor)	Grapefruit products ↑ serum concentrations of nilotinib	Due to effect of grapefruit juice as an inhibitor of CYP3A4	The dose of nilotinib should not exceed 400 mg once daily (a dose ↓ to half the usual daily dose)
GRAPEFRUIT JUICE	TAMOXIFEN	Likely interaction	Due to inhibition of CYP3A4-mediated metabolism of tamoxifen. Clinical significance is not yet known as the interaction has not been scientifically tested	Be aware. Advise patients to ↓ intake of foods and beverages containing bioflavonoids
GRAPEFRUIT JUICE	VINBLASTINE, VINCRISTINE	↑ adverse effects of vinblastine and vincristine	Inhibition of CYP3A4-mediated metabolism. Also inhibition of intestinal P-gp efflux of vinblastine. Quercetin constituent of grapefruit juice enhances the phosphorylation of P-gp	Advice patients to ↓ intake foods and beverages containing bioflavonoids. Monitor FBC and watch for early features of toxicity (pain, numbness, tingling in the fingers and toes, jaw pain, abdominal pain, constipation, paralytic ileus). Consider selecting an alternative drug
GRAPEFRUIT JUICE	**HORMONES AND HORMONE ANTAGONISTS**			
GRAPEFRUIT JUICE	TOREMIFENE	↑ plasma concentrations of toremifene	Due to inhibition of metabolism of toremifene by the CYP3A4 isoenzymes by grapefruit juice	Clinical relevance is uncertain. Necessary to monitor for clinical toxicities
GRAPEFRUIT JUICE	**IMMUNOMODULATING DRUGS**			
GRAPEFRUIT JUICE	CICLOSPORIN	↑ plasma concentrations of ciclosporin, with risk of nephrotoxicity, myelosuppression, neurotoxicity, excessive immunosuppression and post-transplant lymphoproliferative disease	Inhibition of CYP3A4-mediated metabolism of ciclosporin; these inhibitors vary in potency. Grapefruit juice is classified as a potent inhibitor	Avoid grapefruit juice while taking ciclosporin

MISCELLANEOUS GRAPEFRUIT JUICE

GRAPEFRUIT JUICE	CORTICOSTEROIDS	↑ adrenal suppressive effects of corticosteroids, which may ↑ risk of infections and produce an inadequate response to stress scenarios (e.g. septic shock). However, studies have shown only moderate ↑ plasma concentrations of methylprednisolone and minimal or no changes with prednisolone	Due to inhibition of metabolism of corticosteroids	Monitor cortisol levels and warn patients to report symptoms such as fever and sore throat
GRAPEFRUIT JUICE	SIROLIMUS, TACROLIMUS	Possibly ↑ efficacy and ↑ adverse effects of sirolimus	Possibly ↑ bioavailability via inhibition of intestinal CYP3A4 and effects of P-gp	Avoid concomitant use
GRAPEFRUIT JUICE	ANTICOAGULANTS – ORAL	↑ efficacy and ↑ adverse effects of warfarin, e.g. ↑ INR, haemorrhage	Unclear. Possibly via inhibition of intestinal CYP3A4	Monitor INR more closely. Avoid concomitant use if unstable INR
GRAPEFRUIT JUICE	**ANTIDEPRESSANTS**			
GRAPEFRUIT JUICE	FLUVOXAMINE, SERTRALINE	Possibly ↑ efficacy and ↑ adverse effects due to ↑ plasma concentrations	Possibly ↓ metabolism	Clinical significance unclear
GRAPEFRUIT JUICE	CLOMIPRAMINE	↑ risk of clomipramine toxicity. Not known whether ↑ plasma concentration is sustained	Clomipramine metabolism involves several CYP isoenzymes (e.g. CYP1A2, CYP3A4, ↓ CYP2D6)	Be aware
GRAPEFRUIT JUICE	ANTIDIABETIC DRUGS – REPAGLINIDE	Possibly ↑ repaglinide levels	Due to inhibition of CYP3A4 isoenzymes, which metabolize repaglinide	Uncertain if clinically significant. May need to monitor blood glucose more closely

MISCELLANEOUS GRAPEFRUIT JUICE

MISCELLANEOUS GRAPEFRUIT JUICE

Primary drug	Secondary drug	Effect	Mechanism	Precautions
GRAPEFRUIT JUICE	ANTIEPILEPTICS – CARBAMAZEPINE	↑ in plasma concentrations of carbamazepine (AUC ↑ 1.4-fold, maximum concentration ↑), which is of clinical significance because of the narrow therapeutic index of carbamazepine; thus, toxic effects are likely. ↑ efficacy and ↑ adverse effects	Grapefruit juice irreversibly inhibits intestinal CYP3A4. Transport via P-gp and MRP-2 efflux pumps is also inhibited	Monitor for ↑ side-effects/toxicity and check carbamazepine levels weekly. If levels or control of fits are variable, remove grapefruit and grapefruit juice from the diet
GRAPEFRUIT JUICE	**ANTIFUNGALS**			
GRAPEFRUIT JUICE	ITRACONAZOLE	Co-administration of grapefruit juice ↓ AUC and maximum concentration of itraconazole by 47% and 35% respectively	↓ absorption, possibly by inhibition of intestinal CYP3A4, affecting P-gp or lowering duodenal pH. Effect appears to be greater in females	Clinical significance is unknown. The effect of the interaction may vary between capsules and oral liquid preparations
GRAPEFRUIT JUICE	IVABRADINE	↑ levels with grapefruit juice	Uncertain	Avoid co-administration
GRAPEFRUIT JUICE	**ANTIHISTAMINES/ANTI-ALLERGY DRUGS**			
GRAPEFRUIT JUICE	ASTEMIZOLE	Likely ↑ in cardiotoxicity. Likely ↑ in Q–Tc interval	Due to effects of grapefruit juice grapefruit juice on CYP isoenzymes and P-gp	Do not co-administer as there are suitable alternatives that are less harmful, e.g. loratidine, cetrizine, desloratidine
GRAPEFRUIT JUICE	FEXOFENADINE	↓ plasma concentrations of fexofenadine (AUC <2.7-fold, maximum concentration <2.1-fold). Risk of lack of therapeutic effects. Possibly ↓ efficacy	↓ absorption, possibly by affecting P-gp and direct inhibition of uptake by intestinal OATP1A2	Clinical significance unclear. No clinically significant changes in ECG parameters were observed in the study. Suitable alternatives are available
GRAPEFRUIT JUICE	RUPATADINE	↑ risk of cardiac toxicity due to threefold ↑ plasma concentrations of rupatadine	Due to effects of grapefruit juice on CYP isoenzymes and P-gp	Do not co-administer as there are suitable alternatives that are less harmful, e.g. loratidine, cetrizine, desloratidine

GRAPEFRUIT JUICE	TERFENADINE	Statistically ↑ Q–T interval prolongation, hence the risk of cardiac toxicity. ↑ in AUC, maximum concentration and T max. Two-fold ↑ half-life. Possibly ↑ efficacy and ↑ adverse effects, e.g. torsade de pointes	Altered metabolism so the parent drug accumulates. Due to effects of grapefruit juice on CYP isoenzymes and P-gp	Avoid concomitant intake. Suitable alternatives that are less harmful are available, e.g. loratidine (which is also metabolized by CYP2D6), cetrizine, desloratidine. This is despite a report that no significant cardiotoxicity is likely in normal subjects
GRAPEFRUIT JUICE	**ANTIMALARIALS**			
GRAPEFRUIT JUICE	ARTEMETHER (WITH LUMEFANTRINE)	↑ plasma concentrations of artemether (AUC by 2.5-fold, maximum concentration >twofold. There were no signs of bradycardia or evidence of Q–Tc prolongation	Very likely to be due to inhibition of intestinal CYP3A4 by grapefruit juice, which suggests a role for the presystemic metabolism of artemether	Monitor more closely. No ECG changes were seen in the study. Be aware
GRAPEFRUIT JUICE	CHLOROQUINE	↑ plasma concentrations of chloroquine (AUC ↑ 1.3-fold, ↑ maximum concentration). The interaction has not been studied in patients with malaria	Due to inhibition of metabolism of chloroquine	Be aware
GRAPEFRUIT JUICE	HALOFANTRINE	Markedly ↑ plasma concentrations of halofantrine (AUC ↑ 2.8-fold, maximum concentration ↑ 3.2-fold). Maximum Q–Tc prolongation was ↑ from 17 msec to 31 msec, thus giving a risk of cardiotoxicity	Due to inhibition of metabolism of CYP3A4-mediated metabolism of halofantrine	Do not co-administer because of Q–Tc interval prolongation effects
GRAPEFRUIT JUICE	QUININE	Report of ↓ heart rate and PR that returned to normal 4–6 hours after intake of quinine. Not considered to be clinically significant	Due to inhibition of metabolism of CYP3A4-mediated metabolism. However, metabolism of quinine is predominantly hepatic and thus unaffected by grapefruit juice	Be aware

Primary drug	Secondary drug	Effect	Mechanism	Precautions
GRAPEFRUIT JUICE	ANTIOBESITY DRUGS – SIBUTRAMINE	Possibly ↑ efficacy and ↑ adverse effects, e.g. higher BP and raised heart rate	Unclear	Monitor PR and BP
GRAPEFRUIT JUICE	ANTIPSYCHOTICS – PIMOZIDE	Possibly ↑ efficacy and ↑ adverse effects. Interaction may occur rapidly, but clinical significance is uncertain	Not evaluated in clinical trials	Avoid concomitant use. No interaction was observed with haloperidol
GRAPEFRUIT JUICE	**ANTIVIRALS**			
GRAPEFRUIT JUICE	EFAVIRENZ	Possibly ↑ efficacy and ↑ adverse effects	Unclear	Monitor more closely
GRAPEFRUIT JUICE	SAQUINAVIR (Invirase hard capsules)	Possibly ↑ efficacy with oral (and not when administered intravenous) preparations. The AUC of oral saquinavir ↑ by 50%, but maximum concentration, T max and terminal half-life were not significantly altered in one study	Possibly ↑ bioavailability; ↓ pre-systemic metabolism. Constituents of grapefruit juice and grapefruit irreversibly inhibit intestinal cytochrome CYP3A4. Transport via P-gp and MRP-2 efflux pumps is also inhibited	No dose adjustment is advised. Oral bioavailability is very low and is enhanced beneficially with grapefruit juice or grapefruit. Soft gel capsules have greater bioavailability so may interact to a lesser degree. No dose adjustments are recommended by manufacturers for indinavir
GRAPEFRUIT JUICE	**ANXIOLYTICS AND HYPNOTICS**			
GRAPEFRUIT JUICE	BUSPIRONE– ORAL	Significant ↑ pharmacodynamic effects. AUC ↑ 9.2-fold and maximum concentration 4.3-fold, with ↑ in T max. Possibly ↑ efficacy and ↑ adverse effects, e.g. sedation, CNS depression	Possibly ↑ bioavailability; ↓ presystemic metabolism. Constituents of grapefruit juice irreversibly inhibit intestinal cytochrome CYP3A4. Transport via P-gp and MRP-2 efflux pumps is also inhibited	Avoid concomitant use. Be particularly vigilant in elderly patients or those with impaired liver function. Consider an alternative, e.g. temazepam

GRAPEFRUIT JUICE	BZDs – MIDAZOLAM TRIAZOLAM QUAZEPAM DIAZEPAM ALPRAZOLAM	A slight but statistically significant ↑ drowsiness due to a 1.5-fold ↑ in AUC and a 1.3-fold ↑ in maximum concentration with triazolam that was accompanied by a ↑ in reaching peak effects (from 1.6 to 2.5 hours). There is ↑ AUC, maximum concentration and T max of quazepam and its active metabolite 2-oxoquazepam. No change is seen in psychomotor function with alprazolam, while with diazepam there was ↑ maximum concentration. With midazolam, there was minor ↑ reaction time (and minor ↑ digital symbol substitution test results)	With alprazolam, due to its inherent high bioavailability, grapefruit juice is unlikely to produce a significant change, in contrast to midazolam and triazolam. There is less contribution to presystemic metabolism by intestinal CYP3A4 for alprazolam. Grapefruit juice caused ↓ CYP3A12 activity in the liver and ↑ CYP3A12 activity in the intestine when tested with diazepam. This was attributed to the bergamotton constituent of grapefruit juice	Alprazolam is probably the BZD least affected by grapefruit juice, although many consider that the effect of grapefruit juice on midazolam is unlikely to be clinically important with 300 mL of juice. ↑ plasma concentrations of diazepam are considered to be clinically insignificant – be aware of impaired cognition
GRAPEFRUIT JUICE	BETA-BLOCKERS – CELIPROLOL (not available in USA)	Very likely to be ineffective therapeutically due to a great ↓ plasma concentrations (AUC ↓ by 85% and maximum concentration by 95%)	Attributed mainly to marked ↓ absorption. This may be due to physicochemical factors or due to an inhibition of drug uptake transporters	Do not co-administer
GRAPEFRUIT JUICE	BRONCHODILATORS – THEOPHYLLINES	Possibly ↓ efficacy	Unclear. ↓ bio-availability (significant from 1 to 4 hours)	Avoid concomitant intake if slow-release theophylline preparations are used. Monitor levels and clinical state weekly if intake of grapefruit is altered

Primary drug	Secondary drug	Effect	Mechanism	Precautions
GRAPEFRUIT JUICE	CALCIUM CHANNEL BLOCKERS			
GRAPEFRUIT JUICE	CALCIUM CHANNEL BLOCKERS	↑ risk of systemic hypotension. ↑ bioavailability of felodipine and nisoldipine (with reports of adverse effects), and ↑ bioavailability of isradipine, lacidipine, lercanidipine, nicardipine, nifedipine, nimodipine (threefold ↑ bioavailability) and verapamil (without reported adverse clinical effects)	Postulated that flavonoids in grapefruit juice (and possibly Seville oranges and limes), inhibit intestinal (but not hepatic) CYP3A4. Further grapefruit juice limits apical to basal transport by P-gp and MRP-2, which limits drug excretion of and ↑ bioavailability of drugs, e.g. verapamil, nimodipine	Be aware. Avoid concurrent use of felodipine, nimodipine or nisoldipine and grapefruit juice. However, there is considerable interindividual variation, and if concomitant use is necessary, be aware of interaction, the severity of which may vary between drugs
GRAPEFRUIT JUICE	AZELNIDIPINE	↑ in plasma concentrations of azelnidipine 2.5-fold, and ↑ AUC 3.3-fold. Risk of azelnidipine toxicity	Azelnidipine is metabolized by CYP3A4 isoenzymes in the intestinal wall, and this metabolism is inhibited by grapefruit juice	
GRAPEFRUIT JUICE	CANDESARTAN, EPROSARTAN, TELMISARTAN, VALSARTAN	Likely interaction. Clinical significance is uncertain and not confirmed by scientific testing	These angiotensin II receptor blockers have low bioavailability, attributed to P-gp, which is inhibited by grapefruit juice. Thus ↑ bioavailability is likely	Be aware
GRAPEFRUIT JUICE	CARDIAC GLYCOSIDES – DIGOXIN	Possible ↑ efficacy and ↑ adverse effects	Possibly via altered absorption	Most patients were unaffected. Consider if unexpected bradycardia or heart block with digoxin. Rationale is based on the theoretical concept that digoxin is a substrate of P-gp
GRAPEFRUIT JUICE	CISAPRIDE	↑ plasma concentrations and likely ↑ risk of adverse effects (e.g. cardiotoxicity, Q–T prolongation, torsade de pointes)	↑ oral bioavailability and slight but significant ↑ elimination half-life	Although a study in volunteers did not show any changes in heart rate, PR or Q–T prolongation, avoid concurrent use

MISCELLANEOUS GRAPEFRUIT JUICE

GRAPEFRUIT JUICE	ERGOT ALKALOIDS – ERGOTAMINE	Possibly ↑ efficacy and ↑ adverse effects, e.g. vasospasm, ergotism, peripheral vasoconstriction, gangrene	Oral administration only. ↑ bioavailability; ↓ presystemic metabolism. Constituents of grapefruit juice and grapefruit irreversibly inhibit intestinal cytochrome CYP3A4. Transport via P-gp and MRP-2 efflux pumps is also inhibited	Monitor for ↑ side-effects; stop intake of grapefruit preparations if side-effects occur
GRAPEFRUIT JUICE	5-HT1 AGONISTS – ALMOTRIPTAN, ELETRIPTAN	↑ plasma concentrations of almotriptan and eletriptan, with risk of toxic effects, e.g. flushing, sensations of tingling, heat, heaviness, pressure or tightness of any part of body including the throat and chest, dizziness	Almotriptan and eletriptan are metabolized mainly by CYP3A4 isoenzymes. Most CYP isoenzymes are inhibited by grapefruit juice to varying degrees, and since there is an alternative pathway of metabolism by MAOA, toxicity responses vary between individuals	The CSM has advised that if chest tightness or pressure is intense, the triptan should be discontinued immediately and the patient investigated for ischaemic heart disease by measuring cardiac enzymes and doing an ECG. Avoid concomitant use in patients with coronary artery disease and in those with severe or uncontrolled hypertension
GRAPEFRUIT JUICE	LIPID-LOWERING DRUGS – ATORVASTATIN, SIMVASTATIN	Grapefruit juice ↑ plasma levels of simvastatin 16-fold, and the 3-hydroxy-3-methyl-glutaryl-CoA reductase inhibition was also ↑. ↑ levels with simvastatin, and a slight rise with atorvastatin. ↑ risk of adverse effects such as myopathy. Threefold ↑ AUC for atorvastatin and atorvastatin lactone	Constituent of grapefruit juice inhibits CYP3A4-mediated metabolism of simvastatin and atorvastatin. CYP3A4 plays only a minor role in the metabolism of fluvastatin	Patients taking simvastatin and atorvastatin should avoid grapefruit juice. Use an alternative statin not influenced by CYP3A4 activity, e.g. rosuvastatin

MISCELLANEOUS GRAPEFRUIT JUICE

Primary drug	Secondary drug	Effect	Mechanism	Precautions
GRAPEFRUIT JUICE	NICOTINE	Significant ↑ renal clearance of nicotine	Grapefruit juice inhibits the formation of cotinine from nicotine, ↑ renal clearance of cotinine and ↓ plasma concentrations of cotinine by 15%	Be aware in patients using varying forms of nicotine replacement therapy for stopping smoking
GRAPEFRUIT JUICE	OESTROGENS – ESTRADIOL, POSSIBLY ETHINYLESTRADIOL	↑ efficacy and ↑ adverse effects	Oral administration only. ↑ bioavailability; ↓ presystemic metabolism. Constituents of grapefruit juice and grapefruit irreversibly inhibit intestinal cytochrome CYP3A4. Transport via P-gp and MRP-2 efflux pumps is also inhibited	Monitor for ↑ side-effects
GRAPEFRUIT JUICE	PHOSPHODIESTERASE TYPE 5 INHIBITORS (e.g. sidenafil, tadalafil, vardenafil)	Possibly ↑ efficacy and ↑ adverse effects, e.g. hypotension	Small ↑ bioavailability. ↑ variability in pharmacokinetics, i.e. interindividual variations in metabolism	Safest to advise against intake of grapefruit juice for at least 48 hours prior to intending to take any of these preparations. When necessary, the starting dose of sildenafil should not exceed 25–50 mg and that of tadalafil 10 mg. Avoid co-administration with vardenafil

MINERALS				
CALCIUM				
CALCIUM	ANALGESICS – ASPIRIN	May ↓ calcium levels in blood and body	Attributed to aspirin ↑ excretion	Be aware
CALCIUM	ANTIBIOTICS – QUINOLONES (CIPROFLOXACIN) TETRACYCLINES	↓ antibiotic levels	↓ absorption due to formation of unabsorbable chelates	Separate doses by at least 2 hours
CALCIUM	**ANTICANCER AND IMMUNOMODULATING DRUGS**			
CALCIUM	CORTICOSTEROIDS	↓ calcium levels	↓ intestinal absorption and ↑ excretion	Separate doses as much as possible
CALCIUM AND DAIRY PRODUCTS	ESTRAMUSTINE	↓ plasma concentrations of estramustine and risk of poor therapeutic response	Due to ↓ absorption of estramustine due to the formation of a calcium phosphate complex	Administer estramustine 1 hour before or 2 hours after dairy products or calcium supplements
CALCIUM	ANTIEPILEPTIC DRUGS	↓ plasma/body concentrations of calcium	A direct ↓ effect on absorption and also by ↓ vitamin D	Be aware
CALCIUM	BISPHOSPHONATES	↓ bisphosphonate levels	↓ absorption	Separate doses by at least 30 minutes
CALCIUM	CARDIAC GLYCOSIDES – DIGOXIN	Risk of cardiac arrhythmias with large intravenous doses of calcium	Uncertain. It is known that calcium levels directly correlate with the action of digoxin; therefore, high levels, even if transient, may increase the chance of toxicity	It is recommended that the parenteral administration of calcium should be avoided in patients taking digoxin. If this is not possible, administer calcium slowly and in small aliquots
CALCIUM	DIURETICS – THIAZIDES	Risk of hypercalcaemia with high-dose calcium	↓ renal excretion of calcium by thiazides	Monitor calcium levels closely
CALCIUM	FLUORIDE	↓ efficacy of fluoride	↓ absorption	Separate doses by 2–3 hours

Primary drug	Secondary drug	Effect	Mechanism	Precautions
CALCIUM	IRON – ORAL	↓ iron levels when iron is given orally. Possibly ↓ calcium levels	↓ absorption. These two minerals compete for absorption	Separate doses as much as possible; monitor FBC closely. Monitor plasma calcium levels
CALCIUM COMPOUNDS	SYMPATHOMIMETICS	Parenteral calcium administration may ↓ positive inotropic effects of epinephrine and dobutamine	Uncertain; postulated that calcium modulates signal transmission from the receptor	Monitor BP closely; watch for poor response to these inotropes
CALCIUM	THYROID HORMONES – LEVOTHYROXINE	↓ levothyroxine levels	↓ absorption due to formation of unabsorbable chelates	Separate doses by at least 4 hours. Monitor TFTs regularly and consider ↑ dose of levothyroxine
CALCIUM	ZINC	↓ efficacy of zinc	Unknown	Separate doses by 2–3 hours
CINACALCET				
CINACALCET	BUPROPION	↑ plasma concentrations of these substrates, with risk of toxic effects	Bupropion and its metabolite hydroxybupropion inhibit CYP2D6	Initiate therapy of these drugs, particularly those with a narrow therapeutic index, at the lowest effective dose. Interaction is likely to be important with substrates for which CYP2D6 is considered the only metabolic pathway (e.g. hydrocodone, oxycodone, desipramine, paroxetine, chlorpheniramine, mesoridazine, alprenolol, amphetamines, atomoxetine)
FLUORIDE				
FLUORIDE	CALCIUM	↓ efficacy of fluoride	↓ absorption	Separate doses by 2–3 hours
MAGNESIUM				
MAGNESIUM (PARENTERAL)	ANAESTHETICS – LOCAL – PROCAINE SOLUTIONS	Precipitation of drugs, which may not be immediately apparent	A pharmaceutical interaction	Do not mix in the same infusion or syringe
MAGNESIUM	ANALGESICS – ASPIRIN	May ↓ effects of magnesium in the body	Attributed to an antagonistic effect; mechanism is uncertain	Be aware

MAGNESIUM (PARENTERAL)	CALCIUM CHANNEL BLOCKERS	Case reports of profound muscular weakness when nifedipine was given with parenteral magnesium	Both drugs inhibit calcium influx across cell membranes, and magnesium promotes the movement of calcium into the sarcoplasmic reticulum; this results in muscular paralysis	Do not administer calcium channel blockers during parenteral magnesium therapy
MAGNESIUM (PARENTERAL)	MUSCLE RELAXANTS – DEPOLARIZING, NON-DEPOLARIZING	↑ efficacy of these muscle relaxants, with risk of prolonged neuromuscular blockade	Additive effect; magnesium inhibits ACh release and ↓ postsynaptic receptor sensitivity	Monitor nerve blockade closely
MAGNESIUM	HORMONE REPLACEMENT THERAPY	May cause magnesium depletion	Mg levels tend to ↓ during menopause. Risk–benefit ratios need to be considered on an individual basis as there are suggestions that magnesium can counteract the alleged ↑ risk of heart attacks and strokes in patients on hormone replacement therapy	Be aware
MAGNESIUM	ORAL CONTRACEPTIVES	May cause magnesium depletion	Oral contraceptives tend to increase copper levels, which when high results in ↓ magnesium levels	Be aware
MAGNESIUM	PENICILLAMINE	May cause magnesium depletion	Penicillamine ↓ absorption of several minerals, including magnesium	Be aware and separate the oral intake. Parenteral magnesium is unlikely to be affected
POLYSTYRENE SULPHONATE RESINS				
SODIUM POLYSTYRENE SULPHONATE	ANTACIDS – MAGNESIUM-CONTAINING	Cases of metabolic alkalosis	Uncertain; possibly ↑ absorption of bicarbonate due to its abnormal neutralization in the stomach	Consider an alternative antacid or administer sodium polystyrene sulphonate as an enema. If both need to be co-administered orally, monitor U&Es and blood gases closely

Primary drug	Secondary drug	Effect	Mechanism	Precautions
SODIUM POLYSTYRENE SULPHONATE	THYROID HORMONES	↓ levothyroxine levels	↓ absorption	Monitor TFTs regularly, and consider ↑ dose of levothyroxine
POTASSIUM				
Warn patients to avoid salt substitutes that contain potassium. OTC preparations of minerals and vitamins are unlikely to contain a potentially harmful content of potassium. However, a quarter of a teaspoon of salt substitute with potassium may contain 650 mg of potassium, compared with a prescription potassium tablet of 20 mEq, which contains 750 mg				
POTASSIUM	ALISKIREN	Risk of hyperkalaemia	Additive effect	Avoid co-administration
POTASSIUM	**ANALGESICS**			
POTASSIUM	ASPIRIN	Risk of hypokalaemia	Aspirin is considered to ↑ excretion of potassium	Be aware, particularly in people on long-term aspirin therapy, although it is uncertain whether 75–100 mg doses of aspirin cause significant effects
POTASSIUM	NSAIDs	↑ risk of hyperkalaemia	Additive effect	➢ ***For signs and symptoms of hyperkalaemia, see Clinical Features of Some Adverse Drug Interactions, Hyperkalaemia***
POTASSIUM CITRATE	ANTIBIOTICS – METHENAMINE	↓ methenamine levels	Citrate alkalinizes the urine, which ↑ excretion of methenamine	Avoid co-administration
POTASSIUM	**ANTICANCER AND IMMUNOMODULATING DRUGS**			
POTASSIUM	CICLOSPORIN	↑ risk of hyperkalaemia	Additive effect	➢ ***For signs and symptoms of hyperkalaemia, see Clinical Features of Some Adverse Drug Interactions, Hyperkalaemia***
POTASSIUM	CORTICOSTEROIDS	Risk of hypokalaemia	Most corticosteroids (cortisone, prednisone) ↑ loss of potassium	Be aware and monitor serum potassium levels, particularly in patients on long-term therapy with steroids
POTASSIUM	TACROLIMUS	Risk of hyperkalaemia	Additive effect	Monitor potassium levels closely

POTASSIUM	ANTIHYPERTENSIVES AND HEART FAILURE DRUGS – ACE INHIBITORS, ANGIOTENSIN II RECEPTOR ANTAGONISTS	↑ risk of hyperkalaemia	Retention of potassium by ACE inhibitors and additional intake of potassium	Monitor serum potassium daily
POTASSIUM	DIURETICS – POTASSIUM-SPARING	Risk of hyperkalaemia	Additive effect	Monitor potassium levels closely
POTASSIUM	LAXATIVES	Long-term use of laxatives may cause hypokalaemia. Laxatives may cause ↓ plasma/body concentrations of several minerals	Due to ↑ intestinal loss of potassium. Long-term use may cause ↓ absorption of several minerals	Be aware
SEVELAMER				
SEVELAMER	ANTIBIOTICS – CIPROFLOXACIN	↓ plasma concentrations of ciprofloxacin	↓ absorption	Separate the doses as much as possible
SEVELAMER	MYCOPHENOLATE	↓ plasma concentrations of mycophenolate	Attributed to binding of mycophenolate to calcium free phosphate binders	Separate administration by at least 2 hours
VITAMINS				
VITAMIN A	RETINOIDS	Risk of vitamin A toxicity	Additive effect; tretinoin is a form of vitamin A	Avoid co-administration
VITAMIN B6	ANTIEPILEPTICS – PHENOBARBITONE, PHENYTOIN	↓ plasma concentrations of these antiepileptics	Uncertain	Watch for poor response to these antiepileptics if large doses of vitamin B6 are given

Primary drug	Secondary drug	Effect	Mechanism	Precautions
VITAMIN B6	ANTIPARKINSON'S DRUGS – LEVODOPA	↓ efficacy of levodopa (in the absence of a dopa decarboxylase inhibitor)	A derivative of vitamin B6 is a co-factor in the peripheral conversion of levodopa to dopamine, which ↓ amount available for conversion in the CNS. Dopa decarboxylase inhibitors inhibit this peripheral reaction	Avoid co-administration of levodopa with vitamin B6; co-administration of vitamin B6 with co-beneldopa or co-careldopa is acceptable
VITAMIN B12	ANTIBIOTICS – CHLORAMPHENICOL	↓ efficacy of hydroxycobalamin	Chloramphenicol depresses the bone marrow; this opposes the action of vitamin B12	Be aware; monitor FBC and vitamin B12 levels closely
VITAMIN C	ANTACIDS CONTAINING ALUMINIUM	↑ aluminium levels, with risk of encephalopathy in patients with renal failure	Uncertain; possibly ↑ absorption due to the ascorbic acid in the presence of ↓ renal excretion	Avoid co-ingestion in patients with renal failure
VITAMIN C	ASPIRIN	May ↓ vitamin C levels	Attributed to aspirin 'blocking' the absorption of vitamin C. Aspirin has been found to ↑ elimination of vitamin C and all B vitamins	Be aware
VITAMIN D	ANTIEPILEPTICS – PHENYTOIN, CARBAMAZEPINE, PRIMIDONE , BARBITURATES	↓ efficacy of vitamin D	Attributed to induction of vitamin D metabolism	Be aware; consider ↑ dose of vitamin D
VITAMIN D	DIURETICS – THIAZIDES	Risk of hypercalcaemia with vitamin D	↓ renal excretion of calcium by thiazides	Monitor calcium levels closely
VITAMIN D	MAGNESIUM	↑ plasma concentrations of magnesium	Due to ↑ absorption	Be aware
VITAMIN E	ANTICOAGULANTS – ORAL	Case of ↑ anticoagulant effect	Uncertain	Monitor INR closely for 1–2 weeks after starting and stopping vitamin E

ZINC				
ZINC	ANTIBIOTICS – CIPROFLOXACIN, TETRACYCLINES	↓ antibiotic levels; doxycycline is less of a problem than the other tetracyclines	↓ absorption	Separate doses by at least 2 hours
ZINC	ANTICANCER AND IMMUNOMODULATING DRUGS – PENICILLAMINE	↓ penicillamine and zinc levels	Mutual ↓ absorption	Avoid co-administration
ZINC	CALCIUM	↓ efficacy of zinc	Unknown	Separate doses by 2–3 hours
ZINC	IRON – ORAL	↓ iron levels when iron is given orally	↓ absorption	Separate doses as much as possible – monitor FBC closely
ZINC	TRIENTINE	↓ zinc and trientine levels	Mutually ↓ absorption	Separate doses by at least 2 hours
OTHER DRUG–MINERAL INTERACTIONS				
ALLOPURINOL	COPPER	↓ plasma concentration of copper	Allopurinol chelates copper	Be aware and separate oral intake by at least 2 hours
ANTACIDS				
ANTACIDS	COPPER	↓ plasma concentration of copper	Most antacids will ↓ absorption of copper	If antacids are used in the long term, consider copper supplements of 1–2 mg/day
H2 ANTAGONISTS	COPPER AND IRON	↓ plasma and body concentrations of copper, iron, zinc and calcium	As a class, H2 antagonists act as free radical scavengers and cause depletion of calcium, iron and zinc. Cimetidine in particular binds to copper and iron, and these minerals are not made available for free radical production	Be aware and separate oral intake by 2 hours
ANTIBIOTICS				
AZITHROMYCIN	MAGNESIUM	↓ plasma/body concentrations of magnesium	Due to ↓ absorption	Be aware

Primary drug	Secondary drug	Effect	Mechanism	Precautions
CIPROFLOXACIN	MINERALS – CALCIUM, MAGNESIUM, IRON, ZINC, COPPER	↓ plasma/body levels of calcium, magnesium, iron and zinc	↓ absorption due to formation of unabsorbable chelates	Separate oral intake by at least 2 hours
OFLOXACIN	MINERALS – CALCIUM, MAGNESIUM, IRON, ZINC	↓ absorption of iron and zinc	Due to formation of unabsorbable chelates	Separate oral intake by at least 2 hours
LEVOFLOXACIN	MAGNESIUM, IRON	↓ plasma/body levels of magnesium and iron	↓ absorption due to formation of unabsorbable chelates	Separate oral intake by at least 2 hours
NITROFURANTOIN	MAGNESIUM	↓ plasma/body concentrations of magnesium	Due to ↓ absorption	Be aware
TETRACYCLINES	MINERALS – CALCIUM, MAGNESIUM, IRON, ZINC	↓ plasma/body levels of calcium, magnesium, iron and zinc	↓ absorption due to formation of unabsorbable chelates	Separate oral intake by at least 2 hours
ANTIDIABETIC DRUGS				
GLIPIZIDE	MAGNESIUM	↓ plasma/body concentrations of magnesium	Due to ↓ absorption	Be aware
HYPOGLYCAEMIC DRUGS	CHROMIUM	Chromium supplements may ↑ risk of hypoglycaemia	Chromium is necessary for the production of insulin	Be aware
ANTIEPILEPTICS				
CARBAMAZEPINE PHENYTOIN BARBITURATES PRIMIDONE	COPPER AND ZINC	↓ plasma concentrations of copper and zinc	Attributed to ↓ absorption	Be aware
VALPROIC ACID	SELENIUM	↓ selenium levels	Uncertain	Be aware
ANTIPSYCHOTIC DRUGS – CLOZAPINE	SELENIUM	↓ selenium levels	Uncertain	Be aware
COLESTYRAMINE, COLESTIPOL	IRON	↓ plasma/body concentrations of iron	Due to ↓ absorption	Be aware and do an FBC at least 2-weekly if on long-term therapy. Separate oral intake by 2 hours

CORTICOSTEROIDS				
CORTICOSTEROIDS	SELENIUM, CHROMIUM	↓ selenium and chromium levels	Attributed to ↑ loss of selenium and chromium	Be aware
PREDNISONE, CORTISONE	ZINC, CALCIUM, CHROMIUM, MAGNESIUM, SELENIUM	↓ plasma/body concentrations of these minerals	Attributed to ↑ loss and/or ↓ absorption	Be aware and monitor plasma concentrations of these minerals; provide supplements
ETHAMBUTOL	COPPER	↓ plasma concentration of copper	Ethambutol binds to copper	Be aware and separate oral intake by at least 2 hours
LEVODOPA, METHYLDOPA	IRON-CONTAINING COMPOUNDS	↓ plasma concentrations of methyldopa (peak levels ↓ by 55%) and levodopa, with risk of therapeutic failure	Iron preparations impair the absorption of methyldopa and levodopa	Be aware and separate oral intake by at least 2 hours
PENICILLAMINE	ZINC, IRON AND OTHER MINERALS	↓ plasma concentrations of several minerals	Due to formation of unabsorbable chelates	Separate oral intake by at least 2 hours
PROTON PUMP INHIBITORS	IRON	↓ plasma concentrations of iron	Proton pump inhibitors inhibit the absorption of iron	Consider use of parenteral iron in patients on proton pump inhibitors treatment
WARFARIN	MAGNESIUM, IRON, ZINC	↓ plasma/body concentrations of magnesium, iron and zinc	Due to ↓ absorption	Be aware
ZIDOVUDINE	ZINC	↓ plasma/body concentrations of zinc	Due to ↓ absorption	Be aware

Herbal drug	Allopathic drug	Clinical effects	Probable mechanism of interaction	Precautions
HERBAL DRUGS				
Herbs that may ↑ risk of bleeding				
1. Arnica 2. Bilberry leaf 3. Black cohosh 4. Boldo 5. *Capsicum* spp. (chilli pepper) 6. Chamomile 7. Chinese wolfberry (*Lycium barbarum*) 8. Clove 9. Cranberry juice 10. Curbicin (containing pumpkin seed – *Cucurbita pepo*) 11. Dan shen (*Salvia miitiorrhiza*) 12. Devil's claw 13. Dong quai 14. Evening primrose oil 15. Fenugreek 16. Feverfew 17. Garlic (*Allium sativum*) 18. Ginger 19. Ginkgo biloba 20. Ginseng 21. Goldenseal 22. Horse chestnut 23. Kangen-karyu (a mixture containing dan shen, saussurea root, cnidium, cyperus rhizomes) 24. Lycium 25. Melilot (sweet clover) 26. Papaya 27. Prickly ash 28. Quassia 29. Saw palmetto 30. Senna 31. Soy/soya 32. Tonka beans 33. Sweet woodruff 34. Tamarind 35. Umbelliferae 36. Willow 37. Woodruff	1. Aspirin 2. Clopidogrel 3. Ticlopidine 4. Dipyridamole 5. Warfarin 6. Heparin	May cause easy bruising and excessive bleeding from minor injuries. Reports of haemorrhage with concomitant use of warfarin and dan shen. INR may not always be altered. Case report with ginseng of normal coagulation studies during postoperative bleeding	• Antiplatelet effect (bilberry leaf, evening primrose, garlic, ginger, gingko biloba, ginseng). Clove contains eugenol derivatives, which inhibit platelets • Inhibit the metabolizing isoenzyme (CYP2C9) of warfarin (cranberry juice, dan shen, ginseng, lycium, soy/soya) • Coumarin constituents (black cohosh, chamomile, fenugreek, horse chestnut, sweet melilot, tonka beans, sweet woodruff). Naturally occurring coumarins are only weakly anticoagulant, but improper storage causes the production of dicoumarol by microbial transformation. Woodruff may contain constituents of warfarin • ↑ fibrinolytic activity (capsicum) • Unknown mechanisms (arnica, boldo, cucurbita, devil's claw, dong quai, kangen-karyu, papaya, saw palmetto) • ↓ vitamin K absorption (senna) • Other: tamarind ↑ bioavailability of aspirin. Meadow sweet and willow bark contain salicylates leading to ↑ effects of aspirin. Feverfew is considered to inhibit the release of serotonin from platelets	Inform physicians if either drug is introduced. Avoid changes in dosage of the herb. Monitor INR closely. If maintenance of the desired INR is difficult, avoid the herb. Monitor for ↑ tendency to bleed (petechiae, bruising, bleeding). Avoid concomitant use if possible

Herbs that may ↓ anticoagulant or antiplatelet effects				
1. Asian ginseng 2. Avocado 3. American ginseng 4. Goldenseal 5. Green tea 6. Psyllium seed (*Plantago psyllium*) 7. Ispaghula husk 8. Yarrow	1. Aspirin 2. Clopidogrel 3. Ticlopidine 4. Dipyridamole 5. Warfarin 6. Heparin	May ↓ effect of warfarin with ↓ INR, ↓ antiplatelet effects and antithrombotic effects	• ↓ absorption of warfarin (avocado, psyllium seed, ispaghula husk) • Unknown (ginseng, goldenseal) • Contains vitamin K, which antagonizes the action of warfarin (green tea). Poyphenols in tea (consumed in larger quantities) may inhibit the absorption of warfarin. Yarrow has been found to be a coagulant in vivo	Inform physicians if either drug is introduced. Avoid changes in dosage of the herb. Monitor INR closely. If maintenance of the desired INR is difficult, avoid the herb. Avoid concomitant use if possible
Herbs that may cause ↓ sedation				
1. Bai zhi 2. Calamus 3. Catnip 4. Elecampane 5. Jamaican dogwood 6. German chamomile 7. Hops 8. Kava kava 9. Passion flower 10. Valerian	BZDs and barbiturates 1. Alprazolam 2. Clobazam 3. Clonazepam 4. Diazepam 5. Midazolam 6. Nitrazepam 7. Triazolam 8. Quazepam 9. Flunitrazepam 10. Phenobarbitone 11. Primidone	↑ sedative effects	• Inhibits the metabolizing enzyme CYP3A4 (bai zhi, German chamomile) • Contains additive sedative action. May possess the ability to mediate GABA (catnip, German chamomile, hops, kava kava, passion flower, valerian)	Avoid driving and actions that need fine movements if either drug is added. ↓ dose of the herb if the patient is excessively sleepy
Herbs that may ↓ sedative action of sedatives				
1. Ginkgo biloba	BZDs and barbiturates as above	May antagonize the sedative action of these drugs	Induces the metabolizing enzyme CYP3A4: gingko weakly induces CYP2D6, which metabolizes alprazolam	Avoid concomitant use if possible. If the sedative action is impaired, discontinue the herb

Herbal drug	Allopathic drug	Clinical effects	Probable mechanism of interaction	Precautions
Herbs that may ↓ blood levels of anti-HIV drugs				
1. Garlic 2. Ginger 3. Milk thistle	1. Indinavir, 2. Lamivudine 3. Amprenavir 4. Saquinavir 5. Nelfinavir 6. Lopinavir 7. Efavirenz 8. Nevirapine	↓ blood levels of these drugs. Blood levels of saquinavir may be ↓ by garlic and ginger. Milk thistle ↓ blood levels of indinavir. Garlic ↑ gastrointestinal side-effects of ritonavir	• Induces metabolizing enzymes (CYP3A4). Garlic and ginger ↓ blood levels of saquinavir • Unknown mechanism (milk thistle) • Induction of transport protein P-gp (St John's wort)	Avoid concomitant use
Herbs that may ↑ blood levels of anti-HIV drugs				
1. *Piper longum* 2. *Hypoxis hemerocallidea*	1. Nevirapine	↑ blood levels, with potential risk of side-effects	• Inhibits metabolizing CYP450 isoenzyme (nevirapine) • Inhibits both CYP3A4 and P-gp (*Hypoxis hemerocallidea*)	If either drug is introduced, monitor closely for side-effects
Herbs that may ↑ effects of drugs used in blood sugar control				
1. Angelica dahurica 2. Aloe 3. Asian ginseng 4. Bai zhi 5. Garlic 6. Gingko biloba 7. Guarana 8. Karela (bitter melon) 9. Ma huang (*Ephedra sinica*) 10. Neem 11. Rosemary 12. Sage 13. Milk thistle	1. Tolbutamide 2. Metformin 3. Glimepiride 4. Glipizide 5. Glipizide 6. Glyburide 7. Insulin 8. Pioglitazone 9. Nateglinide 10. Repaglinide	May run the risk of low blood sugar	• ↓ absorption of sugar (aloe) • Unknown (Asian ginseng, garlic, karela, neem) • Inhibits CYP2E1 isoenzyme (bai zhi). Gingko biloba induces metabolism of tolbutamide) • May ↑ serum insulin level (rosemary ↑ insulin in rats)	Monitor blood glucose regularly when either drug is introduced. Once the blood sugar has been stabilized, avoid sudden changes of doses of either form of drug. Use alternative antidiabetic drugs metabolized less through CYP2E1 (pioglitazone, rosiglitazone, netoglitazone, repaglinide) when indicated. Avoid using longer-acting oral hypoglycaemic drugs such as glibenclamide, especially in elderly people. Report symptoms such as light-headedness, lethargy and sweating to the physician

Herbs that may ↓ effects of drugs used in blood sugar control				
1. Guar gum	1. Metformin 2. Glibenclamide	May lead to ↑ blood sugar levels	• ↓ absorption of metformin and glibenclamide	Avoid concomitant use. Monitor blood sugar closely if either drug is introduced
Herbs that may ↑ blood levels of antiepileptic medications or ↑ potency of antiepileptic medications				
1. Piper longum *2. Piper nigrum* 3. Willow 4. Valerian 5. Passion flower 6. Kava 7. Shankapushpi	1. Phenytoin 2. Carbamazepine 3. Valproate 4. Lamotrigine 5. Gabapentin	↑ phenytoin levels, which may lead to ↑ side-effects. Valerian, passion flower and kava kava may theoretically potentiate antiepileptic drugs as animal experiments have revealed antiseizure activity. Valerian constituents inhibit breakdown of GABA and enhance BZD binding, which could potentiate the effects of carbamazepine	• Inhibition of transport (P-gp) and metabolizing enzymes (CYP2C9 and CYP3A4). Piperine found in *Piper nigrum* (black pepper) and *Piper longum* ↑ bioavailability of phenytoin • Displaces from protein binding (salicylate contained in willow displaces phenytoin from binding sites) • Passion flower contains chrysin, which is a partial agonist at GABA receptors and shows antiseizure effects	Closely monitor for side effects of phenytoin if *Piper nigrum* is introduced. Avoid sudden withdrawal of the herb after stabilization to avoid breakthrough seizures
Herbs that may ↓ plasma levels of antiepileptic drugs or ↓ seizure threshold				
1. Borage oil 2. Ginkgo biloba 3. Evening primrose oil 4. Plantain 5. Sage 6. Shankapushpi 7. Guarana, cola (contain caffeine) 8. Volatile oils, e.g. rosemary, sage, hyssop, fennel	1. Valproate 2. Carbamazepine	↓ valproate and carbamazepine levels and may precipitate seizures. Evening primrose oil and borage oil contain gamolenic acid, which is reported to ↓ seizure threshold. Report of tonic-clonic seizures in subjects without a prior history of epilepsy after using essential oils transdermally and orally	• Unknown mechanism (ginkgo biloba ↓ valproate levels) • ↓ seizure threshold (evening primrose oil, shankhapushpi) • Plantain ↓ absorption of valproate • Caffeine is known to ↓ seizure threshold and exacerbate seizures in animals. Volatile oils contain epileptogenic compounds (e.g. cineole, camphor, fenchone), which can be absorbed through the skin during aromatherapy. Sage is known to cause seizures in large doses	Avoid concomitant use if possible. Avoid eating plantains 30 minutes before and after carbamazepine. Avoid concomitant use of St John's wort, especially in patients with poor seizure control. Avoid driving and work with machinery if either drug is introduced

MISCELLANEOUS HERBAL DRUGS

Herbal drug	Allopathic drug	Clinical effects	Probable mechanism of interaction	Precautions
Herbs that may ↑ cardiac glycoside effects or levels				
1. Adonis 2. Aloe 3. Ashwagandha 4. Asian ginseng 5. Broom 6. Cascara 7. Dan shen (*Salvia mitiorrhiza)* 8. Devil's claw 9. Echinacea 10. Ginger 11. Ginkgo biloba 12. Ginseng 13. Ginseng (Siberian) 14. Hawthorn 15. Kyushin 16. Liquorice 17. Plantain 18. Oleander 19. Rhubarb 20. Squill 21. Uzara root	1. Digoxin 2. Digitoxin 3. Ouabain 4. Deslanoside	May worsen the adverse effects of cardiac glycosides. May give rise to falsely ↑ or ↓ digoxin levels	• Contains cardiac glycosides or cardioactive substances (adonis, broom, devil's claw, ginger, hawthorn, oleander, squill) • Lowers serum potassium (aloe, cascara, liquorice, rhubarb) • Interferes with digoxin assay using fluorescence polarization immunoassay (ashwagandha, ginseng and Siberian ginseng falsely elevate, Asian ginseng and dan shen ↑ or ↓ levels) • Inhibits P-gp (echinacea, ginkgo biloba) • ↑ levels due to unknown mechanism (ginseng)	Avoid the concomitant use of herbs that contain cardiac glycosides with these drugs. Monitor serum potassium, and administer potassium supplements orally if indicated. Take drugs 1 hour before or 2 hours after herbal products. Avoid taking ashwagandha and Asian ginseng at least a week before digoxin assay
Herbs that may ↓ cardiac glycoside levels				
1. Guar gum 2. Senna	1. Digoxin 2. Digitoxin 3. Ouabain 4. Deslanoside	May lower therapeutic effect	• May lower the absorption of these drugs (guar gum, senna) • Induces P-gp (St John's wort)	Avoid concomitant use. Monitor for worsening of therapeutic effects if the herb is introduced. If used concomitantly, take herbs at least 1 hour before and after these drugs
Herbs that may ↑ antibiotic blood levels				
1. *Piper nigrum* and *Piper longum*	1. Amoxicillin 2. Cefotaxime 3. Rifampicin 4. Erythromycin 5. Telithromycin	↑ blood levels of these antibiotics	• Attributed to inhibition of metabolism and of P-gp, e.g. *Piper longum*	Be aware that toxic effects of antibiotics may occur, particularly when the prescriber/dispenser is unaware of the intake of herbal medicines

MISCELLANEOUS HERBAL DRUGS

Herbs that may ↓ antibiotic blood levels				
1. Dandelion 2. Fennel 3. Guar gum 4. Khat 5. Yohimbine	1. Ciprofloxacin 2. Amoxicillin 3. Penicillin 4. Tetracycline	↓ blood levels may potentially ↓ antibacterial potential	• Unknown mechanism (dandelion ↓ ciprofloxacin levels in rats; khat ↓ absorption and thus blood levels of ampicillin and amoxicillin, possibly due to the formation of a tannin–antibiotic complex; guar gum ↓ absorption of penicillin) • Other mechanism (yohimbine chelates tetracyclines). Fennel extracts are considered to chelate with ciprofloxacin	Be aware. Discontinue the herb during the course of antibiotic therapy. Penicillins should be taken on an empty stomach
Herbs that may ↓ immunosuppressant effects				
1. Astralagus 2. Echinacea 3. Liquorice 4. Milk thistle 5. Neem 6. Sea buckthorn	1. Ciclosporin 2. Azathioprine 3. Methotrexate 4. Tacrolimus 5. Daclizumab 6. Cyclophosphamide	Possibility of graft rejection	• ↓ blood level; unknown mechanism (astralagus). • Other mechanisms:alkyl amides from echinacea modulate tumour necrosis factor alpha mRNA expression in human monocytes/macrophages via the cannabinoid type 2 receptor • Unknown mechanism (milk thistle is known to ↓ cyclosporine levels; neem ↓ effects of azathioprine, prednisolone and daclizumab; sea buckthorn may ↓ effect of cyclophosphamide) • Induces metabolizing enzymes, CYP3A4 and P-gp (St John's wort ↓ ciclosporin and tacrolimus levels)	Avoid concomitant use of the herb

Herbal drug	Allopathic drug	Clinical effects	Probable mechanism of interaction	Precautions
Herbs that may ↑ immunosuppressant effects				
1. Black cohosh 2. Geum chiloense 3. Liquorice	1. Cisplatin 2. Azathioprine 3. Ciclosporin 4. Prednisolone	↑ cytotoxic properties. Geum ↑ plasma ciclosporin levels 6–8-fold	• Unknown mechanism (black cohosh) • Inhibits metabolizing enzymes. Glycyrrhizin present in liquorice inhibits the metabolizing enzyme of prednisolone, 11 beta-hydroxysteroid dehydrogenase, which converts the active metabolite to an inactive form. ↓ clearance of prednisolone in healthy individuals	Be aware. Advice is to avoid echinacea with immunosuppressants
Herbs that may ↓ effects of anticancer medication				
1. Aloe 2. Soy/soya 3. Red clover 4. Kava kava 5. Ginseng 6. Garlic 7. Echinacea 8. Beta-carotene 9. Quercetin	1. Cisplatin 2. Tamoxifen	Lower the anticancer activity of these drugs. Most oncolytic drugs have a narrow therapeutic window	• Red clover and soya contain oestrogenic isoflavonoids. Unknown mechanism with aloe • Induces the metabolizing enzyme (soy induces CYP isoenzymes that metabolize tamoxifen)	It is best to avoid the concomitant use of herbs with hormonal effects (includes dong quai, chasteberry, black cohosh) in patients with hormone-dependent cancers, e.g. breast cancer
Herbs that may ↑ effects of anticancer medication				
1. Black cohosh 2. Caffeine 3. Evening primrose oil *4. Scutellaria baicalensis* 5. Starflower (borage)	1. Docetaxel 2. Paclitaxel 3. Doxorubicin 4. Tamoxifen 5. Cisplatin 6. Vinorelbine	↑ cytotoxic properties	• Unknown mechanism (black cohosh). Caffeine ↑ cytotoxic effects of cisplatin; wogonin present in *Scutellaria* enhances etoposide-induced apoptosis. Gamolenic acid found in evening primrose oil and borage potentiated the in vitro toxicity of paclitaxel and vinorelbine, attributed to an unsaturated fatty acid as modulators of tumour cell chemosensitivity	Be aware and avoid concomitant use

Herbs that may interact with MAOIs				
1. Anise 2. Asian ginseng 3. Cereus 4. Ephedra 5. Ginseng 6. Parsley 7. Shepherds purse 8. Verbena (vervain) 9. Capsicum	1. Phenelzine 2. Tranylcypromine 3. Moclobemide	May cause ↑ blood pressure with anise and ephedra. ↑ risk of side-effects such as psychosis and hallucinations with Asian ginseng. Headache, tremulousness and manic episodes have been reported with ginseng and phenelzine	• Unknown mechanism (anise, Asian ginseng) • Inhibits metabolism of ephedra (MAOIs inhibit the metabolism of ephedra)	Avoid concomitant use
Herbs that may ↓ effects of diuretics				
1. Aloe 2. Dandelion 3. Elder 4. Liquorice 5. Nettle 6. Rhubarb	1. Bendroflumethiazide 2. Bumetanide 3. Chlortalidone 4. Hydrochlorothiazide 5. Indapamide 6. Furosemide 7. Torasemide	Low body potassium, which may give rise to lethargy and muscle weakness	• ↑ potassium loss from the gut (aloe, liquorice) • Possess diuretic properties (dandelion, elder, nettle, rhubarb)	Avoid concomitant use. Provide potassium supplements orally. Use a potassium-sparing diuretic such as spironolactone or amiloride
Herbs that may ↑ effects of diuretics				
1. Couchgrass 2. Ginkgo biloba 3. Ginseng 4. Guar gum 5. Comfrey	1. Bendroflumethiazide 2. Bumetanide 3. Chlortalidone 4. Hydrochlorothiazide 5. Torasemide	Poor blood pressure control and diuresis	• Unknown (ginkgo biloba ↓ effect of thiazide diuretics; ginseng) • ↓ absorption (guar gum has been shown to ↓ absorption of bumetanide)	Avoid concomitant use of the herb if blood pressure control is poor

Herbal drug	Allopathic drug	Clinical effects	Probable mechanism of interaction	Precautions
Herbs that may interfere with antihypertension medication				
1. Betel nut *2. Piper longum*/*Piper nigrum* 3. Black cohosh 4. Capsicum 5. Cowslip 6. Ginkgo biloba 7. Gingseng 8. Hawthorn 9. Indian snakeroot 10. Liquorice (*Glycyrrhiza glabra*) 11. Parsley	1. Beta-blockers (atenolol, acebutolol, bisoprolol, carvedilol, esmolol, labetolol, metoprolol, nadolol, nebivolol, pindolol, sotalol, timolol) 2. Calcium channel blockers (amlodipine, diltiazem, felodipine, isradipine, lacidipine, nicardipine, nifedipine, nimodipine, nisoldipine, verapamil) 3. ACE inhibitors and angiotensin II receptor blockers (captopril, lisinopril, enalapril, verapamil, losartan , candesartan)	Has been known to worsen bradycardia and hypotension. May worsen cough associated with ACE inhibitors	• Betel nut causes bradycardia and hawthorn ↓ blood pressure through unknown mechanisms. Piperine, a constituent of black pepper and other species (e.g. *Piper nigrum*), ↑ bioavailability of propranolol. Indian snakeroot was found to contain a 'reserpine'-like constituent • Inhibits the metabolizing enzymes. *Piper longum* inhibits CYP1A1 and CYPA2, which metabolize propranolol. Ginkgo inhibits metabolism of nifedipine, nicardipine (CYP3A4) and propranolol (CYP1A2) enzymes. Gingseng inhibits CYP3A4 and ↑ nifedipine levels. Goldenseal inhibits losartan's metabolizing enzyme. Grapefruit inhibits the metabolizing enzyme (CYP3A4) of felodipine, nicardipine, nifedipine, nisoldipine or nitrendipine. Grapefruit juice may also inhibit the metabolism of verapamil and losartan • Unknown (black cohosh) • Other mechanisms (capsicum depletes substance P; cowslip has demonstrated hypotensive properties in animals)	Inform physicians if either drug is introduced. Avoid sudden changes of the herb dose. Monitor PR and blood pressure closely if either drug is introduced. Discontinue the herb if side-effects worsen. Use alternative antihypertensive medications if possible (e.g. replace beta-blockers and calcium channel blockers with ACE inhibitors or angiotensin II receptor blockers if bradycardia is worsened, and replace ACE inhibitors with angiotensin II receptor blockers if cough is worsened)

MISCELLANEOUS HERBAL DRUGS

Herbs that may ↓ effect of antihypertension medication				
1. Broom 2. Ephedra 3. Glycyrrhizin (liquorice) 4. Ma huang 5. Sage 6. Yohimbe	The antihypertensive drugs mentioned above	Poor control of hypertension	• Causes peripheral vasoconstriction (broom) • Contains vasoconstrictive alkaloids (ephedrine). Ma huang (a constituent of slimming pills, decongestants and antiasthma drugs) contains ephedrine • Pseudoaldosteronism (glycyrrhizin causes pseudaldosteronism and antagonises the effect of ACE inhibitors) • Yohimbe bark contains yohimbine, which is a presynaptic alpha-2 adrenoceptor agonist (and possibly an MAOI)	Avoid concomitant use
Herbs that may ↑ effect of anti arrhythmic medication				
1. Adonis 2. Guarana 3. Liquorice 4. Milk thistle 5. Scopolia 6. Squill	1. Quinidine 2. Amiodarone 3. Adenosine 4. Procainamide	May cause ↑ adverse effects of quinidine and amiodarone. ↑ risk of prolonged Q–T interval on ECG	• Additive inotropic effects of the constituent cardiac glycosides of the herb (adonis and squill) • Inhibits metabolizing enzymes (grapefruit juice inhibits CYP3A4, which metabolizes amiodarone and quinidine; milk thistle inhibits the metabolizing enzyme of amiodarone (CYP3A4) • Unknown (liquorice, scopolia)	Avoid concomitant use. Monitor for side-effects of amiodarone if the herb is introduced. Inform physicians if used concomitantly. Monitor Q–T interval
Herbs that may ↓ effect of antiarrhythmic medication				
1. Guar gum	1. Adenosine	↓ blood levels and therapeutic effects	• Unknown	Be aware

MISCELLANEOUS HERBAL DRUGS

Herbal drug	Allopathic drug	Clinical effects	Probable mechanism of interaction	Precautions
Herbs that may ↑ effects of antidepressant medication				
1. Broom 2. Ginkgo biloba 3. Scopolia 4. Yohimbine	1. TCAs (e.g. amitriptyline, nortriptyline, clomipramine) 2. SSRIs (e.g. fluvoxamine fluoxetine, paroxetine) 3. Venlafaxine 4. Trazodone	May develop cardiac arrhythmias and side-effects such as dryness of the mouth, retention of urine and tachycardia. ↑ sedation	• Broom contains cardioactive alkalamines such as sparteine • Inhibits metabolizing enzymes • Anticholinergic properties (hyoscine present in scopolia may worsen side-effects of TCAs-additive antimuscarinic effects) • Yohimbine alone can cause hypertension, but lower doses cause hypertension when combined with TCAs • Unknown mechanism (ginkgo ↑ sedative effects of trazodone) • St John's wort inhibits the uptake of serotonin and thereby ↑ serotonin levels	Avoid concomitant use. An SSRI may be a better alternative to be used with broom
Herbs that may ↑ effects of antipsychotic medication				
1. Betel nut 2. Caffeine 3. Ephedra 4. Ginkgo biloba 5. Hops 6. Kava kava 7. Valerian	1. Phenothiazines (e.g. chlorpromazine, promazine, levomepromazine, pericyazine, pipotiazine, fluphenazine, perphenazine, trifluphenazine) 2. Clozapine 3. Lithium 4. Haloperidol 5. Risperidone	Worsening of side-effects such as slowness, stiffness and tremor. ↑ blood levels. A single case report of priapism induced by a ginkgo–risperidone combination. Hyperthermia	• Unknown mechanism (betel nut worsens the side-effects of flupentixol and fluphenazine). Ginkgo may ↑ haloperidol effects. Kava kava ↑ side-effects of haloperidol and risperidone • Inhibits metabolizing enzymes (caffeine inhibits CYP1A2, which metabolizes clozapine). Inhibition of CYP by ginkgo ↑ alpha-1 effects of risperidone. Valerian may worsen the sedative properties of haloperidol. Hops and phenothiazine have been associated with hyperthermia in dogs • Worsens the cardiovascular effects of phenothiazines (ephedra)	Be aware. Discontinue the herb if the side-effects of these drugs ↑

Herbs that may ↓ effects of antipsychotic medication				
1. Caffeine 2. Chaste tree 3. Green tea 4. Plantain (*Plantain orata, Plantain psyllium*) 5. Ispaghula (*psyllium*)	1. Lithium 2. Phenothiazines (e.g. chlorpromazine, promazine, levomepromazine, pericyazine, pipotiazine, fluphenazine, perphenazine, trifluphenazine) 3. Clozapine	↓ blood lithium levels with ↓ clinical effects with ispaghula and psyllium. ↓ effects of phenothiazines. Herbal diuretics contained in a mixture of juniper, buchu, horsetail, corn silk, bearberry, parsley, bromelain and paprika caused lithium toxicity	• Unknown mechanism (caffeine) • Contains dopamine agonists (chaste tree) • Induction of metabolizing enzymes (green tea may induce CYP1A2, which metabolizes clozapine) • ↓ absorption from the gut (plantain, psyllium and ispaghula may ↓ absorption of lithium, or preparations may have high a sodium content in the form of sodium bicarbonate to aid their dispersal in water before ingestion). Herbal diuretics are weak compared with their allopathic counterparts. This may be due to diuresis or other factors, e.g. enzyme inhibition	Be aware. Caffeine withdrawal may precipitate lithium toxicity, so avoid sudden caffeine withdrawal. Avoid concomitant use if possible
Herbs that may interact with melatonin				
1. Ashwagandha 2. Celery 3. Chamomile 4. German chamomile 5. Goldenseal 6. Hops 7. Kava kava 8. Valerian	1. Melatonin	May cause ↑ sedation	Unknown mechanism	Be aware

Herbal drug	Allopathic drug	Clinical effects	Probable mechanism of interaction	Precautions
Herbs that may ↑ risk of theophylline adverse effects				
1. *Piper longum* 2. Caffeine 3. Capsicum 4. Dan shen 5. Ephedra 6. Green tea 7. Guarana 8. Squill	1. Theophylline	↑ plasma level of theophylline and may potentiate side-effects. Ephedra, caffeine, squill and green tea may worsen tachycardia and palpitation	• Inhibition of CYP 450 enzymes (*Piper longum*, dan shen) • Additive sympathetic stimulation (caffeine, ephedra, green tea, guarana) • May ↑ absorption (capsicum) • Unknown mechanism (squill)	Inform physicians if either drug is introduced. Avoid sudden changes of the herb dose. Discontinue the herb if side-effects worsen
Herbs that may interfere with general anaesthetic medication				
1. Black cohosh 2. Kava kava 3. Ginkgo 4. Ginseng 5. Garlic 6. Goldenseal 7. Ma huang 8. Echinacea 9. Aloe 10. Ephedra 11. Sage 12. Sassafras 13. Valerian 14. Wild carrot	Anaesthetic medication, including drugs used in premedication, induction, maintenance of anaesthesia, muscle relaxation, analgesia (intra- and postoperative), bleeding and recovery	These effects are attributed to herbs that may have sedating properties (e.g. valerian, kava kava) or cause ↑ bleeding (e.g. garlic, ginger, gingko), or those that may cause changes in blood pressure (often unpredictable), e.g. black cohosh, ma huang, ephedra. Also mentioned are herbs that may interfere with healing (e.g. echinacea). Aloe vera ↓ prostaglandin synthesis and inhibits aggregations of platelets, while sevoflurane inhibits thromboxane A2 formation, resulting in ↑ blood loss	Herbal preparations are known to: • ↑ intra- and postoperative bleeding • ↑ CNS effects of drugs used in anaesthesia • cause unpredictable changes in blood pressure and PR • cause unpredictable effects on the excretions of drugs used during anaesthesia	The American Society of Anaesthesiologists has recommended that all herbal medications be stopped 2–3 weeks prior to an elective surgical procedure. Employ stringent measures related to discontinuing ginkgo, ginseng and garlic because of ↑ risk of bleeding. Discontinue black cohosh 2 weeks before surgery. Inform the anaesthetist before the procedure
Herbs that may interact with phosphodiesterase inhibitors use for impotence				
1. Squill	1. Sildenafil 2. Tadalafil 3. Vardenafil	↑ blood levels of the drug, leading to serious vasodilatation. ↑ risk of cardiac arrhythmia	• Inhibits CYP3A4, which metabolizes these drugs (grapefruit juice) • Unknown mechanism (squill)	Avoid concomitant use. Avoid the combination of grapefruit juice and nitrates with these medications

Herbs that may ↑ side-effects of lipid-lowering agents				
1. Goldenseal	1. Atorvastatin 2. Simvastatin 3. Lovastatin	↑ blood levels of atorvastatin (grapefruit juice) and lovastatin (goldenseal), with ↑ risk of side-effects (e.g. muscle pain due to rhabdomyolysis)	• Possibly through inhibition of P-gp. Also through the inhibition of CYP3A4. Goldenseal inhibits CYP3A4	Avoid concomitant use. Report muscle pain to physicians. Suitable alternatives are pravastatin, rosuvastatin and fluvastatin, which interact less with P-gp. Pravastatin and rosuvastatin are mainly excreted unchanged, and fluvastatin (CYP2C9) is not metabolized through CYP3A4
Herbs that may interfere with ACh receptor antagonists				
1. Areca nut	1 Procyclidine (used to control extrapyramidal – parkinsonian – with antipsychotic medications)	Caused severe rigidity and jaw tremor. This is an established and clinically significant interaction	• Procyclidine is an antimuscarinic agent, i.e. antagonizes the effects of ACh in one set of ACh receptors. Thus, herbal products used culturally with effects similar to ACh, e.g. areca nut, will produce enhanced effects at other – nicotinic – receptors to produce adverse effects	Avoid chewing betel nut (also found in prepared 'pan masala')
Herbs that may ↓ effects of antidepressant medications				
1. St John's wort	1. TCAs (e.g. amitryptyline, nortryptiline, clomipramine) 2. SSRIs (e.g. fluvoxamine, fluoxetine) 3. Venlafaxine	Low blood amitriptyline levels (<20%). May potentially ↓ therapeutic effects. Nortriptyline levels may be ↓ by 50%. St John's wort ↑ sedative effects (weakness, lethargy, fatigue, slow movements, incoherence) of SSRIs	• Due to induction of metabolizing CYP3A4 enzyme and P-gp transport proteins • St John's wort inhibits uptake of serotonin and thereby ↑ serotonin levels	Avoid concomitant use

Herbal drug	Allopathic drug	Clinical effects	Probable mechanism of interaction	Precautions
Herbs that may ↑ effects of antipsychotic medication				
1. Betel nut 2. Caffeine 3. Ephedra 4. Ginkgo biloba 5. Hops 6. Kava kava 7. Valerian	1, Phenothiazines (e.g. chlorpromazine, promazine, levomepromazine, pericyazine, pipotiazine, fluphenazine, perphenazine, trifluphenazine) 2. Clozapine 3. Lithium 4. Haloperidol 5. Risperidone	Worsen side-effects such as slowness, stiffness and tremor. ↑ blood levels. A single case report of priapism induced by a ginkgo–risperidone combination. Hyperthermia	• Unknown mechanism (betel nut worsens the side-effects of flupentixol and fluphenazine). Ginkgo may ↑ haloperidol effects. Kava kava ↑ side-effects of haloperidol and risperidone • Inhibits metabolizing enzymes (caffeine inhibits CYP1A2, which metabolizes clozapine). Inhibition of CYP by ginkgo ↑ alpha-1 effects of risperidone. Valerian may worsen the sedative properties of haloperidol. Hops and phenothiazine have been associated with hyperthermia in dogs • Worsens the cardiovascular effects of phenothiazines (ephedra)	Be aware. Discontinue the herb if the side-effects of these drugs ↑
Herbs that may ↓ effects of antipsychotic medication				
1. Caffeine 2. Chaste tree 3. Green tea 4. Plantain	1. Lithium 2. Phenothiazines (e.g. chlorpromazine, promazine, levomepromazine, pericyazine, pipotiazine, fluphenazine, perphenazine, trifluphenazine) 3. Clozapine	↓ blood lithium levels with ↓ clinical effects. ↓ effects of phenothiazines	• Unknown mechanism (caffeine) • Contains dopamine agonists (chaste tree) • Induction of metabolizing enzymes (green tea may induce CYP1A2, which metabolizes clozapine) • ↓ absorption from the gut (plantain may ↓ absorption of lithium)	Be aware. Caffeine withdrawal may precipitate lithium toxicity, so avoid sudden caffeine withdrawal. Avoid concomitant use if possible

Herbs that may interact with melatonin				
1. Ashwagandha 2. Celery 3. Chamomile 4. German chamomile 5. Goldenseal 6. Hops 7. Kava kava 8. Valerian	1. Melatonin	May cause ↑ sedation	• Unknown mechanism	Be aware
Herbs that may ↑ risk of theophylline side-effects				
1. Piper longum 2. Caffeine 3. Capsicum 4. Dan shen 5. Ephedra 6. Green tea 7. Guarana 8. Squill	1. Theophylline	↑ plasma level of theophylline and may potentiate side-effects Ephedra, caffeine, squill and green tea may worsen tachycardia and palpitation	• Inhibition of CYP450 enzymes (*Piper longum*, dan shen) • Additive sympathetic stimulation (caffeine, ephedra, green tea, guarana) • May ↑ absorption (capsicum) • Unknown mechanism (squill)	Inform physicians if either drug is introduced. Avoid sudden changes of the herb dose. Discontinue the herb if side-effects worsen
Herbs that may ↓ effect of theophylline				
1. St John's wort 2. Royal jelly	1. Theophylline	↓ theophylline levels and risk of therapeutic failure	• Due to activation of metabolizing CYP1A2 enzymes, which metabolize theophylline	Discontinue St John's wort if the therapeutic effects of theophylline ↓
Herbs that may interact with phosphodiesterase inhibitors used for impotence				
1. Grapefruit juice 2. Squill	1. Sildenafil 2. Tadalafil 3. Vardenafil	↑ blood levels of the medication, leading to serious vasodilatation. ↑ risk of cardiac arrhythmia	• Inhibits CYP3A4, which metabolizes these drugs (grapefruit juice) • Unknown mechanism (squill)	Avoid concomitant use. Avoid the combination of grapefruit juice and nitrates with these medications

MISCELLANEOUS HERBAL DRUGS

Herbal drug	Allopathic drug	Clinical effects	Probable mechanism of interaction	Precautions
Herbs that may ↑ adverse effects of lipid-lowering agents				
1. Grapefruit juice 2. Goldenseal	1. Atorvastatin 2. Simvastatin 3. Lovastatin	↑ blood levels of atorvastatin (grapefruit juice) and lovastatin (goldenseal) with ↑ risk of side-effects (e.g. muscle pain due to rhabdomyolysis)	• Possibly through inhibition of P-gp. Also through inhibition of CYP3A4 (grapefruit juice). Goldenseal inhibits CYP3A4	Avoid concomitant use. Report muscle pain to physicians. Suitable alternatives are pravastatin, rosuvastatin and fluvastatin, which interact less with P-gp. Pravastatin and rosuvastatin are mainly excreted unchanged, while fluvastatin (CYP2C9) is not metabolized through CYP3A4
Herbs that may ↓ effects of lipid-lowering agents				
1. St John's wort	1. Atorvastatin 2. Simvastatin 3. Lovastatin	↓ blood levels and lipid-lowering effect	• Induction of metabolizing CYP3A4 enzymes, which metabolize simvastatin	Avoid concomitant use if possible. Monitor response to simvastatin closely. Avoid sudden changes of the herb dosage
Herbs that may interfere with oral contraceptive medication				
1. St John's wort 2. Red clover 3. Saw palmetto	1. Oral contraceptives	Failure of contraception. Theoretically, saw palmetto could interfere with oral contraception and hormone replacement therapy	St John's wort preparations induce metabolizing CYP3A4 enzymes and glycoprotein drug transporters of these medications	Avoid concomitant use. Use an alternative contraceptive methods (barrier methods) if the herb is introduced
Herbs that may cause additive hepatotoxicity				
1. Echinacea	1. Hepatotoxic drugs, e.g. anabolic steroids 2. amiodarone 3. Methotrexate 4. Ketoconazole	Risk of additive hepatotoxicity	• Use of echinacea for over 8 weeks can cause hepatotoxicity	Be aware and use drugs with a potential to cause hypertonicity cautiously, monitoring clinically and biochemically for any early signs of hepatic dysfunction

MISCELLANEOUS HERBAL DRUGS

Herbs that may cause additive endocrine effects				
1. Ginseng 2. Saw palmetto 3. Kelp 4. Sage	1. Corticosteroids 2. Oestrogens 3. Androgens (e.g. finasteride, flutamide) 4. Thyroid replacement therapy	Risk of additive/antagonistic hormonal effects. Kelp may interfere with thyroid therapy. Saw palmetto interferes with male hormones and oestrogen-containing therapies	• Additive/antagonistic hormonal effects. Kelp is a source of iodine. Sage may increase TSH levels	Be aware
Herbs that may ↓ absorption of co-administered drugs				
1. St John's wort 2. Saw palmetto	1. Iron	↓ absorption of co-administered iron	• Due to tannic acid content	Be aware and separate oral intake by at least 2 hours
Herbs that may interfere with drugs used in the treatment of migraine				
1. Feverfew	1. Antimigraine drugs, e.g. sumatriptan	↑ risk of episodes of tachycardia and hypertension (may be dangerous)	The parthenolide constituent of feverfew has been shown to inhibit the release of serotonin and prostaglandins. Sumatriptan is an SSRI	Avoid concomitant use
Herbs that may interfere with drugs used in the treatment of Alzheimer's disease				
	1. Donepezil 2. Galant-amine 3. Memantine	May be ↑ anticholinergic effects	Sage possesses some anticholinergic effects, such as that on sweating	Be aware

Part 18 OVER-THE-COUNTER DRUGS

More OTC drugs have been introduced to encourage self-care for minor ailments and for patients to take greater responsibility for their own health. This section gives an overview of the constituents of OTC drugs that could be involved in adverse drug interactions.

Also considered are drugs available for purchase online. An important difference between OTC drugs and those available online is that approval for drugs available OTC has undergone a rather rigorous assessment by regulatory bodies such as the Medicines and HealthCare Products Regulatory Agency in the UK, while drugs available online include drugs that are available only on prescription in the UK (e.g. diazepam, sildenafil) and include a wide range of hallucinogens and similar drugs affecting the CNS, which are often illegal in a particular country or state (as in the USA).

The FDA's Consumer Health Information Web page (www.fda.gov/consumer), updated on 27th February 2009, warns consumers about the possible dangers of buying medicines over the Internet. This provides the opportunity for drug interactions to occur that may not be reported, especially with traditional remedies, or may not be detected because of the anonymity that consumers desire when purchasing drugs online. In addition, any increase in the number of preparations taken by an individual, including medications of varying composition bought from multiple online sites, increases the likelihood of potential interactions. The delay in identifying these potential interactions may have severe, even life-threatening consequences.

In simple terms, 'rogue websites' often sell unapproved drugs. In the USA, the FDA states that counterfeit drugs (fake or copycat products) may:

- be contaminated with dangerous ingredients;
- not provide the desired therapeutic response;
- cause serious side-effects;
- contain the wrong active ingredient;
- be made with the wrong amount of active ingredient (varying from no active ingredient to too much) and be packaged in phoney packaging that looks legitimate.

Some sites that offer prescription drugs without prescription provide assurances of free medical consultations and the services of experienced trusted fully licensed pharmacists. However, the range of drugs available online (some sites offering over 1000 medications) cause severe concerns associated with adverse drug interactions as they include BZDs (e.g. alprazolam, lorazepam), antidepressants (escitalopram, fluoxetine), antimigraine drugs (e.g. sibutramine), hypnotics (e.g. zolpidem), sildenafil, injectable testosterone, human growth hormone and drugs used in the treatment of asthma, skin disorders (e.g. psoriasis) and fungal infections (e.g. itraconazole). The patient's past medical history and current drug armamentarium may also not be fully taken into account.

More and more traditional medicines and nutritional supplements are available. Such preparations have the potential for serious drug interactions (e.g. St John's wort, grapefruit juice, ginseng, ephedra, garlic). Furthermore, traditional medicines in particular may contain heavy metals (e.g. mercury, lead, arsenic) or adulterants (which may be banned in the country of use, e.g. fenfluramine, phenylbutazone). Many online and OTC drugs also contain glucose, sodium and potassium as constituents, so patients with diabetes, renal impairment and heart failure should take extra precautions when using these drugs.

The UK's Medicines Control Agency investigated 24 British websites as, under the Medicines Act of 1968, it is illegal to sell prescription drugs to an individual without a prescription. Unfortunately, as many online pharmacies operate internationally, the Medicines Control Agency has no jurisdiction abroad.

This résumé is intended to warn consumers in particular and also to make doctors and pharmacists aware of the likelihood that people seeking prescriptions or medications will take drugs from online pharmacies and possibly not reveal them to either the doctor or the pharmacist. It is important for healthcare professionals to specifically ask whether the patient uses drugs bought online, as well as asking about prescribed medicines, OTC drugs and supplements, and traditional and herbal remedies.

The following is an overview of interactions that may occur with OTC drugs. The OTC drugs are classified following the classification used in the September 2008 edition of *Guide to OTC Medicines and Diagnostics*.

Analgesics

Although interactions with OTC analgesics are infrequent, there is a common perception among the general public that analgesics are harmless; therefore they may not realize that there is potential for interactions with drugs that cause additive adverse effects on the gastric mucosa, kidney or liver (e.g. **aspirin**, **NSAIDs**). Dangerous interactions with antidepressants (e.g. **MAOIs**) may also occur (from opioids such as **codeine** and **dextromethorphan** in several cough and flu remedies).

In addition, inadvertent overdose may occur if OTC analgesics or analgesic-containing 'cold cures' are taken in addition to prescribed analgesics. For example, systemic toxicity may occur if **paracetamol** is taken in a dose greater than 150 mg/kg body weight per day. It is also important to ensure that an age-appropriate dose for each constituent is dispensed.

Ibuprofen and other NSAIDs, even in therapeutic doses, may precipitate symptoms of heart failure due to fluid retention in susceptible individuals.

Aspirin and NSAIDs

Some interactions that may occur are:

- **Antacids** – decrease the absorption of NSAIDs.
- **Other NSAIDs** – an additive irritant effect on the gastric mucosa.
- **Anticoagulants** – a risk of catastrophic haemorrhage from the gastric mucosa. Remember that other drugs, for example antidepressants such as **SSRIs** and **MAOIs**, may have an anticoagulant side-effect.
- **Antigout drugs** (e.g. probenecid and sulphinpyrazone) decrease the uricosuric effect.
- **Methotrexate**, which is used for several disease states such as rheumatoid arthritis (where OTC analgesics are often taken to relieve pain) or malignant disease, as a cytotoxic (where pain relief also becomes important) – increased methotrexate levels may occur, with risk of toxicity.
- **Diuretics** (commonly referred to as 'water pills'), which are used to treat heart failure and high blood pressure – a decreased effect of these drugs because NSAIDs cause fluid retention.
- **Antiepileptics** – aspirin may cause an elevation and even toxic effects of phenytoin and valproate.
- **Antidiabetic drugs** – high-dose aspirin may cause hypoglycaemia, which may add to the effect of the drugs used to treat diabetes mellitus, thus increasing the risk of hypoglycaemic episodes.

For full details of the potential interactions, see:

- Aspirin – Cardiovascular Drugs, Antiplatelets
- NSAIDs – Analgesics, Non-steroidal anti-inflammatory drugs

Paracetamol

It is necessary to be aware that paracetamol may cause liver damage in overdose; in certain susceptible individuals, the toxic dose is reduced (>75 mg/kg compared with 150 mg/kg for non-susceptible individuals). Malnutrition, chronic alcoholism and HIV infection all make people more susceptible.

The absorption of paracetamol is decreased by anion exchange resins (**colestyramine**), whereas some drugs used to control nausea and vomiting, such as **metoclopramide** and **domperidone**, hasten the absorption of paracetamol.

For full details of potential interactions, see Analgesics, Paracetamol

Opioids

Several OTC pain relievers contain codeine, which can cause additive depression of the CNS when used with other sedative drugs:

- **alcohol**;
- **antihistamines**, which are both prescribable and found in OTC cold and flu preparations, and as treatment for travel sickness;
- **anxiolytics** and **hypnotics** – 'sleeping tablets' such as BZDs or 'Z' drugs;
- **antidepressants**;
- **antipsychotics**.

These interactions impair the performance of tasks that require attention and quick reflexes (e.g. driving motor vehicles and using machinery or sharp instruments). It is necessary to warn consumers in order to prevent injury to themselves and others. Similar CNS effects can occur if subjects are taking antidepressants or antipsychotic drugs – the concurrent consumption of alcohol could be disastrous.

For full details of potential interactions, see Analgesics, Opioids

Topical formulations

Topical analgesics may contain:

- salicylates

See Cardiovascular Drugs, Antiplatelets

- NSAIDs

See Analgesics, Non-steroidal anti-inflammatory drugs

- belladonna alkaloids, for example hyoscyamine

See Drugs acting on the Nervous System, Antiparkinson's drugs section

Please see interactions for each group if in doubt or if there is a possibility of increased systemic absorption (e.g. if applied on damaged skin).

Stomach remedies

Antacids

These include:

- aluminium-containing products, for example Alu-cap, AlternaGel, Amphojel and Basaljel;
- aluminium and magnesium combinations, for example Gelusil, Maalox, Mylanta and Riopan. Sucralfate (e.g. Carafate), which is an antiulcer preparation, also contains aluminium;

- calcium-containing products such as Caltrate, Citrucel, Os-Cal, PhosLo, Titralac and Tums;
- magnesium-containing products, for example Almora, citrate of magnesium, Mag-Ox 400, Milk of Magnesia, Slow-Mag and Uro-Mag.

The above preparations are also referred to as drugs containing divalent and trivalent cations (which also includes preparations containing iron).

Antacids essentially produce the following changes in the stomach:

- *Alter the pH within the stomach*. This may alter the dissolution of some drug formulations, reducing their absorption.
- *Bind to other drugs* that are administered within 1 or 2 hours of the antacid. This process results in reduced availability of the co-administered drug for absorption. For example, the chelation of tetracyclines (e.g. **tetracycline**, **doxycycline**) will decrease their absorption by up to 90%. A very similar process – precipitation – occurs with drugs such as **quinine** with aluminium and magnesium hydroxide preparations, which results in a decreased absorption of quinine. It has to be noted that the absorption of fluoroquinolones (e.g. **ciprofloxacin**, **norfloxacin**, **ofloxacin**, **enoxacin**, **perfloxacin**) will be decreased by 60–75% if they are co-administered with divalent and trivalent cations. Patients are recommended not to take these divalent and trivalent cationic preparations until fluoroquinolone therapy is discontinued. If concomitant intake is absolutely necessary, the intake of the two drugs should be separated by at least 2 hours.

See Drugs Acting on the Gastrointestinal Tract, Antacids; Drugs to Treat Infections, antibiotics sections; Miscellaneous, minerals

- With rapidly absorbed antacids (e.g. sodium bicarbonate), the *pH of the urine* is affected, which will urinary pH.
- *Altering the rate of gastric emptying* and lower gastrointestinal tract transit influences the absorption of any co-administered drugs.
- Inadvertent *overdosing of potassium bicarbonate*-containing indigestion preparations has led to severe metabolic alkalosis and unconsciousness needing intensive care management (Gawarammana et al., 2007). The extraordinarily large intake in that case was certainly not of suicidal intent and can be attributed to insufficient information/knowledge for consumers regarding the dosages, adverse effects and precautions related to OTC drugs.

For full details of the potential interactions, see:

- antacids;

See Drugs Acting on the Gastrointestinal Tract, Antacids

- sodium bicarbonate.

See Urological Drugs, Urinary alkalinization

H2 receptor antagonists

This group of drugs (e.g. cimetidine) is used to relieve gastric acidity and dyspepsia. Cimetidine may cause inhibition of metabolism of a large number of drugs as it inhibits multiple CYP isoenzymes. This affects, for example:

- anticoagulants such as **warfarin**;
- antiepileptics, for example **phenytoin** and **carbamazepine**;
- **theophylline**.

This may potentially cause toxic effects.

Conversely, H2 receptor blockers may reduce the absorption of certain drugs, for example:

- antimalarials – **proguanil**;
- **dipyridamole** – an antiplatelet drug used in patients who have had a stroke, to reduce the risk of further strokes.

For full details of potential interactions, see Drugs Acting on the Gastrointestinal Tract, Antacids

Allergy drugs and cold and flu remedies

OTC drugs available for treating allergies usually contain the following:

- *Sedating antihistamines* (promethazine, e.g. Phenergan; chlorphenamine, e.g. Allercalm, Allerief, Hayleve, Haymine, Piriton, Pollenase; diphenhydramine, e.g. Histergan), which may impair tasks requiring attention (e.g. driving, using machinery). Increased sedation may occur if these drugs are taken with other **sedatives**, including **alcohol**.
- *Non-sedating antihistamines* (e.g. loratidine, e.g. Clarityn; cetirizine, e.g. Benadryl, Piriteze, Zirtek; clemastine), which can cause dangerous arrhythmias with antifungal agents (**itraconazole**, **ketoconazole**), antibiotics (**erythromycin**, **clarithromycin**) and drugs used to counteract acidity (e.g. **H2 antagonists** – for cimetidine).
- *Sympathomimetics* (pseudoephedrine, e.g. Sudafed; phenylephrine, e.g. Fenox; oxymetazoline, e.g. Lemsip, Otrivine, Vicks), which should not be used if taking **antidepressants**, particularly MAOIs and TCAs because of the risk of life-threatening episodes of high blood pressure (hypertensive crisis) and adverse effects on the CNS. These drugs need to be used cautiously by patients with heart disease and those on treatment for high blood pressure.

The groups of drugs used in remedies for colds and flu usually contain:

- pain relievers (analgesics) – aspirin, paracetamol, NSAIDs;
- antihistamines – see above;
- sympathomimetics – see above;
- dextromethorphan and pholcodine, which are opioid cough suppressants – these may cause sedation if taken with other sedatives – see below;
- caffeine – which may cause tremor or arrhythmias.

Cough suppressants

Opioids

- *Dextromethorphan* is probably the most common constituent of OTC cough remedies and is chemically related to morphine. It is a substrate of CYP2B6 (minor), CYP2C8/9 (minor), CYP2C19 (minor), CYP2D6 (major), CYP2E1 (minor) and CYP3A4 (minor), and inhibits CYP2D6 (weak effect).
- *Pholcodine*, a related drug (opioid), is relatively selective in its depressive effect on the cough centre (affecting the respiratory centre less).
- *Codeine*, another common constituent of several OTC drugs, is also an opioid and is converted to morphine in the body.

Codeine and pholcodine are generally considered more potent depressants than dextromethorphan. Several OTC cough suppressants also contain guaifenesin, a mucolytic agent.

For full details of potential interactions, see Analgesics, Opioids

Drugs for heart disease

The OTC drugs available are:

- aspirin (usually enteric coated in 75 mg doses) – see above;
- statins (simvastatin).

The most serious adverse effect of simvastatin is myopathy, which rarely may progress to rhabdomyolysis. Abnormalities of liver function may also occur. These effects are dose-dependent, and a number of drugs and foods may inhibit the metabolism of simvastatin, thereby increasing its toxicity. Examples of these are **grapefruit juice** and **erythromycin**, both of which should be avoided in patients taking simvastatin.

For full details of potential interactions, see Cardiovascular Drugs, Lipid-lowering drugs

Drugs acting on the central nervous system – hypnotics 'sleeping tablets'

OTC drugs available may contain sedating **antihistamines** – see above.

Travel sickness medications

The OTC drugs available may contain:

- antihistamines – see above;
- hyoscine.

Hyoscine has antimuscarinic side-effects that may add to the effect of a wide range of prescribable medications such as **TCAs**. Also, the antimuscarinic effect may reduce the efficacy of sublingual **GTN** tablets.

> For full details of potential interactions, see Drugs Acting on the Nervous System, Antiparkinson's drugs

Medications to treat a sore throat

OTC drugs available may contain:

- NSAIDs – see above;
- local anaesthetics, for example benzocaine and lidocaine

> See Anaesthetic Drugs, Anaesthetics – local

- antiseptics such as amylmetacresol, hexylresorcinol, chlorhexidine, benzalkonium chloride, cetylpyridium and dequalinium.

Treatment for menstrual disorders

OTC drugs available may contain:

- pain relievers (analgesics) such as aspirin and NSAIDs – see above;
- ammonium chloride

> See Urological Drugs, Urinary alkalinization

- caffeine.

Antidiarrhoeal preparations

The OTC drugs available may contain:

- opioids such as morphine and codeine – see above;
- adsorbents, for example kaolin.

Kaolin can reduce the absorption and efficacy of other drugs, notably drugs acting on the heart, such as **digoxin** and **beta-blockers**.

> For full details of potential interactions, see Drugs Acting on the Gastrointestinal Tract, Antidiarrhoeals

Drugs for irritable bowel syndrome

OTC drugs available may contain:

- antispasmodics, for example alverine citrate and mebeverine (no known interactions)
- anticholinergic antimuscarinics, such as hyoscine

See Drugs Acting on the Nervous System, Antiparkinson's drugs

- carminatives and antispasmodics such as peppermint oil (no known interactions)

Nutritional supplements

OTC drugs available include the following vitamins:

- A – retinol;
- B1 – thiamin;
- B2 – riboflavin;
- B6 – pyridoxine;
- B12 – cyanocobalamine;
- nicotinic acid – a constituent of the vitamin B complex;
- folic acid – a constituent of the vitamin B complex, whose concentrations and activity can be decreased by **antiepileptics**;
- C – ascorbic acid, the absorption of which is reduced by **aspirin**;
- D – calciferol, levels of which are reduced by **phenytoin**;
- E – tocopherol;
- K – phytomenadione.

For full details of potential interactions, see Miscellaneous, Minerals section

Minerals and electrolytes are also available in OTC preparations:

- iodine, which increases the risk of hypothyroidism;
- iron;
- calcium;
- magnesium;
- potassium;
- phosphorus;
- zinc.

Potassium supplements are associated with an increased risk of hyperkalaemia with **ACE inhibitors** and **potassium-sparing diuretics**. Salt substitutes (which may be recommended for patients with hypertension) contain potassium, so patients taking ACE inhibitors should be advised not to use salt substitutes.

For full details of potential interactions, see Cardiovascular drugs, Antihypertensive and heart failure drugs, Duiretics

Oral contraceptives

See Drugs Used in Obstetrics and Gynaecology

Drugs to treat constipation

The main adverse drug interactions are associated with abuse, which leads to hypokalaemia and in some instances to decreased absorption of other orally administered drugs.

The following OTC laxative preparations are available:

- senna derivatives;
- bisacodyl sodium;
- picosulphate;
- lactulose;
- docusate sodium;
- glycerin suppositories;
- ispaghula husk;
- methylcellulose;
- sterculia.

Preparations for haemorrhoids

OTC drugs available contain:

- *local anaesthetics*, for example lidocaine, benzocaine and cinchocaine;

See Anaesthetic Drugs, Anaesthetics – Local

- corticosteroids such as hydrocortisone;

Anticancer and Immunomodulating Drugs, Other immunomodulating drugs

- astringents such as zinc oxide, bismuth, aloe, balsam and hamamelis (no known interactions).

Medications for worm infestations

The OTC drugs available contain anthelmintics, such as mebendazole and piperazine (no known interactions).

For interactions of mebendazole, See Drugs to Treat Infections, Other antiprotozoals

Medications for colic in children

OTC drugs available may contain:

- sodium bicarbonate;

See Urological Drugs, Urinary alkalinization

- dimeticone (no known interactions);
- aromatic oils, such as dill, caraway and ginger.

Preparations for skin disorders

OTC drugs available may contain:

- corticosteroids, for example hydrocortisone and clobetasone (no known interactions);
- local anaesthetics, such as lidocaine and lauromacrogols;

See Anaesthetic Drugs, Anaesthetics – local

- coal tar (no known interactions);
- dithranol;
- aluminium chloride;

See Urological Drugs, Urinary alkalinization

- antifungals, for example oral fluconazole. Fluconazole decreases the metabolism of a wide range of drugs including **warfarin**, antidiabetic drugs such as **sulphonylureas**, antiepileptics such as **phenytoin**, **astemizole**, **terfenadine** (high concentrations of these two drugs would cause life-threatening ventricular arrhythmias with torsades des pointes) and **theophylline**. The diuretic **hydrochlorothiazide** decreases the metabolism of fluconazole and may cause toxic effects of fluconazole. The antibiotic **rifampicin** increases the metabolism of fluconazole and thus reduces its efficacy.

See Drugs to Treat Infections, Antifungal drugs

Antiasthma preparations containing theophylline

Several drugs, for example the **oral contraceptive pill**, **viloxazine**, **thiabendazole**, **aminoglutethimide**, antiepileptics (**carbamazepine**, **phenytoin**, **barbiturates**) and the antibiotic **rifampicin** decrease plasma concentrations of theophylline.

Allopurinol and some **antibiotics** increase plasma concentrations of theophylline and increase the risk of adverse effects of theophylline.

See section on theophylline interactions.

Treatments for scalp disorders

The OTC drugs available may contain antihypertensive such as minoxidil.

See Cardiovascular Drugs, Antihypertensives and heart failure drugs

Preparations for dandruff – dermatitis

The OTC drugs available may contain:

- antifungals such as ketoconazole;

See Drugs to Treat Infections, Antifungal drugs

- zinc pyrithione;
- selenium sulphide;
- coal tar (no known interactions).

Head louse preparations

The OTC drugs available may contain:

- insecticides such as malathion (no known interactions);
- phenothrin (no known interactions);
- permethrin (no known interactions);
- dimeticone (no known interactions).

Information sources

Chemist and Druggist. *Guide to OTC Medicines and Diagnostics: for Pharmacists and Pharmacy Assistants*, 33rd edn. Tonbridge: CMPMedica, 2008.

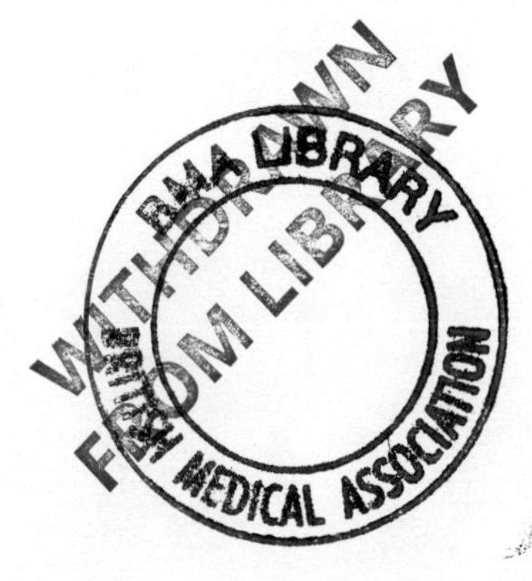
BMA LIBRARY
BRITISH MEDICAL ASSOCIATION
WITHDRAWN
FROM LIBRARY